Building Effective Physical Education Programs

Deborah Tannehill, PhD

University of Limerick

Hans van der Mars, PhD

Arizona State University

Ann MacPhail, PhD

University of Limerick

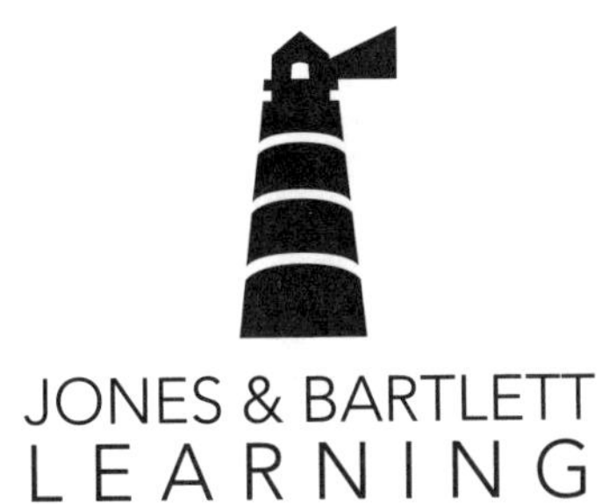

JONES & BARTLETT
LEARNING

World Headquarters
Jones & Bartlett Learning
5 Wall Street
Burlington, MA 01803
978-443-5000
info@jblearning.com
www.jblearning.com

Jones & Bartlett Learning books and products are available through most bookstores and online booksellers. To contact Jones & Bartlett Learning directly, call 800-832-0034, fax 978-443-8000, or visit our website, www.jblearning.com.

Substantial discounts on bulk quantities of Jones & Bartlett Learning publications are available to corporations, professional associations, and other qualified organizations. For details and specific discount information, contact the special sales department at Jones & Bartlett Learning via the above contact information or send an email to specialsales@jblearning.com.

Production Credits
Executive Publisher: William Brottmiller
Acquisitions Editor: Ryan Angel
Editorial Assistant: Kayla Dos Santos
Production Editor: Jessica Steele Newfell
Senior Marketing Manager: Andrea DeFronzo
VP, Manufacturing and Inventory Control: Therese Connell
Composition: Cenveo® Publisher Services
Cover Design: Kristin E. Parker
Photo Research and Permissions Coordinator: Amy Rathburn
Cover Images: (curved lines) © pzAxe/ShutterStock, Inc.; (triangles) © theromb/ShutterStock, Inc.
Printing and Binding: Edwards Brothers Malloy
Cover Printing: Edwards Brothers Malloy

To order this product, use ISBN: 978-1-284-02110-3

Library of Congress Cataloging-in-Publication Data
Tannehill, Deborah.
Building effective physical education programs / by Deborah Tannehill, Hans van der Mars, and Ann MacPhail.
Includes bibliographical references and index.
ISBN 978-1-4496-4635-6 — ISBN 1-4496-4635-2
1. Physical education and training—Administration. 2. Sports administration. 3. School sports—Management.
I. Van der Mars, Hans, 1955- II. MacPhail, Ann. III. Title.
GV343.5.T36 2015
372.86—dc23

2013027710

6048

Printed in the United States of America
17 16 15 14 13 10 9 8 7 6 5 4 3 2 1

Brief Contents

Contents

Introduction

Tannehill, van der Mars, and MacPhail have produced a comprehensive textbook that provides a series of approaches that together clearly describe strategies for physical education teachers to deliver high-quality physical education programs. The various sections of *Building Effective Physical Education Programs* are clearly written with numerous examples that describe the details of the teaching strategies that lead to desired outcomes.

Section I, *Broadening Perspectives of Physical Education in Changing Contexts*, includes important information about how beginning teachers throughout the world can continue to develop their teaching skills and how they can learn to deal with the many issues that physical education teachers inevitably experience with their students, fellow teachers, and parents. The authors have provided a useful section on the "hidden dimensions" of teaching physical education and how to develop and promote a Comprehensive School Physical Education Program.

In Section II, *Developing Responsible Learners*, the authors provide teaching strategies for managing groups of children and youths as they participate in physical education classes, with the goal that students learn how to self-manage their participation and with the outcome leading to physical education classes that move forward without having to deal with management issues. They emphasize the importance of building a relationship with learners as the key step in developing a positive and caring learning environment and discuss the implications for designing a discipline plan to allow and support maintenance of this environment.

Section III, *Designing an Instructionally Aligned Physical Education Program*, highlights the concept of aligning the goals of physical education with the appropriate choice of curriculum model, instructional models, teaching strategies, and, ultimately, assessment. The text provides clear explanations of high-quality physical education curriculum models and how teachers can introduce these models and follow through with classes that achieve the intended outcomes of the various models. The authors provide clear explanations of effective teaching practices, ranging from creating unit and lesson plans to delivering a series of lessons through which students achieve the goals of the unit. Chapter 17 provides ample strategies for the use of technology in teaching physical education.

Section IV, *The Reality of Teaching Physical Education*, helps preservice and practicing teachers recognize that learning to teach is not something that is completed during a teacher education program but, rather, is a lifelong process. This section help readers understand the importance of continuing professional development to their personal growth and the role of advocacy in the growth and development of physical education itself.

Daryl Siedentop

Professor Emeritus, Sport and Exercise Science

The Ohio State University

Preface

Our intent in *Building Effective Physical Education Programs* is to provide a view of physical education from a global perspective. We believe that it is essential today to learn more about the many different contexts and practices used in different countries. We also believe that we have much to gain from one another—in fact, we have more in common in education worldwide than we have differences. However, we also believe that every country has chosen to respond to various physical education issues in different ways depending on their context and, from each of those, we may draw insight to influence our own practices. While the majority of this text is based on the North American context, we have attempted to share examples and policies from various parts of the world to allow teachers and teacher educators to draw from others' effective practices.

What does it take to plan and teach an effective, meaningful, and relevant physical education program in the context of today's schools? This text explores possible answers to that question. We focus on learning to teach with the intent that you become, what Dewey (1904) called, critical and continuous *students of teaching*. We contend that, for teachers to design and teach a diverse group of young people a physical education program that is worthwhile, meaningful and relevant requires the (1) knowledge to design and plan a meaningful curriculum, (2) managerial and instructional skills to implement those curricula, (3) ongoing assessment of students' progress and the program's impact, (4) administrative skill to produce an organizational structure within school time that optimizes the impact of the program, and (5) creative energy to link the school program to opportunities for children and youth outside of the school. Effective physical education, therefore, lies at the point where curriculum, assessment, instruction, organization, and program extension come together.

It is not easy to plan and teach effective physical education—it takes time and energy as well as the desire to help young people choose to be physically active across their life span and gain the skills and knowledge to be successful. Drawing on the insights of teachers, teacher educators, and researchers in physical education, we are now in a better position to achieve effective physical education than ever before. Physical education has several widely replicated curriculum models that have been well received by students, school administrators, and parents. We know more about classroom management and how to help young people take responsibility for their own learning and behavior. Instructional models, aligned teaching strategies, and assessment for learning have been developed to assist teachers in facilitating student learning and enjoying that learning. There are growing signs that different school and class organizational structures can improve the achievement of important learning outcomes, especially when housed within a positive and caring learning environment. We include many examples of how school physical education programs can link to community efforts to positively impact the physical activity habits of children and youth. *Building Effective Physical Education Programs* highlights and shares what we know about these topics and how the reader, as a teacher, can gain practice and skill in developing, implementing, and maintaining them.

We build upon and extend the work of Daryl Siedentop, *Developing Teaching Skills in Physical Education* (1983; 1991) and Daryl Siedentop and Deborah Tannehill, *Developing Teaching Skills in Physical Education* (2000). We developed the strengths from earlier texts on physical education and integrated key aspects of teaching and learning more thoroughly, drawing ideas and insight from physical education teacher education programs and research internationally. In addition to this international perspective, we include chapters on the three pillars of physical education, physical activity and sport outside of school, Comprehensive School Physical Education Programs, educational reform, technology, professional development, and advocacy.

We have made every effort to present knowledge about issues as well as the skills necessary to put this knowledge to work—not only to consider what contexts encourage students to learn and in what way but also how teachers and teacher educators can impact that learning. We emphasize how key skills can be practiced, how they can be observed, and what kinds of feedback are necessary to improve them. We continue to base our suggestions on what research tells us, and we have relied primarily on research conducted in schools under typical conditions. We take positions, but we do not advocate a singular approach to teaching or curriculum. With respect to teaching skills and strategies, our position is that the characteristics of effective teaching can be found in many different instructional models. With respect to curriculum, our position is that many different approaches can be successful if they are well-planned and appropriately implemented, but that successful curricula typically focus on meaningful outcomes and allow time to achieve these outcomes. Regardless of whether teachers choose to deliver a program that is primarily fitness-oriented, sport-oriented, or outdoor pursuits-oriented (or a blend), each requires thorough planning, strong content knowledge, skillful instruction, and a commitment to continuously ask the question "How do I know that my efforts are impacting my students as desired?"

We believe effective teachers are consistently reflective, although we also recognize the daily demands on teachers are such that reflection often comes in small spurts and stolen moments. We suggest throughout *Building Effective Physical Education Programs* that reflection can be aided substantially by data gathered through observation, and we discuss many ways to accomplish this task.

Book Structure

Building Effective Physical Education Programs is evidence-based and composed of 19 chapters divided into four sections:

- Section I, *Broadening Perspectives of Physical Education in Changing Contexts*
- Section II, *Developing Responsible Learners*
- Section III, *Designing an Instructionally Aligned Physical Education Program*
- Section IV, *The Reality of Teaching Physical Education*

Sections are introduced prior to the set of chapters that make up each section cluster. The chapters are built on a set of concepts and principles linked to research that shows an impact on teaching and learning in physical education. Each chapter begins with an overall chapter outcome followed by learning outcomes, an inspirational quote, and a box of key terms related to the chapter's content.

Within the main body of each chapter are learning experiences that challenge the reader to investigate a particular concept, area of knowledge, or strategy and to apply it to your own practice—we also challenge the reader to observe and analyze that concept in a school setting. In closing, each chapter has a summary that highlights the key points we emphasized and want the reader to remember.

About the Authors

Deborah Tannehill, PhD, is a Senior Lecturer in the Department of Physical Education and Sport Sciences and Co-Director of the Physical Education, Physical Activity, and Youth Sport (PEPAYS) Research Centre at the University of Limerick.

Hans van der Mars, PhD, is Professor and Program Director in Physical Education Teacher Education, Mary Lou Fulton Teachers College at Arizona State University.

Ann MacPhail, PhD, is Senior Lecturer and Head of the Department of Physical Education and Sport Sciences at the University of Limerick.

Acknowledgments

Becoming a student of teaching—whether a novice teacher just entering the workforce, a practicing teacher intent on improving his or her skills through professional development, or a teacher educator striving to design new and innovative education—is not done in isolation. The three authors of *Building Effective Physical Education Programs* are fortunate to have worked with skilled and knowledgeable colleagues at various institutions in the United States, Ireland and the United Kingdom over a number of years. We have been privileged to work closely with undergraduate and practicing teachers committed to physical education for young people and focused on designing and delivering programs that make a difference in the lives of these young people. Over the years, we have advised many exemplary post-graduate students who have conducted research related to physical education, physical activity and coaching that influenced and informed practice. We want to thank all of them for their unwavering commitment to excellence in teaching physical education, their professionalism, and their willingness to share their insights.

Writing a text such as this one requires the assistance from a good publisher. The support and guidance we received from Jones & Bartlett Learning was first rate. Specifically we would like to acknowledge the contributions made by Ryan Angel, Acquisitions Editor; Kayla Dos Santos, Editorial Assistant; and Jess Newfell, Production Editor. Finally, we would like to thank the many reviewers who provided thoughtful and insightful comments on the chapters of this book as they evolved.

Reviewers

Helena Baert, PhD
State University of New York–Cortland
Cortland, New York

William W. Ballard
Florida Atlantic University
Boca Raton, Florida

Janice Bibik
University of Delaware
Newark, Delaware

Christine E.W. Brett
University of Pennsylvania–East Stroudsburg
Easton, Pennsylvania

Rebecca Bryan
Sonoma State University
Rohnert Park, California

Charles Duncan, PhD
University of Louisiana
Lafayette, Louisiana

Lorna Gillespie
University of Waikato, New Zealand

Dr. Gregory Green
Fort Valley University
Fort Valley, Georgia

Dr. Michelle Hsiu-Chen Liu
Averett University
Danville, Virigina

Jayne M. Jenkins
University of Wyoming
Laramie, Wyoming

Ingrid L. Johnson, PhD
Grand Valley State University
Allendale, Michigan

Dr. Robert Martin
Delaware State University
Oxford, Pennsylvania

Timothy Mirtz, DC, PhD
Indiana Institute of Technology
Fort Wayne, Indiana

Pilvikki Heikinaro-Johansson
University of Jyväskylä, Finland

Dr. Jesse Rhoades
University of North Dakota
Grand Forks, North Dakota

Scott Ronspies, PhD
Eastern Illinois University
Charleston, Illinois

Paula J. Scraba, PhD
St. Bonaventure University
Saint Bonaventure, New York

Nancy Magee Speed
The University of Southern Mississippi
Hattiesburg, Mississippi

SECTION I Broadening Perspectives of Physical Education in Changing Contexts

Introduction

We live in a global society, and thus have an opportunity to learn and grow through input, interaction, and consultation with other countries around the world. As you will see in this section, there are perhaps more similarities internationally than differences in terms of education, and more specifically physical education, physical activity, and sport. With this in mind, we have chosen to provide a broad perspective in these introductory chapters with the intent of broadening the insights of physical education teacher educators, and physical educators at the preservice, novice, and veteran levels. If physical education is going to have an impact on the health and well-being of society and influence policy and practice at local, national, and international levels, then everyone in the physical education, physical activity, and sport community must be knowledgeable and prepared to serve as change agents in this global world.

The chapters in this section highlight the place of physical education in school programs and communities, outline physical education's unique contribution to the development of young people, and present the current status of physical education programs. Moreover, in this section we will introduce a broader definition of the central role that the physical education program plays within the school environment. Currently, physical education teacher education (PETE) programs seek to prepare new specialists to deliver quality physical education lessons. It is our goal to help PETE faculty prepare future professionals who are skilled to go beyond that, and have specialists see the need for promotion of physical activity throughout the school day and beyond. All the while, the central message will be that if we want children and youth to make physical activity truly part of every day (in whatever form—e.g., sport, fitness, dance, outdoor pursuits), we must do so by making physical activity an enjoyable process that leads to competence and stronger self-efficacy toward physical activity in general and certain activities in particular.

CHAPTER 1 The Role of the Physical Educator in and Beyond the School

Overall Chapter Outcome

To examine the role of the physical educator in encouraging young people to engage with physical activity and sport beyond the school physical education environment

Learning Outcomes

The learner will:

- Appreciate that to enable physical education to encourage the development of a physically educated person, it is essential that physical education enhances not only the physical development but also the emotional, cognitive, and social development of individuals
- Describe the relationship among school physical education, extracurricular sport, and community and club sport
- Consider what is feasible as regards effective school physical education contributing to an increase in young people's physical activity levels through extracurricular sport and community and club sport
- Enunciate the necessary relationships between physical education teachers and other teaching and physical activity professions to increase young people's physical activity levels
- Discuss opportunities for physical education teachers to engage with a range of professional organizations interested in increasing young people's activity levels
- Consider the feasibility of online physical education

We acknowledge that a significant amount of time is required to successfully physically educate young people (i.e., to enhance their physical, emotional, cognitive, and social development). Therefore, **physical education** lessons, and by association physical educators, cannot be solely responsible for increasing the **physical activity** levels of young people. If physical educators are to be central to increasing physical activity levels in young people, then it may be more appropriate to consider in what other contexts, in addition to school physical education, they can advocate and/or contribute in a bid to pursue the desired outcome. These other contexts include the school campus (i.e., **extracurricular sport**) and the surrounding communities (i.e., **community and club sport**). Physical educators do have a responsibility to help engage young people with physical activity and **sport** beyond the physical education environment, providing young people with potential pathways that can help them maintain involvement in physical activity. That is not to say that physical educators need to take on additional roles in the delivery of all physical activity content (i.e., take responsibility for physical

BOX 1.1 Key Terms in This Chapter

- *Community and club sport:* Sport and physical activity (including dance) within the framework of a sport club or community organization.
- *Extracurricular sport:* Competitive and noncompetitive physical activities (including dance) outside of the formal physical education curriculum but offered within the institutional framework of school.
- *Physical activity:* Any movement activity undertaken in daily life, ranging from normal active living conditions to intentional moderate physical activities, to structured physical fitness and training sessions (including dance).
- *Physical education:* Competitive and noncompetitive physical activities (including dance) taught as part of a formal school curriculum intended for every student attending school. Physical education applies a holistic approach to the concept of physical activity for young people, recognizing the physical, emotional, cognitive, and social dimensions of human movement.
- *Sport:* All forms of physical activity (including dance) that, through casual or regular participation, expresses or improves physical fitness and mental well-being and forms social relationships.

education, extracurricular sport, and community sport) but rather that physical educators need to think beyond their lessons and school teams regarding how best to advocate for and prepare young people to undertake a life of autonomous well-being. Physical educators must link meaningfully with young people and be aware of their engagement in extracurricular and community and club sport by collaborating with the providers of those opportunities. Those who provide physical education and/or physical activity opportunities in or around school settings should ensure that the young people they are working with are receiving consistent messages and quality experiences not only regarding participation in physical activity but also in becoming physically educated. A collaborative and consistent approach to physical education, physical activity, and sport has the potential to be influential in a young person's holistic learning and development. Such an approach locates physical education within the ecology of the young person's lived experience, not just as a subject to be studied at school.

This chapter begins by presenting the roles and objectives of school physical education and what it means to be a professional physical educator. We then introduce and examine the relationship between physical education, extracurricular sport, and community and club sport. The changing context of school physical education is then discussed to contextualize the relationship and tensions among physical education, extracurricular sport, and community and club sport. Making connections with other professionals involved in the promotion of physical activity leads to the sharing of a number of programs that specifically encourage physical education teachers to be central in supporting a cooperative structure across physical education, extracurricular sport, and community and club sport. It is not the intention of the chapter to state the extent to which such programs have been effective; this requires an understanding of the culture and context in which they operate, something that we are unable to address due to space limitations. Rather, they are introduced to provide the reader with possible structures that they may consider the relevance to, and the potential reconfiguring for, their own particular student, school, community, and country context. The chapter concludes by introducing the practice of online physical education, where, it can be argued, students who do not attend the traditionally timetabled physical education school lessons can be reached through an online program.

Roles and Objectives of School Physical Education

There is general agreement on what the roles and objectives of school physical education should be (Bailey et al., 2009). To enable physical education to encourage the development of a physically educated person, it is essential that physical education (1) enhances physical, emotional, cognitive, and social development; (2) develops physical creativity, competence, and confidence to perform a variety of physical activities; (3) examines human movement from different key perspectives; (4) encourages young people to work as individuals, with partners, in groups, and as part of a team, in both competitive and noncompetitive situations; and (5) encourages an appreciation of physical activities and promotes a positive attitude towards establishing, sustaining, and supporting an active and healthy lifestyle. In a meta-analysis of international studies pertaining to physical activity and cognition in young people, Sibley and Etnier (2003) report that there is some evidence that physical activity may be related to improved cognitive performance and academic achievement. This provides evidence for the argument that physical activity (potentially provided by physical

BOX 1.2 NASPE Outcomes for the Physically Educated Person

The physically educated person

Has learned the skills necessary to perform a variety of physical activities

1. Moves using concepts of body awareness, space awareness, effort, and relationships
2. Demonstrates competence in a variety of manipulative, locomotor, and non-locomotor skills
3. Demonstrates competence in combinations of manipulative, locomotor, and non-locomotor skills performed individually and with others
4. Demonstrates competence in many different forms of physical activity
5. Demonstrates proficiency in at least a few forms of physical activity
6. Has learned how to learn new skills

Is physically fit

7. Assesses, achieves, and maintains physical fitness
8. Designs safe personal fitness programs in accordance with principles of training and conditioning

Does participate regularly in physical activity

9. Participates in health-enhancing physical activity at least three times a week
10. Selects and regularly participates in lifetime physical activities

Knows the implications of and the benefits from involvement in physical activities

11. Identifies the benefits, costs, and obligations associated with regular participation in physical activity
12. Recognizes the risk and safety factors associated with regular participation in physical activity
13. Applies concepts and principles to the development of motor skills
14. Understands that wellness involves more than being physically fit
15. Knows the rules, strategies, and appropriate behaviors for selected physical activities
16. Recognizes that participation in physical activity can lead to multicultural and international understanding
17. Understands that physical activity provides the opportunity for enjoyment, self-expression, and communication

Values physical activity and its contributions to a healthy lifestyle

18. Appreciates the relationships with others that result from participation in physical activity
19. Respects the role that regular physical activity plays in the pursuit of lifelong health and well-being
20. Cherishes the feelings that result from regular participation in physical activity

Reproduced with permission from NASPE. (2004). *Moving into the Future: National Standards for Physical Education* (2nd ed.). Reston, VA: NASPE.

education) should be part of the school day for both its physical and cognitive benefits. Differences in the extent to which countries expand and refine what a physically educated person looks like are evident in examining the National Association of Sport and Physical Education of the American Alliance for Health, Physical Education, Recreation, and Dance (NASPE and AAHPERD) outcomes of quality physical education programs (see **Box 1.2**), and Physical and Health Education (PHE) Canada's (PHE Canada, 2009) and the United Kingdom's Association for Physical Education's (afPE) manifesto for a world-class system of physical education (afPE, 2008).

What It Means to Be a Professional Physical Educator

Historically, the role of the physical education teacher has been one of overseeing the administration of physical education classes in school settings. In most European countries, the teacher would deliver physical education lessons during the day, and might have a coaching role in a sport club context that would be separate from the school. In the United States, sport is perhaps more intertwined in the secondary (or postprimary) school culture than anywhere else in the world. Here, teachers are generally expected to take on the role of coach of one (or more) sports at a school. In sports such as basketball and American football, with the trends toward early specialization and year-round strength conditioning, teacher–coaches sometimes have difficulty balancing the two roles, often resulting in a role conflict (Siedentop & van der Mars, 2012).

The discussion on what it means to be a professional physical educator in today's society incorporates the consideration of a number of roles that challenge the previous expectation that a physical educator did not deviate from teaching physical education full-time in one school. There are now examples around the world where qualified physical educators can (1) teach physical education half-time and coach in community clubs half-time, (2) teach physical education in postprimary half-time and in feeder primary schools half-time, (3) teach physical education half-time and teach/coach extracurricular activities half-time, and (4) be employed full-time within a school physical education program that functions with strong links to the community and other sporting and physical activity organizations. Even in instances where physical educators do not have a formalized position to share their time across physical education and another area of responsibility, it is common for them to report the responsibility that is embedded within their physical education role to accommodate extracurricular sport:

> *I am also left to reflect on the position of the PE teacher in schools. . . . I do spend more time than nearly all other teachers helping out with teams at lunchtime and after-school. I really enjoy helping young people to participate in physical activity and get a great "buzz" from the social side of being involved with teams. However I must be careful for the future to ensure that I do not suffer from burnout. . . . It seems that the PE teacher is expected to coach teams of all sports after school.*[1]

Increasingly, particularly in the United States, physical education is expected to play an important role in increasing physical activity levels in young people and promoting lifelong physical activity as part of the broader efforts to reverse trends in the percentages of children and youth who are overweight/obese (Pate et al., 2007). However, there needs to be some consideration of what is feasible as regards physical education contributing to an increase in young people's physical activity levels when limited time is allocated to physical education in the school week. In examining the status of physical education in schools worldwide, timetable allocation for school physical education has in general stabilized (Hardman, n.d.). It is evident that there is an international trend of time allocation for physical education reducing with increasing age, especially the final years of schooling, when it either becomes an optional subject or disappears from the timetable (Hardman, n.d.). We acknowledge that the time afforded to physical education teachers is already limited as regards the potential to effectively produce a physically educated person (i.e., physical, mental, emotional, cognitive, and social development). As a consequence, we believe that the physical educator should advocate for young people to access complementary opportunities in which to further develop such attributes and, perhaps more so, an increase in physical activity levels.

Physical education lessons cannot be solely responsible for increasing the physical activity levels of young people. If physical educators are to be central to increasing physical activity levels in young people, then it may be more appropriate to consider in what other contexts, in addition to physical education classes, they can contribute in a bid to pursue the desired outcome. These other contexts would include the school campus and the surrounding communities. Complementary is the investigation in the Netherlands of the physical education teacher functioning in the school as a "new style professional" (Broeke, van Dalfsen, Bax, Rijpstra, & Schouten, 2008), that is, a physical educator with an *acknowledged* responsibility for additional sport and physical activity opportunities.

In the United States, the mission of the National Association for Sport and Physical Education (NASPE) is to enhance knowledge, improve professional practice, and increase support for high-quality physical education, sport, and physical activity programs. Recently, NASPE initiated a campaign to reconceptualize the role of physical educators as "physical activity leaders" within the context of the new Comprehensive School Physical Activity Program (CSPAP) (NASPE, 2008; see www.letsmoveschools.org). Within the CSPAP framework, beyond delivering quality physical education lessons, physical activity leaders would (1) coordinate the programming and facilitation of physical activity opportunities for students throughout the school day on campus (i.e., before school, recess and lunch periods, after school), (2) encourage teachers of classroom subjects to infuse their lessons with physical activity breaks, (3) create opportunities for the school's teaching and support staff, and (4) create opportunities for members of the surrounding communities.

[1] Reproduced with permission from Hartley, T. (2011). Preparing physical education teachers for the reality of teaching in schools: The case of one physical education teacher education (PETE) programme. Master's thesis, University of Limerick, Ireland.

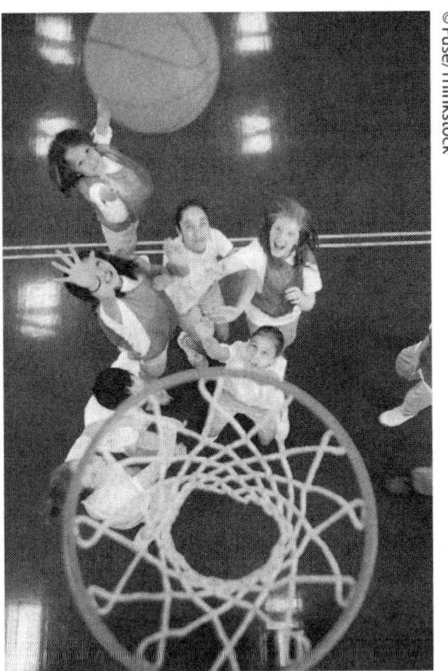
© Fuse/Thinkstock

Before moving on to further consider and interrogate the relationship among school physical education, extracurricular sport and activity, and community and club sport, it is important to establish what each is likely to entail in different parts of the world.

The Three Pillars of School Physical Education, Extracurricular Sport, and Community and Club Sport

Providing young people with sport and physical activity has been characterized in Ireland as resting on three pillars (Fahey, Delaney, & Gannon, 2005): (1) physical education curriculum in schools, (2) extracurricular sport played in the school, and (3) sport played outside the school in sport clubs or other organized contexts. Clive Pope (2011) warns that as physical educators we need to review how physical education and sport should be positioned for ensuing generations of students, "Unless educators focus more attention on how sport and physical education is presented to young people it could become an increasingly irrelevant part of many of their lives. The retention of traditional and contemporary physical education programmes should be evaluated against the needs of today's students" (p. 280). Fry and McNeill (2011) warn that although school sport has gained a significant national and political profile in Singapore, physical education has not.

School physical education incorporates competitive and noncompetitive physical activities taught as part of a formal school curriculum intended for every pupil attending school, with a preference for delivery by qualified physical education teachers in postprimary schools. The United States has national standards for physical education that direct physical education teachers in the development of physical education curricula, instruction, and assessment (NASPE, 2013). Specialist physical education teachers are employed in primary schools in the United States and Scotland but are not found in Australia, Cyprus, France, or Ireland. However, through the Physical Education, School Sport and Club Sport (PESSCL) initiative in England and Wales (Department for Education and Skills & Department for Culture, Media and Sport, 2003), qualified secondary physical education teachers were obliged to teach physical education in feeder primary schools (i.e., primary schools where the students were likely to move on to the physical education teacher's postprimary school). In some countries it is considered desirable for the classroom primary teacher to up-skill to teach physical education rather than employing a physical education specialist who has no classroom experience (Wright, 2002). Such an argument is made on the basis that the classroom primary teacher can enhance cross-curricular links if teaching all subject areas and integrate the use of curriculum and instructional models for wider classroom practice (e.g., enacting working in teams, an essential component of Sport Education, across the whole curriculum). There is general agreement on certain factors that affect the delivery of school physical education across the world, such as staffing levels, time allocation, and subject status (Hardman, 2008).

Extracurricular sport and physical activity in Australia and Europe tend to provide competitive and noncompetitive physical activities outside of the formal physical education curriculum but offered within the institutional framework of school. That is, extracurricular is "extra" and is undertaken outside of the timetabled day, not taking time from the curriculum. Students choose to participate in extracurricular sport during lunchtime, before and/or after school, and in some instances on weekends. The extracurricular sport and physical activity opportunities in the United States tend to be much narrower due to student participation in such programs being the basis for college scholarships in a particular sport. In instances where extracurricular is not extra, physical education teachers arrange games/matches during the school day, resulting in physical education classes being cancelled or covered by someone other than the physical education teacher responsible for the class. This has repercussions for students missing other school classes in addition to physical education and potentially sends the message that sport and physical activity opportunities favor those who are more physically able. Extracurricular sport programs that are marked as recreational are less competitive in nature and have the potential to accommodate a wider range of young people who are perhaps not interested in participating in competitive sport. Peer culture continues to grow as an important aspect of adolescents' physical activity, with more young people choosing to be active outside of formalized extracurricular or community and club sport and taking part in a wide range of physical activities (Wright, Macdonald, &

Groom, 2003). Such "unorganized" sport or physical activity can include jogging, skiing, biking, and skateboarding.

Community and club sport provides young people with opportunities to maintain an involvement in sport or physical activity within the framework of a community organization or sport club, and again can vary considerably depending on the country. For example, formalized community and club sport in Ireland is very strong through the Gaelic Athletic Association (GAA), which is a 32-county sporting and cultural organization. It is a community-based organization that promotes multiple leagues and competitions in Gaelic games such as camogie, Gaelic football, Gaelic handball, hurling, and rounders. Although the GAA should be commended on its strong club structure (there is at least one GAA club in every parish in Ireland), schools naturally feed into such a structure with the result that there is a resounding dominance of invasion games in Ireland (Woods, Tannehill, Quinlan, Moyna, & Walsh, 2010). In the United States, community sport tends to be more focused on recreational activities (e.g., cycling, walking) than on competition.

Learning Experience 1.1

Before reading further, construct an argument for or against the development of a solid relationship among the school physical education curriculum, extracurricular sport, and community and club sport and the associated role of the physical education teacher.

- To what extent are the three pillars practiced as discrete opportunities to be physically active in your context? Is there a blurring of boundaries when distinguishing the practices of each pillar? If so, how can this be addressed?
- Consider the tensions among the school physical education curriculum, extracurricular sport, and community and club sport. Consider what the shared expectations of the role of the physical education teacher across all three might be.

Although the three pillars are contextually different, they each have the potential to contribute to the health of young people by encouraging them to acquire and develop the affective, cognitive, and psychomotor skills that allow them to be physically active. That is, they are concerned with having a positive influence not only on young people's physical activity levels but also on their knowledge, understanding, and attitudes towards lifelong physical activity. Although acknowledging the shared focus on engaging young people in physical activity, there are differences in the way in which each pillar is implemented in different countries and continents. There also are likely to be some tensions among the three pillars in instances where those involved in facilitating each convey different values and philosophies on how best to encourage young people to be, and maintain an interest in being, physically active. We revisit the connections among physical education teachers, other teachers, and physical activity professionals later in the chapter.

International Similarities Across the Pillars as Regards to Physical Activity Engagement

There is strong consensus on what influences young people's interaction, participation, and performance in the three pillars (MacPhail, 2011). More personalized influences that affect young people's disposition to being physically active include gender, physical skill ability, (dis) ability, socioeconomic status, and ethnicity (Kirk, 2005). Maturation differences and hereditary factors should also be considered. There are further issues we should be cognizant of when providing and delivering opportunities to be physically active as we strive to be an effective and appropriate teacher or coach. These include (1) the relevance of what is being offered to young people's lives and its contribution to health, (2) an opportunity to share their physical activity preferences through providing variety and choice, (3) encouraging social interaction and allowing space for making friends, (4) providing opportunities for enjoyment, (5) providing opportunity for developing/perceiving physical and social competence, (6) ensuring young people feel included, and (7) providing encouragement through positive feedback and reinforcement. There are other competing interests, such as exposure to media representations of being (or not) physically active, the power of peer culture (alluded to earlier), and the increasing demand for computer games, that we may find difficult to address with respect to the impact they have on young people's interest in being physically active.

Physical educators need to be critical consumers of media agendas and discuss the agendas with young people to avoid instances, for example, where young people may use physical activity to lose weight and then cease being active once they have achieved a desired body weight. Physical educators need to be critical of the way in which young people's health, activity levels, and obesity levels are reported in the popular media. Researchers suggest that when there is an uncritical and uneducated focus on obesity and related norm-referencing testing, this can contribute to (not cause) the etiology of disordered eating (Neumark-Sztainer et al., 2006).

Physical Education's Changing Context

Physical Education Curriculum

It is suggested that specialist postprimary school programs in their traditional form have had limited impact in terms of transferring knowledge learned in school to adult life

(Kirk, 2005). Tannehill (2007, 2011) challenges physical education teachers to reconsider the physical education program and how such a program can make meaningful connections between the context of the school and local community. Providing young people with physical activity options that are important and meaningful to them may encourage participation in both school physical education and physical activity opportunities outside of school: "We need to do things differently, move away from curricula that mirror only what has been done in the past, and build programmes that reflect the desires and needs of young people so that they might persist in their efforts to develop physically active lifestyles" (Tannehill, 2007, p. 3).

Young people need to acquire skills that will allow them to be involved in the three pillars as something other than a player when and where appropriate. This is the main premise of Daryl Siedentop's Sport Education (1994) curriculum and instructional model, where "players" learn how to perform various nonplaying roles such as team coach, game official, team publicist, team scout, and team manager.

Over time the physical education curriculum has tended to evolve and change in line with dominant and popularized notions of what constitutes worthwhile and meaningful physical activity and sporting opportunities. The United States has always focused on fitness as an element of school physical education; the dramatic increase in the potential health implications associated with being physically active, and by association addressing the number of overweight and obese children and young people, has begun to impact school physical education programs internationally. *Physical well-being*, including the components of physical fitness and health, have become more prominent in teaching school physical education, as has an increasing interest in the notion of health-based physical education programs, with countries such as Australia, Canada, and New Zealand including Health and Physical Education as a curriculum area.

The key role that physical education teachers play in determining young people's attitudes and feelings towards physical education can be heightened when the teacher is further involved in extracurricular sport and community and club sport, provides young people with information on how to access physical activity out of school, and/or develops links between physical education and community programs.

School Physical Education's Influence on Extracurricular Sport and Community and Club Sport

A positive and powerful relationship among physical education, extracurricular sport, and community and club sport can result in young people being disposed to involvement in physical activity and, by association, conveying a positive and proactive attitude towards physical education during adolescence and physical activity in young adulthood. Alternatively, in instances where schools are under pressure to produce competitive and skillful players to compete in extracurricular sport, the relationship between physical education and extracurricular sport is somewhat forced. Positioning physical education in this way could result in physical education being seen as a precursor to the school sports program and the foundation of the elite sport pyramid (Kirk & Gorely, 2000, cited in Pope, 2011). Physical education should not be viewed as supplying the raw fodder for extracurricular clubs, where week one of class in the new academic year is about fitness testing pupils and then streaming them into more- and less-able groups as a precursor to initially identifying those with a talent in a particular sport.

The relationship between physical education and community and club sport can also be powerful. A 10-year Norwegian longitudinal study has examined the relationship between participation in organized youth sport and attitude to physical education during adolescence and physical activity in young adulthood (Kjønniksen, Fjørtoft, & Wold, 2009). Participation in organized sport was found to be the strongest predictor of physical activity at age 23 years in males, whereas attitude to physical education was the strongest predictor in females. The authors concluded that participation in sport and physical activity in different arenas during adolescence may affect participation differently in young adult men and women. It is therefore imperative that physical education teachers consider the impact that physical education can have on young people's future involvement in maintaining active lifestyles as well as the positive reciprocal relationship between young people's attitude to physical education and participation in organized sports during adolescence.

Extracurricular Sport and Community and Club Sport

There is a strong possibility that the activities young people choose to play through extracurricular sport are also the activities they undertake in a community and sport club setting. This then poses a challenge to the physical education teacher, if they are involved in providing extracurricular sport, as to how best to provide and promote an extracurricular provision that interfaces between physical education and community and sport club contexts. In producing a database of physical activity, physical education, and sport participation levels of children and youth in Ireland, Woods and colleagues (2010) found that participation in extracurricular sport increased the likelihood of postprimary students' involvement in community and club sport (what they termed extraschool sport) by 99%.

There is also the possibility that young people may like to have access to different kinds of extracurricular sport and physical activity opportunities beyond the more traditional choices available to them. For example, young people have been exposed in recent years to increasing recreational participation in activities—such as dance, BMX, and martial arts—that have achieved popular status through media exposure. Such activities do not, however, challenge the continuing dominance of games being taught in physical education programs (Hardman, 2008).

An Example of a Challenge Set by the Three Pillars

Referencing Ireland as a case study example, the link between physical activities offered in school and what is available in the community varies, with some activities having better pathways and being more successful at recruiting and engaging young people than others (Woods et al., 2010). **Table 1.1** and **Table 1.2** show the postprimary participation rates across all three pillars of physical activity in an Irish context. Table 1.1 conveys that for Irish postprimary males, a number of activities that they participate in during physical education are either not provided for as extracurricular sport or community and club sport (extraschool sport) or students choose not to continue participation outside of school. Such activities include basketball, badminton, and gymnastics. Table 1.2 conveys a similar trend for Irish postprimary girls, with basketball, athletics, and badminton being some of the activities that a significant number of girls are exposed to during physical education but do not engage with as extracurricular sport or community and club sport (extraschool sport).

Although this example is based on data from Ireland, there may be similar patterns internationally of concern as regards the difference in participation levels across the three pillars for particular physical activities. It was alluded

TABLE 1.1 Participation Levels in Extraschool Sport/Activity, Extracurricular Sport/Activity, and Physical Education Among Postprimary Males

Activity	Extraschool (%)	Extracurricular (%)	Physical Education (%)
Soccer	32	17	62
Gaelic football	27	12	32
Hurling	17	8	15
Rugby	12	7	26
Weight training	12	3	14
Swimming	12	3	14
Athletics	9	7	38
Basketball	6	9	47
Martial arts	6	5	5
Tennis	5	3	17
Baseball/rounders	4	4	35
Badminton	4	5	38
Dance	4	2	12
Cross country running	4	3	13
Adventure activities	3	2	22
Handball	3	3	24
Horse riding	3	1	3
Hockey	2	2	20
Aerobics/exercise class	2	2	17
Gymnastics	1	2	21
Camogie	1	1	4
Squash	1	2	6
Any other sport	10	3	6

Reproduced from Woods, C. B., Tannehill D., Quinlan, A., Moyna, N., & Walsh, J. (2010). *Children's sport participation and physical activity study (CSPPA).* Research Report No 1. School of Health and Human Performance, Dublin City University and The Irish Sports Council, Dublin, Ireland. Table 35, page 108. Used with permission of The Irish Sports Council.

TABLE 1.2 Participation Levels in Extraschool Sport/Activity, Extracurricular Sport/Activity, and Physical Education Among Postprimary Females

Activity	Extraschool (%)	Extracurricular (%)	Physical Education (%)
Dance	23	6	35
Swimming	19	4	15
Gaelic football	17	9	27
Camogie	11	6	12
Soccer	10	7	46
Horse riding	9	2	5
Athletics	8	9	48
Basketball	7	14	63
Tennis	7	5	29
Aerobics/exercise class	6	4	31
Baseball/rounders	6	5	57
Cross country running	5	5	16
Gymnastics	5	3	34
Hurling	5	3	9
Adventure activities	4	2	26
Badminton	4	6	53
Hockey	4	6	34
Martial arts	4	4	8
Rugby	3	3	20
Weight training	3	1	7
Handball	2	2	21
Squash	2	1	6
Any other sport	10	3	7

Reproduced from Woods, C. B., Tannehill D., Quinlan, A., Moyna, N., & Walsh, J. (2010). *Children's sport participation and physical activity study (CSPPA).* Research Report No 1. School of Health and Human Performance, Dublin City University and The Irish Sports Council, Dublin, Ireland. Table 36, page 109. Used with permission of The Irish Sports Council.

to earlier in the chapter that physical education should not solely set out to promote physical activities that young people are involved in as an extracurricular sport and/or community and club sport. Rather, physical education should be seen as an opportunity to gain the appropriate and necessary skills that will allow young people to access physical activities in their local community, and also introduce them to organized physical activities not available in their local community but that may enhance their chances of being physically active into the future (e.g., dance). We are not suggesting that the physical education curriculum and extracurricular content be based solely on what is available outside of school. This could potentially lead to a narrowing of experiences for young people and maintaining the status quo of prevailing sporting opportunities (e.g., team sports/games).

Learning Experience 1.2

In your own context, which physical activities offered in school also are available in the community? What activities are offered in the community but not in physical education? Which are offered in physical education but not in the community? Which physical activities do young people seem to stop participating in beyond physical education?

Connection with Other Physical Activity Professionals

One would hope that those involved in promoting physical activity (e.g., physical education teachers, youth sport trainers and coaches, youth sport coordinators, volunteers, youth workers, parents, other subject teachers, representatives of sport federations/sport development officers) would share a relatively common understanding of the role of physical education, sport, and physical activity in the lives of young people. However, it is likely that there will be instances where the values and philosophies towards each will differ. The challenge is to develop partnerships across the professions, hoping that such differences do not compromise the young person's exposure to meaningful and worthwhile opportunities to be physically active. There can be little doubt that those involved in promoting a lifelong physically active and healthy lifestyle need to work together to meet the challenge of providing physical activities and sports that meet the needs and interests of young people.

In England, the PE and Sport Strategy for Young People initiative (PESSYP) encourages those involved in promoting physical education and community sport to work together to offer all young people ages 5 to 16 years the opportunity to participate in 5 hours of physical education and sport each week. The *Guide to Delivering the Five-Hour Offer* (Sport England/YST/PE & Sport for Young People, 2009) outlines a vision for the strategy, and in particular the 5-hour offer (see **Box 1.3**), providing case-study examples illustrating how the school and community can interact to provide the 5 hours of physical education and sport (see **Box 1.4**). There is an acknowledgement that the roles and responsibilities of the providers need to be shared, and that providers should make physical education and sport more accessible, attractive, affordable, and appropriate to the needs of young people (MacPhail, 2011).

BOX 1.3 Vision for the PE and Sport Strategy for Young People

For 5- to 16-year-olds, the expectation is that schools will provide 3 of the 5 hours; 2 hours through high quality PE within the curriculum and at least 1 hour a week of sport for all young people beyond the curriculum (out of school hours on school sites). Community and club providers will seek to ensure that an additional 2 hours a week are available.

For 16- to 19-year-olds in school, schools/colleges will be expected to work in partnership with community groups and clubs to ensure an appropriate 3-hour offer is available. For those young people not in the educational system, hiring and training community providers in partnership with local authorities will be expected to provide access to affordable opportunities to take part in sport.

As part of this, every young person should have the following:

- Access to regular competitive sport
- Coaching to improve their skills and enjoyment
- A choice of different sports
- Pathways to club and elite sport
- Opportunities to lead and volunteer in sport

Each young person is likely to access their 5 hours in a range of different settings. We have identified five environments where most activity will take place:

1. *School:* This includes all PE plus sport-related specialty courses that lead to a qualification (e.g., GCSE, A Level, BTEC). It includes structured changing time but not break times, lunchtimes, or travel time.
2. *School/college:* This includes all sporting activity that is managed and coordinated by the school/college or school/college bodies outside of curriculum time.
3. *Structured community sports clubs:* These are sports or dance clubs where a membership fee is generally paid. This will mainly (but not exclusively) be those sports with a national governing body (NGB). This does not include generic membership in, for example, a local community center, which is covered in the following point.
4. *Community sport settings (not in clubs):* This is sporting activity where a conscious decision has been made to participate or train but not in a constituted club environment. It includes activities such as "pay and play" sport, free swimming, and classes/lessons that are paid for on a regular basis.
5. *Community settings where sport is part of a wider range of activity:* This is sporting activity in settings where sport is part of a varied menu of activity. This can include the youth club sectors, such as uniformed organizations and youth clubs as well as kids clubs operated by organizations such as local authorities.

Reproduced from Sport England/Youth Sport Trust/PE & Sport for Young People. (2009). *The PE and sport strategy for young people: A guide to delivering the five-hour offer* (pp. 6–9). Loughborough, UK: Youth Sports Trust.

BOX 1.4 Examples of Personalized Five-Hour Offers for Young People

Case Study 1: Shanwaz, a 6-Year-Old Student at a Primary School

School and school sport partnership:

- Shanwaz participates in 75 minutes of PE every Thursday morning and another 75 minutes on Thursday afternoon.
- Every Friday at lunchtime, he takes part in a 30-minute organized session of playground activity led by Year 6 (fifth-grade) students from his school, and on Monday evenings he attends a 45-minute dance club at the school.

Club and community:

- Shanwaz has swimming lessons on Saturday mornings at his local club. Once he can swim 50 meters, he is looking forward to joining the improver group on Monday evenings for 1 hour a week.
- On Friday evenings Shanwaz goes with his brother and dad to a family fun sports session at his local community center.

Case Study 2: Ellie, a 13-Year-Old Student at a Secondary School

School and school sport partnership:

- Ellie's school operates a 2-week timetable/schedule. In the first week she participates in 2 hours of PE, and in the second week this increases to 3 hours.
- Ellie was identified by her school a year ago as someone who wasn't fully engaging in PE. She was invited to attend an active lifestyle club at lunch on Thursdays. This helped to build her confidence, and she now participates fully in PE and still attends the club, joining in activity and supporting Year 7 and 8 (sixth- and seventh-grade) students.

Club and community:

- Through her attendance at a local youth club, Ellie heard about a 10-week trampolining program offered at a local community/leisure center. After attending eight sessions, she decided to take it up more regularly and has joined a local gymnastics club, attending for 2 hours a week.
- Through her involvement in the trampolining session, Ellie met two new friends at the community/leisure center and now meets up with them every Friday night at the center to do a 1-hour aerobics session.

Reproduced from Sport England/Youth Sport Trust/PE & Sport for Young People. (2009). *The PE and sport strategy for young people: A guide to delivering the five-hour offer* (pp. 22–23). Loughborough, UK: Youth Sports Trust.

In the United States, the National Plan for Physical Activity was unveiled in 2010 (see www.physicalactivityplan.org), bringing together eight societal sectors with the central objective of increasing access to and opportunity for physical activity for all Americans. The participating sectors are education; parks, recreation, fitness, and sports; public health; health care; business and industry; mass media; transportation, land use, and community design; and volunteer and nonprofit organizations. Each sector developed general strategies with accompanying tactics. **Box 1.5** shows the education sector's overall strategies and related tactics. Since its unveiling, an implementation guide has been published with information about implementation priorities and suggested resources to aid organizations such as schools in implementing the strategies and tactics.

The following section provides examples of programs that encourage consideration of physical educators' changing context, and by association working in partnership with other professionals interested in increasing young people's exposure to physical activity.

Examples of Programs and Related Partnerships

Numerous suggestions have been made in recent years on how best to support schools' potential for effectively providing and promoting physical activity within the physical education program, throughout the school day and beyond the school campus (Broeke, van Dalfsen, Bax, Rijpstra, & Schouten, 2008; NASPE, 2008; Pate et al., 2007). De Knop, Engstrom, and Skirstad's (1996) comment remains somewhat true to this day:

> *Perhaps one of the greatest challenges facing youth sport now and in the near future is to set up a cooperative and coordinated approach by schools and clubs*

BOX 1.5 National Physical Activity Plan: Education Sector Strategies and Related Tactics

Strategy 1

Provide access to and opportunities for high-quality, comprehensive physical activity programs, anchored by physical education, in pre-kindergarten through grade 12 educational settings. Ensure that the programs are physically active, inclusive, safe, and developmentally and culturally appropriate.

Tactics:

- Advocate for increased federal funding of programs such as the Carol White Physical Education for Progress (PEP) grant program.
- Include in funding criteria the development of state-of-the-art, comprehensive physical activity demonstration programs and pilot projects, and effective evaluation of those programs.
- Include a preference for adoption of physical education (PE) and physical activity (PA) programs demonstrated to provide high amounts of physical activity.
- Widely disseminate successful demonstration and pilot programs and those with practice-based evidence. Work with states to identify areas of great need, prioritizing funding efforts toward lower-resourced communities.
- Provide adequate funding for research that advances this strategy and all other education sector strategies.
- Require pre-service and continuing education for physical education and elementary classroom teachers to deliver high-quality physical education and physical activity programs.
- Provide continuing education classes and seminars for all teachers on state-of-the-art physical activities for children that provide information on adapting activities for children with disabilities, in classrooms and physical education settings.
- Encourage higher education institutions to train future teachers and school personnel on the importance of physical activity to academic achievement and success for students from pre-kindergarten through grade 12.

Strategy 2

Develop and implement state and school district policies requiring school accountability for the quality and quantity of physical education and physical activity programs.

Tactics:

- Advocate for binding requirements for PreK–12 standards-based physical education that address state standards, curriculum time, class size, and employment of certified, highly qualified physical education teachers in accordance with national standards and guidelines, such as those published by the National Association for Sport and Physical Education (NASPE).
- Advocate for local, state, and national standards that emphasize provision of high levels of physical activity in physical education (e.g., 50% of class time in moderate-to-vigorous activity).
- Enact federal legislation, such as the FIT Kids Act, to require school accountability for the quality and quantity of physical education and physical activity programs.
- Provide local, state, and national funding to ensure that schools have the resources (e.g., facilities, equipment, appropriately trained staff) to provide high-quality physical education and activity programming. Designate the largest portion of funding for schools that are under-resourced. Work with states to identify areas of greatest need.
- Develop and implement state-level policies that require school districts to report on the quality and quantity of physical education and physical activity programs.
- Develop and implement a measurement and reporting system to determine the progress of states toward meeting this strategy. Include in this measurement and reporting system data to monitor the benefits and adaptations made or needed for children with disabilities.
- Require school districts to annually collect, monitor, and track students' health-related fitness data, including Body Mass Index.

BOX 1.5 National Physical Activity Plan: Education Sector Strategies and Related Tactics (*Continued*)

Strategy 3

Develop partnerships with other sectors for the purpose of linking youth with physical activity opportunities in schools and communities.

Tactics:

- Develop plans at local levels for leadership and collaboration across sectors, such as education, youth serving organizations, and parks and recreation.
- Develop and institute local policies and joint use agreements that facilitate shared use of physical activity facilities, such as school gyms and community recreation centers and programming.
- Prioritize efforts to target communities and schools by working with states to identify areas of greatest need.
- Develop partnerships with organizations that encourage citizen involvement, community mobilization, and volunteerism to link to and sustain community opportunities for physical activity.

Strategy 4

Ensure that early childhood education settings for children ages 0 to 5 years promote and facilitate physical activity.

Tactics:

- Develop policies that clearly define physical activity components for Head Start and other early childhood program providers.
- Develop and institute state-level standards for early childhood education programs that require the delivery of safe and appropriate physical activity programming.
- Work with community college systems to include physical activity training as part of childcare certification and early childhood training programs.
- Advocate for physical activity policies at childcare facilities that address the developmental needs of all children, including children with disabilities, those classified as obese, or children at high risk of inactivity.

Strategy 5

Provide access to and opportunities for physical activity before and after school.

Tactics:

- Support Safe Routes to School efforts to increase active transportation to and from school and support accommodations for children with disabilities.
- Encourage states to adopt standards for the inclusion of physical activity in after-school programs.
- Require a physical activity component in all state and federally funded after-school programs, including 21st Century Community Learning Centers.
- Work with community college systems to include physical activity training as part of early childhood and school-age childcare preparation programs.
- Subsidize the transportation and program costs of after-school programs through local, state, and federal sources.
- Provide resources for innovative pilot projects in the after-school setting.
- Encourage states to abide by national after-school accreditation standards on physical activity as applicable, and advance state licensure requirements in alignment with those standards.

Strategy 6

Encourage post-secondary institutions to provide access to physical activity opportunities, including physical activity courses, robust club and intramural programs, and adequate physical activity and recreation facilities.

(*continues*)

BOX 1.5 National Physical Activity Plan: Education Sector Strategies and Related Tactics (*Continued*)

Tactics:

- Advocate for state and federal funding to ensure that post-secondary institutions have resources (e.g., facilities, equipment, staff) to provide quality physical activity programming.
- Develop and implement local policies and joint use agreements that allow students in post-secondary institutions to have access to physical activity facilities, such as school gyms and community recreation centers.
- Encourage USDE/CHEA accrediting agencies to require all institutions receiving Federal (Title IV) funding to hold a class focusing on the impact of physical inactivity, resources and opportunities for physical activity, and positive health behaviors such as an institutional graduation requirement.

Strategy 7

Encourage post-secondary institutions to incorporate population-focused physical activity promotion training in a range of disciplinary degree and certificate programs.

Tactics:

- Fund the development and pilot testing of population-based physical activity promotion curricula for relevant disciplines such as nursing, medicine, physical therapy, urban planning, education, library science, and lay health advisor.
- Incorporate modules of population-based physical activity into Board exams.

Courtesy of the National Physical Activity Plan.

with the purpose of offering sports as an educational environment for all children that will enable them to develop at their own speed according to their own interests.[2]

We focus now on a number of programs that specifically encourage physical education teachers to be central in supporting a cooperative structure across physical education, extracurricular sport, and community and club sport. We acknowledge that in some countries partnerships among schools, clubs, and associations have a short history or are a result of local or random circumstances (i.e., are specific rather than institutionalized); in other instances collaboration is not obvious. We also are conscious that the extent to which individual governments prioritize the promotion and development of sport and physical education differs. Central points of reference are available for those who wish to further examine how different European and other countries practice and extend the delivery of physical education (Klein & Hardman, 2008; Puhse & Gerber, 2005).

Active Schools

The Active Schools Acceleration Project (ASAP) in the United States seeks to increase quality physical activity in schools as a means to promote healthy, active living and to evoke beneficial behavioral and academic outcomes. The project is committed to facilitating cross-sector collaboration to reverse the trend of childhood obesity within one generation's time. The initiative is to unfold in four phases: (1) identifying innovation, (2) replicating best practices in diverse environments, (3) scaling up nationally, and (4) achieving long-term sustainability. A principal tool for innovation discovery is a national innovation competition, funded by a consortium of the nation's leading health plans. The innovation competition is composed of two categories that solicit entries from distinct audiences to unearth the best strategies for increasing physical activity. The first category is newly developed technologies and/or unique applications of existing technologies that can increase quality physical activity in school and beyond. The second category is on-the-ground physical activity programs underway in schools across the country (see www.activeschoolsasap.org/about/asap).

The aims of the Active Schools initiative (popular in Australia, New Zealand, and Scotland) are to increase awareness, skills, and education regarding quality physical activity opportunities and physical education within the communities surrounding the school, and to enhance student physical activity and overall well-being. Related

[2] Reprinted, with permission, from De Knop, P., Engstrom, L. M., & Skirstad, B. (1996). *Worldwide trends in youth sport*. Champaign, IL: Human Kinetics. p. 281.

opportunities have included active commuting to school and providing the coaching for recreational activities. In one example from Scotland, the Active Schools team was able to create after-school girls-only dance clubs in each of the five secondary schools in the local authority. These clubs ran throughout two terms during the school year and were delivered by professional dance teachers from clubs in the local area. The Dance Project culminated in the very first regional Dance Festival at one of the schools. *Sport and Recreation* (formerly known as SPARC) New Zealand has produced an Active Schools Toolkit resource to help schools develop a culture of physical activity through (1) offering ideas for physical activity and activity-based learning across the curriculum, (2) providing easy ways to increase physical activity in co-curriculum areas, and (3) encouraging physical activity as a part of daily life in the school community (see www.sportnz.org.nz/en-nz/young-people/Ages-5-12-Years/Active-Schools-Toolkit).

The Active School Flag initiative in Ireland is a noncompetitive initiative that seeks to recognize schools that strive to achieve a physically active and physically educated school community. To be awarded the Active School Flag, schools must (1) commit to a process of self-evaluation in terms of the physical education programs and physical opportunities that they offer, and (2) plan and implement a series of changes that will enhance physical education and extracurricular provision and promote physical activity. The initiative encourages a partnership approach, empowering schools to become more proactive in approaching groups to help and support them to develop their physical education programs and to promote physical activity. Activities that schools have undertaken to bolster their chances of being awarded an Active School Flag include (1) introducing physical activity events for children, their parents, and school staff; (2) mini sport tournaments; (3) sport taster days where students try an activity for the first time; (4) orienteering in the local public park; (5) visits to local sports facilities; and (6) guest speakers to include local sport role models, referees, and physical activity coordinators/advisers.

In the United States, a Comprehensive School Physical Activity Program (CSPAP) is an approach by which school districts and schools utilize all opportunities for school-based physical activity to develop physically educated students (defined previously in the chapter) who participate in the nationally recommended 60+ minutes of physical activity each day and develop the knowledge, skills, and confidence to be physically active for a lifetime. The goals of a CSPAP and the five related components are listed in **Box 1.6**.

BOX 1.6 A Comprehensive School Physical Activity Program (CSPAP)

The goal of a CSPAP is two-fold.

- Provide a variety of school-based physical activity opportunities that enable all students to participate in at least 60 minutes of moderate-to-vigorous physical activity each day.
- Provide coordination among the CSPAP components to maximize understanding, application, and practice of the knowledge and skills learned in physical education so that all students will be fully physically educated and well-equipped for a lifetime of physical activity.

The five related components are:

1. *Physical education:* Physical education is the foundation of a comprehensive school physical activity program. It is an academic subject that uses a planned, sequential program of curricula and instruction, based on state and/or national physical education standards, which results in all students, including those with disabilities, developing the knowledge, skills, and confidence needed to adopt and maintain a physically activity lifestyle. Physical education should be taught by state-certified physical education teachers.
2. *Physical activity during school:* Physical activity during school provides opportunities for all students, including those with disabilities, to practice what they've learned in physical education, work towards the nationally recommended 60+ minutes of daily moderate-vigorous physical activity, and prepare the brain for learning. Opportunities include:
   - Physical activity integrated into classroom lessons
   - Physical activity breaks in the classroom
   - Recess (elementary school)
   - Drop-in physical activity (e.g., after eating lunch) (middle and high school)

(continues)

BOX 1.6 A Comprehensive School Physical Activity Program (CSPAP) (*Continued*)

3. *Physical activity before and after school:* Physical activity before and after school provides opportunities for all students, including those with disabilities, to practice what they've learned in physical education, work towards the nationally recommended 60+ minutes of daily moderate-vigorous physical activity, and prepare the brain for learning. Additional benefits include social interaction and engagement of students in safe, supervised activities. Opportunities include:
   - Walk and bike to school and implementation of a comprehensive Safe Routes to School program
   - Informal recreation or play on school grounds
   - Physical activity in school-based child-care
   - Physical activity clubs and intramural sports
   - Interscholastic sports
4. *Staff involvement:* High-level support from school administrators is critical to successful comprehensive school physical activity programs. Staff involvement in school-based physical activity provides two key benefits:
   - School employee wellness programs have been shown to improve staff health, increase physical activity levels, and be cost effective.
   - When school staff are personally committed to good health practices, they are positive role models for students and may show increased support for student participation.
5. *Family and community involvement:* Family and community involvement in school-based physical activity provides numerous benefits. Research shows that youth participation in physical activity is influenced by participation and support of parents and siblings. When families are active together, they spend additional time together and experience health benefits. Families can support a comprehensive school physical activity program by participating in evening/weekend special events and parents/guardians serving as physical education/activity volunteers. Community involvement allows maximum use of school and community resources (e.g., facilities, personnel) and creates a connection between school- and community-based physical activity opportunities. Joint-use agreements are an example of a formal school–community collaboration.

The Active and Healthy Schools program (AHS) in the United States is designed to improve the overall health and increase the activity levels of students by making changes to the whole school environment. Acknowledging that the implementation of new concepts may result in teachers feeling overwhelmed, the program consists of many small initiatives as a series of manageable tasks, such as forming an AHS committee and generating interest among parents and administrators. Core goals are identified in three key program areas and are listed in **Box 1.7**.

Healthy Schools

Schools across numerous countries (e.g., Australia, Canada, New Zealand, United States) are supported in their efforts to create environments where physical activity and healthy eating are accessible and encouraged. Collaboration among students, a school's teaching and nonteaching staff, families, and health professionals is encouraged to transform schools into healthy campuses. Associated initiatives that have been introduced to schools include improving the nutritional value of school meals, allowing access to school facilities after school and on weekends, increasing the amount of afterschool program time for physical activity opportunities, and increasing the length of recess breaks. Such initiatives are included in the Healthy Schools Program Framework (Alliance for a Healthier Generation, 2009), which provides criteria for developing a healthier school environment.

In the United States, Coordinated School Health (CSH) is recommended by the Centers for Disease Control and Prevention as a strategy for improving students' health and learning in schools, acknowledging that after the family, the school is the primary institution responsible for the development of young people in the United States. A CSPAP (discussed previously) is part of a larger school health framework called Coordinated School Health (CSH). A summary of the key goals and strategies for CSH is available in **Box 1.8**.

The initiative is viewed as perhaps one of the most efficient means to prevent or reduce risk behaviors and prevent serious health problems among students. Effective school health policies and programs may also increase academic

BOX 1.7 Active and Healthy Schools Program Goals

Active school day:

- Provide 15+ minutes of recess daily.
- Offer 20+ minutes or more for physical activity after lunchtime.
- Hold at least three activity breaks of 3 to 5 minutes in length throughout the school day (not including recess or lunchtime).
- Provide a PE program that meets two or more days each week.
- Offer students the opportunity to earn the President's Challenge Active Lifestyle Award.
- Provide a physical activity program to teachers and staff.
- Post activity prompts and signs promoting activity throughout the school.

Active after school:

- Establish an after-school activity program (playground or gym facilities should be open and available).
- Zone playground for safety, according to AHS guidelines.
- Create an AHS message center (bulletin board) highlighting after-school activities, rules, news, and activity directions.
- Focus on recreational (rather than competitive) activities.
- Offer after-school field trips.

Nutrition:

- Create a Food and Nutrition Team to oversee breakfast, snacks, lunch, celebrations, and fundraisers.
- Promote awareness of food groups, calories, and balance of activity and nutrition.
- Post Point-of-Decision signs to encouraging healthy food choices.
- Offer healthy breakfast and lunch menus.
- Offer incentives for making healthy food choices.
- Provide take-home information about healthy food choices.

BOX 1.8 A Summary of the Key Goals and Strategies of School Health Programs

1. *Increase health knowledge, attitudes, and skills.*
   - School health instruction helps young people improve their health knowledge. For example, students learn nutrition facts and how to read product labels so they can make healthy eating choices.
   - School health instruction helps young people develop related life skills, including communication and interpersonal skills, decision making and critical thinking skills, and coping and self-management skills. For example, students learn a variety of ways to refuse alcohol or tobacco and practice those skills.
   - Improved communication and life skills can positively affect students' health decisions and behaviors and promote effective citizenship.
2. *Increase positive health behaviors and health outcomes.*
   - School health programs can be designed to help youth avoid specific risk behaviors, including those that contribute to the leading causes of injury, illness, social problems, and death in the United States; alcohol and other drug use; tobacco use; injury and violence; unhealthy eating; physical inactivity; and sexual risk behaviors. These behaviors, often established during childhood and early adolescence, are interrelated and can persist into adulthood.
   - Specific school health interventions have proven effective in significantly reducing these risk behaviors, improving health promoting behaviors, and improving health outcomes.
   - School health programs can also create safer schools and positive social environments that contribute to improved health and learning.

(continues)

BOX 1.8 A Summary of the Key Goals and Strategies of School Health Programs (*Continued*)

3. *Improve education outcomes.*
   - Students who are healthy are more likely to learn than those who are unhealthy. School health programs can appraise, protect, and improve the health of students, thus reducing tardiness and absenteeism and increasing academic achievement.
   - Students who acquire more years of education ultimately become healthier adults and practice fewer of the health risk behaviors most likely to lead to premature illness and death.
4. *Improve social outcomes.*
   - School health programs can provide opportunities to build positive social interactions and foster the development of students' respect, tolerance, and self-discipline. For example, conflict resolution and peer mediation programs help students learn how to listen and solve problems.
   - School health programs can reduce delinquency, drug use, and teen pregnancy, increasing the likelihood that young people will become productive, well-adjusted members of their communities.
   - School health programs can provide access to community programs and services that can help students contribute positively to their family, school, and community.

Courtesy of Centers for Disease Control and Prevention. Adapted from Kolbe, L. (2002). Education reform and the goals of modern school health programs. *The State Education Standard*, 3(4), 4–11. Available from www.cdc.gov/healthyyouth/cshp/goals.htm

achievement through the reduction of health-risk behaviors such as substance use and physical inactivity. The reason for coordinating school health is to address the different expectations (and in some cases duplication) that arise through policies and programs targeted at a school and the associated range of regulations, initiatives, and funding. Coordinating the many parts of school health into a systematic approach can enable schools to (1) eliminate gaps and reduce redundancies across the many initiatives and funding streams; (2) build partnerships and teamwork among school health and education professionals in the school; (3) build collaboration and enhance communication among public health, school health, and other education and health professionals in the community; and (4) focus efforts on helping students engage in protective, health-enhancing behaviors and avoid risk behaviors (see www.cdc.gov/healthyyouth/cshp/case.htm).

The framework for planning and coordinating school health activities centers around eight critical, interrelated components: health education, physical education, health services, mental health and social services, nutrition services, healthy and safe environment, family involvement, and community involvement (see www.cdc.gov/healthyyouth/cshp/components.htm). A success story from New Mexico on how schools are helping students be healthy is noted in **Box 1.9**.

In the United States, SPARK (Sports, Play and Active Recreation for Kids) is dedicated to creating, implementing, and evaluating programs that promote lifelong wellness. A review of completed research on the SPARK program has been completed by McKenzie, Sallis, and Rosengard (2009). SPARK strives to improve the health of children, adolescents, and adults by disseminating evidence-based physical education, after school, early childhood, and coordinated school health programs to teachers and recreation leaders serving all school-aged children (see www.sparkpe.org/what-is-spark). Each SPARK program fosters environmental and behavioral change by providing a coordinated package of highly active curriculum, on-site teacher training, extensive follow-up support, and content-matched equipment. SPARK is a commercial enterprise in which curriculum, training, and equipment related to the program are purchased by those who wish to introduce the initiative. One success story from SPARK is noted in **Box 1.10**.

Olympic Day/Mini Olympic Games

Many countries (Cyprus, Czech Republic, Estonia, Lithuania) report a number of initiatives based on publicizing the Olympic movement, involving schools planning and implementing Olympic Day festivals (Klein & Hardman, 2008). Such festivals include teachers from different subject areas working in cooperation in the school curriculum as well as making connections with physical education teacher associations, relevant government departments, sport federations, and the national Olympic committee. The Olympic program tends not to focus only on the performance of athletic competitions but also acknowledges students' engagement with the principles of the Olympics (e.g., fair play) as well as meeting with Olympic athletes.

BOX 1.9 New Mexico: Strengthening Health Education Through Graduation Requirements

More than half of the states have recognized the importance of teaching health education (HE) in middle or high school and have implemented an HE requirement for graduation. In 2009, New Mexico did not have a state-level HE requirement for graduation. At the district level, only 34 of 89 school districts were teaching HE as a stand-alone class. School districts integrated HE into a variety of other classes, did not require an HE class to graduate, or did not require that the class be taught by a state-licensed health educator.

Although legislative efforts in 2009 did not result in HE being mandated as a graduation requirement in New Mexico, the Senate Education Committee recommended further study to determine the level of need and public support for this change. The New Mexico Public Education Department (NMPED) convened a workgroup that included representatives from the NMPED (including a CDC-supported coordinator for the HIV Prevention Education Program), the state health department, higher education institutions, community groups, and the legislative education study committee as well as school superintendents and educators.

The workgroup researched best practices for delivering HE and conducted extensive surveys to determine support for making HE a graduation requirement. Finding strong evidence and support for including a stand-alone HE class in the state's graduation requirements, the workgroup presented that recommendation to the Senate Education Committee.

In 2010, New Mexico passed a new law that went into effect during the 2012–2013 school year. The law will:

- Require a class in HE for graduation from a public school.
- Allow school districts to determine if the class will be taught in middle school or high school.
- Require that HE be taught in a stand-alone class by a licensed health educator.

Requiring HE as a graduation requirement is a major step toward ensuring that New Mexico's youth receive

- Evidence-based health information to guide their decision-making.
- More opportunities to learn about and practice healthy lifestyle habits, including healthy eating and physical activity, which can lower the risk of becoming obese.
- More skills-based instruction focused on reducing health risk behaviors, including sexual risk behaviors.

A CDC-supported program coordinator is helping to train curriculum directors, school administrators, and health educators to implement the new requirement. The coordinator also will review school districts' implementation plans to ensure compliance with state HE standards. The NMPED will use CDC's School Health Profiles, a survey that can be used to assess school health policies and practices, to monitor the effect of the new requirement.

Courtesy of Centers for Disease Control and Prevention. (2011). Reproduced from School health programs: How states are helping students be healthy. Available from www.cdc.gov/chronicdisease/resources/publications/aag/pdf/2011/School_Health_success_stories.pdf

BOX 1.10 A Public Health Success Story

Highmark Healthy High 5 is a 5-year, $100 million investment of the Highmark Foundation. Through Healthy High 5, the Highmark Foundation strives to improve the health and well-being of children and create a brighter future for us all.

Highmark chose SPARK as their partner to improve the quantity and quality of physical activity in after school programs. The SPARK After School Program provides research-based content (the "what" to teach), professional development (the "how" to teach) and age-appropriate equipment (the "tools" needed to teach). These coordinated components, along with extensive follow up support from SPARK and Highmark, are provided to schools in the counties Highmark serves in Pennsylvania and West Virginia.

Working closely with Highmark, the SPARK staff listened to their vision and prescribed a dissemination plan that built capacity, utilized economy of scale, and was sustainable. SPARK also consulted on assessment and evaluation so the results could be measured and outcomes authentically demonstrated. To date, SPARK has provided training for 6 different Highmark staff with physical activity backgrounds. These dynamic professionals were taught the SPARK After School Program via workshops, Institutes, and a train the trainer model, then practiced teaching it to children, and now are SPARK Certified Trainers able to conduct effective and inspirational SPARK workshops for the Healthy High 5 initiative. The after school programs that participate in training also receive SPARK curriculum, equipment and follow up support so their programs work and last! To date, dozens of sites and hundreds of youth leaders have become trained and their after school programs are lighting up children's lives throughout Pennsylvania!

Initiatives such as Olympic day and mini Olympic games are grounded in the Sport for All movement. Sport for All promotes the Olympic ideal that sport is a human right for all individuals regardless of race, social class, and sex. The movement encourages sports activities that can be exercised by people of all ages, both sexes, and different social and economic conditions. The intention is that the goal can be achieved through cooperation via international sports federations, national Olympic committees, and national sports organizations (see www.olympic.org/sport-for-all-commission?tab=mission).

School Sport Associations

In the Czech Republic, school sport clubs are encouraged to become affiliated with the Association of School Sport Clubs, which organizes interclass and interschool contests. The association's events are open to all students and promote a friendly atmosphere, the spirit of fair play, and the maintenance of an active lifestyle. Meetings of school teams are a typical feature of the association's competitions, and members of a team have to be students from the same school. In Hungary, School Sport Games provide a framework for organizing sports competitions in which students can participate.

Relative to the within-school competitions, the program mirrors in part the intramural program that historically has been a part of many physical education programs in the United States. Intramural programs are regarded as an extension of the regular physical education lessons. Students at the school form teams and sign up for a tournament of games that are typically played during lunch recess periods. Unfortunately, in recent years many programs have eliminated the intramural program as a consequence of, for example, budget cutbacks and reductions in time available for lunch.

Annual Sport Festivals

In France, public authorities coordinate with schools and sport clubs to run annual sport festivals in a variety of sports as a means to promote an active lifestyle among students. Teachers and students can be involved in seeking financial support for such festivals from local authorities and sponsors.

Partnership Opportunities with Sporting Federations

In many European countries, sporting federations visit schools to promote their particular sport, bringing with them the appropriate equipment for students to try out and also local club athletes to mentor those interested in participating in the sport. The Wibbel an Dribbel (Moves and Dribble) initiative in Luxembourg invites all 10-year-old students to gather for one day in the Sport and Cultural National Center to take part in 30-minute workshops for 10 new activities presented by a number of sporting federations.

Learning Experience 1.3

Choose one example from the programs listed in the previous section and consider (1) how the program could be reconfigured to suit your local context, (2) who you would need to establish partnerships with to deliver the program, (3) how you would establish such partnerships, and (4) how you would propose to initiate such a program.

Revisit the programs listed and consider those programs that you either do not support the practices of or do not see being possible in your particular teaching context.

Online Physical Education: The Way Forward or the Demise of Physical Education?

Peter was nearly finished high school and was finding it hard to complete his physical education requirement while balancing studies, sports, and a social life. Through the Minneapolis school system's online physical education, Peter could fulfill his physical education credit after school by playing on the Ultimate Frisbee team. The Minneapolis school system's online physical education allows students to choose a physical activity they enjoy, do it for 30 minutes three times a week—on their own time—while keeping an online journal. A parent or coach must confirm the student did the activities.

Learning Experience 1.4

Complete a physical activity timeline. On an 8 1/2 by 11, landscape piece of paper, draw a line from left to right in the bottom third of the paper. Working from left to right on the line, denote intervals of 5 years (e.g., 5 years old, 10 years old). Note (1) the physical activities and sport you participated in during each interval, (2) who facilitated the activities, and (3) where they took place. In what way does your timeline provide support (or not) for online physical education that accounts for the time you spend being physically active outside of school physical education?

The number of online physical education programs has grown over the past few years, particularly in the United States (Mosier, 2010). Arguments have been made that online physical education programs help students make the transition into lifelong healthy fitness habits, encouraging self-responsibility, with the view that students who do not attend the traditionally timetabled physical education school lessons can be reached through an online program. Online programs also report a shift from the team sport emphasis (common in physical education) to personal fitness, health, and wellness. Students choose the activities they wish to take part in and have been reported as choosing activities that they could continue into their adult lives, including skateboarding, training for a triathlon, and Ultimate Frisbee. Some programs require that students perform better at the end of the online program on fitness tests than they did at the start to pass the program.

The National Association for Sport and Physical Education (NASPE) is cautious about supporting online physical education, noting that there is a need for further research on such programs, and in particular the effectiveness of online physical education courses on student learning. They surmise that many physical educators still advocate face-to-face teaching to ensure that learning takes place and that motor movements and exercises are performed efficiently, correctly, and safely. NASPE has produced a document, *Initial Guidelines for Online Physical Education* (NASPE, 2007), intended for those who are considering the multitude of implications for preparing and teaching online physical education courses at the high school level. To assist teachers in determining the quality and effectiveness of online physical education courses, the guidelines prompt teachers to consider student, teacher, and curriculum prerequisites; assessment; class size; time allocation; availability of community facilities; equipment and technology systems; program evaluation; and students with special needs.

Learning Experience 1.5

What are your thoughts regarding online physical education, and how would you propose to address the limitations of the likely self-reported mechanisms supported by online physical education? What concerns would you have for physical education as a school subject if sports clubs provided all the physical activity requirements for online physical education? How would you go about creating a quality online physical education program?

CHAPTER SUMMARY

This chapter encouraged physical educators to consider their responsibility in helping young people engage with physical activity and sport beyond the physical education environment, providing young people with potential pathways for maintaining an involvement in physical activity. We would hope that such a responsibility is considered as physical educators (1) strive to design positive learning environments, (2) deliver instructionally aligned physical education programs, and (3) sustain high-quality physical education programs. That is, as physical educators, you continually think beyond your physical education lessons and school teams to how best to advocate for, and prepare young people to undertake, a life of autonomous well-being.

1. Physical education lessons alone, and by association physical educators, cannot be solely responsible for increasing the physical activity levels of young people.
2. Physical educators have a responsibility to help engage young people with physical activity and sport beyond the physical education environment, providing young people with potential pathways for maintaining an involvement in physical activity.
3. Although there is a general level of consensus on what the roles and objectives of school physical education should be, differences exist in the extent to which countries expand and refine what a physically educated person looks like.
4. The historical expectation that a physical educator does not deviate from teaching physical education full-time in one school is now being challenged. Examples around the world encourage physical educators to be somewhat involved in school extracurricular sport and physical activities throughout the school day as well as enhance links between the school and community sporting and physical activity opportunities.
5. School physical education provision appears to be more similar than different in its delivery across numerous countries. What constitutes extracurricular sport and physical activity and community and club sport across countries is noticeably different.
6. As a physical educator, one has to consider the extent to which sports and physical activities experienced in the physical education program encourage involvement in extracurricular and community and club sport and physical activity.
7. Numerous initiatives are now up and running that develop partnerships across the professions involved in promoting sport and physical activity to young people. There is an acknowledgment that the shared roles and responsibilities of providers are to make physical education and sport more accessible, attractive, affordable, and appropriate to the needs of young people.
8. The role of the physical educator to encourage "active" schools has been developed to incorporate activity as an element of "healthy" schools. The focus here is on developing a healthier school environment, looking to prevent or reduce risk behaviors and prevent serious health problems among students.
9. Arguments have been made that the development of online physical education programs helps students make the transition into lifelong healthy fitness habits, encouraging self-responsibility, with the view that students who do not attend the traditionally timetabled physical education school lessons can be reached through an online program.

REFERENCES

Alliance for a Healthier Generation. (2009). *Healthy schools program framework. Criteria for developing a healthier school environment*. Portland, OR: Alliance for a Healthier Generation.

Association for Physical Education (afPE). (2008). Manifesto for a world class system of physical education, 2008. Available from www.afpe.org.uk/images/stories/Manifesto.pdf

Bailey, R., Armour, K., Kirk, D., Jess, M., Pickup, I., Sandford, R., & BERA Physical Education and Sport Pedagogy Special Interest Group. (2009). The educational benefits claimed for physical education and school sport: An academic review. *Research Papers in Education, 24*(1), 1–27.

Broeke, A., van Dalfsen, G., Bax, H., Rijpstra, J., & Schouten, M. (2008). Physical education and sport education in the Netherlands. In G. Klein & K. Hardman (Eds.), *Physical education and sport education in the European Union* (pp. 298–314). Paris: Editions Revue EP.S.

De Knop, P., Engstrom, L. M., & Skirstad, B. (1996). *Worldwide trends in youth sport*. Champaign, IL: Human Kinetics.

Department for Education and Skills & Department for Culture, Media and Sport. (2003). *Learning through PE and sport. A guide to the physical education, school sport and club links strategy*. Nottingham, England: DfES.

Fahey, T., Delaney, L., & Gannon, B. (2005). *School children and sport in Ireland*. Dublin: Irish Sports Council.

Fry, J. M., & McNeill, M. (2011). "In the nation's good": Physical education and school sport in Singapore. *European Physical Education Review, 17*, 287–300.

Hardman, K. (2008). Physical education in schools: A global perspective. *Kinesiology, 40*(1), 5–28.

Hardman, K. (n.d.). An up-date on the status of physical education in schools worldwide: Technical report for the World Health Organisation. Available from www.icsspe.org/sites/default/files/Kenneth%20Hardman%20update%20on%20physical%20education%20in%20schools%20worldwide.pdf

Hartley, T. (2011). Preparing physical education teachers for the reality of teaching in schools: The case of one physical education teacher education (PETE) programme. Master's thesis, University of Limerick, Ireland.

Kirk, D. (2005). Physical education, youth sport and lifelong participation: The importance of early learning experiences. *European Physical Education Review, 11*, 239–255.

Kirk, D., & Gorely, T. (2000). Challenging thinking about the relationship between school physical education and sports performance. *European Physical Education Review, 6*(2), 119–133.

Kjønniksen, L., Fjørtoft, I., & Wold, B. (2009). Attitude to physical education and participation in organized youth sports during adolescence related to physical activity in young adulthood: A 10-year longitudinal study. *European Physical Education Review, 15*, 139–154.

Klein, G., & Hardman, K. (Eds.). (2008). *Physical education and sport education in the European Union*. Paris: Editions Revue EP.S.

Kolbe, L. (2002). Education reform and the goals of modern school health programs. *State Education Standard, 3*(4), 4–11.

MacPhail, A. (2011). Youth voices in physical education and sport: What are they telling us? In K. Armour (ed.), *Sport pedagogy: An introduction for teaching and coaching* (pp. 105–116). Harrow, England: Prentice Hall.

McKenzie, T. L., Sallis, J. F., & Rosengard, P. (2009). Beyond the stucco tower: Design, development, and dissemination of the SPARK physical education programs. *Quest, 61*(1), 114–127.

Mosier, B. (2010). A descriptive study of Florida virtual school's physical education students: An initial exploration. PhD dissertation, Florida State University.

National Association for Sport and Physical Education. (2013). Minutes of the 2013 NASPE Board Meeting.

National Association for Sport and Physical Education. (2007). *Initial guidelines for online physical education* [Position statement]. Reston, VA: National Association for Sport and Physical Education.

National Association for Sport and Physical Education. (2008). *Comprehensive school physical activity programs* [Position statement]. Reston, VA: National Association for Sport and Physical Education.

Neumark-Sztainer, D., Wall, M., Guo, J., Story, M., Haines, J., & Eisenberg, M. (2006). Obesity, disordered eating, and eating disorders in a longitudinal study of adolescents: How do dieters fare 5 years later? *Journal of the American Dietetic Association, 106*(4), 559–568.

Pate, R. R., Davis, M. G., Robinson, T. N., Stone, E. J., McKenzie, T. L., & Young, J. C. (2007). Promoting physical activity in children and youth: A leadership role for schools. *Circulation, 114*, 1214–1224.

Physical and Health Education (PHE) Canada. (2009). What is the relationship between physical education and physical literacy? Available from www.phecanada.ca/sites/default/files/Physical_Literacy_Brochure_2010.pdf

Pope, C. (2011). The physical education and sport interface: Models, maxims and maelstrom. *European Physical Education Review, 17*, 273–285.

Puhse, U., & Gerber, M. (Eds.). (2005). *International comparison of physical education*. Oxford: Meyer & Meyer Sport.

Sibley, B. A., & Etnier, J. L. (2003). The relationship between physical activity and cognition in children: A meta-analysis. *Pediatric Exercise Science, 15*, 243–256.

Siedentop, D. (1994). *Sport education: Quality PE through positive sport experiences*. Champaign, IL: Human Kinetics.

Siedentop, D., & van der Mars, H. (2012). *Introduction to physical education, fitness, and sport* (8th ed.). New York: McGraw-Hill.

Sport England/YST/PE & Sport for Young People. (2009). *The PE and Sport strategy for young people: Guide to delivering the five-hour offer*. Loughborough, UK: Youth Sports Trust.

Tannehill, D. (2007, Oct.). *Involving teachers in the design of a coherent physical education curriculum*. Paper presented at the Physical Education Association of Ireland (PEAI) Annual Conference, University of Limerick, Ireland.

Tannehill, D. (2011). Physical education for all: The impact of curriculum on student choice. In S. Dagkas & K. Armour (Eds.), *Inclusion and exclusion through youth sport*. Loughborough, UK: Continuum Press.

Woods, C. B., Tannehill, D., Quinlan, A., Moyna, N., & Walsh, J. (2010). *The children's sport participation and physical activity study (CSPPA)*. Research Report No 1. Dublin, Ireland: School of Health and Human Performance, Dublin City University and the Irish Sports Council.

Wright, J., Macdonald, D., & Groom, L. (2003). Physical activity and young people: Beyond participation. *Sport, Education and Society, 8*(1), 17–33.

Wright, L. (2002). Rescuing primary physical education and saving those values that matter most. *British Journal of Teaching Physical Education, 33*(1), 37–38.

Wright, P. M., & Li, W. (2009). Exploring the relevance of positive youth development in urban physical education. *Physical Education and Sport Pedagogy, 14*(3), 241–251.

CHAPTER 2 Comprehensive School Physical Activity Programs

Overall Chapter Outcome

To develop understanding of the key features of Comprehensive School Physical Activity Programs (CSPAPs), develop the skills and knowledge to help schools maximize physical activity opportunities for all students throughout the school day, and make school campuses a hub for physical activity for not just students on campus but also the school's staff, parents, and the surrounding community members

Learning Outcomes

The learner will:

- Demonstrate understanding of the five components of CSPAPs and how they are related
- Demonstrate understanding of why the school environment is a central setting for promoting physical activity for children and youth
- Understand the underlying factors that have given rise to CSPAPs
- Articulate the role of physical educators as Physical Activity Leaders and the various associated roles and responsibilities
- Explain the evidence supporting the implementation of CSPAPs
- Identify and develop skills and knowledge needed for implementing a CSPAP
- Understand and be able to employ CSPAP implementation strategies
- Explain how CSPAPs are part of the broader societal efforts to improve public health

In this chapter, we will focus on a relatively new trend that is signaling a fundamental shift in how school physical education is being conceptualized in several different countries, namely the **Comprehensive School Physical Activity Program (CSPAP)**. In virtually all developed countries, opportunities for physical activity beyond physical education lessons lie beyond the school's campus in the form of sport clubs. People of wide-ranging ages and skill levels can join a club and participate at a level of competition where they can be successful. It is common for most sport clubs to have more than one team compete within each age bracket. This is regarded as an inclusionary model of delivering organized sport experiences. It is common as well for adults to continue playing well into their 40s.

In the United States, the physical education program historically has been composed of regular physical education lessons, intramurals, and interscholastic after-school sport programs. The intramural program provides opportunities for students to hone their skills and engage in competitive activities beyond the regular physical education program but within the confines of school campus. Siedentop and van der Mars (2012) noted that in contrast to the rising popularity of intramural and club sport programs on college and university campuses (with their expansive recreational facilities), in most post-primary schools the intramural program has all but disappeared. This can be attributed to various factors including schools lacking the resources to hire personnel to oversee such programs, and full-time teachers viewing intramurals

BOX 2.1 Key Terms in This Chapter

- *Academic achievement:* Performance on a formal test covering academic content (e.g., math, science, social studies).
- *Classroom activity break:* Time allocated for physical activity during instruction of academic subjects in classrooms, with the goal of increasing total daily physical activity and/or integrating physical activity into academic content.
- *Common content knowledge (CCK):* Knowledge needed to perform an activity (e.g., soccer, dance). Typically acquired in the process of learning to play and playing a game/performing an activity.
- *Comprehensive School Physical Activity Program (CSPAP):* A program, overseen and directed by the physical education teacher, aimed at maximizing physical activity opportunities for all students, school staff members, and students' families and members of the surrounding community.
- *Employee fitness/wellness programs:* Programs developed for improving employees' health and wellness in a school system. Program sessions are typically held during after-school hours. Participation may involve incentive programs that result in a reduction in employees' health insurance premiums.
- *Health-optimizing physical activity:* Any physical activity that requires the energy equivalent to or more than that needed for a brisk walk.
- *Recess:* Time during the school day allocated for free play by students. Typically scheduled during mid-morning and mid-afternoon.
- *Sedentary behavior:* Time spent lying down, sitting, or standing still.
- *Shared-use agreements:* Formal agreements between a school (or school system) and an outside organization that stipulate the use of a school's physical activity facility during nonschool hours (i.e., evenings and/or weekends).
- *Social marketing:* Use of commercial marketing strategies with the goal to change people's health behavior to improve personal welfare and that of society.
- *Specialized content knowledge (SCK):* Knowledge needed to teach an activity (e.g., aerobics, strength conditioning). Typically not acquired through playing/performing.

as an excessive workload. Transportation has also become a significant barrier to participation in intramurals for many students today because over the last few decades the distance to and from school has increased substantially. This example is but one that shows how school environments often will include barriers that suppress or prevent physical activity opportunities for many students.

Conversely, the interscholastic sport program has grown into arguably the most dominant and recognizable feature of U.S. post-primary schools. Interscholastic sport programs focus on fostering the highly talented athletes in the school. Consequently, if a student is "not good enough," she or he is excluded from participation. Thus, interscholastic sport programs reflect an exclusionary model of delivering sport opportunities. With the increased emphasis and dominance, today's teacher/coaches experience significant pressure, which often results in role conflict. A common consequence of this role conflict is that teacher/coaches focus more on their coaching responsibilities. As part of this, they may become more aggressive in controlling the use of and access to the school's various activity venues. Teacher/coaches may actually encroach on the instructional spaces during the school day by scheduling team practices during lunch periods, thereby restricting other students from accessing such venues (see **Figure 2.1**).

Yet, schools have enormous potential for increasing physical activity opportunities for all students. In 2013, the Institute of Medicine published a report that included several recommendations that would support school-based physical

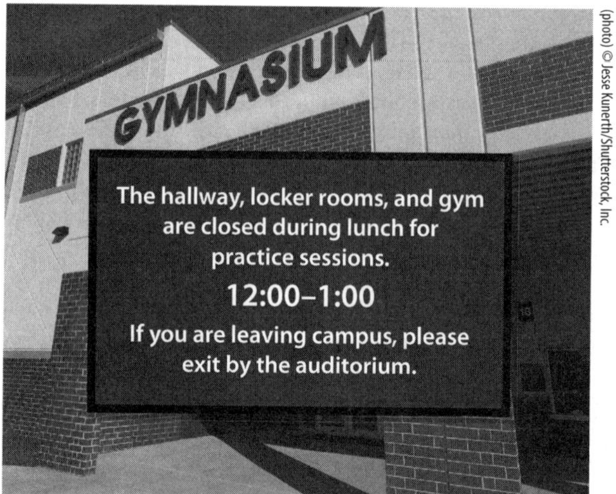

FIGURE 2.1 Physical activity venue restricted during regular school hours.

activity and physical education. The first recommendation called for a "whole-of-school approach" toward accomplishing this:

> *District and school administrators, teachers, and parents should advocate for and create a whole-of-school approach to physical activity that fosters and provides access in the school environment to at least 60 minutes per day of vigorous or moderate-intensity physical activity more than half (> 50 percent) of which should be accomplished during regular school hours.*
>
> - *School districts should provide high-quality curricular physical education during which the students should spend at least half (≥ 50 percent) of the class-time engaged in vigorous or moderate-intensity physical activity. All elementary school students should spend an average of 30 minutes per day and all middle and high school students an average of 45 minutes per day in physical education class. To allow for flexibility in curriculum scheduling, this recommendation is equivalent to 150 minutes per week for elementary school students and 225 minutes per week for middle and high school students.*
> - *Students should engage in additional vigorous or moderate-intensity physical activity throughout the school day through recess, dedicated classroom physical activity time, and other opportunities.*
> - *Additional opportunities for physical activity before and after school hours, including but not limited to active transport, before- and afterschool programming, and intramural and extramural sports, should be made accessible to all students. (IOM, 2013, p. 8-2)*

In this chapter we highlight key information and strategies for gradually building a CSPAP that directly target this recommendation by describing the following:

- Main features of CSPAPs
- Reasons for the rise of CSPAPs
- Redefined role of physical educators as Directors of Physical Activity
- Emerging evidence supporting the implementation of CSPAPs
- Skills, knowledge, and strategies for implementing a CSPAP
- Selected resources in support of creating a CSPAP

Comprehensive School Physical Activity Programs: A Global Trend

CSPAPs constitute a fundamental reconceptualization of the role that school physical education programs play in the broader societal efforts to improve the health of school-aged children and youth, and directly target such national health objectives. The overarching goal of CSPAPs is the development of the skills and understanding necessary for long-term physically active living. This, in turn, can have improved or sustained health as a by-product (e.g., Metzler et al., 2013a). It is not a coincidence that in the United States, the National Physical Activity Plan (see www.physicalactivityplan.org) and Healthy People 2020's physical activity–related health objectives target increased access to school physical activity spaces during nonschool hours for all persons (i.e., before school, after school, and on weekends). It is equally important to understand that the trend towards building CSPAPs is a global trend beyond the United States. Programs with a similar "whole-of-school" approach have been initiated in Ireland, Germany, Switzerland, Finland, France, Poland, and Australia.

For example, in Ireland (see www.activeschoolflag.ie), primary and post-primary schools can apply for *Active School Flag* status (valid for 3 years) by showing that they have: (1) provided the correct physical education timetable provision as per Department of Education and Skills Guidelines, (2) informed and invited the school community to participate in the Active School Flag program, (3) planned and implemented improvements that will enhance physical education and physical activity provision for all students, and (4) committed to conducting formal self-evaluation and reviewing current provisions across 15 performance areas. Following the application, an outside accreditation agent visits the school campus and reviews the quality of the program in place.

In Finland (one of the few countries where the government has mandated increased time for school physical education), the *Schools on the Move* program was started in 2010, with the main goal to increase physical activity levels of Finnish students throughout the school day. The central goal of Schools on the Move is to ensure that physical activity is and remains " . . . a natural part of a young person's life and to ensure that all young people participate in the recommended amount of daily physical activity" (Heikinaro-Johansson, Lyyra, & McEvoy, 2012, p. 291). Physical activity is now being integrated into the lessons of various classroom subjects, recess, daily transportation to and from school, and extracurricular (i.e., after-school) activities.

In Australia, the Queensland state government initiated *Smart Moves* in 2007. Again (much like in Finland), different government agencies (e.g., Department of Education, Training and Employment; Department of Communities; Sport and Recreation; and Queensland Health) came together to develop this program, which has similar features as CSPAPs. Smart Moves programs include six components (Queensland Government, n.d.):

1. Allocate required time for physical activity
2. Improve access to resources for physical activity
3. Increase capacity to deliver physical activity
4. Provide professional development in physical activity
5. Build community partnerships to enhance physical activity
6. Be accountable for physical activity

Smart Moves programs are assessed using three basic criteria: (1) an increase in the overall amount of physical activity in schools, (2) the embedding of physical activity across the curriculum, and (3) an increase in access to school facilities by the community.

In France, a partnership among school board members, teachers, recreation professionals, and medical staff, among others, resulted in the development of Intervention Centered on Adolescents' Physical Activity and Sedentary Behavior (ICAPS). The focus of ICAPS is on physical activity promotion with a major emphasis on minimizing barriers during after-school hours. As a result of the program, participating students increased their activity levels and reduced the amount of time they spent in sedentary activities such as watching television and playing computer games (Simon et al., 2004).

Finally, in Germany, the *Bewegte Schule* ("Moving Schools") program has been implemented in various places (Schmidt-Millard, 2003). In Switzerland, the University of Basel has initiated the *Bewegungsfreundliche Schule* ("Activity-Friendly Schools") program (Zahner, Furger, Graber, & Keller, 2012).

Importantly, school physical education programs will likely have difficulty implementing such comprehensive school-based physical activity programs. In Finland, numerous government agencies and other outside groups support these efforts, including the Ministry of Education and Culture; the Ministry of Social Affairs and Health; the National Board of Education; various national sport federations; municipal sport associations; the Center for Economic Development, Transport, and the Environment; and the University of Jyväskylä, among others.

Thus, the common threads in most of these initiatives are (1) the central focus of creating school campuses that promote and support physical activity for all students throughout the full school day, (2) ongoing professional development to support teachers, and (3) support from and collaboration with government and other outside agencies. This does not mean that without the added outside support CSPAP is completely impossible. We have seen many individual teachers being creative in building at least certain portions of CSPAP. However, being able to connect with supportive outside groups and agencies will improve the odds of building and sustaining such programs.

Key Features of a Comprehensive School Physical Activity Program

A CSPAP is a framework by which school systems and/or individual schools aim to accomplish two goals. First, it seeks to maximize the use of all possible school times and physical activity venues on the school campus for all students to engage in a wide variety of physical activities. By doing this, schools make significant contributions to having students meet the recommended **health-optimizing physical activity** levels. Second, CSPAPs form the foundation for developing students' understanding, skillfulness, confidence, and affinity for physical activity so that they are more likely to continue to engage in it as they move into adulthood. In the United States, the National Association for Sport and Physical Education (NASPE, 2008a, 2011d) first unveiled the basic CSPAP framework. As shown in **Figure 2.2**, a CSPAP is composed of five components:

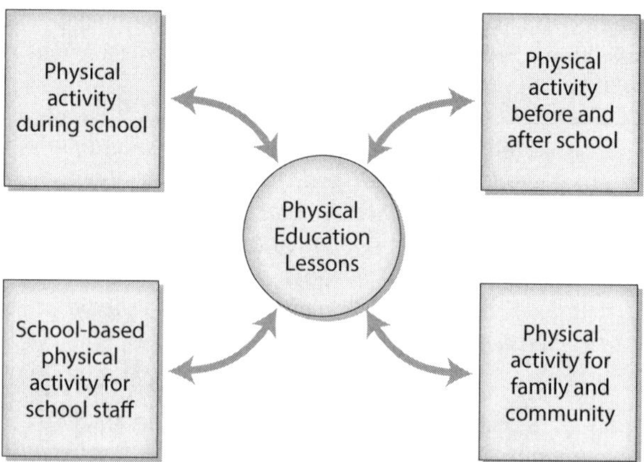

FIGURE 2.2 Comprehensive School Physical Activity Program framework.
Data from National Association for Sport and Physical Education. (2011). Overview of a comprehensive school physical activity program. Available at www.aahperd.org/letsmoveinschool/about/overview.cfm

- Physical education
- Physical activity during school
- Physical activity before and after school
- School-based physical activity for school staff
- Family and community involvement

The American Alliance for Health, Physical Education, Recreation and Dance (AAHPERD, 2011) reported that few primary and post-primary schools have implemented the full CSPAP model, although a substantial number of schools have started up at least some of its features.

Physical Education Lessons

Physical education lessons continue to be the centerpiece component and foundation of a CSPAP. A quality physical education program is one delivered by certified professional physical educators who can provide students with well-planned, sequential, and developmentally appropriate learning experiences that allow all students to meet national and/or local (state)-level physical education standards/outcomes. Consequently, such a program would be expected to develop the needed knowledge, skills, and dispositions in students to make physical activity an integral and natural part of daily life well into adulthood. However, in order for students to become truly "physically educated," the physical education program alone is not enough to provide the needed depth and breadth of physical activity opportunities. To that end, CSPAPs create additional opportunities.

Physical Activity During the School Day

Beyond physical education lessons, there are multiple ways in which physical activity can be made part of the entire school day. They include: (1) building physical activity breaks into academic subject lessons that allow for increased physical activity and possibly integrate academic concepts specific to academic subjects (e.g., language arts, math), (2) morning and afternoon recess in primary schools, and (3) the opportunity for physical activity prior to or after eating lunch. When present in the school, each of these approaches (together with the physical education lessons) can make significant contributions to students accumulating the recommended 60-plus minutes of daily moderate to vigorous physical activity.

Classroom Physical Activity Breaks

Classroom physical activity breaks (also known as "brain breaks") offer an important way of increasing students' physical activity levels. One example of how this is being done in an Irish primary school is that the student body and even teachers are taught a dance (e.g., the Macarena) in the yard/playground at the beginning of each week. Then, every time the Macarena music comes on the school loudspeaker, everyone in the school gets up and does the dance. The dance changes every month.

There is evidence that building physical activity breaks into classroom instruction has multiple benefits. They not only contribute to increasing the overall daily physical activity levels of students but also help students be more focused on academic tasks and less distracted. Moreover, students are less likely to engage in off-task/disruptive behavior (Mahar, 2011; Mahar et al., 2006; Stewart, Dennison, Kohl, & Doyle, 2004).

The importance of periodic classroom physical activity breaks (also called "brain breaks") cannot be underestimated. For this culture of "moving classrooms" to develop, school managers/principals and classroom teachers must come to understand the multiple benefits of physical activity breaks. **Classroom activity breaks** may help increase physical activity levels, but for classroom teachers it is more important that they recognize how such short breaks can help produce higher levels of on-task behavior (i.e., engagement in academic tasks). This is likely a higher priority for them. That such physical activity breaks can contribute to improving academic performance may be the more powerful selling point to school managers and classroom teachers; otherwise, they may not be willing to give up valuable class time to only help increase students' physical activity levels. Understanding these related benefits may help them become more receptive.

Physical educators are the premier professionals in schools who can develop buy-in from both school managers and classroom colleagues. Getting the support from the school manager is perhaps the most important barrier to overcome. If/when the school manager is on board, he or she becomes a key ally in persuading classroom teachers to employ physical activity breaks. Using time during staff meetings held before and/or during the school year, physical educators can develop this buy-in by offering short tutorials on the multiple benefits of classroom activity breaks, followed by additional tutorials on selecting appropriate activity breaks, and how to organize and manage them. With each staff meeting, physical educators can introduce and model one or two new examples of activity breaks. The short tutorials can, in fact, be used as activity breaks for staff meetings. A brief introduction on how to do the activity break would be followed by having the teaching staff do the activity.

A question often asked about trying to convince classroom teachers to incorporate physical activity breaks is, "How do I get the reluctant classroom teachers motivated to start using physical activity breaks?" As with every effort to change existing teaching practices, there are always those who are excited to try something new, those who approach it with some hesitation, and those who may outright refuse to change. Our suggestion is that you focus on those classroom colleagues who are willing to try activity breaks. With some practice and support, they are likely to find success in the form of seeing more focused and on-task students in their classrooms. They then become powerful advocates for implementing physical activity breaks with their classroom colleagues.

Recess Periods

Historically, in primary schools in the United States, **recess** periods have been an integral part of each school day. In the 1950s, it was not unusual for schools to have three recess periods (morning, post-lunch, and afternoon). The unstructured play during recess is generally viewed as a critical time for students not only to be physically active for health reasons but also to develop social skills, creativity, conflict resolution skills, and the like. Even today's school managers generally view recess periods as having multiple important benefits. **Box 2.2** shows some of the key findings from a recent survey by the Robert Wood Johnson Foundation (2010) of U.S. school managers' views on school recess.

BOX 2.2 School Managers' Views on the Role and Importance of School Recess

Of the over 1,950 school managers surveyed:

- 80 percent reported that recess has a positive impact on **academic achievement**.
- 66 percent reported that students listen better after recess and are more focused in class.
- 96 percent noted that recess has a positive impact on students' social development.
- Virtually all (97 percent) believe recess has a positive impact on students' general well-being.
- Almost 8 out of 10 report taking recess away as a form of punishment.

When asked what school managers would like to improve about recess at their particular school, they prioritized the following strategies:

1. Increase the number of staff to supervise recess periods
2. Obtain better equipment for student use
3. Provide playground management training

Data from Robert Wood Johnson Foundation. (2010). *State of play: Gallup survey of principals on school recess*. Princeton, NJ.

Learning Experience 2.1

Visit a primary school, and observe the recess periods of both lower and higher grades. Review the following questions, and answer them based on your observations.

- What are the typical activity patterns of the students in terms of the more prevalent activities in which they engage?
- What activities tend to be more active from an intensity perspective?
- What differences are there in activity choices between boys and girls?
- What activities tend to result in greater amounts of more vigorous student engagement?
- Which students tend to be drawn to certain activities?
- Which students tend to be more sedentary?
- What, if any, conflict emerges among students, and how do they resolve it?
- What possible differences in play patterns are there between the lower and upper grades at that school?
- What is the predominant pattern of behavior among the adult playground supervisors? Who do they interact with?
- Should recess periods be more structured or left up to the students? What is the basis for that position?

Numerous professional organizations and other agencies have published formal position statements strongly advocating for recess to be a regular part of each school day. Most recently, the American Academy of Pediatrics (2013) published a formal policy statement in which it (1) summarized the cognitive/academic, social/emotional, and physical benefits of recess; (2) addressed the emerging issue of whether recess periods should be composed of more structured activities or activities that are children-designed; (3) described the timing and duration of recess; and (4) provided six key recommendations for parents, teachers, school managers, and policy makers pertinent to school recess (see **Box 2.3**).

Physical Activity Before and After School

There are several ways in which students' physical activity can be increased during before- and after-school hours. They include:

- *Active commuting to and from school:* If the neighborhood in which students live is located within 1 mile of the school grounds, walking or using their bicycle should be encouraged.
- *Informal recreation or play on school grounds:* Similar to recess periods during the school day, providing access and equipment during informal play time offers significant physical activity opportunities.
- *Physical activity in school-based after-school programs:* Many schools today offer after-school programming, especially for students whose parent(s) work. Traditionally, such programs have focused primarily on developing academic skills, life skills, and arts and crafts, rather than physical activity.
- *After-school activity clubs and intramural sports:* In many post-primary schools, students may participate in faculty-sponsored clubs across a wide variety of interests (e.g., photography, art). Relative to physical activity–based clubs, students may organize a ballroom dance, table tennis, or salsa club.
- *Interscholastic sports:* School sport is an important cultural phenomenon in many countries. Especially in smaller rural communities, the sport programs in postprimary schools are a binding force.

Learning Experience 2.2

Develop a plan for how you would go about maximizing the use of all physical activity venues and equipment during after-school hours (i.e., approximately between 3 p.m. and 6 p.m.) in ways that make the participation enjoyable for the greatest number of the school's students. Explain what resources you would seek to use.

BOX 2.3 Recommendations for School Recess Periods

From the perspective of educating the whole child, the American Academy of Pediatrics (AAP) made the following recommendations:

- Recess is a necessary break in the day for optimizing a child's social, emotional, physical, and cognitive development. In essence, recess should be considered a child's personal time, and it should not be withheld for academic or punitive reasons.
- Cognitive processing and academic performance depend on regular breaks from concentrated classroom work. This applies equally to adolescents and to younger children. To be effective, the frequency and duration of breaks should be sufficient to allow the student to mentally decompress.
- Recess is a complement to, but not a replacement for, physical education. Physical education is an academic discipline. Whereas both have the potential to promote activity and a healthy lifestyle, only recess (particularly unstructured recess) provides the creative, social, and emotional benefits of play.
- Recess can serve as a counterbalance to sedentary time and contribute to the recommended 60 minutes of moderate to vigorous activity per day, a standard strongly supported by AAP policy as a means to lessen risk of overweight.
- Whether structured or unstructured, recess should be safe and well supervised. Although schools should ban games and activities that are unsafe, they should not discontinue recess altogether just because of concerns connected with child safety. Environmental conditions, well-maintained playground equipment, and well-trained supervisors are the critical components of safe recess.
- Peer interactions during recess are a unique complement to the classroom. The lifelong skills acquired for communication, negotiation, cooperation, sharing, problem solving, and coping are not only foundations for healthy development but also fundamental measures of the school experience.

From American Academy of Pediatrics. (2013). Policy statement: The crucial role of recess in school. *Pediatrics, 131*, 186. DOI: 10.1542/peds.2012-2993

Each year, millions of post-primary school students participate in organized sport programs. Eitzen and Sage (2003) noted some of the benefits of such involvement. They include:

- Improved grades
- Stronger self-concept
- Higher aspirations to further education
- Greater sense of personal control
- Increased likelihood of adopting healthier eating habits
- Lower likelihood of using banned substances (e.g., drugs)

In the United States, sport programs, notably basketball and American football, are increasingly year-round programs in that even when a team is not in season, coaches will keep the teams engaged in various summer leagues and conditioning regimens. Students are expected to specialize in a certain sport and positions within a sport. With this intense level of sustained engagement comes the increased risk of overuse injuries (Siedentop & van der Mars, 2012).

School-Based Physical Activity/Wellness Programming for School Staff

Using the "ounce of prevention is worth a pound of cure" perspective, there is a distinct trend in the healthcare delivery industry to move beyond the traditional reactive/illness treatment–oriented medical model toward providing a more proactive and wellness-oriented healthcare services system, through **employee fitness/wellness programs** (Loeppke, 2008). Much like private companies, schools could offer a similar program for their teachers and support staff because students are not the only ones who spend 7–8 hours a day at school. Over the course of their careers, the millions of primary and post-primary schoolteachers, administrators, and all support staff also spend a large portion of each school day on the school campus. Thus, their health matters as much as that of their students. Especially in post-primary schools, expansive physical activity venues are already in place. These facilities are publicly funded, and thus teachers and all other staff should be able to access them at some point during the workday.

Not unimportant is that school staff members are also important role models for students when they regularly engage in physical activity. Students who see adults being active are more likely to come to see that physical activity is "not just for kids." This positive modeling is thus an important stimulus for school-aged youth. Needless to say, implementation of this particular CSPAP component is dependent on school manager support.

Questions raised when discussing the possibility for after-school staff programs might include:

- After a long workday, will teachers even want to stay after school and do an exercise session?
- Who will deliver/teach the after-school sessions?

- How many and which days of the week would such a program be held?
- Where would such a program be held?

Recently, one of the authors conducted an informal survey targeting staff members (i.e., teachers, school managers, and support staff) at three post-primary schools to gauge their interest and preferences in participating in an after-school physical activity and wellness program to be held at the school site. Respondents reported a high level of interest, with Wednesdays, Thursdays, Tuesdays, and Mondays being the preferred days, in that order. The preferred length and number of sessions per week was between 30 and 60 minutes, twice a week. Staff members were mostly "very interested" and "interested" in session topics such as aerobics, strength conditioning, yoga, and group walks. Not surprisingly, the least preferred activities were team sports. There was also considerable interest in screening opportunities for health markers such as blood pressure, mobile mammography, and body mass index (BMI). The Alliance for a Healthier Generation (see www.HealthierGeneration.org) offers an expansive Employee Wellness Toolkit to assist Physical Activity Leaders in developing a school employee wellness program (Alliance for a Healthier Generation, 2012). With the rising cost of health care in many countries, it is becoming more common to find incentives built into employees' health insurance plans, where regular and sustained involvement in employee fitness programs with a corresponding improvement in health outcomes would result in reductions in health insurance premiums.

Physical educators would not need to deliver such after-school staff health/wellness programs themselves. Rather, they would serve as the facilitator or liaison that brings together the needed expertise from outside, promotes the availability of such programs, and coordinates scheduling of campus and other nearby facilities. Laying the groundwork for after-school programs targeting school staff does require investment of time and energy by physical educators. For example, it includes making connections with local programs, agencies, and healthcare facilities in the community to garner support in the form of providing outside expertise and equipment, coordinating school facility use with others in the school, and promoting the after-school program to the target audience.

Local health/fitness clubs, YMCAs, parks and recreation departments, university programs in physical education/exercise and wellness/exercise science, and local hospitals are powerful partners for schools because they can provide instructors/presenters who can deliver activity sessions and/or present on topics as varied as safe exercise, nutrition, relaxation, and wellness during after-school hours. Group exercise instructors could be recruited from local health clubs to come to the school and lead participating staff members through exercise sessions. Thus, being keenly aware of local community resources places physical educators in a much stronger position to help build after-school programs. Once this groundwork is laid and colleagues in the school start to benefit from such programs, the credibility of the physical educator and the overall program is greatly enhanced.

Physical Activity Involvement by Families and Community

School campuses (especially those located in neighborhoods) are a critical resource in creating opportunities for children, youth, and families to engage in physical activities. In more rural communities and economically disadvantaged neighborhoods, the school is often one of only a few venues for physical activity. In many countries, the taxpayers fund schools, and thus it stands to reason that when schools are not in session, their physical activity venues become an important resource for the members in the surrounding community.

One example of how a well-equipped school campus is an invaluable resource for the surrounding community is Mountain Pointe High School in Ahwatukee, Arizona (a metropolitan area near Phoenix). The school has indoor facilities that include a large gym (14,364 sq. ft.), a smaller second gym (7,676 sq. ft.), two dance studios (2,000 sq. ft. each), a weight room (6,745 sq. ft.), and a wrestling room (5,005 sq. ft.). The outdoor venues include an all-weather 400 m track around a lighted football field, a practice field, two full-sized baseball fields, two full-sized softball fields, eight 4-wall racquetball courts, and eight tennis courts. Although there are several logistical and legal issues to overcome, this school is a precious resource for all in the surrounding neighborhood. **Figure 2.3** shows the density of community members living in close proximity to the school campus. Regardless of how well schools and school systems are outfitted with activity venues, there is no reason why their accessibility and use cannot be maximized.

In most countries, it is common to have outside groups such as sport clubs and other community organizations rent activity spaces in schools for use during after-school hours and weekends. At the heart of such arrangements lie **shared-use agreements** (e.g., Spengler, Connaughton, & Carroll, 2011). Shared- or joint-use agreements are formal agreements between a school (or school system) and an outside organization that stipulate the use of a school's physical activity facility during nonschool hours (i.e., evenings and weekends).

From the perspective of wishing to protect its facilities, many school managers and school systems may be reluctant to let outside groups use the school's facilities, citing legal and logistical barriers such as possible misuse, liability issues, vandalism and crime, and cost incurred for repairs and maintenance (Spengler, 2012). This is evidenced by the fact that between 2:30 and 4:00 p.m., most sport facilities at post-primary schools are largely vacant (Bocarro et al., 2012).

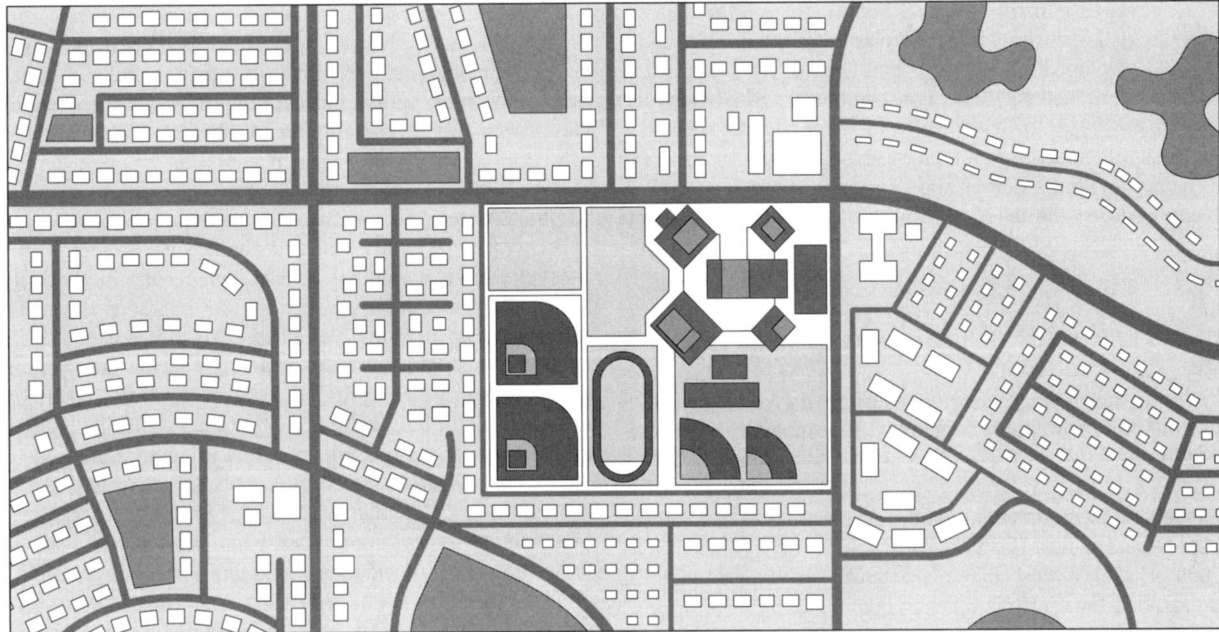

FIGURE 2.3 Population density surrounding a neighborhood school.

Well-designed shared-use agreements can be an excellent means of ensuring that the responsibilities for both parties relative to time and days of use, cleaning, repairs, and the like are stipulated.

Similar to community parks, school physical activity venues that are accessible on weekends are an invaluable resource for promoting physical activity among children, youth, adults, and older adults. We cannot overstate the importance of younger generations seeing adults and older adults modeling health-optimizing physical activity engagement. Moreover, family members can support a CSPAP by participating or volunteering in special evening or weekend events such as after-school fun runs, family fitness and wellness nights, open houses, and/or physical activity–based fundraisers such as walk-a-thons, jog-a-thons, or basketball free-throw challenges. These are vital opportunities to educate adults about the importance and role of the physical education program, active living, and the benefits of healthy choices.

Why Comprehensive School Physical Activity Programs?

The question about what prompted the emergence of the CSPAP model brings together multiple factors, including: (1) the traditional objectives of school physical education programs, (2) the emergence of physical activity behavior as a legitimate program outcome, (3) the status of school physical education programs relative to other school subjects, and (4) the relationship of physical activity (along with physical education) to students' academic achievement. The following sections highlight these topics as they offer an important historic and evidentiary context for CSPAPs.

The Traditional Objectives of School Physical Education Programs

For well over a century, school physical education programs have purported to target multiple objectives/outcomes. A close look will reveal that each time a country has waged war, the fitness levels of its defenders were found to be below acceptable standards. Invariably, school physical education programs received increased attention and were charged with improving the fitness levels of youth (Siedentop & van der Mars, 2012).

Beyond improving students' physical fitness levels, school physical education has also targeted physical skills and cognitive and social outcomes throughout much of the twentieth century (Siedentop & van der Mars, 2012). Even today, learning outcomes internationally continue to clearly reflect the four main foci (i.e., organic education, psychomotor education, character education, intellectual education) of the "new physical education" as proposed by Clark Hetherington back in 1910 (Weston, 1962). However, as Corbin (2002) argued, the field of physical education has tried to be too many things to too many people.

One related issue of this broad focus has been the field's inability to demonstrate that it accomplished what it claimed it could accomplish. A second is how school physical education programs will get students to seek out physical activity for not only health benefits, which Kretchmar (2008) referred to as a utilitarian view of physical education's goals but also find joy and a deeper appreciation in movement itself. Learning to do the latter will improve the odds that young people will come to make physical activity truly a part of daily life.

Physical Activity Behavior as a Central Program Outcome

There is now overwhelming evidence that engaging in health-optimizing physical activity has multiple physical health, mental health, cognitive health, and economic benefits (e.g., Bouchard, Blair, & Haskell, 2012; Gettman, 1996; Landers, 1997; Murtrie & Parfitt, 1998; Strong et al., 2005; U.S. Department of Health and Human Services [USDHHS], 2008). However, most children and youth do not meet the recommended levels of daily health-optimizing physical activity (e.g., Fairclough & Stratton, 2005, 2006; Lee, Burgeson, Fulton, & Spain, 2007; Troiano et al., 2008; USDHHS, 2013; World Health Organization [WHO], 2010). Consequently, this has become a major national health objective in most developed countries (USDHHS, 2000, 2010; WHO, 2010).

Don't Judge People by Their Appearance

A person's fitness level has long been assumed to be closely related to his or her physical activity level. However, at least for school-aged youth (ages 8–17) the two variables barely correlate (e.g., Huang & Malina, 2002; Katzmarzyk, Malina, Song, & Bouchard, 1998; Morrow & Freedson, 1994). It is not until adulthood that physical activity levels impact fitness levels more directly. The key message here is some youngsters who do really well on fitness tests may not be as active in reality as one would think. Conversely, certain youngsters who may be quite active may not do well at all on certain fitness test components. Performance on fitness tests is determined by influential factors other than just physical activity, including other lifestyle behaviors (e.g., dietary habits), one's environment, and heredity. Bouchard (1993) showed that some people will do better on cardiovascular endurance and muscular strength tests than others on account of their genetic makeup, and they do not all respond in the same way to "training." Some may improve little from baseline levels no matter how hard they try, whereas others improve by as much as tenfold (e.g., Bouchard & Rankinen, 2001; Timmons et al., 2010).

This recognition has given rise to a shift away from focusing on improving performance on physical fitness tests (a "product" orientation) to promoting physical activity behavior (a "process" orientation). Corbin, Pangrazi, and Welk (1994) noted that the former had its roots in the exercise physiology research literature (using adults as participants in most cases) and became known as the *Exercise Prescription Model* (EPM). The problem is that this well-evidenced approach to exercise prescription was then generalized to children and youth.

The EPM can be contrasted with the *Lifetime Physical Activity Model* (LPAM), which has a clear health focus. It is defined around promoting activity that results in accumulating sufficient caloric expenditure that has been shown to reduce the risk of chronic diseases. This model is based on two landmark findings that showed (1) how shifting from being sedentary to physical activity at moderate levels of intensity significantly reduced people's risks of dying prematurely, and (2) that the risk reduction in going from moderate to more vigorous levels of activity (i.e., greater caloric expenditure) was smaller than moving from being sedentary to moderate intensity activities (e.g., Blair, 1993; Blair & Bouchard, 1999). In addition, although there is a multitude of environmental, social, economic, and psychological factors that influence people's physical activity behavior, Malina (2001) reported that longitudinally, physical activity patterns track reasonably well from childhood into adulthood; that is, children who are physically active during childhood are more likely to maintain that level as they move through adolescence, young adulthood, and so on.

Learning Experience 2.3

Given the findings discussed in this section, what do you see as the appropriate practices in designing and delivering physical activity experiences? Address the following:

- What types of activities are more likely to attract students to being active beyond your program?
- What can you do to help students of different body types?
- What do you think are highly effective ways of encouraging your students when interacting with them?

Physical Activity Versus Sedentary Behavior

The flip side of the physical activity coin is a person's time spent in **sedentary behavior**. In recent years, there has been extensive interest in determining the consequences of spending excessive time in sedentary behavior (i.e., too much sitting). In today's environment, people may spend many of their waking hours in sedentary behavior such as driving a car, working at a computer, watching television, playing computer games, and the like. Booth and Chakravarthy (2002) referred to sedentary living as a silent enemy, and reported that sedentary lifestyles contributed to the worsening of 23 health conditions (e.g., selected cancers, high blood cholesterol, osteoporosis, type 2 diabetes, depression). Even those who build in a 1-hour period of exercise in the middle of their work, but are largely sedentary throughout most of the rest of the day, are at an increased risk. Owen, Healy, Howard, and Dunstan (2012) refer to them as *active couch potatoes*, and summarized the findings on the consequences of sedentary lifestyles as follows:

> *There is now substantial evidence . . . that higher levels of sedentary time are adversely associated with several adverse functional and clinical health outcomes in the general adult population. These include the presence of risk factors for chronic disease such as large waist circumferences; unhealthy levels of blood glucose, insulin, and blood fat; lower measures of physical functioning; and increased risk for mortality from all-causes, cardiovascular disease, and some cancers. (p. 4)*

Learning Experience 2.4

Over the next 7 consecutive days (not counting your time spent sleeping at night), record the total amount of time that you spent in sedentary activities (e.g., watching television, driving your car, working at a computer). Collect the information so that you can determine the duration of each sedentary episode. Answer the following questions:

- On what days were you more sedentary?
- What was the average amount of consecutive minutes spent sitting each day?
- How were the weekdays different from weekend days?
- What are some possible minor changes you could make to cut down on the extended periods of being sedentary?

The findings on physical activity and sedentary behavior are pertinent to schools in that students spend a significant portion of their formative years at school (approximately 14,000 hours). They spend much of that time in sedentary behavior. Thus, schools have a responsibility to not only ensure that students develop essential academic skills but also attend to their current and future health and well-being. Schools are prime environments for promoting physical activity (e.g., Centers for Disease Control and Prevention [CDC], 2001; National Association of State Boards of Education [NASBE], 2012; Pate et al., 2006; Sallis et al., 2012). Thus, the discoveries discussed regarding physical fitness and physical activity have important implications for how physical educators go about promoting physical activity both during physical education lessons and at other times throughout the school day.

Learning Experience 2.5

Using the evidence presented on physical fitness, physical activity, and sedentary behavior, what specific implications do you see as a physical educator for what content to select, how to design activities, how to differentiate instruction for groups of individual students, what to assess and how to assess it, and what you can do within physical education classes to encourage students' physical activity beyond the lessons?

Status of School Physical Education Relative to Other School Subjects

The notion of school physical education serving an important role in public health has received widespread support within government agencies, professional societies, and the public health community in the form of national guidelines, recommendations, and position statements (e.g., American Heart Association [Pate et al., 2006], CDC [2011], Institute of Medicine [Koplan, Liverman, & Kraak, 2005], International Council of Sport Science and Physical Education [2010], American Academy of Pediatrics [2006], the World Health Organization [2010]). A comprehensive review of the research on the efficacy of multiple interventions aimed at increasing physical activity levels showed school physical education as one of only six interventions to have sufficient evidence (CDC, 2001). Importantly, the parents of youth have also voiced strong support for increasing time allocation for physical education, recess, and interventions targeting other health behaviors in students (see **Figure 2.4**).

Unfortunately, school physical education programs globally continue to be marginalized, with Hardman (2004) noting that:

> *The evidence presented in this Report indicates that many national governments have committed themselves through legislation to making provision for physical education but they have been either slow or reticent in translating this into action i.e. actual implementation and assurance of quality of delivery at the national level. Deficiencies continue to be apparent in curriculum time allocation, subject status, financial, material and human resources (particularly in primary school teacher preparation for physical education teaching), the quality and relevance of the physical*

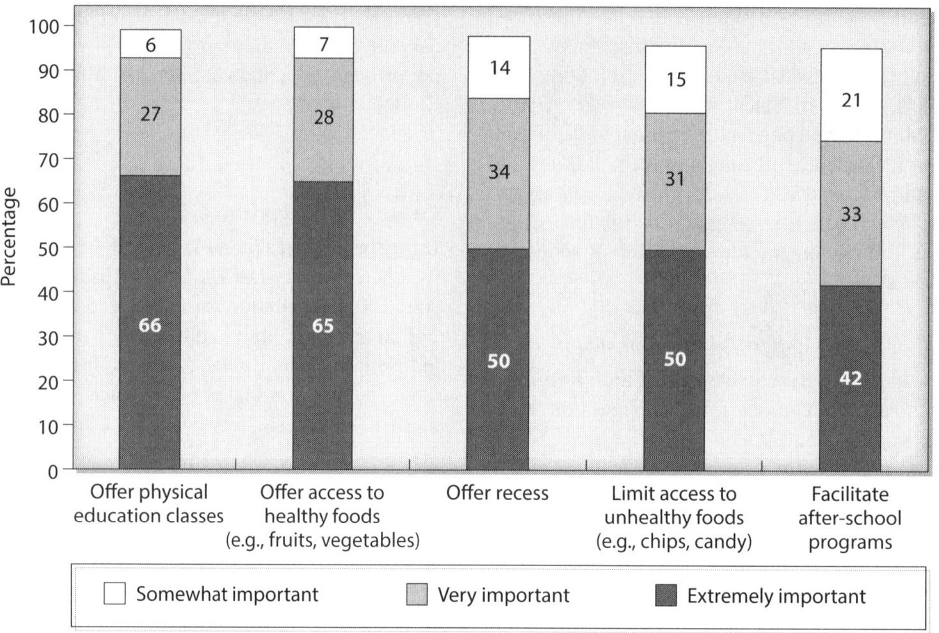

FIGURE 2.4 Parental views on students' access to and opportunity for physical education, recess, and other health behaviors.

Reproduced with permission from Alliance for a Healthier Generation, 2013, www.healthiergeneration.org.

> *education curriculum and its delivery and gender and disability issues. Of particular concern are the considerable inadequacies in facility and equipment supply, frequently associated with under-funding, especially in economically underdeveloped and developing countries and regions.*[1]

In a more recent update, Hardman and Marshall (2009) reported that, despite improvements in some areas, continuing concerns include:

> *. . . insufficient curriculum time allocation, perceived inferior subject status, insufficient competent qualified and/or inadequately trained teachers (particularly in primary schools), inadequate provision of facilities and equipment and teaching materials frequently associated with under-funding, large class sizes and funding cuts and, in some countries, inadequate provision or awareness of pathway links to wider community programmes and facilities outside of schools.*[2]

Relationship of Physical Activity (and Physical Education) with Students' Academic Performance

For several decades, there has been interest in answering the question of whether and how physical activity (along with physical education) affects students' academic performance. Given the extensive focus on educational reform efforts aimed at improving academic achievement in recent years, this interest increased even further (Howie & Pate, 2012). There is now a substantial body of evidence from over 150 published studies, from different countries, using various approaches to answering the question: What is the nature of the relationship between students' time spent in physical activity (which would include physical education lessons) and their academic performance? Rasberry and colleagues (2011) reported that in most studies, students with higher physical activity levels also tended to have higher academic scores and improved concentration.

The knowledge base around this relationship will continue to evolve, and, as is the case with all research, there

[1] Reproduced with permission from Hardman, K. (2004). An update on the status of physical education in schools worldwide: Technical report for the World Health Organization (p. 11). Available from www.icsspe.org/sites/default/files/Kenneth%20Hardman%20update%20on%20physical%20education%20in%20schools%20worldwide.pdf. Accessed March 13, 2013. © Copyright World Health Organization (WHO), 2013. All Rights Reserved.

[2] Reproduced with permission from Hardman, K., & Marshall, J. (2009). Physical education in schools: A global perspective. *Kinesiology, 40*(1), 5.

are always limitations. Moreover, how research projects are designed and interpreted must be taken into account (e.g., remembering to not confuse correlation with causation). However, based on their review of studies on the same relationship, Trost and van der Mars (2009, p. 64) offered the following key take-away messages[3]:

- *Decreasing (or eliminating) the time allotted for physical education in favor of traditional academic subjects does not automatically lead to improved academic performance.*
- *Increasing the number of minutes students spend per week in physical education will not impede their academic performance.*
- *Increasing the amount of time students spend in physical education may make small positive contributions to academic performance, particularly for girls.*
- *Regular physical activity and physical fitness are associated with higher levels of academic performance.*
- *Physical activity is beneficial to general cognitive functioning.*

More Is Not Always Better

A commonly held assumption is that student performance in classroom subjects (e.g., reading and math) will improve when time allocated to physical education, recess, and other subjects like art and music is reduced (or worse, eliminated). Wilkins and colleagues (2003) found that time shifted from physical education (along with art and music) to math and reading did not translate into improved performance in academic subjects. The exact mechanisms that affect this complex relationship are not yet fully understood because there are multiple contextual mediating factors at work (e.g., quality of instruction) that affect this likely curvilinear relationship (see **Figure 2.5**). For example, increased activity helps students concentrate and focus better, which then helps them complete academic tasks with greater success. However, once the amount of time in physical activity increases, students may reach a point of diminishing returns, where it may start to interfere with academic tasks.

The Physical Educator as Director of Physical Activity

Schools have been recognized as a central point of intervention for promoting physical activity to students (e.g., Pate et al., 2006; Wechsler, McKenna, Lee, & Dietz, 2004). Thus, the central question to ask is: Who is better positioned than

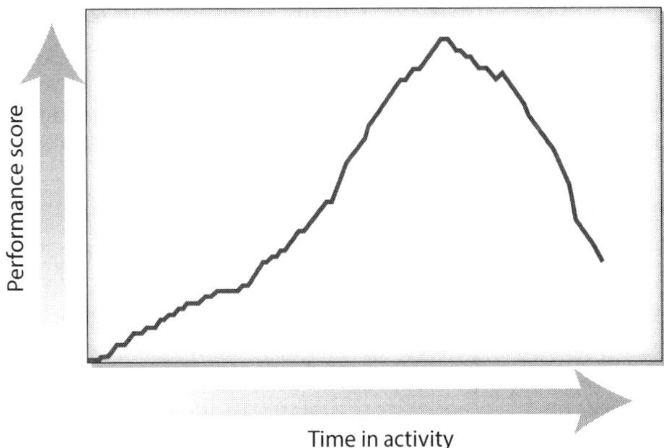

FIGURE 2.5 The relationship between time spent in physical activity and academic performance.

the physical educator to be the lead person for promoting physical activity for all students in schools? However, the emergence of CSPAPs has important implications for physical educators' day-to-day work. In the United States, to support the implementation of CSPAPs, NASPE launched a Director of Physical Activity (DPA) certification program open only to physical educators that targets the skills and knowledge necessary for planning, implementing, and evaluating CSPAPs (Carson, 2012). To become a certified DPA, physical educators would need to:

- View and complete three modules: public health, advocacy, and sustainability
- Complete and pass a certification exam of 35 questions
- Develop, upload, and implement a CSPAP action plan
- Submit artifacts that reflect evidence of program implementation

A similar training program, "Physical Activity Leader (PAL)," is under development to support the recently announced *Let's Move!* Active Schools initiative (see www.letsmoveschools.org). The PAL program is expected to launch in August 2013 with an anticipated target of 20,000 trained PALs by 2018. These efforts are part of a large-scale effort to bring together the resources and programs of public and private sectors to maximize opportunities for physical activity by students, staff, and community members in U.S. schools (Carson, 2013).

First and foremost, PALs will want to get support from their school managers to introduce physical activity promotion

[3] Republished with permission of *Educational Leadership*, from Trost, S., & van der Mars, H. Why we should not cut PE. p. 64, 2009. Permission conveyed through Copyright Clearance Center, Inc.

strategies to classroom teachers during school staff meetings, support an after-school staff wellness program, recognize those classroom teachers who infuse physical activity breaks in the classroom, and so on. Carson (2012) rightly noted that school managers play a key role as well in helping set up a school wellness council. Typically, this council would include the physical education teacher/PAL, a classroom teacher, and representatives from the school's management team, food services, parents, and students. Where possible, persons with expertise in student health and wellness from the community would also be included. This council is advisory, with the task to ensure that the students' physical activity and nutrition needs are met.

The key for the PAL is to show how each CSPAP component complements the physical education lessons (rather than replacing them). Thus, PALs are the lead persons in schools who, in addition to delivering physical education lessons, plan, coordinate, and manage the other CSPAP components (Beighle, Erwin, Castelli, & Ernst, 2009). One of the most often voiced concerns about physical educators taking on the PAL role is that they cannot do all of this because being "just a physical educator" is already a full-time job. As we will show, many of the strategies used to build a CSPAP include recruiting help from others who can assist and take the lead on organizing and delivering the other CSPAP components. Moreover, as with everything, building a successful full-fledged CSPAP takes time. And in certain cases, one particular component may simply not be a reasonable option. For example, local contexts (e.g., rural locations with limited outside support resources in the community) may limit or even prevent implementation of after-school activity/wellness programming for the school's teaching and support staff.

Supporting Evidence for Implementing CSPAP

Increasingly, teachers and school managers are urged to employ evidence-informed practices in order to improve students' learning experiences. Although full-scale implementation of CSPAPs that include all five components is yet to become commonplace (AAHPERD, 2011), there is now substantial empirical evidence on the efficacy of at least some of its individual student-focused components. **Box 2.4** provides a brief overview of the evidence compiled from studies across primary and post-primary grade levels, and from various countries. The full report is accessible at www.activelivingresearch.org/files/Synthesis_Ward_SchoolPolicies_Oct2011_1.pdf.

BOX 2.4 A Summary of the Evidence Base for Various CSPAP Components

1. School physical education programs where teachers employed standardized curricula (e.g., CATCH, SPARK) specifically designed to improve physical activity and supported with sustained/ongoing staff development produced significant increases in students' health-enhancing (i.e., moderate to vigorous) physical activity levels, by as much as 12 minutes per day.
2. Schools that increased opportunities for physical activity across the full school day (i.e., recess, in-classroom physical activity breaks, and after-school activities) saw increased physical activity levels, although differentially between boys and girls.
3. Increased time for supervised recess, coupled with improved access to activity equipment and improvement to play spaces (e.g., playground markings) results in higher physical activity levels among primary school students.
4. In-class physical activity breaks increase students' physical activity, help reduce off-task behavior, increase their on-task behavior, and aid in concentration and focus on learning tasks. This can contribute to improved performance on academic achievement.
5. Well-designed playgrounds and improved open spaces, facilities, and equipment that are available, accessible, and inviting to children encourage more physical activity, both during and after school.
6. After-school programs that include well-designed physical activity opportunities make important contributions to the total day's physical activity levels, and are especially beneficial for students living in economically disadvantaged conditions (e.g., low-income urban and rural environments).
7. Making school grounds accessible through joint-use agreements between schools and communities increases physical activity during after-school hours and weekends, most notably for children and youth whose access to other safe activity spaces and programs are limited.
8. Well-designed policies and/or legislation that require specific daily amounts of time for physical activity in schools can have an important impact on the population of school-aged children.

Data from Ward, D. S. (2011). *School policies on physical education and physical activity: Research synthesis.* San Diego, CA: Active Living Research.

Skills, Knowledge, and Strategies for Implementing CSPAPs

This section focuses on specific strategies that physical educators can employ to bring about the CSPAP components. From the perspective of "If you build it, will they come? And if they come, will they be active?," certain conditions must be met. Based on extensive observations throughout the school day in 24 schools with early post-primary students, McKenzie, Marshall, Sallis, and Conway (2000) concluded that although access to physical activity venues was not a major barrier, "The provision of more supervision, equipment, and organized activities . . . might lead to more students being more physically active" (p. 75).

It is generally accepted now that teachers require specific content knowledge (CK) and pedagogical content knowledge (PCK) to successfully plan, deliver, and evaluate a physical education program. In physical education, CK focuses on what a teacher knows about the subject matter of physical education. The field has long debated what constitutes the specific subject matter of physical education. We agree with Siedentop (2002) that first and foremost our subject matter is that of *physically active motor play* in all its forms, such as dance, fitness and exercise, games, and other leisure activities (e.g., hiking, skiing). NASPE (2008b) also regards a basic understanding of the scientific foundation of human movement, and principles of social, cognitive, and psychological development specific to school-aged youth as part of the required content knowledge.

PCK constitutes the knowledge teachers develop about how to blend their CK with the pedagogical skills and understanding of how to teach the subject matter. However, developing and delivering a CSPAP requires more. Metzler et al. (2013a) targeted the areas discussed in the following sections.

Coordinate Before-, During-, and After-School Physical Activity Programming

As we have noted, a PAL cannot implement a CSPAP alone. Collaborating with others within the school and the surrounding community is a must. **Table 2.1** shows an action plan for building a CSPAP, with a timeline. It shows that creating a quality CSPAP requires thorough planning and does not happen overnight.

TABLE 2.1 Action Plan for Building a CSPAP

Year	CSPAP Component	Primary Tasks	Potential Outside Support Sources/Expertise Sought	Outcome Indicator(s)
2014–2015	Laying the CSPAP groundwork	• Work with physical education staff to divide planning and prep tasks • Develop and present CSPAP plan to school management • Present plan to parent organization • Present plan to the school's wellness council • Present plan to school staff • Develop marketing/promotion plan (i.e., signage, website) • Form student volunteer team/club • Develop/conduct student interest survey on preferred activities, physical activity (PA) barriers • Sample usage of school's PA areas during various parts of the school day	• School management • Parent organization • Physical education teacher • Education program faculty member	• Completed plan presented to various constituents
2015–2016	Lunchtime PA program	• Recruit supervisory staff • Set up dedicated equipment cart • Create activity zone signage • Train supervisory staff • Hold fundraiser for adding equipment • Market and promote the program • Set up activity rotation schedule to refresh activity menu	• Parent volunteers • Interns from local university program	• Improved access to PA venues • Increased number of students engaging in health-optimizing PA

(*continues*)

TABLE 2.1 Action Plan for Building a CSPAP (*Continued*)

Year	CSPAP Component	Primary Tasks	Potential Outside Support Sources/Expertise Sought	Outcome Indicator(s)
2016–2017	Before-school PA program	• Update marketing plan to include new PA opportunities • Set up supervisory rotation schedule for physical education staff and other adults • Set up activity rotation schedule to refresh activity menu	• Interns from local university program • School wellness council • Parent volunteers • Paraprofessionals	• Improved access to PA venues • Increased number of students engaging in health-optimizing PA
2017–2018	Classroom PA breaks	• Find/develop classroom teacher resources • Work with school manager to schedule time for ongoing staff development for classroom teachers • Develop schedule for introducing and modeling PA breaks to staff • Plan and present rationale for infusing PA breaks to classroom staff • Develop and conduct school staff interest survey about after-school staff wellness/activities program (i.e., features, activity preferences, preferred times and days) • Survey expertise among the school's parents for potential instructional/wellness support	• Classroom teacher colleagues • Physical education teacher • Education program faculty member	• Percentage of teachers using PA breaks at least once a day
2018–2019	School staff wellness program	• Meet with school system's human resources office to determine possibility of designing program participation incentive for school staff • Secure/schedule classroom and activity spaces • Develop activity schedule for staff program • Recruit expert activities instructor(s) (e.g., fitness/yoga/strength instructors)	• Community activity experts from health/fitness clubs, etc. • Parents • Local healthcare provider(s) • Interns from university programs in physical education/exercise science	• Percentage of school staff members participating in program at least once a week
2019–2020	Family/community involvement	• Survey school's families on level of interest in having PA program(s) access on school campus, and preferred program types • Determine percentage of families who live within 2 miles of school • Plan calendar of special family events (e.g., family activity night, family fun run, family hike on local mountain trails) • Develop announcement messaging for each event • Schedule busing for off-campus transportation to hiking trailhead • Work with local community program (e.g., parks and recreation) for use of gymnasium on Saturdays and Sundays • Develop shared-use agreement	• Student council members • Parent organization • Classroom colleagues • Community organizations	• Improved access to school's PA venues during nonschool hours and weekends • Delivery of three family events during nonschool hours

Before school, recess, lunch periods, and immediately after school are times when the focus is primarily on promoting physical activity levels of students. For safety and liability reasons, adult supervision is required at all times from when students arrive at school until they leave the school at the end of the school day. Thus, recruiting and training adults to assist with overseeing the various activity venues and time outside of physical education lessons is essential. Support staff, volunteers (i.e., custodians, paraprofessionals, parents), and classroom colleagues can contribute in various ways. For example, classroom teachers and paraprofessionals typically will have scheduled playground supervision duties during recess and lunch periods (on a rotating basis). Moreover, parent volunteers in primary schools may also be available and asked to assist.

As the PAL, the physical educator can organize short professional development training sessions to help the adults take on a new role as physical activity facilitator while supervising. The adults can be shown how and where to move equipment carts at the onset of recess or before-school time, and how to set up the activity zones with signage. Getting the adult volunteers/paraprofessionals engaged in some of the activities and showing them how to play each activity during the professional development sessions enables them to help students get started. As Kretchmar (2012) recently argued, genuine play is something that may be increasingly foreign to many of today's children and youth, to the point where they could be described as having a play disability. They may lack the needed knowledge, skill, and interest in playing even the most common games (e.g., hopscotch, four-square, jump rope games) that historically have been part of the play landscape. Adults can also be trained to help diffuse any conflicts between students that might arise. Beyond reminding students about overall conduct, they can also offer simple conflict resolution strategies when minor activity-specific problems occur (e.g., rock-paper-scissors, do-over).

Recess and lunch periods are generally regarded as times for free play with minimal adult direction. However, adult supervisors can be activity facilitators as well; that is, they can be encouraged to move about the playgrounds and/or gymnasium to approach students and "prompt/encourage" them to come play, and even briefly participate or assist periodically in the students' activity (e.g., turning a long jump rope). In many cases, simply walking over to a group of students with a jump rope or ball and suggesting an activity is all that is needed. Related to this, the adult facilitators are also a powerful source of social reinforcement, by verbally and nonverbally recognizing both "good play" and appropriate conduct by students. The PAL can help the adult facilitators by providing them with 4" by 6" index cards that have multiple examples of verbal and nonverbal positive reinforcement (see **Figure 2.6**). The overarching goal here is not to have highly structured recess but rather a highly active recess.

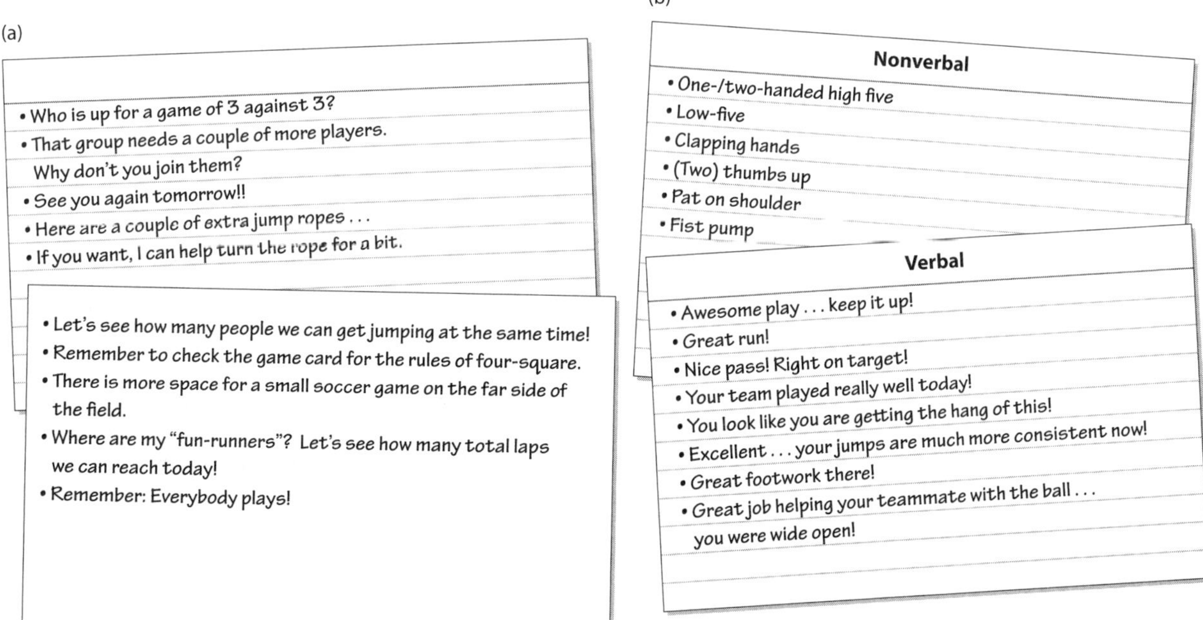

FIGURE 2.6 Sample cue cards for adult facilitator. (a) Sample prompts to encourage students to participate in physical activity. (b) Sample verbal and nonverbal social reinforcement statements.

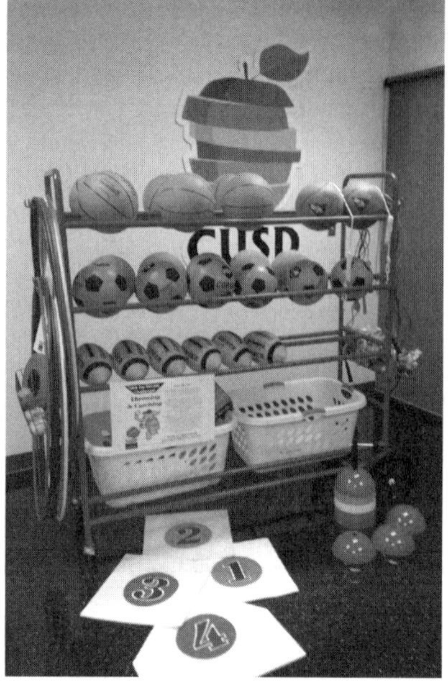

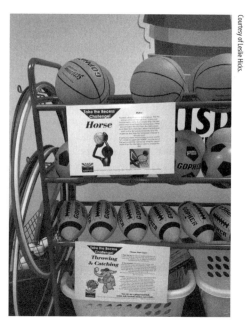

Courtesy of Leslie Hicks.

FIGURE 2.7 Two recess equipment carts with activity cards.

Providing appropriate equipment along with having clean and attractive activity venues can help increase students' physical activity levels. For example, there is good evidence that adding playground markings on primary school playgrounds can significantly increase students' activity levels (e.g., Ridgers, Stratton, Fairclough, & Twisk, 2007; Stratton & Mullan, 2005). In Chandler, Arizona, through grant support, the school district has funded the purchase of equipment and equipment carts dedicated solely for use during recess periods (see **Figure 2.7**). Having activity cards located on the equipment cart during recess can help encourage game play engagement (see Figure 2.6). Especially when introducing new games, students can be directed to review these cards to familiarize themselves with the various activities.

Depending on the size of the school's student population, the type and size of its activity venues, and the number of students present in the venues (i.e., gymnasiums, grass fields, and hardtop areas) the areas may need to be divided into different activity zones. This not only provides students with activity choices but also provides boundaries that will help keep students from interfering with the activity in adjacent areas. By way of clear signage, students will learn to differentiate between the areas designated for different activities. Students will have certain activities that will always be mainstays (e.g., soccer, basketball). However, we suggest that the activity choices be rotated periodically to maintain student interest. Student favorites can be determined by way of a quick informal survey of a sample of the school's students, administered with assistance from classroom teachers.

Relative to before- and after-school times, programs that are developed and organized by the school itself will have "first right" to the use of the facilities. During afternoon and evening hours, the gymnasium may also be used for other already scheduled activities. Thus, working with those who schedule such activities will help ensure that any out-of-class programming finds a place on the schedule.

After-school programs are a potentially large source for physical activity. Many after-school programs may be delivered by outside agencies or private companies that have contracted with the school (or school system). The outside group provides the service of delivering the after-school program in exchange for the use of the school's facility. When connecting with the personnel from the after-school program, the physical educator can first determine the overall focus of the program and the extent to which physical activity is a built-in program component. Based on that assessment, the physical educator can offer guidance and suggestions for how physical activity can be built into the schedule more prominently.

Collaborate with Outside Experts, Organizations, and Agencies

Implementing CSPAPs cannot be successful without tapping into the resources and expertise in the community/

region surrounding the school. Knowing what human and programmatic resources/programs are available and recruiting this expertise is critical for at least two reasons. First, it helps in promoting/encouraging physical activity beyond the school campus in upcoming physical activity–based events and other programs available in the surrounding community. For example, physical educators can announce an upcoming 5K–10K walk–run event, encourage students to join a nature hike with their families in a local nature preserve, or announce the availability of local physical activity–based programs scheduled during the school's vacation periods. One example is the KidSpirit program at Oregon State University. For a nominal fee, KidSpirit offers programs ranging from sessions held on 1-day school holidays to 4-week summer day camps held at the university. Traditionally, most sessions are centered on physical activities; in recent years, however, KidSpirit has infused sessions focusing on related health behaviors (e.g., healthy eating, cooking, nutrition). Similarly, the Sports Arena at the University of Limerick (Ireland) offers activity opportunities for children and youth after school, on weekends, and during school holidays.

Second, it can help the physical educator with recruiting people with the needed qualifications and expertise who can help deliver workshops or classes, or organize special events at the school during after-school hours. For example, if a teacher lacks the content background and/or equipment to teach golf or tennis, local instructors might be interested to offer instruction through workshops for either students or school staff. A parent or fitness instructor at a local club might be interested in offering a weekly fitness activity to the school's teachers and support staff as part of the school's staff wellness program. A local healthcare facility might be recruited to provide periodic health screenings to that same staff.

Depending on the local context, physical educators can draw from the local and regional experts and organizations listed in **Table 2.2**. In many ways, physical educators in their role as PALs become brokers of resources. We do not want to fool you: The outlay of time and energy early on in getting a CSPAP started is high. But utilizing the available resources within and beyond the school to the fullest extent possible will help the physical educator reach the point where he or she can increasingly rely on partners and collaborators.

TABLE 2.2 Community and Regional Expertise That Can Support CSPAPs

School-Based and Outside Expertise and Organizations	Possible Assistance
Other subject-/grade-level teachers	Following some training and professional development, classroom teachers can help increase physical activity by infusing brief 3- to 5-minute physical activity breaks. This is especially critical in schools that use 80- to 95-minute block periods.
Paraprofessionals	Promote physical activity during lunch or recess through prompting, encouragement, and facilitation among all students, including those with special needs; transport physical activity equipment to and from activity areas before, during, and after school.
School/parent organizations	Help advocate for CSPAP efforts at school board meetings and opportunities outside of school; fund new initiatives aimed at promoting physical activity (e.g., purchasing pedometers).
Parents/guardians	Especially in primary schools, parents will volunteer in various ways. Depending on their own background, they can help advocate at school board meetings, assist with school-based fundraisers, serve as representatives on the school wellness council, recruit other experts, assist on playgrounds during recess period, or facilitate physical activity. Some parents may have the expertise to teach certain types of group exercise activities (e.g., Zumba, yoga, Pilates).
School food services staff	Promote physical activity along with healthy eating habits among students, teachers, and school staff; publicize locations, times, and dates of farmers markets in the community; speak at meetings of policy makers.
School and local media	Help inform the public and promote the school's efforts in supporting students' physical activity through feature articles, interviews, and television.
School health experts and local healthcare providers	Promote healthy behavior practices, through presentations and marketing; offer services such as periodic health screening for school staff; speak at meetings of policy makers, etc. For example, local physicians/medical specialists can speak to the need for physical activity for health, and the risks of being sedentary for extended periods of time. Others might help present to the school's parents about the critical role of physical activity and good eating habits in ensuring a better quality of life, or break down the myths of fad diets.

(*continues*)

TABLE 2.2 Community and Regional Expertise That Can Support CSPAPs (*Continued*)

School-Based and Outside Expertise and Organizations	Possible Assistance
School technology specialists	Publicize and market CSPAP efforts through the school website and social media; help with creating web-based prompts to promote physical activity during nonschool hours and weekends.
Community organizations	Offer after-school programming; make presentations at school during special events and staff meetings.
Coaches and instructors from local sport clubs and other recreation programs	Lend expertise during after-school programs; offer sport-specific clinics at school during holiday breaks; help strengthen content knowledge of the physical educator on specific sports; encourage use of the school's physical activity facilities by offering activity programs during evening hours and on weekends.
Community/state health agencies and physical activity advocates	Provide fact sheets; speak in support of school program at meetings with policy makers.
Local fitness club and recreation center staff	Provide content expertise to broaden the options in programming physical activity for students, teachers, school support staff, and parents.
Registered dieticians	Help work with school food service personnel; develop promotional prompts for use at school to promote healthy eating; optimize food choices at school; assess and counsel students and school staff on eating habits (i.e., type and amounts of food and beverage intake); speak to policy makers on issues related to school's food service (e.g., use of vending machines, pros and cons of competitive food contracts).
Disability sport organizations and adapted physical education (APE) experts	Assist in ensuring that physical activity opportunities of students with special needs are promoted and supported as much as those for typically developing peers; offer training to peer tutors and paraprofessionals to assist students with special needs; help organize physical activity–based special events at school for students with special needs.
Physical education teacher education (PETE) faculty	Provide assistance in setting up before-, during-, and after-school physical activity programming; provide unpaid interns who can deliver activity-based sessions for school's students; assess the impact of extended school-based physical activity opportunities.
Exercise science and exercise and wellness experts (e.g., motor learning/ development experts; exercise physiology, exercise psychology)	Provide content knowledge expertise specific to issues related to physical activity; supply unpaid interns who can deliver activity-based information sessions for the school's students, teachers, support staff, and families; speak/advocate for physical activity programming before local and state policy makers.

Learn Sport, Games, Dance, and Other Movement Forms as a Source of Lifelong Physical Activity

Physical educators are expected to have a broad and in-depth knowledge of the subject matter (i.e., physically active motor play). This includes not only the knowledge needed to perform the activities but also the knowledge needed to teach the activities. Ball, Thames, and Phelps (2008) referred to these as **common content knowledge (CCK)** and **specialized content knowledge (SCK)**, respectively. Ward (2011) noted, "While CCK is acquired in the process of learning to play and playing a game; SCK is typically not acquired by playing (i.e., performing)" (p. 64).

Although traditional sports such as basketball and soccer may be popular with many students, other students may be interested in learning a host of other games and activities. In order to attract more students to being active physically, teachers must have a sufficient CCK background in other activities to help them gain beginning competence so that they are more likely to continue to seek it out. Thus, part of building a CSPAP will require developing a reasonably strong CCK and SCK across the various sports, lifetime activities, fitness content, dance content, and so on. Beyond personal participation, formal coursework, membership in professional organizations, conference attendance, and specialized workshops on today's technology afford physical education specialists ample opportunities to gain important knowledge. Ward (2009) proposed that our field's CCK can be classified into the following four domains: (1) rules, etiquette, and safety; (2) technique and tactics; (3) errors; and (4) instructional representations and tasks (i.e., the tasks and progressions used to teach a particular activity). Each of these domains is essential in designing the appropriate types of activity experiences so that participating children, youth, and adults experience success.

Learning Experience 2.6

Strengthening your subject matter knowledge: Select an activity (e.g., swimming, Tae Bo, Ultimate Frisbee, golf, dance, or weight training) of which you have no common content knowledge. Develop a plan of action to help strengthen your common content knowledge. Describe your sources of information and types of experiences you had in gaining this new knowledge. As you go through the process of learning about this activity, describe your experiences as a learner. How might this help you in terms of instructing others in this new activity?

Promote and Market Out-of-Class Physical Activity Programming

In the face of all the ways in which people in most countries have managed to squeeze physical activity out of their daily lives (i.e., escalators, computer games, remote controls, drive-through restaurants), encouraging children and youth to choose fun and health-optimizing physical activity over more sedentary activities is essential. Effective marketing strategies lie at the heart of promoting commercial products, where the overall goal is to make money for the company that sells the product.

Social marketing employs " . . . commercial marketing technologies to the analysis, planning, execution, and evaluation of programs designed to influence voluntary behavior of target audiences in order to improve their personal welfare and that of society" (Andreasen, 1995, p. 7). Social marketing has been employed to change other health behaviors such as preventing/reducing tobacco use and increasing immunizations, and can be used to change the physical activity behavior of children, youth, and adults. The key difference between commercial and social marketing is that the outcome benefits in the former come to the products' sellers, whereas in the latter the benefits come to the people who engage in the behavior. In the case of physical activity (the product), the "consumer" (and the larger society) benefits from its use.

Social marketing offers physical educators several key strategies to help promote and implement a CSPAP. It is essential for physical educators to understand the physical activity interests and needs of student, teachers, and support staff. Key social marketing principles pertinent for physical educators are product, price, place, and promotion.

Product refers to physical activity in all its various forms that can lead to improved health and well-being, from health-related fitness content to lifetime activities (e.g., biking, hiking, rock climbing, golf), sport (e.g., soccer, basketball, tennis, volleyball), and dance (e.g., hip-hop, ballroom, country and western). Metzler, McKenzie, van der Mars, Barrett-Williams, and Ellis (2013b) reminded us that how we present our product will help students decide whether they want more of it or make every effort to avoid it. Across physical education lessons and beyond, our product in its various forms should appeal to all students; it must be fun, developmentally appropriate, provide for success (i.e., the right level of challenge), be inclusive, and provide choices. The key is for physical educators to make the physical activity product as attractive as possible in the physical education lessons and beyond.

Price refers to costs and barriers involved in engaging in the behavior (e.g., money, time, effort, transportation) relative to its benefits. Times before school, recess, and lunch periods are free to all students. Assuming that transportation is not a barrier, access to quality after-school programs that are free, as opposed to fee-based, may attract more students as well. In many cases, if a school's facility is not an option for after-school programming, nearby community/recreation centers may be a viable alternative. The school could partner with and offer access to the center. Such partnerships are especially critical for economically disadvantaged children and youth.

Place refers to establishing the space and time for students to access the physical activity venues. The goal here is to make these easy to find, usable, and accessible throughout the school day. That is, students who typically arrive at school 45 minutes ahead of the first lesson, prior to the start of the first period, would know where they can come to play. Equipment should be out and ready for use. Importantly, the evidence is overwhelming that girls are less active than boys. Thus, it is especially important to ensure that barriers such as access, opportunity, and activity choice are eliminated. It may be useful to designate certain activity areas as "girls only" areas.

Promotion refers to any efforts to let the students know about all opportunities, types of activities, locations, and times when they can come be active. Options for doing so abound. Just like in commercial marketing, visual "points of decision" prompts that encourage physical activity can be provided throughout the school campus, through strategically placed signage located in high traffic areas (e.g., student drop-off areas, in and near changing rooms, in lunch rooms, at school entrances).

Similarly, naming the school's program for increasing physical activity during out-of-class times allows for it to be "branded." Branding is a key principle in commercial marketing (think of company logos) that helps with product/name recognition. This is a key factor in drawing persons to a product. Thus, all signage should include the activity program's name and/or logo (which could be designed by the students themselves).

Auditory prompts can be provided as well by way of daily announcements through the public address (PA) system, closed circuit school TV, and the like. The entire teaching staff in the school can help promote participation with frequent end-of-class reminders. School assemblies and other special events (e.g., open houses, family fitness nights, curriculum night) are another opportunity for such promotion. Local print and television media can be invited to do feature stories on the school's efforts to be an activity-friendly place for all.

Finally, attention can be drawn to all of the school's physical activity programming by way of the various types of technologies. For example the school's and CSPAP's websites are a key source of information for students and families. A web link like this can include information about the times, locations, and days of the week that the program is held as well as information about what new activities might be included in the upcoming week. Facebook and Twitter also offer a way to publicize the programming.

Increase Administrator and School Staff Knowledge of, and Support for, Physical Activity

In many countries today, schools appear increasingly fixated on improving students' academic achievement. School managers appear to lack the needed background knowledge about the importance of physical activity as a learned behavior and the central role that schools play (e.g., Lounsbery, McKenzie, Trost, & Smith, 2011; Lounsbery, McKenzie, Morrow, Monnat, & Holt, 2013; Sallis, 2010). They also likely lack a deep understanding of what a quality physical education program can and should look like (let alone a CSPAP). Thus, it is imperative that they become more informed. The question is: Which person is best positioned to educate them? Physical educators are the experts when it comes to promoting and informing the public about the program, and physical activity in general.

Learning Experience 2.7

Develop a short survey that you would give out to all teachers at your school to determine their knowledge of such aspects as: (1) the role and purpose of physical education, (2) physical activity benefits, (3) their own experiences in physical education when a student, and (4) how physical activity might benefit them in the classroom.

Compile/summarize the survey results. What are the key findings? Do the teachers have a solid understanding of our field and its importance? What is lacking in their knowledge and understanding?

A proactive and ongoing approach to doing this would include providing regular updates about topics such as: (1) quality physical education, (2) physical activity and its many health benefits, (3) the relationship of physical education (and physical activity) and academic achievement, and (4) programmatic efforts to maximize physical activity opportunities. The more informed school managers and teaching colleagues are about this, the more likely they are to begin to view the physical educator and the program as a central and indispensable part of the school.

Inform and Educate Parents, Guardians, Other Family Members, and Members of the Community

Much like the adults within the school, the family of the students and the public in the surrounding community can benefit from having a nearby school be a hub for physical activity and related activities. Unless they are informed about what the CSPAP has to offer, however, they are less likely to view it as an essential part of the community, visit the campus and enjoy the access and opportunity for physical activity, and support it.

Periodic events held at the school that target students and adults are more likely to attract them to the campus. In addition to word of mouth from students to parents, website announcements, school newsletter announcements, promotional campaigns by way of local television stations, the local newspaper, and messaging on the school's marquee board are all ways in which community members can learn about ongoing programming and special events.

Working with Students Versus Adults

There is considerable overlap in the skills and knowledge needed for developing before-, during- and after-school programming for students and a school employee physical activity/wellness program. Both require effective use of generic instructional skills such as being organized and prepared, starting on time, designing appropriate activities using clear demonstrations, using encouragement, and prompting and providing quality performance feedback (both positive and corrective). These are important regardless of the topic or the type of learners.

However, there is a fundamental difference from the perspective of knowing your learner. Adults (in this case the school employees) approach learning differently than do children and youth. Whoever is recruited to work with the school's staff members (the physical educator or outside guest instructors/presenters) will want to be mindful of such differences.

Cercone (2008) suggested the following general instructional principles and strategies when working with adults. First, although adults typically are *more self-directed and motivated*, they become more resistant to learning/participation if they perceive that the instructor tries to impose information, ideas, or actions. Instead, instructors will want to design appropriately paced activities that offer success, and only gradually move from simple (or less demanding) to more complex tasks. In addition, adults will look for the instructor to go out of his or her way to show interest in them, develop rapport, be approachable, and encourage questions. Adults will quickly determine whether the instructor is actually listening to the participants, and they will appreciate encouragement, along with constructive and specific positive and corrective feedback.

Second, adult learners bring with them *a longer history of life experiences*. The instructor/presenter will want to provide ample opportunity to participating employees to use that base of experience as a springboard toward scaffolding the new knowledge/understanding and skills into their personal experience base.

Third, in order to learn the new skills and knowledge, adult learners *need to see the relevance* of it. Getting them to regularly reflect on their experience before they came to the program and how the new skills and knowledge have affected their life can help them see the relevance and importance of the new skills, knowledge, and experiences.

Fourth, compared to children and youth, adults generally are *more goal-oriented*. Physical educators can tap into this readiness to learn by getting the adult learners to recognize the relevance of the new knowledge and skills.

Fifth, adults tend to be *more practical*. Again, because of their life experiences, adult learners are more likely to prefer and relate to hands-on active learning, so they can determine how it would fit in their life's context.

Finally, not unlike students in primary and post-primary schools, adult learners *want to be respected*. Adults come to feel respected if/when they see that the instructor sees them more as colleagues, as opposed to students in the traditional sense. Taking genuine interest in the participating employees, and encouraging them to express their ideas, experiences, concerns, and difficulties whenever possible, are effective strategies for creating that type of relationship.

CSPAPs: Getting Started

We have attempted to show how today's physical education programs are perhaps even more essential to schools and society at large by explaining (1) the features of CSPAPs, (2) why CSPAPs are important to build, (3) how to reconceptualize the position of traditional physical educators as that of Physical Activity Leaders (PALs), (4) the evidence base underlying implementation of the various CSPAP components, and (5) the skills and knowledge needed for implementing a CSPAP, along with suggested teaching strategies.

Box 2.5 provides a sample listing of various resources that physical educators around the world can use to learn about and gradually create a school environment that vigorously supports physical activity for all students during the school day and beyond.

BOX 2.5 Suggested Resources for Creating Activity-Friendly School Environments

Sample Program Descriptions by Country

- Australia: *Smart Moves* (www.education.qld.gov.au/schools/healthy/docs/planning-smart-moves.pdf)
- Ireland: *Active School Flag* (www.activeschoolflag.ie)
- Finland: *Schools on the Move* (www.liikkuvakoulu.fi/filebank/475-Finnish-schools-on-the-move.pdf)
- Switzerland: *Bewegungsfreundliche Schule* (www.bewegungsfreundlicheschule.ch)
- United States: *Comprehensive School Physical Activity Program* (www.aahperd.org/letsmoveinschool/about/overview.cfm?renderforprint=1)

Programmatic Resources

- *Active and Healthy Schools Program:* www.activeandhealthyschools.com
- NASPE (2011a). *Let's move in school physical education teacher toolkit:* www.aahperd.org/letsmoveinschool/tools/peteachers/index.cfm
- NASPE (2011c). *101 Tips for implementing a comprehensive school physical activity program*: www.aahperd.org/naspe/publications/products/newreleases.cfm?renderforprint=1 (fee-based)
- Partnership for Prevention (2008). *School-based physical education: Working with schools to increase physical activity among children and adolescents in physical education classes*: www.prevent.org/The-Community-Health-Promotion-Handbook/School-Based-Physical-Education.aspx
- *SPARK:* www.sparkpe.org
- *SPARK—After School:* www.sparkpe.org/after-school

(continues)

BOX 2.5 Suggested Resources for Creating Activity-Friendly School Environments (*Continued*)

Classroom Physical Activity Break Resources

- *Take10:* www.take10.net
- Mahar, M. T., Kenny, R. K., Shields, A. T., Scales, D. P., & Collins, G. (2004). *Energizers: Classroom-based physical activities.* Raleigh, NC: North Carolina Department of Public Instruction: www.ecu.edu/cs-hhp/exss/apl.cfm
- Mahar, M. T., Kenny, R. K., Scales, D. P., Shields, A. T., & Miller, T. Y. (2006). *Middle school energizers: Classroom-based physical activities.* Raleigh, NC: North Carolina Department of Public Instruction: www.ecu.edu/cs-hhp/exss/apl.cfm
- Pangrazi, R. P., Beighle, A., & Pangrazi, D. (2008). *Promoting physical activity and health in the classroom.* San Francisco: Benjamin Cummings.
- Pangrazi, R. P., Beighle, A., & Pangrazi, D. (2009). *Activity cards for promoting physical activity and health in the classroom.* San Francisco: Benjamin Cummings.
- Rink, J. E., Hall, T. J., & Williams, L. H. (2010). *Schoolwide physical activity: A comprehensive guide to developing and conducting programs.* Champaign, IL: Human Kinetics.

School Employee Wellness Resources

- Directors of Health Promotion and Education. (2005). *School employee wellness: A guide for protecting the assets of our nation's schools.* Washington, DC: Author.
- *School Alliance for a Healthier Generation (requires no-fee membership):* www.healthiergeneration.org
- *Employee Wellness Toolkit:* www.schools.healthiergeneration.org/_asset/n0rrcr/08-439_EWToolkit.pdf
- *Employee Wellness Interest Survey:* www.schools.healthiergeneration.org/_asset/74qhor/07165_EWInterestSurvey.pdf

CHAPTER SUMMARY

In this chapter we have provided an overview of possible programming strategies to promote physical activity for all students throughout the school day. Although much of the focus was on CSPAPs, as proposed by the National Association for Sport and Physical Education in the United States, many of the features and implementation strategies mirror those of similar efforts in other countries. The key is for physical educators anywhere to determine which aspects of the model presented can be built into the existing program. Given the status of the field in many countries, gradually moving toward CSPAP-like programs constitutes a major step toward increasing physical education programs' credibility.

1. Promotion of health-optimizing physical activity among children and youth throughout the school day is the prime focus of comprehensive school physical activity programs (CSPAPs).
2. CSPAP-like initiatives are being implemented in countries around the globe, including Australia, Finland, Ireland, Germany, and Switzerland.
3. A CSPAP is composed of five components: (1) physical education lessons, (2) physical activity during school, (3) physical activity before and after school, (4) school-based physical activity for school staff, and (5) family and community involvement.
4. The centerpiece feature of a CSPAP is the physical education lesson component.
5. Physical activity opportunities during the school day include: (1) classroom physical activity breaks (e.g., during language arts, math, science), (2) morning and afternoon recess in primary schools, and (3) opportunity for physical activity immediately prior to or after eating lunch.
6. Physical activity before and after school opportunities include: (1) active commuting to and from school, (2) informal recreation or play on school grounds, (3) campus-based after-school programs, (4) after-school activity clubs and intramural sports, and (5) interscholastic sport programs.
7. School employees spend much of the workday at school; their health and wellness can be enhanced through school-based physical activity/wellness programming.
8. Parents and adults in the school's surrounding community can benefit from having access to a school's physical activity facilities.
9. CSPAPs emergence is in part a consequence of increasing levels of overweight and obesity across all age groups. This has resulted in health-optimizing physical activity being accepted as a legitimate program outcome for school physical education. Although such programs are receiving widespread support from outside organizations, they remain marginalized relative to other school subjects.
10. Increased physical activity (along with physical education) does not affect academic achievement negatively,

and decreased time in physical education does not automatically translate into improved academic achievement.

11. Physical educators in their role as Physical Activity Leaders would coordinate, oversee, and facilitate the CSPAP.
12. There is substantial empirical evidence that demonstrates the efficacy of student-focused CSPAP components (e.g., classroom activity breaks, active recess and lunch periods).
13. Some of the skills and knowledge needed for delivering quality physical education programs do transfer to planning and implementing a CSPAP, including sound management and organization skills, subject matter content knowledge, and pedagogical content knowledge.
14. CSPAP implementation requires additional skills, including (1) coordinating before-, during-, and after-school physical activity programming through recruitment and training of other school staff and parent volunteers in the promotion of physical activity; (2) recruiting and collaborating with experts, agencies, and organizations in the community; (3) using social marketing techniques to promote physical activity beyond physical education lessons; (4) raising awareness of the importance of physical activity among classroom colleagues and school (system) managers; and (5) informing and educating parents, guardians, other family members, and members of the community about physical activity opportunities and healthy lifestyles.

When working with school staff and other adults in the community, physical educators should be mindful of the unique differences in working with adults compared to children and youth because each approaches the learning of new skills and knowledge in different ways. Adults tend to be more self-directed and motivated, have more life experiences, want to see the relevance of the learning experiences, are more goal-oriented, are practical, and want to be seen more as colleagues of the instructor.

REFERENCES

Alliance for a Healthier Generation. (2012). Employee wellness toolkit. Available from https://schools.healthiergeneration.org/_asset/n0rrcr/08-439_EWToolkit.pdf

American Academy of Pediatrics. (2006). Active healthy living: Prevention of childhood obesity through increased physical activity. *Pediatrics, 117*, 1834–1842.

American Academy of Pediatrics. (2013). Policy statement: The crucial role of recess in school. *Pediatrics, 131*, 183–188. DOI: 10.1542/peds.2012-2993

American Alliance for Health, Physical Education, Recreation and Dance. (2011). *2011 comprehensive school physical activity program (CSPAP) survey report*. Reston, VA: Author.

Andreasen, A. R. (1995). *Marketing social change: Changing behavior to promote health, social development, and the environment*. San Francisco, CA: Jossey-Bass.

Ball, D. L., Thames, M. H., & Phelps, G. (2008). Content knowledge for teaching: What makes it special? *Journal of Teacher Education, 59*, 389–407.

Beighle, A., Erwin, H., Castelli, D., & Ernst, M. (2009). Preparing physical educators for the role of physical activity director. *Journal of Physical Education, Recreation and Dance, 80*(4), 24–29.

Blair, S. N. (1993). C.H. McCloy research lecture: Physical activity, physical fitness, and health. *Research Quarterly for Exercise and Sport, 64*, 365–376.

Blair, S. N., & Bouchard, C. (1999). Physical activity and obesity: American College of Sports Medicine consensus conference. *Medicine and Science in Sports and Exercise, 31*, S497.

Bocarro, J. N., Kanters, M. A., Cerin, E., Floyd, M. F., Casper J. M., Suau, L. J., et al. (2012). School sport policy and school-based physical activity environments and their association with observed physical activity in middle school children. *Health and Place, 18*, 31–38.

Booth, F. W., & Chakravarthy, M. V. (2002). Cost and consequences of sedentary living: New battleground for an old enemy. *President's Council on Physical Fitness and Sports Research Digest, 3*(16), pp. 1–8. Available from www.presidentschallenge.org/informed/digest/docs/200203digest.pdf

Bouchard, C. (1993). Heredity and health-related fitness. *President's Council on Physical Fitness and Sports Research Digest, 1*(4), 1–7. Available from www.presidentschallenge.org/informed/digest/docs/199311digest.pdf

Bouchard, C., Blair, S. N., & Haskell, W. (Eds.). (2012). *Physical activity and health* (2nd ed.). Champaign, IL: Human Kinetics.

Bouchard, C., & Rankinen, T. (2001). Individual differences in response to regular physical activity. *Medicine and Science in Sport and Exercise, 33*, S446–S451.

Carson, R. L. (in press). Calling all practitioners: Encourage and support the creation of active schools and school physical activity champions [Editorial]. *American Journal of Lifestyle Management*.

Carson, R. (2012). Certification and duties of a director of physical activity. *Journal of Physical Education, Recreation & Dance, 83*(6), 16–29.

Carson, R. (June, 2013). *Changing role of the physical educator*. Paper presented at the Southwest District-AAHPERD Convention, Las Vegas, NV.

Centers for Disease Control and Prevention. (2001). Increasing physical activity: A report on recommendations of the Task Force on Community Preventive Services. *Morbidity and Mortality Weekly Report, 50*(RR-18), 1–14.

Centers for Disease Control and Prevention. (2011). School health guidelines to promote healthy eating and physical activity. *Morbidity and Mortality Weekly Report, 60*(5), 1–76. Available from www.cdc.gov/mmwr/pdf/rr/rr6005.pdf

Cercone, K. (2008). Characteristics of adult learners with implications for online learning design. *AACE Journal, 16*(2), 137–159.

Corbin, C. B. (2002). Physical activity for everyone: What every physical educator should know about promoting lifelong physical activity. *Journal of Teaching in Physical Education, 21*, 128–144.

Corbin, C. B., Pangrazi, R. P., & Welk, G. (1994). Toward an understanding of appropriate physical activity levels for youth. *President's Council on Physical Fitness and Sports Research Digest, 1*(8), 1–8. Available from www.presidentschallenge.org/informed/digest/docs/199411digest.pdf

Directors of Health Promotion and Education. (2005). *School employee wellness: A guide for protecting the assets of our nation's schools.* Washington, DC: Author.

Eitzen, S., & Sage, G. (2003). *Sociology of North American sport* (7th ed.). Boston: McGraw-Hill.

Fairclough, S., & Stratton, G. (2005). Physical activity levels in middle and high school physical education: A review. *Pediatric Exercise Science, 17*, 217–236.

Fairclough, S., & Stratton, G. (2006). A review of physical activity levels during elementary school physical education. *Journal of Teaching in Physical Education, 25*, 239–257.

Gettman, L. R. (1996). Economic benefits of physical activity. *President's Council on Physical Fitness and Sports Research Digest, 2*(7), 1–8. Available from www.presidentschallenge.org/informed/digest/docs/199609digest.pdf

Hardman, K. (2004). An update on the status of physical education in schools worldwide: Technical report for the World Health Organization. Available from www.icsspe.org/sites/default/files/Kenneth%20Hardman%20update%20on%20physical%20education%20in%20schools%20worldwide.pdf

Hardman, K., & Marshall, J. (2009). Physical education in schools: A global perspective. *Kinesiology, 40*(1), 5–28.

Heikinaro-Johansson, P., Lyyra, N., & McEvoy, E. (2012). Promoting health through physical education and physical activity in Finnish schools. *Global Journal of Health and Physical Education Pedagogy, 1*, 283–294.

Howie, E. K., & Pate, R. R. (2012). Physical activity and academic achievement in children: A historical perspective. *Journal of Sport and Health Sciences, 1*, 160–169.

Huang, Y. C., & Malina, R. M. (2002). Physical activity and health-related fitness in Taiwanese adolescents. *Journal of Physiological and Anthropological Human Sciences, 21*, 11–19.

Institute of Medicine (IOM). (2013). *Educating the student body: Taking physical activity and physical education to school.* Washington, DC: National Academies Press.

International Council of Sport Science and Physical Education. (2010). *International position statement on physical education.* Berlin, Germany: Author. Available from www.icsspe.org/sites/default/files/International%20Position%20Statement%20on%20Physical%20Education.pdf

Katzmarzyk, P. T., Malina, R. M., Song, T. M. K., & Bouchard, C. (1998). Physical activity and health-related fitness in youth: A multivariate analysis. *Medicine and Science in Sports and Exercise, 30*, 709–714.

Koplan, J. P., Liverman, C. T., & Kraak, V. I. (2005). *Preventing childhood obesity: Health in the balance.* Washington, DC: Institute of Medicine.

Kretchmar, R. S. (2008). The increasing utility of elementary school physical education: A mixed blessing and unique challenge. *Elementary School Journal, 108*, 161–170.

Kretchmar, R. S. (2012). Play disabilities: A reason for physical educators to rethink the boundaries of special education. *Quest, 64*, 79–86.

Landers, D. (1997). The influence of exercise on mental health. *President's Council on Physical Fitness and Sport Research Digest, 2*, 1–8. Available from www.icsspe.org/sites/default/files/International%20Position%20Statement%20on%20Physical%20Education.pdf

Lee, S. M., Burgeson, C. R., Fulton, J. E., & Spain, C. G. (2007). Physical education and physical activity: Results from the school health policies and programs study 2006. *Journal of School Health, 77*, 435–463.

Loeppke, R. (2008). The value of health and the power of prevention. *International Journal of Workplace Health Management, 1*, 95–108.

Lounsbery, M. A. F., McKenzie, T. L., Morrow Jr., J. R., Monnat, S. M., & Holt, K. A. (2013). District and school physical education policies: Implications for physical education and recess time. *Annals of Behavioral Medicine, 45*(Suppl. 1), S131–S141. DOI 10.1007/s12160-012-9427-9

Lounsbery, M. A. F., McKenzie, T. L., Trost, S. G., & Smith, N. J. (2011). Facilitators and barriers to adopting evidence-based physical education in elementary schools. *Journal of Physical Activity and Health, 8*(Suppl. 1), S17–S25.

Mahar, M. T. (2011). Impact of short bouts of physical activity on attention-to-task in elementary school children. *Preventive Medicine, 52*, S60–S64. DOI 10.1016/j.ypmed.2011.01.026

Mahar, M. T., Kenny, R. K., Scales, D. P., Shields, A. T., & Miller, T. Y. (2006). *Middle-school energizers: Classroom-based physical activities.* Raleigh, NC: North Carolina Department of Public Instruction. Available from www.ecu.edu/cs-hhp/exss/apl.cfm

Mahar, M. T., Kenny, R. K., Shields, A. T., Scales, D. P., & Collins, G. (2004). *Energizers: Classroom-based physical activities.* Raleigh, NC: North Carolina Department of Public Instruction. Available from www.ecu.edu/cs-hhp/exss/apl.cfm

Mahar, M. T., Murphy, S. K., Rowe, D. A., Golden, J., Shields, A. T., & Raedeke, T. D. (2006). Effects of a classroom-based program on physical activity and on-task behavior. *Medicine and Science in Sports and Exercise, 38*, 2086–2094.

Malina, R. M. (2001). Tracking of physical activity across the lifespan. *President's Council on Physical Fitness and Sports Research Digest, 3*(14), 1–8. Available from www.presidentschallenge.org/informed/digest/docs/200109digest.pdf

McKenzie, T. L., Marshall, S. J., Sallis, J. F., & Conway, T. L. (2000). Leisure-time physical activity in school environments: An observational study using SOPLAY. *Preventive Medicine, 30*, 70–77. DOI: 10.1006/pmed.1999.059

Metzler, M. W., McKenzie, T. L., van der Mars, H., Williams, L. H., & Ellis, S. R. (2013a). Health Optimizing Physical Education (HOPE): A new curriculum model for school programs. Part 1: Establishing the need and describing the curriculum model. *Journal of Physical Education, Recreation and Dance, 84*(4), 41–47.

Metzler, M. W., McKenzie, T. L., van der Mars, H., Williams, L. H., & Ellis, S. R. (2013b). Health Optimizing Physical Education

(HOPE): A new curriculum model for school programs. Part 2: Teacher knowledge and collaboration for HOPE. *Journal of Physical Education, Recreation and Dance, 84*(5), 25–34.

Morrow, J., & Freedson, P. (1994). Relationship between habitual physical activity and aerobic fitness in adolescents. *Pediatric Exercise Science, 6*, 315–329.

Murtrie, N., & Parfitt, G. (1998). Physical activity and its link with mental, social, and moral health in young people. In S. Biddle, J. Sallis, & N. Caville (Eds.), *Young and active? Young people and health-enhancing physical activity—evidence and implications* (pp. 49–68). London, UK: Health Education Authority.

National Association for Sport and Physical Education. (2008a). *Comprehensive school physical activity programs* [Position statement]. Reston, VA: Author. Available from www.aahperd.org/naspe/standards/upload/Comprehensive-School-Physical-Activity-Programs-2008.pdf

National Association for Sport and Physical Education. (2008b). *National standards and guidelines for physical education teacher education* (3rd ed.). Reston, VA: Author.

National Association for Sport and Physical Education. (2011a). *Let's move in schools—physical education teacher toolkit.* Available from www.aahperd.org/letsmoveinschool/tools/peteachers/index.cfm

National Association for Sport and Physical Education. (2011b). *NASPE Director of Physical Activity (DPA) certification program.* Available from www.aahperd.org/naspe/professionaldevelopment/dpasignup.cfm

National Association for Sport and Physical Education. (2011c). *101 Tips for implementing a comprehensive school physical activity program.* Reston, VA: Author. Available from www.aahperd.org/naspe/publications/products/newreleases.cfm?renderforprint=1

National Association for Sport and Physical Education. (2011d). *Overview of a comprehensive school physical activity program.* Available from www.aahperd.org/letsmoveinschool/about/overview.cfm

National Association of State Boards of Education. (2012). Fit, healthy, and ready to learn: A school health policy guide—Chapter D: Policies to promote physical activity and physical education. Available from www.nasbe.org/wp-content/uploads/FHRTL-D_Physical-Activity-NASBE-November-2012.pdf

Owen, N., Healy, G. N., Howard, B., & Dunstan, D. W. (2012). Too much sitting: Health risks of sedentary behavior and opportunities for change. *President's Council on Fitness, Sports and Nutrition Research Digest, 13*(3), 1–11. Available from www.presidentschallenge.org/informed/digest/docs/201212digest.pdf

Pangrazi, R. P., Beighle, A., & Pangrazi, D. (2008). *Promoting physical activity and health in the classroom.* San Francisco: Benjamin Cummings.

Pangrazi, R. P., Beighle, A., & Pangrazi, D. (2009). *Activity cards for promoting physical activity and health in the classroom.* San Francisco: Benjamin Cummings.

Pate, R. R., Davis, M. G., Robinson, T. N., Stone, E. J., McKenzie, T. L., & Young, J. C. (2006). Promoting physical activity in children and youth: A leadership role for schools: A scientific statement from the American Heart Association Council on Nutrition, Physical Activity, and Metabolism (Physical Activity Committee) in collaboration with the Councils on Cardiovascular Disease in the Young and Cardiovascular Nursing. *Circulation, 114*, 1214–1224.

Queensland Government. (n.d.). Planning for smart moves—guidelines. Available from www.education.qld.gov.au/schools/healthy/docs/planning-smart-moves.pdf

Rasberry, C. N., Lee, S. M., Robin, L., Laris, B. A., Russell, L. A., Coyle, K. K., et al. (2011). The association between school-based physical activity, including physical education, and academic performance: A systematic review of the literature. *Preventive Medicine, 52*, S10–S20.

Ridgers, N. D., Stratton, G., Fairclough, S. J., & Twisk, J. W. R. (2007). Long-term effects of playground markings and physical structures on children's recess physical activity levels. *Preventive Medicine, 44*, 393–397.

Rink, J. E., Hall, T. J., & Williams, L. H. (2010). *Schoolwide physical activity: A comprehensive guide to developing and conducting programs.* Champaign, IL: Human Kinetics.

Robert Wood Johnson Foundation. (2010). *State of play: Gallup survey of principals on school recess.* Princeton, NJ: Author.

Sallis, J. F. (2010). We do not have to sacrifice children's health to achieve academic goals. *Pediatrics, 124*, 696–697.

Sallis, J. F., & McKenzie, T. L. (1991). Physical education's role in public health. *Research Quarterly for Exercise and Sport, 62*, 124–137.

Sallis, J. F., McKenzie, T. L., Beets, M. W., Beighle, A. H., Erwin, H., & Lee, S. (2012). Physical education's role in public health: Steps forward and backward over 20 years and HOPE for the future. *Research Quarterly for Exercise and Sport, 83*, 125–135.

Schmidt-Millard, T. (2003). Perspectives on modern sports pedagogy. *European Journal of Sport Science, 3*(3), 1–7.

Siedentop, D. (2002). Content knowledge for physical education. *Journal of Teaching in Physical Education, 21*, 368–377.

Siedentop, D., & van der Mars, H. (2012). *Introduction to physical education, fitness and sport* (8th ed.). New York: McGraw-Hill.

Simon, C., Wagner, A., DiVita, C., Rauscher, E., Klein-Platat, C., Arveiler, D., et al. (2004). Intervention centered on adolescents' physical activity and sedentary behavior (ICAPS): Concepts and 6-months results. *International Journal of Obesity, 28*, S96–S103.

Spengler, J. O. (2012). *Promoting physical activity through the shared use of school and community recreational resources.* San Diego, CA: Active Living Research. Available from www.activelivingresearch.org/files/ALR_Brief_SharedUse_April2012.pdf

Spengler, J. O., Connaughton, D. P., & Carroll, M. S. (2011). Addressing challenges to the shared use of school recreational facilities. *Journal of Physical Education, Recreation and Dance, 82*(9), 28–33.

Stewart, J. A., Dennison, D. A., Kohl, H. W., & Doyle, J. A., (2004). Exercise level and energy expenditure in the TAKE 10! in-class physical activity program. *Journal of School Health, 74*(10), 387–400.

Stratton, G., & Mullan, E. (2005). The effect of multicolor playground markings on children's physical activity level during recess. *Preventive Medicine, 41*, 828–833.

Strong, W., Malina, R. M., Blimkie, C. J. R., Daniels, S. R., Dishman, R. K., Gutin, B., et al. (2005). Evidence-based physical activity for school-age youth. *Journal of Pediatrics, 146*, 732–737.

Timmons, J. A., Knudsen, S., Rankinen, T., Koch, L. G., Sarzynski, M., Jensen, T., et al. (2010). Using molecular classification to predict gains in maximal aerobic capacity following endurance exercise training in humans. *Journal of Applied Physiology, 108*, 1487–1496. DOI: 10.1152/japplphysiol.01295.2009

Troiano, R. P., Berrigan, D., Didd, K., Masse, L., Tilert, T., & McDowell, M. (2008). Physical activity in the United States measured by accelerometer. *Medicine and Science in Sports and Exercise, 40*, 181–188.

Trost, S., & van der Mars, H. (2009). Why we should not cut PE. *Educational Leadership, 67*, 60–65.

U.S. Department of Health and Human Services (USDHHS). (2000). *Healthy people 2010* (Conference Edition, in Two Volumes). Washington, DC: U.S. Government Printing Office.

U.S. Department of Health and Human Services (USDHHS). (2008). *2008 physical activity guidelines for Americans*. Washington, DC: Author. Available from www.health.gov/PAGuidelines

U.S. Department of Health and Human Services (USDHHS). (2010). *Healthy people 2020*. Washington, DC: Author. Available from www.healthypeople.gov/2020/topicsobjectives2020/pdfs/HP2020objectives.pdf

U.S. Department of Health and Human Services (USDHHS). (2013). *Physical activity guidelines for Americans midcourse report: Strategies to increase physical activity among youth*. Washington, DC: Author. Available from www.health.gov/paguidelines/midcourse/pag-mid-course-report-final.pdf

Ward, D. S. (2011). *School policies on physical education and physical activity. Research synthesis*. San Diego, CA: Active Living Research. Available from www.activelivingresearch.org/files/Synthesis_Ward_SchoolPolicies_Oct2011_1.pdf

Ward, P. (2009). Content matters: Knowledge that alters teaching. In L. D. Housner, M. W. Metzler, P. G. Shempp, & T.J. Templin (Eds.), *Historic traditions and future directions of research on teaching and teacher education in physical education* (pp. 345–356). Morgantown, VA: Fitness Information Technology, West Virginia University.

Ward, P. (2011). The future direction of physical education teacher education: It's all in the details. *Japanese Journal of Sport Education Studies, 30*(2), 63–72.

Wechsler, H., McKenna, M. L., Lee, S. M., & Dietz, W. H. (2004). Role of schools in preventing childhood obesity. *The State Education Standard, 5*(2), 4–12.

Weston, A. (1962). *The making of American physical education*. New York: Appleton-Century-Crofts.

Wilkins, J. L., Graham, G., Parker, S., Westfall, S., Fraser, R. G., & Tembo, M. (2003). Time in the arts and physical education and school achievement. *Journal of Curriculum Studies, 35*, 721–734.

World Health Organization (WHO). (2010). *Global recommendations on physical activity and health*. Geneva, Switzerland: Author. Available from http://whqlibdoc.who.int/publications/2010/9789241599979_eng.pdf

Zahner, L., Furger, R., Graber, M., & Keller, A. (2012). *Bewegungsfreundliche Schule* [activity-friendly schools]. Basel, Switzerland: Universität Basel. DVD.

CHAPTER 3 Educational Reform: Implications for Teaching Physical Education

Overall Chapter Outcome

To introduce educational reform; the standards/outcomes, assessment, and accountability movements; and the implications of these movements for physical education

Learning Outcomes

The learner will:

- Describe the shift in focus of the education reform movement internationally
- Describe the challenges and opportunities facing physical education in this era of standards and accountability
- Discuss why physical educators are considered part of the problem and part of the solution for educational improvement
- Discuss important concepts of the ecological framework
- Explain the relationship between physical education and public health
- Describe the relationship between school physical education and alternative providers of physical education outside of schools
- Clarify what is meant by the "narrowing of the curriculum" and the factors that are responsible

It is sometimes said that people can't see the forest because of all the trees. This chapter provides a view of the "forest." This wider lens of viewing the teaching of physical education will include a glimpse at educational reform and how it has impacted physical education through the assessment, accountability, and standards movements. In addition, we will explore the *ecological model* as the framework for understanding the influence of various outside forces on teaching in schools.

Educational Reform

Education systems around the world are more similar than dissimilar, sharing common core values, policies, functions, and structures. Facing similar problems and challenges, they are choosing comparable solutions and **educational reform** agendas to address these issues. Recent years have been marked by the focus of educational reform moving toward improving both the quality and relevance of education worldwide (Hargreaves & Shirley, 2009). A shift in focus from teaching to learning, emphasizing learners constructing their own knowledge and gaining greater conceptual understanding, has become apparent in the educational systems of a number of countries (e.g., Finland, Ireland). Alternatively, in other countries there is an emphasis on learning through development of common learning outcomes/standards for all learners, which are reinforced through what has become an international focus on accountability (e.g., United States, European Union, China). Holding students, teachers, administrators, and schools responsible for learning outcomes reflects this focus on accountability while lessening the opportunity for learners to construct their own knowledge. It is a bit of a contradiction that all international education

BOX 3.1 Key Terms in This Chapter

- *Accountability:* The oversight mechanisms of a policy or legislative mandate as well as built-in consequences for schools that are not following such rules. Accountability has moved from a focus on what goes into public education (i.e., funding, facilities, equipment, and teacher and staff qualifications) to teachers being held accountable for student achievement.
- *Boundaries:* In terms of a policy, this refers to how tightly or loosely the accountability for implementation is applied and how explicit or ambiguous the requirements are for its implementation.
- *Change agent:* An educator who intentionally or indirectly causes or accelerates social, cultural, or behavioral change in an education setting.
- *Clarity and ambiguity:* Related concepts that refer to the degree of explicitness and consistency in how policy/legislation is written. Poorly written policies/legislation are those that include language that provides more latitude in terms of whether to implement them.
- *Ecology of physical education:* Ecology is typically made up of a number of systems that interact with each other so that a change in one system influences what happens in the other systems. Just as the natural environment we live in can be understood as an ecological system, so too can teaching/learning in physical education.
- *Educational reform:* Five characteristics of educational reform have been identified as (1) standardization in education, (2) focus on basic student knowledge with an emphasis on literacy and numeracy, (3) teaching for predetermined results, (4) the involvement of the business world in designing and implementing educational reform efforts, and (5) high-stakes accountability systems that have evolved internationally.
- *Governing policy:* A statement/guideline set forth to represent a change in the governance system that directly affects the education (and thus physical education) system.
- *Professional development:* Formal and informal learning experiences designed to enhance professional career development.
- *Risk:* Associated with policy, this refers to the interaction among the ambiguity within the policy, the difficulty of implementing it, and the degree of accountability associated with it.

systems are grappling in an effort to provide a strong education for all young people. Finland has rejected the outcomes-based education reform format, whereas European countries are introducing more flexible forms of curriculum; a focus on assessment for learning (assessment that facilitates continued growth and development), as opposed to assessment of learning (summative assessment of outcomes); varied types of accountability; and opportunities for teachers to work collaboratively in developing a critical pedagogy (Tinning, 2008) to promote learning.

Until recently, accountability has tended to focus on what goes into public education, such as funding, facilities, equipment, and qualifications of teachers and staff, as opposed to student outcomes. A new view of accountability places student learning and performance at the pinnacle of public education. Fuhrman (1999) describes this new accountability as marked by teachers held accountable for student achievement, which is publicly shared and reported, with schools considered the unit of analysis and held responsible for continuous improvement and consequences applied for students and schools failing to achieve. The dichotomy, as Gleeson and O'Donnabhain (2011) describe, is that "while the official discourse is replete with references to change and reform, much of the available evidence suggests that little change has occurred in teachers' 'beliefs and values'" (p. 32). They acknowledge that "real change" requires change in the school culture, which must be the focus of educational reform if it is to impact the quality of education.

Preparing teachers to serve as **change agents** is a critical role of initial teacher education, and one that O'Sullivan (2003) would argue is often overlooked. She encourages physical education teacher education (PETE) programs to move outside their narrow focus on developing teachers "able to follow change, rather than lead change." PETE programs must identify strategies that, when employed, will bring about change, and then design learning experiences that allow preservice teachers to practice using these skills. MacPhail and Tannehill (2012) encourage preservice teachers to explore worthwhile teaching and learning strategies through interacting effectively with teachers, working collaboratively as part of a community, and advocating for physical education if they are to persevere in their teaching of physical education.

Teacher change might also be developed through **professional development** opportunities. Professional development in education and physical education has been practiced in most countries for some time, yet is marked by little change in structure or design, and consequently it has produced limited change in teachers, students' learning, or teachers' ability to be leaders in change. Professional development continues to be offered as generic in-service days or one-off workshops that have little connection to previous or subsequent initiatives. It is overseen by experts external to the school setting, and generally intended to provide teachers with a "recipe" that they are expected to accept and implement without question (MacPhail et al., 2012). The result of teachers being outside the planning and decision loop for these initiatives is professional development being "done to teachers" rather than with teachers.

In recent years, teacher professional development has become a key aspect of education reform, yet those responsible for designing professional development opportunities continue to employ outdated and top-down opportunities with which teachers struggle to find relevance. Teacher professional development needs strategies to move professional development forward in a way that will impact teachers, schools, and learners through what Hargreaves and Fullan (2012) call *professional capital*. This is where every teacher in every school has the opportunity to work together in an environment that values teachers, places them at the head of the teaching profession, and provides support to them in their work as a community of professionals.

Sahlberg (2010) identifies five characteristics of educational policy and reform that have been employed worldwide in an effort to improve the quality of education. First is the notion of standardization in education reflected by outcomes-based reforms; setting of performance standards for students, teachers, and schools; external examination to monitor achievement of those standards; and generic reporting of these results. Second is an increased focus on basic student knowledge and skills in core subjects, with an emphasis on literacy and numeracy. The expectation is that this focus will transcend all subject areas. The third characteristic, teaching for predetermined results, has reduced the content taught to youth, and limited the use of alternative pedagogies and experiential types of learning. Fourth is the involvement of the business world in designing and implementing educational reform efforts. Although some useful initiatives have resulted from these partnerships, by taking decisions away from schools and teachers there are drawbacks for teachers in their attempts to learn from their mistakes and successes. It also limits the amount of growth that can be made by sharing and developing as a group of educators. Finally, the fifth characteristic is the high-stakes accountability systems that have evolved internationally. The result of this focus is schools', teachers', and students' performance resting on standardized tests and examinations that merely provide a snapshot of teaching and learning: "The higher the test-result stakes, the lower the degree of freedom in experimentation and risk-taking in classroom learning" (Sahlberg, 2010, p. 12). In countries where high-stakes assessments are the norm, one implication of these practices for the continuum of teacher education is the difficulty in preparing preservice teachers to move beyond didactic teaching, which anticipatory socialization typically dictates in these contexts.

A prime example of how a national government has sought to exert greater control over classroom practices is the 2002 passage of the No Child Left Behind (NCLB) Act in the United States. This landmark legislation is based on the assumption that by developing more stringent student performance standards along with measurable outcomes in core subjects (i.e., reading and math), student achievement could be improved. States that receive funding from the federal government are required to assess students annually on these basic subjects in selected grade levels. A consequence of this national education reform policy has been an enormous shift in how schools allocate their time and other resources to those subjects examined at the state level (mirroring those noted by Sahlberg). In a later section we will show how this has also directly affected the delivery of school physical education programs.

Learning Experience 3.1

If you were asked to describe the educational accountability movement that exists in your country, where might you source such information? To whom might you talk to find out how it is being taken on board by local and regional school administrators?

Reform in Physical Education

To what extent has physical education reformed itself relative to setting student performance standards? And how strong are the accountability systems monitoring physical education worldwide? A limited number of states in the United States have a formal assessment and evaluation system that holds school districts, schools, and teachers accountable for students achieving these standards. According to the National Association of Sport and Physical Education (NASPE) and American Heart Association *Shape of the Nation Report* (2010), 48 U.S. states (96%) have developed content standards that reflect those set by NASPE or locally developed state initiatives. However, only 34 states (68%) require local districts to comply or align with these standards, and only 19 states (38%) mandate some form of student assessment in physical education. In most cases, the administration of the assessments is left to the individual school districts; only five states (10%) forward the assessment data to their respective state department of education.

In England, Wales, and Northern Ireland, the National Curriculum provides a framework for the development and delivery of physical education across primary and post-primary education. It sets attainment targets, outlines content to be taught, and specifies performance assessment and reporting of results across four key phases. This curriculum is intended to be broad and balanced for all young people 5–16 years of age, with physical education being a foundation subject across all four phases. Accountability lies with local education authorities, which results in some flexibility in design and delivery to suit local contexts. With the latest global economic recession issues impacting educational funding, many of these systems have been put on hold. This prompts the question, is there any accountability in education if there is no system in place to enforce it?

Learning Experience 3.2

Source educational reform initiatives in your country and describe how they are impacting physical education content, teachers, and students in your area.

The Ecology of Physical Education Beyond the Classroom

Even though physical educators often may feel they work in isolation, teaching physical education in schools does not occur in a vacuum. As we have just described, there are numerous outside forces at play that directly affect events in individual physical education classes. In this section we introduce a framework that can help you understand how and why some programs accomplish what they set out to do and others do not. That is, decisions made by school principals, school governing bodies, and community boards, as well as local and national government leaders, also influence teachers' day-to-day work. The framework for understanding the influence of the various outside forces at work is called the *ecological model*. In its generic sense, **ecology** refers to the study of the habitat of living objects, the relationships between organisms and their environment. An ecology is typically made up of a number of systems that interact with each other so that a change in one system influences what happens in the other systems. The delicate balance among the systems within the ecology can be upset if or when changes or disruptions occur in one or more of the systems. Just as the natural environment we live in can be understood as an ecological system, so too can teaching/learning in physical education.

Physical education teachers are responsible for designing a learning environment that is conducive for students to learn about physical activity in ways that make students want to seek it out beyond physical education. How teachers arrange their program, manage their students, and select and deliver the content are important factors that influence how this will be accomplished. However, there are numerous outside influences, such as parent beliefs and community attitudes, that are just as important (if not more so) in determining the impact of school physical education programs.

How Policies Help Physical Education Programs Accomplish Their Mission

To understand the ecology of physical education programs at the broader level, you must see how policy-related tasks develop. Ecologically, the school physical education program is a system that functions along with other systems (e.g., other school subjects, governing bodies that oversee schools). The primary task of a physical education program is to provide structured learning experiences for its students. A *task* is defined by a goal and a set of operations to achieve it. The degree to which this task is accomplished is in large part dependent on the influence exerted by other systems.

Important Concepts in the Ecological Framework

Understanding the interplay among four related concepts—accountability, clarity/ambiguity, risk, and boundaries—will help you recognize how policy-related tasks get accomplished. **Accountability** refers to how a policy or legislative mandate includes oversight mechanisms as well as built-in consequences for schools that are not following such rules; that is, without accountability, no matter how well-intended the policy rules set forth, they are not likely to be effective. For example, suppose a governing body institutes a policy requiring schools to provide physical education to all postprimary students for at least 225 minutes per week in each school year. Without any funding support for oversight to ensure implementation by schools (or consequence for not following the new rules), few schools would abide by this. These are typically labeled as *unfunded mandates*, and consequently are difficult, if not impossible, to implement.

Learning Experience 3.3

In classroom subjects (e.g., math, science), students are expected to learn the subject matter. Explain your position on whether students should be held accountable for learning in physical education. Be sure you can defend your position.

Clarity and ambiguity are related concepts that refer to the degree of explicitness and consistency in how policy/legislation is written. Poorly written policies/legislation include language that provides school districts and individual schools with more latitude in terms of whether to implement them. For example, legislation that includes wording like *suggest*, *recommend*, and *encouraged* carry little weight in terms of changing school and teaching practices (McCullick et al., 2012). Conversely, legislation that is very explicit and clear in its expectations will require attention, and, coupled with stronger accountability mechanisms, can make a difference in how physical education is delivered.

There also is possible ***risk*** associated with policies. Risk refers to the interaction among the ambiguity within the policy, the difficulty of implementing it, and the degree of accountability associated with it. Poorly or ambiguously worded policies may initially pose a higher risk for administrators and teachers until they come to realize that either the implementation of the policy is not difficult or there is no real accountability built into the legislation. A more difficult change in practice with strong accountability results in a high degree of risk for school administrators and teachers. For example, a recent trend in education in the United States is teacher evaluation increasingly tied to student performance on academic achievement tests (National Council on Teacher Quality, 2011). This would pose more risk, especially for physical education teachers, given the profession's rather meager history of demonstrating what students have learned while in the program. On the other hand, policies that require little change in practice (or carry little, if any, accountability) would result in less risk for administrators and teachers. In Ireland, for example, the Junior Cycle Physical Education syllabus (National Council for Curriculum and Assessment [NCCA], Department of Education and Sciences, 2003) is based on the recommendation that all students 11–17 years of age be provided 2 hours of physical education each week. Within these 2 hours, a suggested eight physical activity strands should be included in the curriculum—athletics, adventure, aquatics, dance, gymnastics, invasion games, net and fielding games, and health-related activity. Although this legislation was intended to ensure that all students were provided with a broad range of physical activities in an adequate time frame, the terms *recommended* and *should include* only suggest accountability through teacher and school goodwill and recognition of the importance of physical education to a young person's development. You can see how risk and ambiguity are related, especially when policy accountability is strong. Higher ambiguity may produce more risk if there are real expectations for implementing the policy.

Policies also have **boundaries** in terms of what the overseeing governing body will find acceptable in terms of implementation and outcomes. The boundaries of a policy refer to how tightly or loosely the accountability for implementation is applied and how explicit or ambiguous the requirements are for its implementation. Legislation or policies that are explicit with strong accountability built in have tight boundaries; that is, schools and teachers generally would know exactly what the real expectations are within the policy, and will have little if any latitude in terms of implementing it. **Figure 3.1** shows how a policy or legislation that is supposed to be implemented across various levels of oversight in education may or may not impact program and instructional practices. Although education governance may differ structurally in various countries, the same principles would apply.

Strong Policies and Weak Policies

Ecologically, a **governing policy** is set forth and represents a change in the governance system that directly affects the education (and thus physical education) system. The strength of the policy will dictate how well school administrators and teachers will implement it. The type and level of oversight and accountability tied to the policy are the central determinants of whether the policy is followed.

As you learn more about how policies affect physical education programs, you will find that not all governing policies (if they even exist) are created equal. Strong policies are those that include: (1) funding that comes with the policy, (2) stated and explicit stipulations regarding policy oversight (supervision), (3) rules stipulating to report how policy has been implemented, and (4) stated consequences for failing to follow policy guidelines (as in accountability). Strong policies are more explicit and specific in that they dictate what schools and teachers are expected to do; that is, they set clear task boundaries, and are more likely to be followed all the way from the governing authority down to the class level and impact day-to-day practices of (physical education) teachers. Conversely, weak policies or mandates are those that either are written in ambiguous terms, are minimally

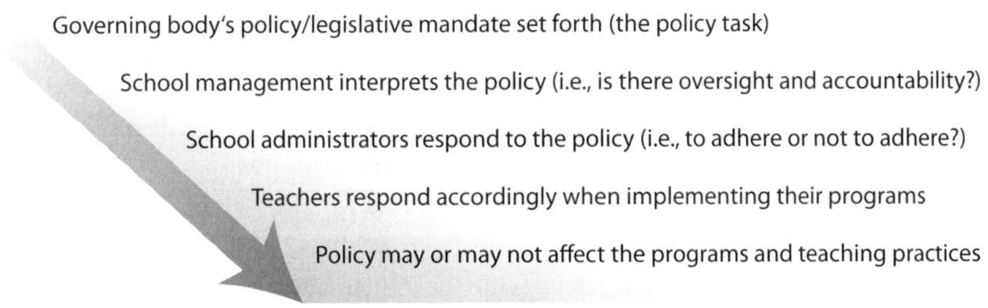

Governing body's policy/legislative mandate set forth (the policy task)

School management interprets the policy (i.e., is there oversight and accountability?)

School administrators respond to the policy (i.e., to adhere or not to adhere?)

Teachers respond accordingly when implementing their programs

Policy may or may not affect the programs and teaching practices

FIGURE 3.1 Contingency-dependent implementation of an educational policy.

funded, or have no built-in mechanisms for oversight and accountability.

You can see how the aforementioned concepts of *risk* and *ambiguity* come into play at the various governance levels. In the state of South Carolina, Dr. Judith Rink and her colleagues have been instrumental in building a strong state policy profile for physical education (Rink & Mitchell, 2003). An outcome is that all schools in South Carolina are required to conduct a formal assessment of student learning outcomes in physical education and report their results to the State. Elementary schools must provide a minimum of 60 minutes of formal physical education per week and an additional 90 minutes of physical activity beyond physical education.

Conversely, weak policies are those that carry little, if any, funding and/or are written in such ambiguous ways that they make oversight and accountability for implementation virtually impossible (McCullick et al., 2012); that is, schools need to pay little, if any, attention to the policy. Consequently, such unfunded mandates carry with them little risk for schools, and thus reflect pseudoaccountability.

Consider the following questions:

- Who or what is holding the individual physical education teacher accountable for designing an up-to-date, exciting physical education program that results in learning among students?
- Who or what is ensuring that the school delivers such a program?
- Who or what is responsible for ensuring that schools follow the policies and mandates in effect to provide quality physical education?
- How can policies and/or legislation that are not specific to physical education still influence this school subject in schools?

Answers to these questions depend in large part on how education at various levels is governed, funded, and overseen. For example, in Canada, the primary responsibility and oversight lies with the individual provinces. Education Scotland (n.d.) is a national governing body responsible for supporting the quality and improvement of learning and teaching from early education to both adult and community learning. In Australia, responsibility for education lies with the states and territories and includes both funding and regulation of public and private primary and secondary schools. In the United States, the structure, organization, and governance of education are left to the individual states (Siedentop, 2009). Although the U.S. federal government has actually been an active player in the last half century through key legislation (e.g., Title IX in 1972, No Child Left Behind in 2001), it is the individual states' boards of education along with state superintendents for public instruction that are responsible for overseeing education by setting the rules and policies for K–12 education (including physical education).

In each country, the policies (or the lack thereof) strongly affect how teachers, principals, and boards of management conduct education on a day-to-day basis. With regard to local policies, for example, the amount of autonomy a school has to determine how much time is allocated to physical education may vary depending on the dominance of the academic profile within the country (e.g., bonus points for math, exam subjects receiving priority). Schools may make accommodations for "priority" subjects by making physical education optional at one level, suggesting that the subject's status is considered as a solution to scheduling problems. As with the ecology in the individual class, the extent to which a school adheres to government policies depends on its *task boundaries*. It is important for you to become intimately familiar with how policies affect your future physical education career.

Learning Experience 3.4

Policy profiles . . . what do you know? Regardless of where you live (e.g., United States, United Kingdom, Canada), what are the answers to the following questions relative to your own context?

- How many minutes of physical education are required weekly across each school level (i.e., elementary/primary and secondary/postprimary schools)?
- What are the minimum number of required minutes of physical activity per week for students across each school level (i.e., elementary/primary schools and secondary/postprimary schools)?
- What is the policy regarding the required minimum number of minutes of recess/physical activity breaks per day in elementary/primary schools?
- What are the secondary/postprimary graduation requirements for physical education?
- What is the policy for use of exemptions/waivers/substitution for physical education?
- What is the required or prescribed curriculum for physical education?
- What is the policy on maximum class sizes allowed across the elementary/primary and secondary/postprimary schools?
- What are the requirements for formal assessment of students in physical education?
- How are student performance data in physical education reported to the public?
- What teaching certification requirements are in place for physical education?

In the last two decades, numerous national and international guidelines and recommendations have been published

BOX 3.2 State Requirements for Physical Education in the United States

- Only five states require physical education in each grade, K–12 (Illinois, Iowa, Massachusetts, New Mexico, and Vermont).
- Forty-three states (86%) mandate elementary school physical education, 40 states (78%) mandate middle-school physical education, and 46 states (90%) mandate high-school physical education.
- Only one state (Alabama) aligns with the nationally recommended 150 minutes per week of physical education in elementary school and 225 minutes per week in middle and high school.
- Forty-eight states (96%) have their own state standards for physical education, but only 34 states (67%) require local districts to comply or align with these standards.
- Only 19 states (37%) require some form of student assessment in physical education.
- Fewer states (14, versus 22 in 2006) require physical education grades to be included in students' grade point averages.
- Only 13 states (25%) require schools to measure body mass index (BMI) and/or height and weight for each student.

Data from National Association for Sport and Physical Education & American Heart Association. (2010). *2010 shape of the nation report: Status of physical education in the USA*. Reston, VA: National Association for Sport and Physical Education.

targeting school physical education and physical activity of children and youth (e.g., NASPE, 2004; National Physical Activity Plan Alliance, 2010; U.S. Department of Health and Human Services [USDHHS], 2008; World Health Organization, 2010). These all are helpful documents that can aid in supporting the cause for quality school physical education; however, they are just that: recommendations and guidelines. By themselves they will not bring about change. For schools to be successful in helping meet such guidelines and recommendations, effective policies need to be put in place. In the United States, the National Association of Sport and Physical Education (NASPE) tracks each state's "policy profile" for K–12 physical education (NASPE, 2010b).

Why a Focus on Policies Is So Important

In a recent analysis of the status of physical education in European countries, Hardman (2008) noted that:

> *[a] "gap" is seen in the rhetoric of official documentation on principles, policies and aims and actual implementation into practice, which exposes a range of deficiencies in PE in schools. . . . There is evidence of general underfunding of PE/school sport as well as the low remuneration of PE/sport teachers in some countries. . . . PE time allocation has been reduced more extensively in central and eastern EU States than in counterpart "western" EU States.*[1]

Similarly, as can be seen in **Box 3.2**, across the United States, states vary widely in their requirements for school physical education.

The good news is that this neglect is slowly being rectified. Internationally, there are efforts underway to improve physical education's policy profile. The efforts in South Carolina are a prime example of success, as is the Physical Education and Sport Strategy for Young People in the UK (see www.ssp-web-solutions.co.uk/PESSYP_small.pdf). A review of related policy documents internationally suggests that several countries are also considering or have passed legislation aimed at increasing physical education requirements in various ways.

Learning Experience 3.5

Schedule an appointment with a principal at a local school (either elementary/primary or secondary/postprimary level). Prepare four interview questions that will help you find out about his or her position regarding the importance of physical education and physical activity for school-age students. Summarize the results in a short paper, and be prepared to present your findings.

Distant Decisions with Local Consequences

Threats to physical education often come with policy decisions made in other areas of education. In the United States, perhaps the best example was the passage of the federal law No Child Left Behind. This landmark law sought to improve students' academic achievement in what were labeled the "core subjects" of language arts and mathematics. Moreover,

[1] Reproduced from Hardman, K. (2008). The situation of physical education in schools: A European perspective. *Human Movement, 9*, 15.

TABLE 3.1 Changes in Instructional Time in Elementary Schools Since No Child Left Behind Was Enacted

Subject	Percentage of Districts Increasing Time	Percentage of Districts Decreasing Time	Average Increase (Minutes Per Week)	Average Decrease (Minutes Per Week)
Language Arts	58		141	
Math	45		89	
Social Studies		36		76
Science		28		75
Art and Music		16		57
Physical Education		9		40
Lunch Recess		5		
Recess		20		50

Reproduced with permission from Center on Education Policy. (2007). *Choices, changes, and challenges: Curriculum and instruction in the NCLB era*. Washington, DC; Center on Education Policy.

it sought to reduce the disparities in academic achievement scores between students from different racial/ethnic groups. If there was ever a doubt that No Child Left Behind would affect school physical education programs, there is now strong evidence that it has had a huge negative impact. **Table 3.1** shows the shifts in instructional time from that allocated to physical education, recess, and lunch recess (as well as other school subjects) to the core subjects targeted in No Child Left Behind (Center on Education Policy, 2008). What is most troublesome for physical education is that this shift has occurred at the same time physical education has never been more important for increasing physical activity opportunities for school-age youth (Siedentop & van der Mars, 2012). From an ecological perspective, this shows how changes in one ecological system in schools can and will affect other systems in the same schools.

As you have seen, there are forces external to the program that directly influence teachers' work at the class level, and the place of physical education in the overall school curriculum. The ecological framework offers a set of lenses through which you can better understand how these forces operate, and what you might do to manage them effectively.

Challenges and Opportunities Facing School Physical Education

Concurrent to the educational reform initiatives taking place internationally, a number of challenges and opportunities are facing physical education. Over the past two decades there has been concern over the perceived decline in the status and inclusion of physical education in schools worldwide (e.g., Hardman, 2008). Concerns range from countries where physical education is not a part of the school curriculum to those where it is not part of the accountability system and thus perceived as less important than the core subjects (Center on Education Policy, 2008). Concerns have been voiced about the lack of qualified teachers, insufficient facilities and equipment, inadequate time allocation for delivering the subject, neglect of inclusion and disability programs, large class sizes, limited curricular focus, an unequal focus on and support for gender, decreasing levels of fitness among the young impacting health risks related to inactivity, and an increase in young people choosing to drop out of sport and physical activity opportunities (e.g., Siedentop & van der Mars, 2012).

On the positive side, numerous initiatives have taken place in support of physical education and its place in international education. In 1999, the Berlin World Summit for Physical Education highlighted physical education as a core subject in a school's curriculum, encouraged promotion of the academic study and the practice of physical education as an important discipline in its own right, and heralded the impact of physical education on physical activity behaviors across the lifespan. In Brussels, the declaration of the Berlin summit in 2011 was revisited and several key points added. The 2011 summit highlighted physical education's contributions to the motor, cognitive, and social development of children, reinforcing the idea that it provides the base for lifelong physical activity. The summit encouraged cooperation among schools, sport clubs, and the local community, with coordination of this effort resting with the physical educator. The summit proposed that only qualified physical educators who possess the theoretical, personal, and practical skills and knowledge required of a good professional should be hired. To reinforce this point, it advised development of a European profile of a professional physical educator to enhance the quality and effectiveness of how physical education is taught in schools.

The European Union declared 2004 as the European Year of Education Through Sport, which resulted in numerous awareness initiatives and opportunities for cooperation among various structures and organizations linked to sport and physical activity. The Toronto Charter for Physical Activity (Global Advocacy Council, 2010) is an international call for action to organizations and individuals interested in promoting healthy lifestyles through physical activity. It was developed in response to the decline in opportunities for physical activity in combination with the growth of sedentary lifestyles in many countries. The charter is intended as an advocacy tool to counteract the negative outcomes of decreased physical activity and to aid in creating authentic and sustainable opportunities for developing physically active lifestyles. It outlines four key actions to increase the social and political commitment of all communities to engage in healthy physically active lifestyles: (1) implement a national policy and action plan, (2) introduce policies that support physical activity, (3) reorient services and funding to prioritize physical activity, and (4) develop partnerships for action.

Challenges Facing Teachers

Teachers are effective when students achieve important learning outcomes in a way that enhances their development as productive citizens and members of society. Nothing is more important to the improvement of schools than an effective, high-quality teaching force. In addition, of all the factors that influence how children learn and grow in schools, the quality of their teachers is most important. What teachers know and can do affects all the experiences students have in schools. Internationally, we have seen convincing evidence to support these assertions (Organisation for Economic Co-Operation and Development [OECD], 2011). This has underscored the importance of ensuring that all children and youth have the opportunity to learn from competent, caring, and qualified teachers. The other side of these assertions suggests that weak teaching is a pervasive problem in schools. This would include teachers without proper certification and licensure, those who are teaching in areas where they have inadequate subject-matter preparation, those who teach content rather than learners, and those who have the certification, caring, and subject-matter preparation but are not working hard and effectively for the betterment of their students. The latter is an approach to teaching that Kretchmar (2006) described as teachers employing "easy street" techniques. Thus, teachers are either part of the cure or part of the problem.

Physical Education and Public Health

From a state, province, national, and international perspective, there is one overarching contribution that physical education can make to the welfare of its populace—the development of citizens who voluntarily seek to sustain healthy, physically active lifestyles. Persons who are physically active and lead reasonably healthy lives not only gain personal benefits but also contribute to important national public goals. Globally, the promotion of physically active, healthy lifestyles has become a major public-health goal because of the enormous costs associated with health care and the increase in health factors associated with inactivity. In recent years, several important public policy documents have appeared that, taken together, have moved the importance of physical activity directly onto the center stage of international concerns: the World Health Organization's 2010 *Global Recommendations on Physical Activity for Health*, the U.S. Department of Health and Human Services' 2008 *Physical Activity Guidelines for Americans* and 2011 *Healthy People 2020 Summary of Objective—Physical Activity*, and the Department of Health and Children's 2009 *Get Ireland Active: The National Guidelines on Physical Activity in Ireland*.

This focus on physically active lifestyles has placed the spotlight squarely on school physical education programs and what they do or do not accomplish. In the United States, the general public has voiced strong support for increasing (1) physical activity opportunities throughout the school day and (2) weekly time allocated for physical education (e.g., Harvard School of Public Health, 2003; NASPE, 2003). Moreover, school physical education programs are a documented, evidence-based approach for increasing the physical activity levels of school-age youth (Centers for Disease Control and Prevention [CDC], 2001).

Similarly in England and Wales, the PE and Sport Strategy for Young People is an attempt to extend the legacy of the 2012 Olympics into the future by designing a world-renowned system for physical education and sport. This strategy aims to provide all young people in England and Wales with 5 hours of quality physical education and sport per week. The central government has acknowledged the contribution of physical education to many aspects of young people's lives, from building self-confidence to improving education outcomes. With this in mind, physical education will deliver at least 2 of the required 5 weekly hours of physical activity.

Is increasing physical activity levels of young people the only goal for physical education? Internationally, we have seen several responses to this question. In the United States, the NASPE outcomes clearly indicate that for children and youth to become physically educated, they must achieve a broad range of goals, including outcomes related to knowledge, participation skills, and valuing. This will not happen without effective teachers. However, as we will show, setting such content outcomes is only one of the three key components of the overall effort to improve the physical education profession. Employing quality assessments and the presence of public policy with strong accountability are the other two key components.

Siedentop and van der Mars (2012) discussed the National Healthy Schools Summit (Action for Healthy Kids, 2002) held in Washington, D.C. They described the summit as attempting to improve children's health and school performance through nutrition and physical activity programs. The summit concluded that responsibility for the healthy lifestyles of young people rests with families, teachers, schools, and the community through well-developed and implemented programs. Like the Irish Active School Flag (see www.activeschoolflag.ie), collaborative efforts that focus on and promote physical activity for young people are essential if we are to achieve healthy and active lives for our youth. The Active School Flag (Mayo Education Centre, n.d.), launched by the Department of Education and Skills in 2009, encourages a partnership approach to planning and implementing changes to enhance physical education and extracurricular programs while promoting physical activity. This initiative encourages schools to achieve a physically active and physically educated school community and empowers them to proactively consult and work with other groups such as national governing bodies, local sport partnerships, the Health Service Executive, regional education centers, and the Professional Development Service for Teachers (PDST).

Learning Experience 3.6

What types of partnerships between schools and the community might be developed to improve the health of young people within your geographic area? What role might physical education teachers play in setting up this partnership?

From the perspective of how school physical education programs might contribute to students' health, Cawley, Meyerhoefer, and Newhouse (2007) demonstrated that policies passed by governments alone might have limited impact. They reported that even when policy makers (national or local) pass mandates for increasing weekly minutes of physical education, it does not guarantee that students will (1) be appreciably more active in class and (2) lose weight or reduce the risk of becoming obese. Cawley et al. (2007) found that in high schools where an extra year of physical education was added to existing requirements (about 200 extra minutes per week), boys and girls increased their amount of in-class physical activity by only 7 and 8 minutes per class, respectively (or about 31 minutes per week). What this also shows is that increased time for physical education alone does not automatically translate into proportional increases in physical activity levels. What teachers do within that available time in terms of their instructional practices is the critical variable. Especially given today's focus on increasing physical activity levels of students during school hours, such findings point to the need for employing curriculum and instructional strategies that motivate students and make "time in physical education" meaningful.

Learning Experience 3.7

To what extent do you agree or disagree with the following statements?

- School physical education should play a central role in contributing to the broader efforts of improving the public health of the nation in which you live.
- School physical education programs should be held accountable for ensuring that all students in school meet the recommended amount of moderate to vigorous physical activity during physical education class.

Be sure you can defend your positions.

Alternative Providers of Physical Education Beyond Schools

Alternative forms of physical education are surfacing internationally. Some schools have designed digital academies that allow young people to take physical education at home using the Nintendo Wii Fit. Designers of these school programs suggest that they allow youth to combine their love of video games with activity, and they are guided by assignments either submitted to the teacher or discussed online. One community offers a swimming program that allows the learner to progress from basic swimming skills, gain their water safety instructor status, and obtain lifeguard certification. This program, designed as an option for physical education, is enhanced by provision of cardiopulmonary resuscitation (CPR) and first aid training. In areas such as those in Africa, where declining numbers of children are attending schools, organized sport activities in urban neighborhoods and rural villages are designed to replace physical education, principally for young people who are not part of the education system. Although not all would agree, these alternative physical education programs are designed to reflect the needs of children and youth in the communities in which they operate.

Inappropriate forms of alternative physical education also exist, and we must strive to replace them. One school district in the United States has exchanged all of its primary physical education teachers with employees from the local YMCA, with no stipulation given to the curriculum they would like delivered to children. In another area there is a move away from innovative and broad coverage of physical activity content in primary physical education, to be replaced with a fitness program led by fitness leaders. The intent is that this new program would emphasize cardiovascular exercise, speed walking, and running, with body mass index (BMI) assessment carried out during the currently administered vision and hearing tests.

A continuing problem in several western countries is the use of exemptions or substitutions for physical education in secondary programs. We see young people being exempt from physical education for being part of an after-school sports team, for military training, or even as a member of a marching band. According to Lee, Burgeson, Fulton, and Spain (2007), more than 20% of U.S. high schools that required physical education allowed exemptions for other school-based activities.

If and when alternative programs are designed because students choose not to take part in the offered physical education, teachers need to examine their programs, their offerings, and their teaching strategies to determine what they are doing, or not doing, to motivate young people to take part. As educated professionals, we need to ask ourselves how we can work with young people in designing worthwhile and meaningful physical education programs that (1) will teach them a broad range of skills and (2) provide them with opportunities that will motivate them to lead physically active lifestyles. If teachers are to achieve this, they must talk to young people, and gain their voice and perspectives on what is most inviting and challenging for them in terms of physical activity, how it is delivered, and types of options available to them. If we are not able to interest young people in physical education in school, then developing options or alternatives outside of school, such as those described that reflect the goal of promoting a physically active lifestyle, might be the only option.

Learning Experience 3.8

As a physical education teacher, outline steps you might take to motivate young people to take part in your program. Discuss why you chose each step and what it means to you and to young people.

Narrowing of the School Curriculum

The increased focus on student knowledge and skills of core subjects, and the emphasis on numeracy and literacy, has had serious consequences for the school curriculum and education of students, from narrowing of the curriculum to timetabling of physical education. Narrowing of the school curriculum is exacerbated by teaching toward predetermined content/outcomes with a focus on an exam rather than the larger scope of the curriculum. In other words, might a high stakes exam at the end of a young person's physical education force them to focus on one or two content areas to an excellent level while neglecting the wider exposure they may now be experiencing? Although the exam may increase the status of physical education in the public's mind, it may reduce students' knowledge of how to develop and maintain a healthy lifestyle and limit opportunities to find physical activities in which they may choose to participate as adults.

A second result of this focus on core subjects, and declining budgets, can be seen as principals in many parts of the world opt to downgrade the status of physical education. Along with a lower status comes neglect of its offerings on the school timetable, with physical education being seriously reduced, eliminated, or in some cases the most frequent subject to be cancelled for other "more academic" elements of the curriculum. What many administrators overlook is the ever-growing evidence reporting the relationship between physical activity (including physical education) and academic achievement (e.g., Active Living Research, 2009; CDC, 2010; Trost & van der Mars, 2009; van der Mars, 2006). The Active Living Research Center (2007) research brief notes that, "the available evidence shows that children who are physically active and fit tend to perform better in the classroom, and that daily physical education does not adversely affect academic performance." The reports highlight that young people who are more active tend to perform better academically. Schools can provide positive and effective physical education, improve the health of youth, and still maintain strong academic success. This, in itself, should warrant reconsideration of curricular choices at all levels.

Learning Experience 3.9

Discuss your views on the following question: Do we want the knowledge that young people take from our programs to be only that which is measureable and part of an exit exam?

CHAPTER SUMMARY

In this chapter we discussed educational reform from an international perspective, providing examples to demonstrate current educational movements related to standards, assessment, and accountability. We provided international policy perspectives on how to increase the proportion of young people leading healthier lives in general and being more physically active. We introduced the notion of an ecological system and how such a system impacts both policy development and its implementation.

1. Education systems internationally are more similar than dissimilar. They share similar problems and challenges and are choosing comparable solutions and educational reform agendas to address these issues.
2. A new view of accountability places student learning and performance at the pinnacle of public education.
3. Sahlberg (2010) identified five characteristics of educational policy and reform that have been employed

worldwide in an effort to improve the quality of education: standardization through outcomes-based reforms, increased focus on basic student knowledge and skills in core subjects with an emphasis on literacy and numeracy, teaching for predetermined results, involvement of the business world in designing and implementing educational reform efforts, and high-stakes accountability systems.

4. Numerous concerns about the status of physical education internationally have been voiced (e.g., a lack of qualified teachers, insufficient facilities and equipment, inadequate time allocation for delivering the subject, neglect of inclusion and disability programs).
5. Numerous initiatives have taken place in support of physical education and its place in international education.
6. Evidence suggests that nothing is more important to the improvement of schools than an effective, high-quality teaching force; however, we also know that teachers are both part of the problem and part of the cure.
7. The physical education ecology is affected by other systems, such as the policy decisions made at the school, state/regional, and/or national governance level. The impact of policies at the different levels depends on the degree to which there is oversight and accountability.
8. Strong policies (i.e., those that come with funding, are explicit, have reporting requirements, and have consequences for lack of adherence) are more likely to impact teaching practices at the local level, whereas weak policies are unlikely to do so.
9. Promotion of physically active and healthy lifestyles has become a major public-health goal in recent years, with several important public policy documents highlighting the significance of physical education as a way to increase physical activity levels internationally.
10. Appropriate and inappropriate forms of physical education outside of schools have been designed to replace or extend what is delivered in the name of physical education in a school context.

REFERENCES

Action for Healthy Kids. (2002). National healthy schools summit. Available from www.actionforhealthykids.org

Active Living Research. (2007). Home page. Available from www.activelivingresearch.org

Active Living Research. (2009). *Active education: Physical education, physical activity and academic performance—Research brief.* San Diego, CA: Author.

Cawley, J., Meyerhoefer, C., & Newhouse, D. (2007). The impact of state physical education requirements on youth physical activity and overweight. *Health Economics, 16*, 1287–1301.

Center on Education Policy. (2008). *Instructional time in elementary schools: A closer look at changes for specific subjects.* Washington, DC: Author.

Centers for Disease Control and Prevention. (2001). Increasing physical activity: A report on recommendations of the Task Force on Community Preventive Services. *Morbidity and Mortality Weekly Report, 50*(RR-18), 1–14.

Centers for Disease Control and Prevention. (2010). *The association between school based physical activity, including physical education, and academic performance.* Atlanta, GA: U.S. Department of Health and Human Services.

Department of Health and Children & Health Service Executive. (2009). Get Ireland active: The national guidelines on physical activity in Ireland. Available from www.getirelandactive.ie/content/wp-content/uploads/2011/12/Get-Ireland-Active-Guidelines-GIA.pdf

Education Scotland. (n.d.). Home page. Available from www.educationscotland.gov.uk

Fuhrman, S. (1999). The new accountability. *Consortium for Policy Research in Education, Policy Briefs, RB-27.*

Gleeson, J., & O'Donnabhain, D. (2011). Strategic planning and accountability in Irish education. *Irish Educational Studies, 28*(1), 27–46.

Global Advocacy for Physical Activity, International Society for Physical Activity and Health. (2010). The Toronto charter for physical activity: A global call to action. Available from www.globalpa.org.uk/charter

Hardman, K. (2008). The situation of physical education in schools: A European perspective. *Human Movement, 9*, 5–18.

Hargreaves, A., & Fullan, M. (2012). *Professional capital: Transforming teaching in every school.* New York: Teachers College Press.

Hargreaves, A., & Shirley, D. (2009). *The fourth way: A new vision for education reform.* Thousand Oaks, CA: Corwin Press.

Harvard School of Public Health. (2003). *Obesity as a public health issue: A look at solutions.* Boston, MA: Author.

Kretchmar, R. S. (2006). Life on easy street: The persistent need for embodied hopes and down-to-earth games. *Quest, 58*, 345–354.

Lee, S., Burgeson, C., Fulton, J., & Spain, C. (2007). Physical education and physical activity: Results from the School Health Policies and Programs Study 2006. *Journal of School Health, 77*, 435–463.

MacPhail, A., Patton, K., Parker, M., & Tannehill, D. (2013). Encouraging physical education teacher educators to lead by example: Involvement in communities of practice. *Quest.*

MacPhail, A., & Tannehill, D. (2012). Helping pre-service and beginning teachers examine and reframe assumptions about themselves as teachers and change agents: "Who is going to listen to you anyway?" *Quest, 64*, 299–312.

Mayo Education Center. (n.d.) Active School Flag. Available from www.activeschoolflag.ie

McCullick, B. A., Baker, T. A., Tomporowski, P. D., Isaac, T., Templin, T., & Lux, K. (2012). An analysis of state physical education policies. *Journal of Teaching in Physical Education, 31*, 200–210.

Miller, D. (2009). *The book whisperer: Awakening the inner reader in every child.* San Francisco, CA: Jossey-Bass.

National Association for Sport and Physical Education. (2003). *Position statement: Physical education is critical for educating the whole child.* Reston, VA: Author.

National Association for Sport and Physical Education. (2004). *Moving into the future: National standards for physical education* (2nd ed.). Reston, VA: Author.

National Association for Sport and Physical Education. (2010). *PE metrics: Assessing national standards 1–6 in elementary school.* Reston, VA: Author.

National Association for Sport and Physical Education & American Heart Association. (2010). *2010 shape of the nation report: Status of physical education in the USA*. Reston, VA: National Association for Sport and Physical Education.

National Council for Curriculum and Assessment. (2003). *Junior cycle: Physical education.* Dublin, Ireland: Author.

National Council on Teacher Quality. (2011). *State of the states: Trends and early lessons on teacher evaluation and effectiveness policies*. Washington, DC: Author.

National Physical Activity Plan Alliance. (2010). Make the move: National physical activity plan. Available from www.physicalactivityplan.org

No Child Left Behind (NCLB) Act of 2001, 20 U.S.C.A. § 6301 *et seq.*

Organisation for Economic Co-operation and Development (OECD). (2011). *Building a high-quality teaching profession: Lessons from around the world.* Background Report for the International Summit on the Teaching Profession. Available from www.oecd.org/publishing

O'Sullivan, M. (2003). Learning to teach physical education. In S. J. Silverman & C. D. Ennis (Eds.), *Student learning in physical education: Applying research to enhance instruction* (2nd ed., pp. 275–294). Champaign, IL: Human Kinetics.

Rink, J., & Mitchell, M. (Eds.). (2003, Oct.). State level assessment in physical education: The South Carolina experience [monograph]. *Journal of Teaching in Physical Education, 22*(5).

Sahlberg, P. (2010, Dec. 2). Global educational reform movement and national educational change. Paper presented at the 2010 EUNEC Conference in Brussels, Belgium.

Siedentop, D. (2009). National plan for physical activity: Education sector. *Journal of Physical Activity and Health, 6*(Suppl. 2), S168–S180.

Siedentop, D., & van der Mars H. (2012). *Introduction to physical education, fitness, and sport* (8th ed.). St. Louis, MO: McGraw-Hill.

Tinning, R. (2008). Pedagogy, sport pedagogy, and the field of kinesiology. *Quest, 60*, 405–424.

Trost, S., & van der Mars, H. (2009). Why we should not cut PE. *Educational Leadership, 67*(4), 60–65.

U.S. Department of Health and Human Services. (2008). *2008 physical activity guidelines for Americans.* Washington, DC: Author. Available from www.health.gov/paguidelines/pdf/paguide.pdf

U.S. Department of Health and Human Services. (2011). *Healthy people 2020 summary of objectives—physical activity.* Washington, DC: Author.

van der Mars, H. (2006). Time and learning in physical education. In D. Kirk, M. M. O'Sullivan, & D. McDonald (Eds.), *The handbook of physical education* (pp. 191–213). Thousand Oaks, CA: Sage.

World Health Organization. (2010). *Global recommendations on physical activity for health.* Geneva, Switzerland: Author.

Youth Sport Trust. (2009). Physical education and sport strategy for young people: A guide to delivering the 5-hour offer. Available from www.ssp-websolutions.co.uk/PESSYP_small.pdf

CHAPTER 4 The Ecology of Teaching Physical Education

Overall Chapter Outcome

Be able to articulate the interrelationships among the three task systems in physical education lessons from the ecological perspective

Learning Outcomes

The learner will:

- Recognize teaching as work and the dual directional influence between teachers and their students
- Articulate the differences among managerial, instructional, and student-social task systems at the individual class level
- Explain the differences among stated, actual, and contingency-developed tasks, and how they are negotiated between teachers and students
- Recognize how accountability, ambiguity, clarity, and risk affect task accomplishments
- Explain how and why supervision and accountability drive task systems
- Be familiar with the results of research in physical education settings on the ecology of teaching in physical education

The ecological framework shows how outside forces affect physical education programs. The same framework also can be used to help understand how all tasks get accomplished at the lesson and program levels. We are most interested in having you develop the essential teaching skills and learn to use them in a way that enables you to more effectively navigate the ever-changing demands and dynamics in your classes. Such skills cannot be applied mechanically, without reference to the particular context of how a group of students (a class) and a particular activity (the subject matter) interact with other factors such as weather, equipment, time of day, how the class session fits in a unit, and where you are in a school year.

Some Common Misconceptions

Two factors are critical to understanding life in the **classroom ecology**. Laypersons, especially those who criticize teachers, most often lack understanding of these factors. First is the understanding that subject-matter work in school classes occurs in groups over long periods of time (Doyle, 1983; Hastie & Siedentop, 2006). To really understand teaching, one has to understand it as work. To be sure, there are clear performance aspects to teaching, and its essential skills and strategies need to be practiced and perfected. Very similar to elite-level performance in sport, music, dance, and drama, it requires deliberate and focused practice day in and day out. However, teaching is first and foremost work. Teachers meet many classes each day, every day of the week, for an entire school year. When one has to teach every class, every day, each week, all year, it becomes work. Unlike professional basketball players who typically get time off between games for rest and relaxation, as a teacher you do not have the luxury of taking time off between classes. In addition, teachers and students have to live together peacefully for all those classes throughout the entire school year. When overlaid onto the

BOX 4.1 Key Terms in This Chapter

- *Accountability:* The practices teachers use to establish and maintain student responsibility for appropriate conduct, task involvement, and outcomes. This comes in different forms, including written or performance tests that students complete for grades, teacher feedback, praise and reprimands, their active supervision, challenges and competitions, public recognition of performance, and keeping records of performance.
- *Active supervision:* The practices teachers use to establish and maintain student responsibility for appropriate conduct, task engagement, and learning outcomes.
- *Classroom ecology:* The study of the behavior of teachers and students within the various systems in their class environment.
- *Competent bystander:* Students who appear to be actively engaged in the instructional tasks but actually avoid most real involvement.
- *Ecology:* An interrelated set of systems in which changes in one system affect the other systems.
- *Instructional task system:* Composed of all the learning tasks that teachers ask students to engage in, such as taking part in skill practice drills, playing in games, doing structured fitness activities, or participating in team building; these activities are designed for more social or affective outcomes coupled with the associated accountability mechanism(s) employed by the teachers.
- *Managerial task system:* Composed of all the different managerial tasks that frequently occur, such as entering the gym, taking roll, transitioning, organizing for instruction, student (re-)grouping, dispersing equipment, staying on task, following the class rules for behavior, and so on, coupled with the associated accountability mechanism(s) employed by the teachers.
- *Members in good standing:* Students who attend class, are on time, wear the appropriate uniform, behave well, and earn a high grade in the class as a consequence.
- *Negotiation between task systems:* Efforts between teachers and students where the demands within one task system are reduced (e.g., the instructional task system) in exchange for student cooperation within another (e.g., student social task system). For example, teachers may allow for certain kinds of student social interaction to gain the necessary cooperation in performing substantive learning tasks.
- *Negotiation within task systems:* Any attempts by students to change the assigned subject matter learning task, to change the conditions under which tasks are performed, or to seek changes in the performance standards by which task completion is judged by making them easier or more challenging.
- *Pseudo-accountability:* Students who are members in good standing and put forth effort to engage in the assigned instructional tasks. The associated level of accountability is directed at effort or participation. Such students get high marks, regardless of the quality of performance.
- *Student-social task system:* All social interactions that students seek with peers during the lesson coupled with the associated accountability mechanism(s) employed by the teachers. (Examples include having fun with a friend during the practice/completion of the learning task and going completely off task with fellow students to engage in some behavior that is social in nature but viewed as disruptive by the teacher.)
- *Supervision:* A central teaching function performed by the teacher throughout the class period. It refers to the practices teachers use to establish and maintain student responsibility for appropriate conduct, task involvement, and learning outcomes.
- *Task:* A set of operations/actions used to achieve a specific goal.
- *Task boundaries:* Refers to how tightly or loosely the teacher applies accountability to task completion and how clear and unambiguous the requirements are for task compliance and completion.
- *Task clarity and ambiguity:* Two interrelated concepts that refer to the degree of explicitness and consistency in how teachers define tasks and the expected performance. A fully explicit task defines (1) the conditions students are to perform under, (2) the performance expected, (3) some standard by which to judge the performance, and (4) the consequences for performance.
- *Task modification:* Any effort by students to change the assigned managerial or subject matter learning task to make it easier if it is too difficult, or more challenging if it appears too easy.
- *Task risk:* The interaction among the ambiguity of the task, its difficulty, and the degree of accountability applied to it. Ambiguous tasks produce increased risk for students until they determine that the tasks are either not difficult or carry little, if any, accountability with them. In contrast, a difficult task with strong accountability results in a high degree of risk for the student.

physical education classroom, the ecological model will help you understand the dynamics of that work setting.

The second most common mistake that most people make when they discuss teaching is to assume that the direction of influence in classes is solely from teacher to student. We understand and accept that teachers are meant to influence students, both in learning gains and in social growth. However, what we have learned is that in the dynamics of class life over time, students exert a strong influence on their teachers as well, and sometimes the influence of students is stronger than that of the teacher. At the individual class level, the ecological model will help you understand the dynamic dual-directional influences between you as the teacher and your students.

The classroom ecological framework, as described in this chapter, was developed from research on real teachers in real classrooms. Originally described by Doyle (1979) and first applied to physical education by Tousignant and Siedentop (1983), it has greatly improved our understanding of the ecology of school physical education. A series of research studies completed at Ohio State University served as the initial foundation for this perspective (e.g., Alexander, 1982; Jones, 1989; Kutame, 1997; Lund, 1992; Marks, 1988; Romar, 1995; Siedentop et al., 1994; Son, 1989; Tinning & Siedentop, 1985).

Since then, additional studies have demonstrated how the ecological perspective can explain student involvement within the dynamics of the various task systems in such contexts as high school sport settings (Griffin, Siedentop, & Tannehill, 1998; Hastie, 1993; Hastie & Saunders, 1992), Sport Education classes (Hastie, 1996, 1998, 2000; Sinelnikov & Hastie, 2008), an outdoor adventure camp (Hastie, 1995), dance classes (Hastie & Pickwell, 1996), free gym times (e.g., lunch times) (Pope & O'Sullivan, 2003), and physical education teacher education programs (Ocansey, 1989).

In this chapter we will show how the same accountability mechanisms in place at the district and government levels also largely determine how much is accomplished by teachers and students in individual lessons.

The Ecology of Task Systems at the Class Level

At the individual class level, teaching/learning in physical education can be viewed as an **ecology** with three primary systems, each of which is developed around a series of tasks to be accomplished. A **task** is defined by a goal and a set of operations to achieve it. Tasks are communicated through "a set of implicit or explicit instructions about what a person is expected to do to cope successfully with a situation" (Doyle, 1981, p. 3). A task system is a regularized pattern for accomplishing tasks. It is composed mostly of the tasks that tend to recur frequently within physical education.

First, there is a **managerial task system**, composed of the many different managerial tasks that recur frequently, such as entering the gym, taking roll, transitioning, organizing for instruction, regrouping, getting equipment out and away, staying on task, obeying rules for behavior, and class closure. A managerial task relates to the organizational and behavioral aspects of physical education—all the non-subject-matter functions necessary for students and teachers to exist together over a period of time. For example, a single managerial task occurs when a teacher says, "When I say 'Go,' find one partner, grab a jump rope, and quickly start practicing a partner jump."

Second is the **instructional task system**, which is composed of all the learning tasks that teachers ask students to engage in, such as taking part in skill practice drills, playing in games, doing structured fitness activities, or team building activities designed for more social or affective outcomes. An instructional task is subject-matter-specific physical education activity intended to foster learning among students through active engagement. For example, a single instructional task occurs when a teacher says, "Work in pairs, 6 feet apart, and keep the volleyball in play by forearm passing to one another."

Third is the **student-social task system**, which is much more difficult than the others to define, because it is less predictable and less easily observed. It is composed of all the individual and group social intentions of the students in a class. In any class of 28 students, there might be a number of different social tasks being pursued by different individuals and groups. The student-social task system is different in that it is typically arranged and directed by students rather than the teacher. Nonetheless, it is clear that students have a social agenda when they come to physical education, and that agenda can be interpreted as a task system. Examples of student-social tasks range from having fun with a friend during the appropriate completion of the instructional volleyball task just described to going completely off task with fellow students to engage in some behavior that is social in nature but viewed as disruptive by the teacher. Contrary to the managerial and instructional tasks, student-social tasks are not announced publicly and then pursued. These tasks are often communicated among students in clever, subtle, and often surreptitious ways. Consequently, the student-social task system can run counter to the other task systems in ways that produce problems for teachers. This is reflected in the numerous ways in which teachers have to spend more time on managing disruptive student behavior.

Learning Experience 4.1

Observe a lesson and carefully listen to each of the teacher's instructional task directions. Include both managerial and instructional task directions. What is your interpretation of what the teacher expects? What, if anything, was not clear? Does your interpretation mirror what you see the students do when following the directions? Were students able to complete the task as stated? Why or why not?

Effective teachers find ways to blend the student-social system into the instructional system. This is typically accomplished through an exciting curriculum that offers students activities they perceive as meaningful and worthwhile. For example, in Sport Education, small groups of students with varying skill levels interact and work together toward a common goal: a season championship.

One group of students may find ways to socialize within the boundaries of the instructional task system. Another group, however, may find their fun in disrupting the instructional task system. This tends to make the student-social task system more variable than either the managerial or instructional task system, and thus more difficult to analyze. However, make no mistake, the student-social task system does operate and does affect what happens in the other two systems.

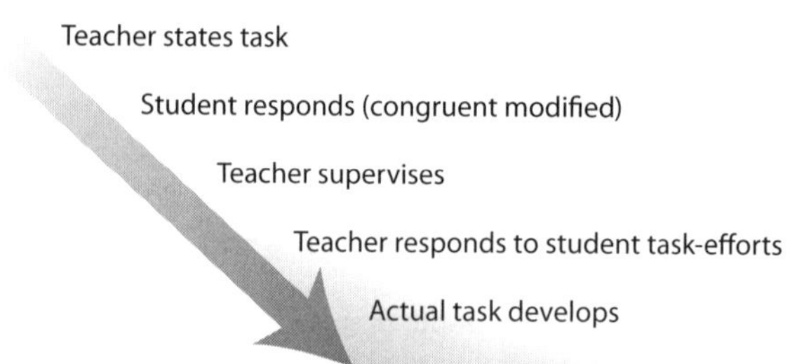

FIGURE 4.1 A contingency-developed task.
Adapted from Alexander, K. (1982). Behavior analysis of tasks and accountability [unpublished doctoral dissertation]. Ohio State University, Columbus, OH.

Learning Experience 4.2

Beyond arriving to class on time and being dressed appropriately, what are 10 managerial tasks that physical education teachers assign to students in a typical class? How do students learn about the "real" expectations that the teacher has regarding these tasks?

How Tasks Develop in Physical Education Lessons

To understand the ecology of physical education at the lesson level, you must be able to see how tasks develop—how the actual task systems develop over time and interact with one another. Managerial and instructional tasks begin as stated tasks that the teacher usually describes verbally. However, the actual managerial and instructional tasks that students develop (i.e., what students actually do when engaging in the activity) over time are primarily a result of how teachers respond to students' performance in executing these tasks, rather than how the tasks were described originally. An "actual" managerial or instructional task tends to develop through the following sequence. The teacher states a task. Students respond to that task. Their responses may or may not be congruent with how the teacher described the task; that is, they may do the task as stated or modify it in some way. As students engage in the learning task, the teacher supervises them, and, on occasion, responds to their task efforts through prompts, corrections, feedback, additional instructions, and so on. It is this cycle of stated task–student response–teacher supervision–teacher response that eventually defines the actual task—what Alexander (1982) described as the contingency developed task system. This pattern that determines the actual task being practiced is shown graphically in **Figure 4.1**. The key variable in how real tasks develop is the manner in which teachers react to students' task efforts. For example, in a tennis unit, assume that the stated task for students is to practice rallying using only the backhand groundstroke. Students will likely start off doing so, but they may then engage in **task modification** by also using forehands and volleys to keep the rally going. If, when supervising the activities, the teacher allows this modification (i.e., by not redirecting the students back to the original task assigned), he or she essentially accepts the students' task modification, and the real task is one where students have set the agenda.

How teachers react is typically also the key to how student socializing develops in class. Although student-social tasks do not begin with a task statement, the development pattern of student socializing is often determined by how their teacher reacts to student efforts to engage in social interactions. When teachers plan, organize, and define managerial or instructional tasks, and incorporate appropriate student socializing in fun ways through the subject matter, the success of the lessons is less dependent on teacher reactions, and the student-social task system is less likely to disrupt the instructional task system. On the other hand, putting students in lines where they spend much of their time waiting and inactive, such as in games like sideline basketball, relay races, or basketball shooting drills, is a perfect recipe for the student-social task system to flourish and dominate. Thus, you want to be very mindful of how you arrange and organize each lesson's learning activities.

Once you recognize how this cycle of task development functions, a number of questions immediately arise. For example, how clearly do teachers state tasks? How different are the actual tasks from those stated originally? How often and in what ways do students modify tasks? How often and how well do teachers supervise students' initial task engagement? Do teachers respond to modified tasks, and if so, how?

How do students learn what is acceptable and unacceptable in any of the three task systems? Possible answers to these questions form the basis for the next section, in which you will learn about four related concepts that are constantly in play during every class.

Important Concepts in the Ecological Framework

Understanding the interplay among the following four related concepts will help you understand how managerial, learning, and student-social tasks get accomplished: accountability, clarity/ambiguity, risk, and task boundaries.

Accountability

This refers to the practices teachers use to establish and maintain student responsibility for appropriate conduct, task involvement, and outcomes. **Accountability** is the driving force behind the instructional task system (Doyle, 1979, 1980, 1986); that is, without accountability, task systems become very loose and sometimes are even suspended. For example, in physical education, if teachers have no real accountability built into the expectations for students to complete managerial and/or general conduct tasks, then their completion is primarily in the hands of the students. Consider the accountability surrounding the countless managerial and behavioral tasks such as getting started quickly on a learning task, transitioning quickly from the gym to outdoor tennis courts, coming to a quick stop on a freeze signal, being attentive during classwide instructions, and so on. If teachers direct students to "hustle" to the tennis courts, and then essentially allow students to merely stroll over there, the students learn very quickly that there is no real need to actually hustle. In subject matter learning tasks such as learning how to return to the center of the court following each stroke in a badminton game, learning how to keep score, or effectively defending space in soccer, accountability plays an equally important role.

Accountability comes in many different forms. Among them are tests that students perform for grades, teacher feedback, teacher praise and reprimands, active teacher supervision, challenges and competitions, public recognition of performance, and keeping records of performance. Eventually, task systems are defined by what teachers hold students accountable for, in both the managerial and instructional systems. In the student-social system, teacher accountability is also a key variable; however, the accountability is typically only for keeping socializing within boundaries defined by the managerial and instructional systems. When socializing among students begins to threaten the stability of those boundaries, then teachers typically intervene to control and redirect it. Relative to accountability, the mantra is, "You get what you accept."

Clarity and Ambiguity

These two related concepts refer to the degree of explicitness and consistency in defining tasks. **Task clarity and ambiguity** are relevant both in the original description of a task (the stated task) and in how the task eventually develops (the actual task). A fully explicit task defines the conditions students are to perform under, the performance expected, some standard by which to judge the performance, and the consequences for performance (Alexander, 1982). An example of an explicit managerial task would be "I want squad 4 to play squad 1 on court A, and squad 2 to play squad 3 on court B. I want you to be in your six-person game formation to begin the game, with the odd-numbered team serving within 15 seconds after I blow my whistle." A task that is less than fully explicit becomes ambiguous for students because there are gaps in information about what the teacher expects, students may not know exactly what to do, under what conditions to do it, how well it needs to be done, or the consequences of doing it well or poorly. Consider, for example, the following subject matter–related task statement in a tennis lesson: "Find a partner, and start warming up." It leaves students with considerable uncertainty as to the teacher's real expectations, and what would be considered acceptable/appropriate.

Clarity and ambiguity in task statements also affect the cycle through which tasks develop. Here, however, the concepts refer to consistency of the teacher's responses to student task efforts. If a teacher accepts one kind of response on one occasion, but not on another, then the task again becomes ambiguous, and student responses are likely to become more varied.

Risk

Task risk refers to the interaction among the ambiguity of the task, its difficulty, and the degree of accountability applied to it. Ambiguous tasks always produce risk for students until they realize either the tasks are not difficult or they will not really be held accountable for successful completion. Conversely, a difficult task with strong accountability results in a high degree of risk for the student.

Learning Experience 4.3

Consider the following task statement by a teacher during the first lesson of a volleyball unit where setting and forearm passing are introduced: "When I say 'Go,' find a partner and start practicing your setting." How would you restate the task expectation to make it more explicit?

Risk and ambiguity are closely related, especially when accountability is strong. That is, if a task is ambiguous, it becomes risky for the student, who will not know what the performance expectations are for completing the task. Effective teachers find ways to organize their content and present it to students as a series of exciting, unambiguous challenges that are reasonably free of risk.

Task Boundaries

Task boundaries refers to how tightly or loosely accountability is applied to task completion, and how clear and unambiguous the requirements are for task compliance and completion. Task systems can have narrow and consistent boundaries. This typically occurs when tasks are explicit and accountability is strong and consistent. For example, in the management task system, teachers in secondary schools are always very specific about their expectations for students being present, on time, and dressed appropriately as well as the consequences for not meeting these expectations. For students there is no wiggle room.

Task systems also can have loose boundaries, which occurs when tasks are ambiguous and accountability is loose, inconsistent, or both (or worse, nonexistent). Again, however, accountability drives the task systems. Weak or inconsistent accountability tends to eliminate risk and makes ambiguity irrelevant; that is, when students know that they will not be held accountable, then trying to cope with an ambiguous task is less of a problem, because it provides little if any risk. For example, in the instructional task system, higher-skilled students are more likely to modify a task to perhaps challenge themselves, or make the task simply more interesting. If the teacher does not insist on them staying with the assigned task, they learn that the task boundary is quite broad and that there is little, if any, accountability in place.

The student-social system is seldom as well defined as the managerial and instructional task systems, thus making it more ambiguous and often riskier. Still, students often persist in trying to see what the boundaries of the student-social system might be in any given class. Adventure Education and Sport Education curriculum models actually accommodate the student-social system within the pursuit of specific learning goals, engage students in meaningful tasks, require student cooperation in the achievement of those tasks, and create a social system that is imbedded within the context of the activities.

Students Influencing Teachers: Negotiation Within Task Systems

As noted earlier, the direction of influence is not a one-way street from teachers to students. Students will also attempt to influence the teachers' agenda for lessons and units. Students learn about the boundaries of task systems in several ways. Some teachers explain the boundaries carefully and hold students accountable quickly and consistently. These accountability strategies can focus on compliance or cooperation. Other teachers may explain boundaries clearly, but their students learn gradually that the *actual* boundaries are different than those explained; that is, the actual boundaries develop contingently through the process described earlier for task development. Still other teachers simply do not explain boundaries clearly or at all. This leaves students to learn through daily experiences what they have to do to stay within the boundaries and what behaviors are considered to be crossing the boundaries and, thus, unacceptable.

Students also bring their own social agendas (along with their history of previous experiences in physical education) with them when they come to your class. Thus, they must learn what kinds of student-social interactions are allowable and under what conditions. Doyle's (1979) initial findings were that students will attempt to negotiate tasks to fix the "ecological balance" of the task systems at a level they can handle and enjoy. This may happen in overt or sometimes more subtle ways.

Negotiation within task systems can be defined as any attempt by students to change tasks, to change the conditions under which tasks are performed, or to change the performance standards by which task completion is judged. How teachers respond to student attempts to negotiate the demands of task systems tends to be the primary factor in determining the ecological balance among the management, instruction, and student-social task systems within a class.

In classrooms, negotiation tends to be verbal, particularly within the instructional task system, with students asking teachers questions or making requests that tend to reduce the risk and ambiguity associated with an assignment. A teacher assigns an instructional task, and students attempt to reduce its ambiguity and risk by verbally negotiating with the teacher. At some point you may have asked questions such as: "How long does the paper have to be?"; "Can it be on this topic rather than the one you assigned?"; "Can I turn my paper in on Tuesday instead of Monday?"; "How much will this assignment count toward our final grade?"; "Will you take off for spelling errors?"; or "Does it have to be typed?" All of these questions serve to negotiate the demands of this particular task. How teachers respond to such questions and how they later assess the products that are turned in will determine the actual task.

In physical education, students negotiate task demands by modifying the assigned task during practice rather than by asking questions. When a teacher describes an instructional task, the students go about doing the task, but often they modify it so that it is somewhat different than the one the teacher described. Next time you observe a class, listen to the specific directions that a teacher provides and then see what students do once they practice.

Learning Experience 4.4

When observing a class, determine how long it takes for students to modify the assigned task. Did they modify it up (i.e., make it more difficult, challenging, or interesting) or down (i.e., easier, simpler)? What, if anything, was the reaction of the teacher?

Students can modify the task upward to make it more challenging than the task described by the teacher, or they can modify it downward to make it easier to do successfully. When the teacher supervises this practice and responds to the modified tasks, what the teacher accepts defines the actual nature of the task. Over time, students learn how much they can modify an assigned task and still be within the boundaries of the instructional task system. Consider the following scenario: A teacher asks her students to organize in pairs with partners 8 feet apart. The task is to forearm pass the volleyball back and forth between partners so that the ball goes over head height with each pass but not more than 3–4 feet over the head. Some of the students in class are on the school volleyball team. For them, this is an easy task, so they modify it by moving farther apart and passing the ball higher. For others, the task is too difficult, so they move a bit closer together and don't pay much attention to the height of the pass. A few other students use sets instead of forearm passes when the ball comes to them at or above shoulder level. The teacher is now supervising this practice. How she responds to each of these modifications will determine the actual task in this case, and it will also provide students with knowledge about the degree to which they can modify assigned tasks and still stay within the boundaries of the instructional task system (e.g., they will know how much they can change the assigned task without being considered off task).

Another example of negotiation within the instructional task system can be seen during a fitness circuit training activity where students are at each fitness station for 45 seconds. The teacher's assignment for students is to engage continuously in the assigned or chosen task while at each station. Students may make the task easier (i.e., less strenuous) by not starting right away, engaging in the task only intermittently during the 45 seconds, or stopping early. The teacher's level of **active supervision**, along with his or her reactions to such modifications, conveys whether the negotiation will be successful.

Students often negotiate in their social task system by trying to pair up with friends or get certain students together on a team. These negotiations often are hidden as instructional negotiations, but they have a clear social emphasis and purpose.

Students Influencing Teachers: Negotiation Between Task Systems

Negotiations also occur among the three task systems that form the ecology of the lessons, which is known as **negotiation between task systems**. For most teachers, the initial and fundamental goal of teaching a class is to gain and maintain student cooperation (Doyle, 1986; Hastie & Siedentop, 2006). Teachers who set clear expectations and boundaries for acceptable student behavior and frequently reinforce these messages, along with actively supervising students for that purpose, have classes in which students are more likely to cooperate and have higher levels of active engagement (Hastie, 1994; Hastie & Siedentop, 2006; Lund, 1992).

Teachers are responsible for many classes each day. Administrators expect them to have control of their classes. For these reasons alone, it is understandable that a teacher's primary concern should be to establish and maintain an orderly class in which students cooperate with good behavior, rather than constantly disrupting the class. Brophy and Good (1986) and Doyle (1986) showed that effective teachers use the first few weeks of each school year to first establish the boundaries of the managerial system.

The issue here is clear. It is understandable that the managerial task system is established quickly and that students learn how to function effectively within the demands of that system to produce a peaceful class throughout the school year. How do teachers negotiate with students to produce consistent compliance with the demands of the managerial task system? Remember, teachers also have to develop an instructional task system, and students have their own social agendas they want to attend to during class. Clearly, several kinds of negotiations might occur among these three systems that form the ecology of the class.

Within the interplay among the managerial, instructional, and student-social task systems, teachers may reduce the demands within the instructional system in exchange for student cooperation within the managerial system. Teachers may allow for certain kinds of student social interaction to gain the necessary cooperation. In some cases, for some students, teachers might simply suspend the instructional task system and allow those students to engage in nondisruptive socializing rather than instructional tasks, as long as they cooperate with the demands of the managerial task system. Each of these negotiations produces a different overall ecology.

Each of these patterns has been identified in research studies. Contextual factors such as class size and student demographics, along with teachers' expectations for students to learn and their skill in effectively employing instructional techniques, will determine the degree to which teachers need to negotiate with their students to produce the necessary balance among the three task systems.

The way in which the managerial, instructional, and student-social task systems interact and influence one another determines the ecology of the gymnasium. The sensitive, effective teacher will understand how these systems interact and work to develop an ecology that students cooperate and behave well within but also is learning oriented and accommodates student-social needs. To develop and maintain this kind of ecology in a typical class in today's schools is not easy. It requires teachers with strong intentions to build this kind of environment and the managerial and instructional skills to make it happen.

For teachers to develop a learning-focused ecology that is enjoyable for all students requires thorough planning around delivering an imaginative curriculum with authentic outcomes. When students get to engage in meaningful activities that bring enjoyment (and include opportunities for social interactions with classmates), there is no need to develop and sustain a student-social system outside the instructional system.

Supervision and Accountability

As noted previously, accountability drives all task systems. Without accountability, the task system is suspended, and whatever happens is attributable solely to student interests and enthusiasms. This is most true for the instructional task system.

All the evidence suggests that accountability is as powerful a force in the ecology of physical education as it is in other classrooms; however, the ecologies of the classroom and the gymnasium operate differently. The primary accountability mechanism in classrooms is what Doyle (1979) called the "performance-grade exchange system." In order for students to earn a higher grade in classroom subjects, they are required to demonstrate their knowledge by way of performing well on quizzes, homework, projects, presentations, and so forth.

The **supervision** performed by teachers throughout every class period is a central teaching function. Supervision refers to the practices teachers use to establish and maintain student responsibility for appropriate conduct, task involvement, and learning outcomes. Teachers use many different forms of accountability—public recognition, verbal interaction, keeping records, challenges, and performance–grade exchanges. They also must actively supervise students to ensure that these accountability mechanisms work.

The most important aspect of supervision is monitoring students' work for a specific purpose. Monitoring means to "observe, record, or detect . . . to watch closely, keep track of" (Merriam-Webster, n.d.). In physical education, the specific purpose would be for the teacher to see if student performance was congruent with the tasks described and assigned in the managerial and instructional task systems. The classroom is smaller than the gymnasium or playing field, and the placement of students within a classroom makes supervising their work easier, whether they are working in a whole-group format or independently at their seats.

Supervision and accountability in physical education classes have unique challenges. Gymnasia and playing fields are quite large, class sizes often are bigger, and students should be moving about engaging in physical activity. This alone makes deliberate supervision of student performance more difficult.

Negotiations in physical education more often occur through students' modifying tasks than asking questions or making requests, which makes negotiations difficult for the teacher to see and respond to. Thus, the supervision and accountability functions of physical education teachers are considerably more complex and difficult to fulfill than for classroom teachers. And when teachers are required to document student learning, it is directly related as well to teachers' effective and ongoing use of formal assessment.

Supervision and accountability may well be the two most important teaching skills in the repertoire of effective physical educators. Consider the following typical example: Joe is teaching basketball to 14-year-old students. He is focusing on the two-person pick and roll strategy that is fundamental to many different basketball offenses. He has the class together as a whole. He describes and demonstrates the main technical points of the pick and roll with the help of several students. The explanation is clear and to the point. The demonstrations are well set up. Joe has the demonstrators show both the correct technical aspects of the pick and roll and the most common errors. Joe then has the students walk through the strategy so that he can be sure they all understand the critical elements—what we refer to as *guided practice*. He provides feedback and answers student questions. Joe then describes clearly how he wants the pick and roll practiced at the several basket areas in the gym. He uses four students to demonstrate how the practice drill should be done, what to emphasize, and what to avoid. Again, he provides feedback and answers questions. He then disperses the students to the basket areas and signals the beginning of the drill—what we refer to as *independent practice*.

Up to that point, it appears that Joe is conducting a terrific lesson. But here, at the critical point where students will *practice* the pick and roll, the lack of any supervision and accountability by Joe has consequences: As students begin practicing independently, Joe makes some notes on a clipboard. He then stays at one end of the gym and watches one of the groups but makes no comments. He sits down to chat with a student who has been ill and did not bring gym clothes for today's lesson. Eight minutes have passed since he dispersed the students. One of the groups has been playing a two-versus-two game with no effort to practice the pick and roll in the drill described. Another group is performing the drill incorrectly. A third group is practicing the drill appropriately but making critical errors in technique each time they do it. Another group, at the far end of the gym, did the drill for a few minutes but has now started a shooting game.

Learning Experience 4.5

Observe a teacher's class (or review a videotape of a class you taught) during the periods of time where students are "in activity." Determine how much of the time the teacher spends silently observing the activities. To what extent was this of help to students? What might be an alternative teaching strategy that the teacher could use to help students? What might be reasons for why the teacher did not employ these strategies?

What would a casual observer (or even a principal) conclude about this teacher and his class? After all, students all appear physically active, seem to be enjoying themselves, and no one is being disruptive. In reality, the instructional task system in Joe's class has been almost completely suspended. Students apparently understand that they will not be supervised carefully. There is little evidence of accountability for performance. Students are not disruptive, so one might assume that there is accountability in the managerial task system. Some students have modified tasks to have more fun, thus accommodating their social agenda within a modified instructional task rather than going off task. All the students are physically active, so one might assume that Joe holds them accountable if they are not physically involved in some task related to the activity, by way of taking away what is commonly referred to as "participation points."

Looking at the same class from the ecological perspective, how would you describe the ecology of this class? Joe knows basketball. He demonstrated and explained the practice drill well. It appears to be a good drill, appropriate to the skill level of the class. At 8 minutes into the practice phase, however, almost nothing is happening that one would consider being good in terms of the assigned practice task. Only a small percentage of students are actually doing the assigned practice task, and an even smaller percentage of them are doing it successfully. In some parts of the gymnasium, the student-social system appears to have taken over completely, even though it is masked by active involvement in basketball. Joe obviously does not supervise actively. There appears to be no accountability for performance except that which comes with his direct physical presence near a practice group. At this rate, few of the students will learn to be good at the pick and roll maneuver in a drill practice context, let alone in a game context.

Learning Experience 4.6

Explain your thoughts regarding the following position: The only learning outcome for which physical education programs should be held accountable is to have students reach high levels of moderate to vigorous physical activity (MVPA). How would you defend your position?

Issues of supervision and accountability appear to be not only related to the teaching of the content. They also are very much related to how the overall physical education curriculum is designed and delivered. *Content-embedded accountability* can be an important factor leading to a learning-focused ecology. For example, when teams are competing in a round-robin league format over an extended period of time, all working to finish as high in the standings as they can, there is accountability embedded in the content. When small groups are planning a half-day bicycle field trip and then actually taking the trip to reach a destination successfully, there is accountability embedded in the content. When a health-fitness class has established collective goals to achieve by the end of a semester, there are regular weekly progress checks toward those goals, and some rewards and celebrations are planned when and if they are achieved, there is accountability embedded in the content. The more accountability that is naturally embedded in how content is organized and presented and how students are organized to pursue the content goals, the less teachers will need to supervise for cooperation, and the less they themselves will have to be the major accountability mechanism in the system.

The Evidence Surrounding the Ecological Task Systems in Physical Education

The usefulness of the classroom ecological model is that it provides a framework within which teachers can interpret what goes on in their classes and generate solutions to problems that arise. It helps teachers to be able to understand the ongoing events in their classes within a framework that takes into account the two-way influence between them and their students. The major purpose of this chapter has been to explain the ecological framework at the class level through which physical education teachers can interpret the managerial, instructional, and social dimensions of their classes.

What follows is a short summary of results from a series of research projects completed on school physical education in the 1980s and 1990s that utilized the ecological framework

(Hastie & Siedentop 2006). Although what is described is typical of the results of those studies, there is no doubt variation from teacher to teacher, and we do not intend to suggest that these results are typical of all physical education teachers:

- The managerial task system tends to be more explicitly described and more carefully supervised than the instructional task system.
- Teachers apply accountability for compliance in the managerial system more quickly and consistently. Thus, its boundaries are more narrow and consistent than those of the instructional system.
- Actual instructional tasks tend to develop contingently and often differ from stated tasks. Students modify tasks to make them more or less difficult or to make them more fun. How teachers react to these modified tasks sets the boundaries of the instructional task system, which is typically less consistent and broader than the managerial system.
- When teachers do not supervise actively and monitor student task responses, the instructional task system becomes very loose, allowing students to modify the tasks at will and, on occasion, to cease engaging in them completely.
- Instructional tasks are seldom described in fully explicit terms. The conditions tasks are to be practiced under often are not described fully, nor are the criteria for judging their completion. Students learn these aspects of the task, if they learn them at all, through the way the teacher reacts to their responses.
- Rather than paying attention to the teacher's instructional task explanations, students will often ask fellow students about what is expected during the transition from instruction to practice or by watching students begin the practice task. Students learn quickly how much or how little attention they have to pay to the teacher's task descriptions.
- Managerial tasks are typically a set of routines. They become established structures and require less teacher attention, especially in the classes of effective teachers. Students are held accountable for compliance with these routines. Rules are typically made clear and enforced. Teachers who need to interact frequently to keep students well behaved are typically less effective managers because they have failed to establish a routine managerial task system.
- In a well-supervised instructional task system, students will modify tasks to make them either more challenging (modify them up) or easier (modify them down). Teachers tend to set the limits to these modifications through their reactions to student task responses. Some teachers sanction these modifications in the way they initially describe tasks to students.
- In a poorly supervised instructional task system, students modify tasks both for the previous reasons and also to engage in social interactions with their peers.
- Cooperation with the demands of the managerial task system appears to be the most important and most immediate goal of the teacher (just as in classrooms). Teachers in physical education appear to accomplish this goal by trading cooperation within the managerial task system for demands in the instructional system. That is, if students attend class, arrive on time, wear the appropriate uniform, and behave well, they can earn a high grade in the class. Thus, the first goal of the teacher (and sometimes the only goal) is for the student to be what Tousignant and Siedentop (1983) called a **member in good standing** of the class.
- Other teachers may require that students be not only members in good standing but also make a visible effort to engage in the assigned instructional tasks. This level of accountability is directed at effort or participation. Thus, students perceived to be consistently engaged in tasks get high grades, no matter the quality of their performance. This would, in essence, be a form of **pseudo-accountability**.
- Accountability systems that require actual skill or knowledge performance to earn high grades occur less frequently than do the systems described previously.
- Some students find clever ways to hide within the instructional task system. They appear to be actively engaged in the instructional tasks, however, they actually avoid most real involvement. They are referred to as **competent bystanders** (see **Box 4.2**).
- Some students may engage in the instructional system appropriately for a while and then shift their engagement so that it is more social, even though they appear to be on task (see **Box 4.3**).
- Instructional task systems that seem to be highly on task and intended to produce skill outcomes are characterized by consistent accountability measures, although few of these can be characterized as performance–grade exchanges.
- Effective teachers hold students accountable informally through appropriate task challenges (e.g., How long can you keep a rally going using just the forehand?), public performances (e.g., in dance classes), frequent task-related feedback, and frequent prompting for on-task behavior. Elementary physical education teachers also use many informal accountability mechanisms, such as point systems, posters, and challenge systems.
- The accountability becomes formal when teachers record the performances and link them directly with students' grades.
- Most physical education classes appear to be highly social. The differences among them seem to lie in whether the

BOX 4.2 The Competent Bystander

In her analysis of task systems in middle and high school physical education classes, Tousignant (1981) observed student strategies for hiding nonparticipation in the instructional task system but doing so in such a clever way that the teacher did not notice. She called students who used these strategies *competent bystanders*. The competent bystander always behaves well in terms of the managerial task system. This is what teachers would call a well-behaved student. Yet the same student cleverly avoids participation in the instructional task system without the teacher noticing. For example, when organized in lines, competent bystanders are always in line, move from fourth to third to second place but then reinsert themselves so that they avoid being first and having to take a turn, especially in tasks they perceive to carry a high degree of risk. In game play, competent bystanders will attach themselves to better players, knowing that the latter will perform the necessary action when the ball comes to them.

Remember, this is a competent bystander. When asked about such students' involvement, teachers will typically respond that they are fairly well skilled and actively engaged. As long as students remain within the boundaries of the managerial task system, teachers will perceive them as "good." The key is how deliberate teachers are in observing the actual engagement during activities.

Next time you observe a basketball or team handball class, see if you can spot the competent bystanders. They cruise up and down the court but somehow manage to stay away from all the action involving the ball.

BOX 4.3 Hiding Social Engagement Within Instructional Tasks

Son (1989) studied the task-system dynamics in South Korean high school physical education. He found a particularly interesting kind of engagement pattern among some highly skilled students.

A teacher would describe an instructional task. The highly skilled student would very successfully perform the task exactly as described. The student would proceed to do four to six repetitions of the task. Then, however, a curious change would occur. The student would modify the task to make it easier and then engage in it but in an unsuccessful manner. What could explain this task modification and unsuccessful engagement with a highly skilled student?

Clearly, the student knew that he could do the task and, indeed, did it successfully several times. Then it was time to do a little socializing but to do so in a way that was hidden within the instructional task system. This was accomplished by modifying the task to make it easier and then to engage in that task but with little thought to success. Instead, the student's attention was diverted from task success to socializing with a fellow student. If the teacher saw the students, he would see task engagement, albeit on a slightly modified task and without high success. Although the teacher might provide some feedback, it would no doubt be related to the instructional task performance rather than to the socializing. Typically, however, because the students were on task, the teacher would not intervene, and the students would have successfully hidden their pursuit of their own social goals within the instructional task system.

student socialization takes place in ways that disrupt or suspend the instructional task system or whether teachers find ways for students to socialize while still taking part appropriately in the instructional task system. Hastie and Pickwell (1996) showed that boys in a dance unit developed specific strategies to avoid participating in instructional tasks they believed were uninviting or lacked importance, just so they could attend to their social agenda.

- Conversely, some curricular models, such as Sport Education, have strong content-embedded accountability that engages students and results in highly task-oriented behavior that is, at the same time, a strong social system. Teachers who used this model (and others such as Adventure Education) report that they no longer have to act primarily as a traffic director or cop. Instead, it affords them the chance to interact with students about the activities and help them get better at doing them. More importantly, in such models the social system will come to support the instructional and managerial task systems because of the strong focus on team members working together to accomplish common goals.

- Management systems can be developed in which students participate in developing rules, routines, and consequences. For example, teachers can employ the use of a *full value contract* (see www.pa.org). When used effectively, it helps achieve buy-in from students to achieve the goals of the managerial system, and they themselves assist in sustaining the system.

Hastie and Siedentop (2006) noted that the strength of using the ecological framework lies in the fact that:

> *. . . it presents a realistic description of "life in the gym". It highlights that considerable negotiation takes place within many classes, where teachers trade off a reduction in the demands of the instructional system and any rigorous accountability for cooperation in the management system. The student social system is generally allowed to flourish, as teachers are more concerned with creating and maintaining a classroom environment where they and their students can live peacefully throughout the year.*[1]

CHAPTER SUMMARY

In this chapter we showed how the ecological framework can be used to explain how teachers and students accomplish the multitude of managerial and instructional tasks in any given lesson. Moreover, we showed how the students' social agenda influences how well the instructional and managerial tasks are accomplished. Finally, we demonstrated how teachers' supervision and accountability are the two main driving forces behind task accomplishment.

1. Teaching needs to be understood as work in which there is a two-way influence between teachers and students.
2. An ecology is an interrelated set of systems in which changes in one system affect the other systems.
3. The managerial, instructional, and student-oriented systems comprise the ecology of physical education.
4. Tasks in physical education lessons begin as stated tasks, but the tasks students actually perform are typically contingency developed.
5. Accountability refers to practices teachers use to establish and maintain student responsibility for appropriate conduct, task involvement, and outcomes.
6. Clarity, risk, and ambiguity of tasks interact to affect the degree to which students negotiate or avoid task involvement.
7. Task boundaries can be tight or loose, depending on task clarity and accountability.
8. Students in physical education typically negotiate tasks by modifying them and seeing how teachers respond to the modifications.
9. Some teachers trade lowered demands in the instructional system for compliance with the managerial system. The first goal of teachers is to gain and maintain the cooperation of students.
10. Supervision and accountability drive task systems.
11. Research has revealed many features of physical education ecologies, including information about task explicitness, contingency-developed systems, task routinization, patterns of involvement, tactics of noninvolvement, accountability formats, and curricular attractiveness.

REFERENCES

Alexander, K. (1982). Behavior analysis of tasks and accountability [unpublished doctoral dissertation]. Ohio State University, Columbus, OH.

Brophy, J., & Good, T. (1986). Teacher behavior and student achievement. In M. C. Wittrock (Ed.), *Handbook of research on teaching* (3rd ed., pp. 328–375). New York: Macmillan.

Doyle, W. (1979). Classroom tasks and students' abilities. In P. Peterson & H. Walberg (Eds.), *Research on teaching: Concepts, findings, and implications* (pp. 183–209). Berkeley, CA: McCutchan.

Doyle, W. (1980). *Student mediating responses in teaching effectiveness.* Denton, TX: North Texas State University. (ERIC No. ED 187698)

Doyle, W. (1981). Research on classroom contexts. *Journal of Teacher Education, 32*(6), 3–6.

Doyle, W. (1983). Academic work. *Review of Educational Research, 53*, 159–199.

Doyle, W. (1986). Classroom organization and management. In M. C. Wittrock (Ed.), *Handbook of research on teaching* (3rd ed., pp. 392–431). New York: Macmillan.

Griffin, L. L., Siedentop, D., & Tannehill, D. (1998). Instructional ecology of a high school volleyball team. *Journal of Teaching in Physical Education, 17*, 404–420.

Hastie, P. A. (1993). Players' perceptions of accountability in school sports settings. *Research Quarterly for Exercise and Sport, 64*, 158–166.

Hastie, P. A. (1994). The development of monitoring skills in physical education: A case study in student teaching. *Journal of Classroom Interaction, 29*(2), 11–20.

Hastie, P. A. (1995). An ecology of a secondary school outdoor adventure camp. *Journal of Teaching in Physical Education, 15*, 79–97.

[1] Reproduced from Hastie, P., & Siedentop, D. (2006). The classroom ecology paradigm. In D. Kirk, D. Macdonald, & M. O'Sullivan (Eds.), *The handbook of physical education* (p. 223). London: Sage.

Hastie, P. A. (1996). Student role involvement during a unit of sport education. *Journal of Teaching in Physical Education, 16*, 88–103.

Hastie, P. A. (1998). The participation and perceptions of girls during a unit of sport education. *Journal of Teaching in Physical Education, 18*, 157–171.

Hastie, P. A. (2000). An ecological analysis of a sport education season. *Journal of Teaching in Physical Education, 19*, 355–373.

Hastie, P. A., & Pickwell, A. (1996). A description of a student social system in a secondary school dance class. *Journal of Teaching in Physical Education, 15*, 171–187.

Hastie, P., & Saunders, J. E. (1992). A study of task systems and accountability in an elite junior sports setting. *Journal of Teaching in Physical Education, 11*, 376–388.

Hastie, P., & Siedentop, D. (2006). The classroom ecology paradigm. In D. Kirk, D. Macdonald, & M. O'Sullivan (Eds.), *The handbook of physical education* (pp. 214–225). London: Sage.

Jones, D. (1989). Analysis of task structures in elementary physical education classes [unpublished doctoral dissertation]. Ohio State University, Columbus, OH.

Kutame, M. (1997). Teacher knowledge and its relationship to student success in learning a gymnastics skill [doctoral dissertation]. Ohio State University, Columbus, OH. *Dissertation Abstracts International, 58*(1637). (University Microfilms No. 9731661)

Lund, J. (1992). Assessment and accountability in secondary physical education. *QUEST, 44*, 352–360.

Marks, M. (1988). Development of a system for the observation of task structures in physical education [unpublished doctoral dissertation]. Ohio State University, Columbus, OH.

Merriam-Webster Dictionary. (n.d.). Available from www.merriam-webster.com

Ocansey, R. (1989). A systematic approach to organizing data generated during monitoring sessions in student teaching. *Journal of Teaching in Physical Education, 8*, 312–317.

Pope, C. C., & O'Sullivan, M. (2003). Darwinism in the gym. *Journal of Teaching in Physical Education, 22*, 311–327.

Romar, J. E. (1995). *Case studies of Finnish physical education teachers: Espoused and enacted theories of action*. Abo, Finland: Abo Akademic University Press.

Siedentop, D., Doutis, P., Tsangaridou, N., Ward, P., & Rauschenbach, J. (1994). Don't sweat gym: An analysis of curriculum and instruction. *Journal on Teaching in Physical Education, 13*, 375–394.

Sinelnikov, O., & Hastie, P. (2008). Teaching sport education to Russian students: An ecological analysis. *European Physical Education Review, 14*, 203–222.

Son, C-T. (1989). Descriptive analysis of task congruence in Korean middle school physical education classes [unpublished doctoral dissertation]. Ohio State University, Columbus, OH.

Tinning, R., & Siedentop, D. (1985). The characteristics of tasks and accountability in student teaching. *Journal of Teaching in Physical Education, 4*, 286–299.

Tousignant, M., & Siedentop, D. (1983). A qualitative analysis of task structures in required secondary physical education classes. *Journal of Teaching in Physical Education, 3*, 47–57.

CHAPTER 5 The Hidden Dimensions of Teaching Physical Education

Overall Chapter Outcome

Be able to recognize and engage in the various non-instructional roles and responsibilities that physical educators have in their daily work

Learning Outcomes

The learner will:

- Explain how teaching physical education encompasses many non-instructional roles and responsibilities
- Explain the teacher's role in managing and organizing physical education programs, including the teacher's central role in program, unit, and lesson planning, and representing the program when interacting with other constituents such as other classroom teachers, school and regional administrators, and parents
- Understand the responsibility of physical educators to contribute to the smooth functioning of the overall school
- Understand the limits of their position when counseling on personal matters (i.e., those unrelated to the physical education program)
- Understand the role of continuing professional development
- Articulate the role of being a strong advocate and representative for the physical education program and the profession

What teachers do day in and day out is work. And if you try to do it well, then it is hard work. There is no evidence that the general public has a clear and accurate conception of the physical and mental demands placed on schoolteachers to not only manage large and highly diverse groups of students 5 days a week but also then help them learn and get excited about what they learn.

There are two related factors that make the first years of teaching often overwhelming. First is your initial conception of what it is like to be a schoolteacher. Second are the countless responsibilities and roles performed by teachers that are not so readily visible to the general public and pre-service teachers (PSTs) when casually observing teachers in action.

Learning Experience 5.1

Choosing your preferred school level, imagine you are a full-time physical educator. Describe in detail what you believe your typical day at work as a physical educator most likely would look like, with particular reference to the associated roles and responsibilities you will be expected to perform. Be detailed and thorough.

Incoming Conceptions of Teaching Physical Education

By the time pre-service physical educators start in their physical education teacher preparation program, they will have

BOX 5.1 Key Terms in This Chapter

- *Apprenticeship of observation:* A theory developed by Lortie (2002) that posits that among prospective teachers, conceptions of teaching as work begin to emerge during the primary and post-primary years of schooling. These conceptions may well contribute to entrenching traditional teaching practices, while at the same time preventing deliberate and informed changes in practice.
- *Bullying:* Unwanted, aggressive behavior among school-age children that involves a real or perceived power imbalance. The behavior is repeated, or has the potential to be repeated, over time (www.stopbullying.gov). This can include actions such as threats, physical/verbal attacks, spreading rumors, or public embarrassment.
- *Cyber-bullying:* A newer form of bullying using various technologies such as texting, the Internet, and social media.
- *Non-instructional responsibilities:* Required tasks and activities, beyond teaching the scheduled classes, that teachers are expected to complete that contribute to the school's mission.
- *Paraprofessional:* Also referred to as an aide or a para-educator, this is an adult assistant who is not a certified teacher, but who performs many duties in support of a teacher, ranging from helping individual students to assisting with organizational tasks. Commonly assigned to individual students with special needs.

witnessed countless teachers at work for long periods of time. As they contemplate a career in teaching physical education, former primary and post-primary teachers and sport coaches likely were influential in this career decision-making process, and sport coaching continues to be the primary reason for entering the physical education profession (Dodds et al., 1992; McCullick, Lux, Belcher, & Davies, 2012). Together, all interactions, experiences, and observations help shape pre-service physical educators' personal, albeit general, views of what teaching must be like. Moreover, they will have developed personal views of what makes for good and poor teaching (Schempp, 1987). This learning is often referred to as the **apprenticeship of observation** (Lortie, 2002).

There is great value in having seen others at work. It clearly does help in giving pre-service teachers (PSTs) certain ideas about what teachers do on a daily basis. However, the conceptions formed are typically incomplete, and may lack accuracy. As we will show, there is an inherent risk in clinging to such views. The values, beliefs, and conceptions of teaching developed prior to joining a teacher preparation program can become quite entrenched, and they filter both compatible and incompatible ideas about teaching as presented within the physical education teacher education (PETE) program (e.g., Holt-Reynolds, 1992; O'Sullivan, MacPhail, & Tannehill, 2009; Timken & van der Mars, 2009). No matter how strong the empirical support, any suggested approaches to teaching that deviate from those incoming beliefs might be dismissed.

Confronting Personal Beliefs and Assumptions

Surely you would not want to drive a car that lacks the most recent safety measures, or have a surgeon repair your damaged knee using surgical techniques from the 1960s? It is important that as you progress through the teacher preparation program you are open to reflecting on your existing values and beliefs about teaching physical education. Just like in other fields, new approaches are developed, and issues that affect school physical education change over time. In order for physical education to have a positive impact on the development of children and youth, physical educators need to continuously seek out ways to improve the quality of programming for students. Thus, as you learn more about teaching within your teacher preparation program, you will find that some of your current conceptions of teaching and learning are indeed incomplete and/or inaccurate. Beginning teachers who are willing to consider other ideas and new approaches, and adjust their opinions, beliefs, and actual teaching practices, are more likely to develop into successful teachers. Thus, we encourage you to continuously reflect on your perspectives about your work as a physical educator. This will likely work better if you (1) continuously consider the recent developments, trends, and key issues that affect school physical education, and (2) remain open to developing the skills and knowledge that may or may not align with your current beliefs and perspectives on teaching. Today's children and youth deserve to be taught in programs that reflect the best available knowledge regarding quality physical education.

Metaphors about teaching are one way for PSTs to recognize their preexisting beliefs about teaching and learning, and they can assist them in reflecting on and examining these beliefs and how they impact their own teaching practices and the learning of their students. Examining their own PSTs' teaching metaphors, Tannehill and MacPhail (2012) found that in some cases these PSTs' metaphors were problematic, contradictory, and/or portrayed implausible narratives. Many were able to identify the contradictions in their initial metaphor when revisiting it following teaching practice; others

BOX 5.2 A Sample Teaching Metaphor

I am the school with doors open as the sun rises each day welcoming all, never closing to anyone who wants to partake in this adventure of life that awaits them. I am a school, sturdy and strong in its foundation made by the sweat of those who took the time to lay the bricks and the grime. I am a school that started new but ripened through the years, only becoming better as different people entered the doors, leaving an everlasting impression on my walls throughout the halls. I am a school with so much pride for the students who sing my school song, for it will be the anthem that echoes through the halls like the veins that lead to my heart that cares about each of them. As the night falls and I must let all go, don't worry, sleep tightly for surely come sunrise my doors will be wide open to all.

realized that their initial metaphors were way too optimistic, yet through peer interaction and discussion were able to make them more achievable. Still others appeared not to have any interest in designing a metaphor to portray their beliefs about teaching and learning. One young man developed the teaching metaphor shown in **Box 5.2**.

The Hidden Dimensions of Physical Educators' Work

Professional physical educators have numerous roles and responsibilities beyond teaching classes. Students in primary and post-primary schools likely only recognize what teachers do when they see teachers at work during regular classes. Consider the following two vignettes (see **Box 5.3** and **Box 5.4**) of two physical educators that can be best described as "A Week in the Life of Physical Educators." Both teach physical education in a post-primary school setting.

Learning Experience 5.2

The teachers in the vignettes highlighted many activities and duties that do not include the actual teaching of lessons. Make contact with a teacher, and request to shadow this teacher for 1 day from the moment he or she arrives on the school campus until the end of the school day. Mark down all the activities that this teacher engages in beyond teaching classes. Ask the teacher to note any school-related activities engaged in at home.

- To what extent do this teacher's activities mirror the vignettes noted in the boxes?
- What might be the reasons that they are similar or different?

As the vignettes show, teachers spend a significant portion of a typical day engaged in activities that do not always directly involve their students. Importantly, there are numerous forces at play in schools that directly affect teachers' day-to-day work, over which they have no control. Examples of such forces include rules, regulations, and laws set forth by principals, school systems, and government; the organizational structure of the school; administrative practices; politics; students' home lives; parents; and more. We want to highlight a number of responsibilities and activities that teachers can influence. We have grouped these various **non-instructional responsibilities** as follows: (1) contributing to the broader school mission; (2) planning and administering the program; (3) managing your resources; (4) collaborating with others; (5) counseling students; (6) continuing your professional development; (7) representing yourself, the school, and the profession; and (8) proactively advocating for your program and profession.

Contributing to the Broader School Mission

As a physical educator, you are part of a larger organization that is responsible for educating future generations. Schools are complex organizations, where teachers, building administrators, and support staff have a common mission: Have the school be a well-organized, pleasant, and smooth running community that makes learning by students possible. Moreover, it should be a positive workplace for you as an employee. Outside of your normal teaching assignments (i.e., teaching schedule), you can expect to have many non-instructional roles that help ensure this common mission is accomplished. A myriad of before-school, lunchtime, and after-school duties are typically assigned to teachers. They may include bus duty and lunchroom duty. In the United States, where many students are bused to and from school, you will be expected to help monitor safety and smooth arrival and departure of school buses. During lunch periods, you will likely have a similar oversight role. In post-primary schools you may be expected to provide oversight during special evening events on the school's campus.

Schools have regular staff meetings. You are not only required to attend them, but you should expect to actively participate in them even if it pertains to matters that only marginally (if at all) affect your own physical education program. For example, if your school is looking to improve students' writing skills, you might be expected to assist classroom teachers with the grading of student writing samples. When schools are trying to improve students' performance in mathematics, you may be expected to participate in training sessions aimed at helping infuse mathematics throughout other subjects (such as physical education).

It also suggests we consider how to help teachers in other subject areas build physical education into their content area, and not just vice versa. For example, in the Irish

BOX 5.3 A Week in the Life of a Physical Educator: Dani

Dani has been a post-primary physical education teacher for 16 years, in a small rural town. In addition to teaching her regular physical education classes, she coaches the school's girl's tennis team. She teaches with two other male teachers, and the program blends the Sport Education and Fitness for Life curriculum models. In addition, she includes team-building content with her first-year classes. She regularly attends and presents at professional workshops and conferences in an effort to stay up-to-date with professional development opportunities.

Sunday:

- Spend 2–4 hours grading, preparing Moodle website (this is where students can access missed work or make up quizzes for my "lifelong fitness" class), and getting ready for the week.

Monday and Friday:

- Arrive 30 minutes before required to disinfect wrestling mats. (This is where we do yoga for my spinning and yoga class.)
- Leave lunch 10 minutes early to set up web-linked whiteboard (also known as a smartboard) for lifelong class and get the quiz ready for students to take review quiz.
- Required to be at school until 3:30 (class gets out at 2:40 p.m.) to have students come in and ask for locker combinations, stolen clothes, and missing assignments.
- Organize the day. (I teach in four different rooms in the school so I have to bring back all my work and organize it in my office.)

Tuesday and Thursday:

- Missed lunch because students needed to talk to me on both days. Went up to office to do a mandatory report because of what the students discussed with me. If it does not require a mandatory report, I talk with a counselor to help students. (Not necessarily a weekly occurrence but at least monthly.)
- Skipped my afternoon break to clean the mats for yoga class at the end of the day.
- End of the day looks the same as my Mondays.

Wednesday:

- Come to work at least 45 minutes early for PLC (Professional Learning Communities) department meetings to write department goals, common assessments, or planning time, or for once-a-month staff meetings. Leave meeting and go clean mats for yoga. End of the day looks the same as Mondays and Fridays.

Other duties and more random activities:

- I have been on the school's Site Council (an advisory council representing teachers, parents, and school administrators), I am the Physical Education Department Chair, and I have been on several other school and regional-level committees. I went to a conference this summer for 3 days learning about how to engage students.
- Throughout every day (often right before class when I try to get ready for it) students will text me, needing to talk to me. This typically takes up at least 3 hours a week.
- As Department Chair, I order all equipment for my teachers. I have one prep period per day, so most of the time I get caught up with what I need to accomplish after school, in the evenings, or on weekends.

education system, numeracy and literacy are a current focus where every subject area is expected to plan for and build these content areas into their lessons; this has huge implications for work with young people. In the United States, the Common Core movement is spreading across the country with a similar focus on preparing primary and post-primary school students to be successful in their university education and/or careers (see www.corestandards.org). Currently, Common Core standards consist of only mathematics and English language arts. Physical educators also are expected to be key players in making contributions.

Physical educators can also expect to be asked to volunteer to serve on various school-level committees. Examples of such committees are the School Improvement Committee, Active School Flag, School Management Team, School Self-Evaluation Committee, or School Site Council. As you gain more experience, you will likely do the same at other education levels beyond your own school. How you contribute

BOX 5.4 A Week in the Life of a Physical Educator: Trevor

Trevor is an experienced post-primary physical educator in the United States who is Board Certified through the National Board of Professional Teaching Standards (NBPTS) and former National Association for Sport and Physical Education (NASPE) National Teacher of the Year. Together with his colleagues, he has developed a cutting-edge program that provides students with a wide range of health-enhancing physical activity experiences, ranging from sport to outdoor education, and health-related fitness. Moreover, his program is increasingly linked with other subject matter areas within the school as well as programs and organizations in the surrounding community. The following shows an actual recount of a week's worth of activities outside of teaching his classes:

Sunday:

- 8:15–8:50 a.m.: Skyped with David Patterson regarding new NASPE standards, providing feedback.
- 6:45–8:15 p.m.: Wrote letter of recommendation for Ashley McFadden.

Monday:

- 7:15 a.m.: Ordered 20 badminton racquets, turned in purchase order after getting it signed off.
- 9:08 a.m.: Contacted King County Parks to confirm location of tomorrow's tree planting event by students.
- 9:10 a.m.: Contacted district transportation office to confirm buses for tomorrow's field experience.
- 10–10:15 a.m.: Met with a student to discuss their senior project progress.
- 2:30–3:00 p.m.: Met with the district health and fitness supervisor about the new independent study curriculum during my planning period.
- 3:15–4:30 p.m.: Along with two other teachers, I met for an hour and 15 minutes after school with a graduate from 2 years ago about getting themselves back on track.
- 4:40–5:00 p.m.: Met with our school's video production teacher about filming my class later in the week.

Tuesday:

- 6:30–7 a.m.: Prepared for field trip to the Log Cabin Reach site for tree planting.
- 3–4 p.m.: Met with two representatives from the Washington Trail Association about developing a partnership for next school year.
- 7–7:45 p.m.: FaceTime meeting with Sam Johnson about presentation for upcoming national conference.
- 8:00–9:15 p.m.: Read three class sets of my students' top three stressors assignment.

Wednesday:

- 7–7:40 a.m.: Phone call with NASPE representative about the Teacher of the Year selection committee.
- 7:40–7:45 a.m.: Quick conversation with school's choir teacher about use of the gym for next week's district concert.
- 7:45–8:10 a.m.: School staff meeting for state testing preparation.
- 11:15–11:45 a.m.: Lunch with two other teachers and a student we have been counseling.
- 2:00–2:40 p.m.: FaceTime with Sam Johnson about presentation.
- 3–4:30 p.m.: Joint Leadership Team committee meeting.
- 7–8:15 p.m.: Read two more class sets of stressor assignment.

Thursday:

- 7:15–7:45 a.m.: Led Physical Education Department meeting.
- 11:15 a.m.: Called Vertical World to set up next month's rock climbing field experience.
- 11:20–11:30 a.m.: Put together waiver forms and field trip form.
- 11:30–11:45 a.m.: Lunch with our district tech support person about how I can use Google forms in class with my iPad.
- 1:00–2:10 p.m.: Planning period meeting to discuss random walk-throughs and discussion about what we observed related to learning goals other teachers communicate to their students.
- 2:35–2:55 p.m.: Phone survey with American Alliance for Health, Physical Education, Recreation and Dance (AAHPERD) about physical education programs.
- 3:00–4:00 p.m.: Three 20-minute student mentee meetings right after school.
- 4:00–4:45 p.m.: Edited video of my class.
- 4:45 p.m.: Spoke with former student who is doing student teaching at another school about their experience and provided a few resources.

to the work of such committees will affect how those around you view you, your program, and physical education in general.

Successful schools are those in which principals create a culture of community and teamwork where the teaching staff really works together toward the same goals. Physical educators should be part of that, and need to do all they can to actively contribute to these efforts. However, in many cases, physical educators can be working as the only physical educator in the school and/or teach only one subject. They are physically separated from the rest of the school's activities and their colleagues. They have their own facility, and often they may not leave that facility during the day. In fact, they may prefer to physically "hide" in their own area on campus because it creates a sense of independence and freedom. However, this may also increase a sense of psychological isolation, and physical educators may feel ignored. To other teachers and building administrators, the physical education teacher may appear invisible.

Physical educators will want to avoid this isolation at all costs and do everything possible to make themselves (and their program) highly visible and credible at all times. As a professional physical educator you will want to be a team player as much as the other teaching staff. Colleagues who see you actively participate, offer suggestions during discussions, show willingness to help out on special projects, and so on are more likely to view you as an important and valued contributor, compared to teachers who sit through meetings appearing detached, uninterested, and uninvolved.

Planning and Administering the Program

One of the core functions of physical educators is to manage and administer the physical education program. This includes such tasks as scheduling the yearly plan of activities to be taught, planning units of instruction and individual lessons, conducting program reviews, revising the curriculum, doing equipment inventories, maintaining equipment, keeping equipment storage spaces organized and safe, and checking for facility safety. In primary schools with a physical education specialist, you must be vigilant in ensuring input on the physical education class schedule because it usually is closely intertwined with other school subjects (i.e., art and music). In post-primary schools, a physical education department head most often oversees this task; however, other teachers in the department should be included in designing and scheduling the yearly plans.

Financial support for school physical education varies widely across countries. In countries where the program is provided an annual budget, it typically is very minimal. For example, a program may get as little as $1,000, or worse, simply not have a budget, and physical educators have to ask for financial support from their administrators/managers. Given this context, you can understand why physical educators must be vigilant in maximizing the life of existing equipment. However, many teachers have been successful in supplementing their equipment inventory through grant writing and creative fundraising. For example, since 2002, the U.S. federal government has had the Carol M. White Physical Education Program (also known as the PEP Grant Program, www2.ed.gov/programs/whitephysed/index.html) where local schools and other community-based organizations can apply for multiyear grants to initiate, expand, or enhance physical education programs, including after-school programs, for students in primary and post-primary schools. Larger school systems may have support personnel who can assist with preparing grant proposals. In addition, the school's Parent Teacher Association (PTA) is another potential source of funding. As long as teachers can provide a coherent rationale for the funding request, showing how the funds will help the students' experiences, the associations generally will provide the support.

In other countries it is more common that government departments disperse monies. For example, in 2010 the Department of Education and Skills in Ireland launched a grant scheme for physical education equipment in all post-primary schools where the same basic grant was awarded to each school with an additional sum per student.

Good teachers find many other national, regional, and local grant programs through private foundations and other organizations. Members of professional associations (e.g., National Association for Sport and Physical Education [NASPE] in the United States; Australian Council for Health, Physical Education and Recreation [ACHPER] in Australia) will have free access to web links specifically dedicated to sharing grant program information. Schools' PTAs and/or boards of management may also have funding available for teachers or be interested in raising funds for a particular cause. A persuasive rationale and clear need/impact statement often are all that are needed to secure the extra funding.

In addition, physical education teachers will have many other managerial roles to play. Some are aimed at promoting the program, whereas others target increasing the program's impact and effectiveness. Three examples include: (1) organizing special events, (2) promoting physical activity during nonclass times (e.g., recess in primary schools), and (3) working with **paraprofessionals**/special educational needs assistants/support staff.

Managing Your Resources

Most physical educators have to be frugal when it comes to their resources, which include small annual budgets and material resources such as their facility and equipment. Oftentimes, equipment for students is lacking or in poor or damaged condition. The same goes for the state of the school's physical activity venues. Teachers who are hired when a new school is opened may have the luxury to have at least some input in the type and quantity of equipment to be purchased. However, from that point forward, annual budgets for additional purchases and upgrades will be very small. The degree to and care with which you manage your existing resources is reflected in part in how well you keep your equipment storage area clean and organized.

Typical tasks include maintaining an accurate inventory of equipment, periodically determining the state of the equipment and facility, ordering new equipment, and the like. Decisions on what equipment should be added or replaced should be based on defensible rationales. Some factors that should be considered when purchasing equipment include (1) developmental appropriateness, (2) alignment with the program's overall mission, (3) instructional approaches to be used, and (4) the balance between cost versus use (i.e., is it worth it to purchase one very expensive piece of equipment if you will only use it sporadically?). For example, it is appropriate for each child to have his or her own playground ball or jump rope in an early primary lesson to practice fundamental skills from the perspective of maximizing individual participation. However, in a post-primary program, having class sizes of 35 students does not automatically imply that you should invest in getting 40 soccer balls, volleyballs, and basketballs (especially if you prefer to employ game-based approaches to teaching such sports!).

Another example may be where you are looking to help students develop behavior change techniques such as goal setting and behavior monitoring as part of a program with a strong focus on developing health-related fitness habits. Pedometers now are considered a household teaching tool, as they have been shown to be reliable and effective in helping students monitor their own physical activity levels over time as well as helping physical educators determine program impact through formative tracking of physical activity. However, there is no reason why every student has to have one. Teachers could rotate a set of six to eight pedometers among groups of students throughout the year and collect samples of the group's physical activity levels. Thus, be mindful of what you invest in and why you invest in it for each particular piece of equipment.

Because of the often-limited budgets, teachers may prefer to purchase equipment that is cheaper (and, thus, greater quantities). The adage of "you get what you pay for" will hold true. Especially with equipment that is used often, the normal wear and tear will likely affect cheaper equipment more so, so make sure to check with colleagues on their experience with the same type of equipment.

Finally, there are countless opportunities to obtain supplementary funding for the purpose of getting more equipment resources, through either fundraising or straight donations. Organizations may have small grant programs. Such grant programs typically require only some time investment in that you will be asked to offer (1) what you request, (2) a clear rationale as to why the equipment is necessary or important to obtain, and (3) a cost overview. Moreover, parent organizations also are prepared to support teachers in their efforts through funding support. Finally, local businesses may be open to periodically donating in-kind resources.

Learning Experience 5.3

As a physical educator, you have been asked to present a budget plan for purchasing new equipment for your program. You have $10,000 available. Using reliable and trustworthy equipment suppliers, your task is to develop a list of equipment you would like to purchase. The equipment request should be accompanied by the following:

- A clearly stated mission statement
- A program content outline (i.e., a listing of the annual units of work/instruction)
- A detailed rationale for each equipment line item that shows how its purchase will contribute to meeting the program's mission

Also, make sure you break down the list of equipment in the following categories:

- Critical to successful program delivery (i.e., "must have")
- Important to have
- Would be great to have but not essential

Collaborating with Others

It should be abundantly clear that physical educators must be effective in collaborating with many parties in order to deliver a successful program. They have to develop strong working relationships with their classroom colleagues, the school's support staff, their school administrators, and parents, as well as physical activity professionals in the community, policy makers, and university faculty members. These relationships are reciprocal—both sides derive benefits. Moreover, it is essential that you become aware of the many support resources that a school and community have available. **Box 5.5** provides an example of an assignment that PSTs undertake prior to their teaching practice placement in one Irish teacher education program. It has proven useful for having future physical educators develop the skills needed to learn about key aspects of the school environment, students, teachers, and the community in which they will teach.

Building strong collaborative relationships with other classroom teachers can pay important dividends. For example, in primary schools with physical education specialists, you want your classroom colleagues to bring their students to your physical education class on time so students do not

BOX 5.5 School Ethnography Assignment

The school ethnography is to include:

- Community mapping assignment
- Case study of a teacher (teacher shadowing assignment)
- Case study of two pupils (pupil shadow assignment)
- Review of the school ethos (policies, mission statement, climate of school)

Community Mapping

The task: "Mapping" the neighbourhood with a camera, observing the neighbourhood, and interacting with the people who work and live in the neighbourhood should allow you to see the community with new lenses. You will map the local area (size should be walkable if in a city/town), collecting information and talking to people. You will create a map of your journey and experiences.

Case Study of a Teacher Assignment

The task: Identify a teacher with a reputation as a highly effective teacher and obtain permission to observe his or her teaching. Observe at least one class and talk to him or her before and after your observation. Design a set of questions that you wish to ask the teacher so you can be sure to use time efficiently. Think beyond physical education so you begin to know other teachers and courses in the school.

Case Study of a Pupil Assignment

The task: Identify at least four pupils and obtain permission to attend some of their classes and conduct a focus group interview with them. Pick pupils you find interesting and with different backgrounds from your own. Take notes that will help you to recall significant events or comments during the day. Do your best to get to know the pupils and understand their feelings about the school and teachers. Design a set of questions that you wish to ask the pupils.

School Ethos (Policies, Mission Statement, Climate of School)

The task: Talk with members of the school staff including teachers, secretaries, and administrators. Examine teacher handbooks, materials provided to pupils and parents, and any written documentation that portrays a picture of the school and its environment. Attempt to identify what makes the school tick. In other words, develop your understanding of the school ethos and climate and the role of teachers, administrators, and pupils in developing it. Reflect upon the implications of this school ethos for your own teaching at this site.

get short-changed. The same applies to physical educators because classroom teachers expect to have their students back in the classroom on time. Professional classroom teachers and physical educators also keep each other abreast of any issues or circumstances surrounding individual students.

From the perspective of enhancing student learning, physical educators can team up with classroom colleagues to integrate classroom subjects (e.g., language arts, mathematics) into their lessons (e.g., Siedentop, Hastie, & van der Mars, 2011). Developing such links also can help build program credibility with classroom teachers.

Building collaborative working relationships with school maintenance, custodial, and office staff is essential as well. Without their help, developing and maintaining your facility, equipment, and program becomes more difficult. When the gymnasium space is used for other purposes (e.g., lunch, science fair, special events, sport club team practices in the evenings) it likely needs to be cleaned. Such staff will work for you in these circumstances. They will come through for you (especially in minor emergencies) but only if you have shown that you work well with others.

A primary responsibility for school administrators/managers is to ensure that teachers have the necessary resources to effectively deliver their programs. In addition, they address staffing and curricular issues, and evaluate teachers, among many other duties. Physical educators not only must demonstrate to their administrators that they are capable of managing and teaching their classes, but also have to show they can work with colleagues, participate in other school functions, show commitment to students, resolve problems, address parents' concerns, and so on. Administrators are much more likely to view you as a truly professional teacher if/when you act proactively, are organized, focus on solving problems, and demonstrate care and concern for students, colleagues, support staff, parents, and other outsiders.

Beginning physical educators may assume that school administrators/managers (1) have a clear understanding of what quality physical education should look like and (2) are familiar and up-to-date relative to the issues, trends, and developments in our field. This is a dangerous assumption to make, especially given the typical job demands of a school administrator/manager. It is virtually impossible to expect a principal to be current in all individual school subjects. Moreover, their own experiences in physical education as school-age students will directly shape administrators'/managers' perceptions of what physical education is and their level of commitment to support the physical education program. There is evidence that administrators are, in fact, largely unaware of the recent developments in school physical education (Lounsbery, McKenzie, Trost, & Smith, 2011; McKenzie & Lounsbery, 2009; Sallis, 2010). Thus, it is essential that physical educators make time to educate and inform their administrators/managers. This should be done both informally and formally through one-on-one meetings and presentations at staff meetings. For example, as part of your efforts to increase physical activity levels throughout the school day, you could offer to train classroom teachers to include physical activity breaks into their daily lessons. Likely, you will need to first educate and persuade your principal in terms of the benefits, need, efficacy, and logistics of doing so.

Physical educators will also want to seek out potential collaboration opportunities with other physical activity professionals and organizations in the surrounding community. In most countries there are multiple pillars that support and promote physical activity in all its forms, including club sports, fitness and health clubs, and other forms of active recreation. All play a central role in creating the overall infrastructure for physical activity across all population groups (Siedentop & van der Mars, 2012). Many physical educators have raised the program's recognition in the community by building formal partnerships with local golf courses, karate clubs, bowling alleys, fitness centers, national sport governing bodies, sports stores, adventure centers, and the like. Instructors from the local sport clubs and governing bodies can be invited to do guest workshops within the physical education programs, or can assist in developing new units of instruction. School-age students could be given discounts when taking additional lessons at programs and facilities in the community. Local sports stores that also rent equipment for use on weekends are always looking to increase the number of future customers, and so may be interested in working with local physical education programs and offer reduced rental rates for outdoor equipment (e.g., inline skates, skis, hiking equipment). Building such partnerships will take time and energy but will help members of the community see your physical education program as much more central to the school's mission.

A final group of colleagues that can be a strong source of collaboration are physical education teacher education (PETE) faculty members at nearby universities. Working with PETE faculty members can take multiple forms. For example, you may be invited to serve as a mentor/cooperating teacher for a prospective physical education intern completing a practicum or student teaching placement. Or the PETE faculty member may be interested in doing a formal research project with you and/or your students. Finally, in several countries, PETE faculty members are expected to serve physical education programs in the surrounding communities. In many schools, teachers will be expected to attend full- or half-day professional development workshops/in-services. For many years we have listened to school physical educators lament that these in-service sessions focus mostly on classroom subjects, and thus have little relevance to them. Together with PETE faculty, physical educators can build stronger programs for children and youth (Siedentop & Locke, 1997) if they recognize and value each other's strengths. In some countries we see learning communities being developed where teachers rotate workshops sharing their expertise and programs that work in physical education settings, and providing substantive help to colleagues who may be struggling with a given content area. The following sections describe three common out-of-class activities in which quality physical educators engage on a regular basis.

Working with Paraprofessionals/Special Needs Assistants/Support Staff

In many countries, schools increasingly employ additional staff such as paraprofessionals and special needs assistants (and/or volunteers) to assist students with special needs when placed in regular classrooms. Unfortunately, such staff may have little (if any) background in providing sound instruction in physical education settings to students with special needs. In many cases, physical educators may feel they need to take full responsibility for the instruction, thereby wasting a valuable support resource. Moreover, there is some evidence that physical educators and support staff are unclear about each other's formal roles and responsibilities (Bryan, McCubbin, & van der Mars, 2013). To ensure worthwhile and enjoyable physical activity experiences for students with special needs, adult support personnel will likely require training sessions during before-school or after-school hours. Sometimes they will have to work with the physical education teacher during their regular classes.

Physical education's teaching spaces often are used for other out-of-school purposes as well, from community badminton tournaments in some countries to political voting sites in others. School-based activities such as music performances, science fairs, high stakes examinations, after-school sport, and breakfast or lunch service often involve the use of the physical education teaching spaces. Physical educators have to be vigilant to stay abreast of the many possible disruptions in the facility schedule. This points to another key role and responsibility for physical educators less well recognized by the casual observer—ongoing collaboration with countless others within and beyond the school.

Promoting Physical Activity During Non-class Times

The increasing emphasis on creating physical activity opportunities for students beyond regular physical education classes (e.g., before school, recess/activity breaks, after school, classroom physical activity breaks) will require planning and training of other adults at the school. First you will need to persuade both the school's administration and classroom teachers that increasing physical activity opportunities during those times are vital to students' academic success. Next, you will need to organize training sessions to help classroom teachers implement the physical activity breaks in their classrooms. In addition, playground supervisory personnel are a key support to encourage physical activity during recess and lunch break periods. They, too, will require some training and support so they can assist in such efforts. Seemingly simple tasks such as the transport and dispersal of equipment at the outset of recess/activity breaks and lunch times as well as its collection at the end of such sessions can be routinized but still require teachers to oversee. Encouraging students to join in the activities and getting activities started are another critical aspect of promoting physical activity throughout the school day. A school's support staff is a great resource to assist physical educators in such efforts.

Organizing Special Events

Special events such as family fitness nights, after-school fun runs, joint school culminating events (often referred to as rich tasks), or a fundraising event are important ways of promoting the physical education program and making it visible to the broader school community and surrounding neighborhoods. Generally, the physical education teacher will serve as lead manager for such events. Event planning requires good organization and volunteer assistance. Teachers will need to recruit and manage the volunteers and set up an advertising campaign to spread the word about the event. Today, technologies such as email and school or program websites make this latter task easier, but it still can be time-consuming. Good teachers develop event scripts and mark adjustments to the script following the event to improve the planning and organization the next time they need to plan the same event.

Counseling Students

Perhaps more so in post-primary schools, physical education teachers can expect to be approached by students seeking support on issues that are often unrelated to how they do in class. Rather, they may seek advice (or simply look for a teacher to be a sounding board) on personal issues ranging from selecting a college program to problems with friends or parents, drug abuse, alcohol abuse, eating disorders, pregnancy, or sexual orientation. If you have demonstrated care, interest, and concern for students, as well as trustworthiness, they are more likely to seek you out. However, you must be cautious in how you respond to and engage with issues beyond physical education.

Although providing advice on what college program to select is relatively safe, providing counsel on more delicate issues must, in almost all cases, be left to persons specifically trained to address such matters. Thus, you should become familiar with the available programs, agencies, and resources within the school and surrounding community. Indirectly related to this, if teachers suspect abuse (physical or otherwise), they are generally required by law to report this to the proper authorities. Thus, although it reflects positively on you that a student might seek your advice, you should be mindful of your limitations in how you can (or are allowed to) handle such situations. You will need to balance the need to maintain the relationship with the students and your responsibilities as a professional.

Bullying

In recent years, **bullying** among students has received increased attention. Most people agree that bullying is a problem in schools. Although the word *bullying* may conjure up instances of physical abuse, it is important to realize that bullying can take many different forms. The multiple means of communicating with each other beyond confronting each other face to face, such as texting and **cyber-bullying**, have brought about new ways of bullying. Schools are trying to address bullying in various ways. Most students have likely either signed pledges not to bully, watched different videos aimed at making them more aware of the issues surrounding bullying (i.e., what it is, how it manifests itself, its consequences, and strategies to avoid/deal with bullies), or had to learn about new school rules set forth by the school. Most have installed elaborate security camera systems both on the outside of the school building and inside the facility.

Two problems become apparent. First, there is no real agreement about what constitutes bullying. Second, there is even less agreement on what to do about the bullying problem. Moreover, there are several myths that surround bullying. Some frequently asked questions and concerns voiced about bullying include:

- Is the amount of bullying worse today than years ago?
- Does a school system that publicly espouses having zero tolerance for bullying have the means to monitor and address instances of bullying?

- Do the various media make the problem seem worse by hyping instances of bullying?
- What separates bullying from what would be considered normal developmental conflict between students?

While you may not have personally experienced any bullying, it is essential that you become aware of not only the many types of bullying but also what the key indicators are, and what effective strategies are to reduce its occurrence. **Box 5.6** offers additional considerations related to bullying.

Learning Experience 5.4

Using the Kinder and Braver World resources (see **Box 5.6**) as well as any others specific to the topic of bullying, develop a one-page fact sheet about bullying. Select a particular audience that would benefit from this information. It could be other teachers in the school, the school board, students, or parents. Determine an effective way of getting the fact sheet to the target audience you selected.

Continuing Professional Development

Virtually all professions (e.g., medicine, law, psychology) have a stated expectation that those working in it stay current with the most recent developments, trends, and critical issues in the profession. For example, as technology improves in the world of medicine, approaches toward preventing disease, managing disease, and rehabilitation change and improve. Physicians, nurses, and surgeons are expected to be current with the requisite knowledge and skills. That is what the public expects. Although education often is criticized as lagging behind, continuing professional development (CPD) is an integral part of one's work as a teacher. Chambers (2007) likened the process of developing as a teacher over the course of a career to embarking on a climb of Mount Everest. The initial training in a PETE program prepares teachers to reach the mountain's basecamp. Engaging in professional development activities throughout one's career reflects a gradual ascent towards the top of the mountain. Reaching the top reflects being a career-long professional physical educator. In some countries, ongoing professional development is embedded in standards for both beginning and advanced teachers in physical education.

BOX 5.6 Bullying: Fact or Fiction?

Following are five commonly heard statements when people discuss bullying. We suggest you try to seek out the facts surrounding these claims:

- *Students engage in bullying because they suffer from low self-esteem.* Could it be, in fact, the opposite? Could it be that they actually have an excessively high self-esteem?
- *Having a zero-tolerance policy for bullying will result in less bullying.* Similar to addressing drug use, sexual harassment, and violence, the zero-tolerance approach to addressing bullying typically results in students being removed from school altogether. Has this resulted in fewer incidences of bullying? Does this approach address the need for helping students learn to be more compassionate?
- *Students having access to new types of technology is the real culprit. Cyber-bullying is the most prevalent form of bullying these days.* The Internet, social media, and smartphones certainly have changed the ways in which today's youth communicate. Such technologies can now extend bullying that might have started during a face-to-face encounter well beyond school campuses. But is it really the primary means of bullying?
- *Everyone is going to be bullied at some point in time.* Consider the following questions related to this claim: Have you been bullied? What are the likely risk factors for a student to get bullied (i.e., which type of student is more likely to be bullied?)? When are kids more likely to be bullied?
- *Being bullied is a major cause of school violence and students choosing to commit suicide.* Certainly there have been several horrific incidents in recent years in which bullying resulted in students taking it out on others in very deadly ways. However, one must consider the following: Has the extensive coverage by the media played a role in creating this connection?

Harvard University's Berkman Center for Internet and Society has developed a series of papers that bring together the latest evidence on topics such as cyber-bullying, the state of legislative efforts to reduce bullying, how to implement anti-bullying programs, and more. The series of papers are part of *The Kinder and Braver World Project: Research Series.* Use the following web address to access these important resources: www.cyber.law.harvard.edu/node/7491.

Effective continuing professional development (CPD), both formal and informal, is an essential means of remaining stimulated professionally and maintaining the passion and enthusiasm that teachers bring with them as they enter the profession (Armour & Yelling, 2007). CPD can take many different forms, including regularly attending workshops and annual professional conferences, participating in staff-development programs, reading professional journals and books, pursuing an advanced degree, and maintaining professional contacts at other schools and in the community.

Representing Yourself, Your School, and Your Profession

Teaching physical education can in some ways be a lonely profession, especially for those in primary schools. However, teachers are also public figures. For example, teachers who also coach an athletic team within the school or community will become well known to the public. Moreover, teachers represent their school and profession, even when they are not performing a school function. Most likely you have seen the ways in which physical education teachers are portrayed in movies and on television. There is evidence that such stereotypical portrayals persist in the mind of the public (McCullick, Belcher, Hardin, & Hardin, 2003). They perpetuate the often-negative perceptions of the profession and those within it. Thus, physical educators must do everything possible to change this perception and make students, parents, other teachers, school administrators, and the like come to realize that they are well informed and truly qualified professionals. This is, of course, a never-ending process that takes many forms. First and foremost, delivering a quality and evidence-based physical education program that reflects current curricular and instructional approaches is one important step towards changing such negative perceptions. Other steps include continuing to engage in professional development throughout one's career, and being a strong voice for the profession through advocacy (see the following section).

In many ways, physical educators have to educate not only their students but also the students' parents. Physical educators can share their expertise and knowledge about physical activity, sport, fitness, nutrition, and active lifestyles in many ways. They include school newsletters (often web-based), the Parent Teacher Organization, and the physical education program's website, among others. How teachers share their expertise and portray their program (and themselves) in these efforts can help to change the public's perception about our field.

Schoolteachers are also expected to behave in ways consistent with a professional role. This refers to how teachers behave when out in public and the relationships they build with students. Especially in smaller, more rural communities, teachers may feel they are under a microscope when they go out into the community. Therefore, teachers want to be mindful of how their actions are perceived by others.

Teachers are well aware of the need to develop positive and supportive relationships with their students because this is a necessary condition for student learning. It goes without saying that developing positive relationships with students while at school for the purpose of supporting their education is critical. However, this is not the same as befriending students. For example, today's social media technology (e.g., Facebook) forms an extraordinary way of connecting with others. Teachers in post-primary schools can expect to get friend requests from some of their students. From a professional conduct perspective, teachers should decline such invitations. Moreover, future and current teachers should be mindful in terms of the type of language they use as well as the photos they post on public websites such as Facebook.

Proactively Advocating for Your Program and Profession

Advocating for the program and the health of students is perhaps the most critical noninstructional function for physical educators in today's education environment. Advocacy occurs both formally and informally. Making presentations at school staff meetings, speaking before school policy makers, and serving on an advisory board of local youth organizations are all examples of formal opportunities to advocate for the importance of the program. They are key in showing that physical educators are informed and knowledgeable about matters related to programming physical education for the school's students. Informal opportunities arise every time physical educators interact with teaching colleagues, school administrators, parents, and decision makers while at school or out in the community. The same will occur informally.

School physical education is in a position where it must do all it can to demonstrate how it is a core subject within the broader mission of schools. Effective advocacy is one important process through which the public (i.e., students, parents, school administrators/managers, policy makers) can be informed about what good programs in school physical education can do. Advocacy is not just the responsibility of individual teachers. Those involved in preparing physical educators, as well as professional organizations, are key players in this effort. In fact, as we show in **Box 5.7**, globally there is broad support from local, regional, and national organizations and government agencies (e.g., Daugbjerg et al., 2009). Many countries now have policy statements, position statements, and/or national recommendations that directly target promotion of physical activity, and many include support for increasing the quantity and quality of school physical education.

BOX 5.7 Sample Organizations and Agencies Supporting Promotion of Physical Education and Physical Activity in Children and Youth

Australia

- *Australian Government:* www.health.gov.au/internet/main/publishing.nsf/Content/health-pubhlth-strateg-active-index.htm

England

- *PE and Sport Strategy for Young People:* www.ssp-websolutions.co.uk/PESSYP_small.pdf
- *Association for Physical Education:* www.afpe.org.uk
- *UK Physical Activity Guidelines:* www.gov.uk/government/publications/uk-physical-activity-guidelines

Ireland

- *Active School Flag:* www.activeschoolflag.ie
- *Irish Sports Council:* www.irishsportscouncil.ie/Participation/Local_Sports_Partnerships
- *National Governing Bodies:* www.coachingireland.com
- *Get Ireland Active:* www.getirelandactive.ie/get-info/links
- *PE PAYS Research Centre:* www.ul.ie/pepays
- *Physical Education Association of Ireland:* www.peai.ie

Scotland

- *Physical Activity and Health Alliance:* www.paha.org.uk/Home
- *Let's Make Scotland More Active:* www.scotland.gov.uk/Publications/2003/02/16324/17895

United States

- *Action for Healthy Kids:* www.actionforhealthykids.org
- *Institute of Medicine:* www.iom.edu
- *President's Council on Fitness, Sports and Nutrition:* www.fitness.gov
- *Alliance for a Healthier Generation:* www.healthiergeneration.org
- *Obesity Society:* www.obesity.org
- *Centers for Disease Control and Prevention, Division of Nutrition, Physical Activity, and Obesity:* www.cdc.gov/nccdphp/dnpao
- *National Coalition for Promoting Physical Activity:* www.ncppa.org

Global

- *World Health Organization:* www.who.int/dietphysicalactivity/en

Learning Experience 5.5

Develop a list of professional organizations, research associations, private foundations, and/or government agencies (along with the contact information) and retrieve the formal policy statement and/or formal recommendations for your country specific to the delivery of physical education. Read them with care and prepare a 4-minute, coherent presentation for local constituents (e.g., parents, school administrators) highlighting the document(s) content and why school physical education should play a central role. Also, develop a one-page summary of the document(s) that provides your audience with the key messages.

Program advocacy is not organizing an event such as a family fitness night and saying "I have done my advocacy for the year." We have to come to see advocacy as an ongoing process, with a strong proactive approach. Moreover, within the school region teachers can be more effective in such efforts if they work together with other physical educators, and plan for a deliberate and ongoing advocacy campaign targeting the key constituents. In addition, by collaborating with other organizations that also focus on the health and well-being of children and youth, the field of physical education can form a more united front to bring about new (or change existing) policies that support physical education. School administrators/managers, who never hear from physical educators about the importance of the subject until proposals are considered for reductions in staff and/or time for physical education, will likely interpret any last-minute effort to "save" the physical education program as simply a way for physical educators to save their teaching jobs.

CHAPTER SUMMARY

1. Prospective physical education teachers have established conceptions of teaching physical education, based on the apprenticeship of observation.
2. Beyond teaching their classes, physical educators have numerous noninstructional roles and responsibilities.
3. Physical educators are part of the broader educational mission of a school. They have a responsibility to contribute to this mission.
4. For school physical education programs to be coherent in their goals and implementation, teachers need to spend significant time and energy on planning, administering, and reviewing the program.
5. Delivering physical education effectively requires extensive collaboration with multiple outside people and programs. They include other teachers, school administrators/managers, principals, community organizations/programs, and university faculty members.
6. Although teachers will frequently serve as surrogate parents for students who wish to discuss more personal matters, they must be mindful about the boundaries and legal obligations surrounding such efforts.
7. Bullying among students is a problem in schools that comes in various forms (e.g., cyber-bullying). Media play a role in shaping people's perceptions about the prevalence of bullying.
8. Bullying is not easily defined nor easily differentiated from normal developmental youth conflicts.
9. Over the course of teachers' careers, continuing professional development (CPD) is an essential element of remaining professionally stimulated and up-to-date on the latest developments in the physical education field.
10. Program advocacy is central to ensuring that school physical education becomes viewed as a core subject in schools.
11. Teachers have a responsibility to serve as informed and knowledgeable professionals when interacting with all audiences in both formal and informal settings. Moreover, when developing relationships with students they must balance their professional responsibilities.

REFERENCES

Armour, K. M., & Yelling, M. (2007). Effective professional development for physical education teachers: The role of informal, collaborative learning. *Journal of Teaching in Physical Education, 26*, 177–200.

Bryan, R. R., McCubbin, J. A., & van der Mars, H. (2013). The ambiguous role of the paraeducator in the general physical education environment. *Adapted Physical Activity Quarterly, 29*, 164–183.

Chambers, F. (2007, May). *How do we prepare physical education teachers for an unknown future?* Seminar presented at the University College Cork, Cork, Ireland.

Daugbjerg, S. B., Kahlmeier, S., Racioppi, S., Martin-Diener, E., Martin, B., Oja, P., et al. (2009). Promotion of physical activity in the European region: Content analysis of 27 national policy documents. *Journal of Physical Activity and Health, 6*, 805–817.

Dodds, P., Placek, J. H., Doolittle, S., Pinkham, K. M., Ratliffe, T. A., & Portman, P. A. (1992). Teacher/coach recruits: Background profiles, occupational decision factors, and comparisons with recruits into other physical education occupations. *Journal of Teaching in Physical Education, 11*, 161–176.

Holt-Reynolds, D. (1992). Personal history-based beliefs as relevant prior knowledge in course work. *American Educational Research Journal, 29*, 325–349.

Lambros, J. (2011). Personal communication.

Lortie, D. C. (2002). *Schoolteacher: A sociological study* (2nd ed.). Chicago: University Of Chicago Press.

Lounsbery, M. A., McKenzie, T. L., Trost. S. G., & Smith, N. J. (2011). Facilitators and barriers to adopting evidence-based physical education in elementary schools. *Journal of Physical Activity & Health, 8*(Suppl. 1), S17–S25.

McCullick, B., Belcher, D., Hardin, B., & Hardin, M. (2003). Butches, bullies and buffoons: Images of physical education teachers in the movies. *Sport, Education and Society, 8*, 3–16.

McCullick, B. A., Lux, K. M., Belcher, D. G., & Davies, N. (2012). A portrait of the PETE major: Re-touched for the early twenty-first century. *Physical Education and Sport Pedagogy, 17*, 177–193.

McKenzie, T. L., & Lounsbery, M. A. F. (2009). School physical education: The pill not taken. *American Journal of Lifestyle Medicine*, 3, 219–225.

O'Sullivan, M., MacPhail, A., & Tannehill, D. (2009). A career in teaching: Decisions of the heart rather than the head. *Irish Educational Studies, 28*, 171–191.

Sallis, J. F. (2010). We do not have to sacrifice children's health to achieve academic goals. *Journal of Pediatrics, 156*, 696–697. doi:10.1016/j.peds.2010.01.001

Schempp, P. (1987, April). *A study of Lortie's "apprenticeship of observation" theory in physical education*. Paper presented at the annual meeting of the American Educational Research Association, Washington, DC.

Siedentop, D., Hastie, P., & van der Mars, H. (2011). *Complete guide to sport education* (2nd ed.). Champaign, IL: Human Kinetics.

Siedentop, D., & Locke, L. F. (1997). Making a difference for physical education: What professors and practitioners must build together. *Journal of Physical Education, Recreation and Dance, 68*(4), 25–33.

Siedentop, D., & van der Mars, H. (2012). *Introduction to physical education, fitness, and sport* (8th ed.). St. Louis, MO: McGraw-Hill.

Tannehill, D., & MacPhail, A. (2012). What examining teaching metaphors tells us about pre-service teachers' developing beliefs about teaching and learning, *Physical Education and Sport Pedagogy*, doi:10.1080/17408989.2012.732056

Timken, G. L., & van der Mars, H. (2009). The effect of case methods on pre-service physical education teachers' value orientations. *Physical Education and Sport Pedagogy, 14*, 169–188.

SECTION II Developing Responsible Learners

Introduction

Most women and men who enter the teaching profession do so because they enjoy teaching and want to help children and youth learn and grow. Most want to learn about teaching skills and strategies to apply them. Most teachers who fail do so because they lack class management skills, which makes it difficult for them to build and maintain a productive learning environment. They tend to have too many discipline problems. In some cases, in order to gain student cooperation, they reduce demands in their instructional system; that is, they make "treaties" that prevent them from sustaining a productive learning environment. If you believe that you simply have to teach well and then all the management and discipline problems will take care of themselves, you are simply wrong!

The chapters in Section II describe the relationship among class management, discipline, and instruction. They also identify skills and strategies you can use to develop a cooperative class and to eventually work toward building a learning community in which students are fully invested in achieving the learning goals of the class. You will learn the importance of preventive strategies and how these, combined with clear and consistent discipline strategies, can form the foundation from which you can work toward developing a community of learners, including all learners in a diverse school population.

Regardless of one's curricular orientation and views of learning, teachers who fail to employ effective class management are doomed to have programs that will not provide students with sufficient opportunities to learn. This area of sport pedagogy probably has the most well-developed empirical base. The focus in this section will be on ensuring that future physical educators become knowledgeable and skilled in employing the kinds of classroom management skills and interpersonal interaction skills that optimize students' opportunity to learn.

CHAPTER 6 Building and Sustaining Student Learning Communities Through Caring and Equitable Pedagogy

Overall Chapter Outcome

To convey the extent to which the caring and equitable pedagogy of the teacher can build and sustain a student (and teacher) learning community in physical education classes

Learning Outcomes

The learner will:

- Outline the dimensions of a caring pedagogy
- Consider an equitable, culturally relevant education for all students
- Describe the Teaching Personal and Social Responsibility model and its relationship to the establishment and maintenance of learning communities
- Consider how prejudices and biases of the student and teacher can affect expectations of a learning community
- Define learning communities
- Describe six characteristics of learning communities
- Identify the potential roles that students and teachers can play in establishing and maintaining a learning community

This chapter engages with what caring pedagogy looks like, appreciating that caring is a way to develop the context within which many positive things can happen for young people in terms of both personal growth and academic achievement. In particular, the chapter focuses on the related aspects of (1) an equitable, culturally relevant education for all students; (2) the ways in which teachers can build a consensus among their students of the necessary behaviors for building and maintaining a productive class environment; and (3) the consideration of prejudices and bias. These aspects, related to a caring pedagogy, are essential before a teacher can effectively encourage students to consider involvement in a learning community that shares similar values and is committed to each other's learning, growth, and welfare.

Physical Education Teachers Who Care

One of the most important educational movements of recent times has been the focus on a **caring pedagogy** (Noddings, 1992). Caring is an umbrella concept that is revealed in many ways as teachers and students interact and as students interact with each other. A caring school and a caring pedagogy protect children and youth and invest in their ongoing development (Chaskin & Mendley-Rauner, 1995). A caring pedagogy also creates the conditions within which children and youth protect the rights and interests of classmates and behave in ways toward their peers that show caring and respect. Caring is not so much a set of specific tools to achieve specific goals as a way to develop the context within which many good things can happen, in terms of both personal growth and academic achievement.

BOX 6.1 Key Terms in This Chapter

- *Antibias teaching:* Achieved by the application of effective, caring teaching skills that allow students to understand that they bring differences to the setting. The goal of antibias teaching is to address these disparities in ways that allow for a growing tolerance, respect, and appreciation of diverse perspectives.
- *Caring pedagogy:* Protects children and youth and invests in their ongoing development. Creates the conditions within which children and youth protect the rights and interests of classmates and behave in ways toward their peers that show caring and respect.
- *Culturally relevant education:* Provides students with the opportunity to engage in activities that prepare them to live in a culturally diverse society. Includes a curriculum that cultivates meaningful, affirming, and equitable learning environments, whereby all students are valued members of the educational community.
- *Learning community:* Exists when students feel valued and supported by their teacher and classmates, are connected to one another, and are committed to each other's learning, growth, and welfare. Students eventually grow to care about each other's successes and failures.
- *Primary prevention:* For physical educators, this means helping children and youth learn how to be responsible for their own behavior and then to act responsibly and helpfully toward their classmates.
- *Teaching personal and social responsibility:* Teachers build a consensus among their students that certain behaviors are necessary for building and maintaining a productive class environment.

The dimensions of caring shown by teachers are remarkably consistent with many of the characteristics of effective teachers. Bosworth (1995) described the following teaching practices that convey caring: (1) helping students with class assignments, (2) valuing students as individuals, (3) treating students respectfully, (4) being tolerant, (5) explaining class tasks and checking for understanding, (6) encouraging and supporting students, and (7) planning class activities that are fun as well as challenging. Teachers who care also show personal attributes such as being nice, liking to help students, being success oriented, and being involved in students' lives, both within and outside of class.

These suggestions are strongly congruent with what Wentzel (1997) found when she investigated the differences between teachers whom students described as "caring" and "not caring." Teachers who were perceived not to care were described as teaching boring classes, ignoring students, embarrassing students, forgetting names, not answering questions, and not correcting work. However, caring does not mean that teachers become overly friendly with students. Teachers are adults and have professional and legal responsibilities for the students under their care.

The Expression, Implementation, and Achievement of Expectations

When we advocate a caring pedagogy, we are not suggesting that social and personal growth (i.e., students feeling good about themselves) be substitutes for a strong focus on learning and performance. We agree with Lipsitz (1995, p. 666), who argued that "the issue is not whether we uphold expectations for our children, but what those expectations will be, how they will be expressed and implemented, and whose shared responsibility it will be to make sure that they are achieved." Teachers do not truly care about students when they fail to offer a challenging and interesting curriculum or fail to translate that curriculum into meaningful class activities. A caring pedagogy certainly is about personal and social growth, but it is also about achievement. Indeed, some evidence (Goodman, Sutton, & Harkavy, 1995; Gorard & See, 2011) suggests that a learning climate characterized by caring and respect promotes learning and performance no matter what instructional strategy or model is used.

We must try to create a synergy between the learning goals and the students' social agendas in physical education. To achieve this, teachers must truly care that their students learn and improve. If the students feel respected and accepted by their teacher and classmates, they are more likely to apply themselves during learning tasks. A caring pedagogy does not avoid challenge, constructive criticism, or mistakes but rather creates a climate in which such features are expected and respected.

Believing that all students can learn, and trying to act on that belief, does not mean all students learn in the same way or should achieve the same outcomes. Children and youth are different in their talents, previous experiences, interests, and expectations. To the extent possible, within the demands of class size, facilities, and equipment, caring teachers make every effort to accommodate these differences.

The Influence of the Teacher's Personal Biography on Caring for Students

The personal biography of a teacher has been found to have a strong influence on teachers caring for their students (Lortie, 2002). Larson and Silverman (2005) more recently supported this concept with respect to physical education teachers. They examined four caring physical education teachers' rationale(s) for exhibiting caring behaviors towards their students. Through formal and informal interviews, along with observations of teaching, these teachers ascribed their conduct to a strong desire to develop and maintain relationships with their students such that growth and/or well-being was fostered. As Larson and Silverman report, "In large part this was due to their personal biography—the positive physical activity experiences they had while growing up and the role models they encountered—and their recognition of how this contributed to their development of positive self-esteem and feeling of self-worth, and their subsequent interest in ensuring that those in their charge could garner the same benefits" (p. 188). Larson (2006) extended her work by exploring student perceptions of caring teaching in physical education. **Box 6.2** lists students' responses around clusters that reflected teachers' demonstration of caring. Of the incidences of caring analyzed, 56% of the in-class incidents were content-related, and 42% were non-content-related. Further analysis of the clusters in Box 6.2 resulted in the emergence of three subcategories of behaviors that pertained to the phenomenon of caring teaching behavior: (1) recognize me, (2) help me learn, and (3) trust/respect me. The main category for all the results was suggested as "pay attention to me," acknowledging that students are particularly perceptive and appreciative of instances where teachers recognize, respect, and notice some aspect of their individuality or learning progress, and foster learning achievement.

BOX 6.2 Clusters of Behavior of Physical Education Teachers Identified as Caring by Students

- Showed me how to do a skill
- Honored my request
- Gave me a compliment
- Confronted my behavior
- Inquired about my health
- Attended to me when I was injured
- Allowed me to redo my test
- Motivated me
- Played/participated with me during class
- Persuaded me
- Showed concern for my future health

Reproduced from Larson, A. (2006). Student perception of caring teaching in physical education. *Sport, Education and Society, 11*, 4. Taylor & Francis Ltd., reprinted by permission of the publisher (Taylor & Francis Ltd, www.tandf.co.uk/journals).

Learning Experience 6.1

Revisit the cluster of behaviors listed in Box 6.2 that students identified as caring behavior of physical education teachers. As you gain opportunities to teach in your program of study or in a school setting, consider the extent to which you convey such behaviors in a teaching episode. What determines your enactment of such behaviors? Do you tend to rely on one or two behaviors at the expense of others?

A Culturally Relevant Education

Individuals preparing to become teachers need to acquire the knowledge and skills to work effectively with all students, and they need to strengthen their predisposition to use their knowledge and skill to provide an equitable, **culturally relevant education** for all students. The Cultural Studies curriculum model responds to changing cultural and social circumstances with respect to sport in society. The model "attempts to offer physical educators an opportunity to help students appreciate and critique the role of physical activity and sport in their own lives, the life of their schools, their community, and the wider society" (O'Sullivan & Kinchin, 2010, p. 104).

What is absolutely clear is that (1) students in schools are increasingly diverse; (2) our society has historic inequities that prevent us from achieving the ideal of a democratic, humane, and just society; and (3) the global community is increasingly interconnected (Osler, 2005; Wan, 2008).

Not all students attend schools that are culturally diverse, but those who attend essentially mono-cultural schools will have to work and live in a culturally diverse society. Their education will be incomplete if they are not prepared to do this. The goal described at the start of this section (i.e., to give teachers the knowledge, skills, and predispositions to provide an equitable, culturally relevant education) is not easy to achieve for teachers or teachers in training who expect to teach students who are much like themselves and have little experience with students who are different (Young, 1998). We are not suggesting that teachers are intentionally biased or mean-spirited toward those different from themselves. However, the evidence suggests that knowledge of, and attitudes toward, diverse students are typically based on stereotypical images held by families and communities and strongly fostered by the media (Coakley, 2008; Lester & Ross, 2011). This is what one might expect when persons have not had the opportunity to learn from close, personal relationships with diverse children and youth. It is thus no wonder

BOX 6.3 Am I Ready to Be Effective in a Diverse Class?

- Am I knowledgeable about the cultural, linguistic, and socioeconomic backgrounds of the students I teach and the community from which they come?
- In my own behavior, do I model respect for, and inclusion of, persons who are different from myself?
- Do students perceive me to be sincerely interested in and respectful of contributions made by minority groups and individuals?
- Have I used, or do I know where to find, resources to help me combat and confront bias based on gender, race, religion, or socioeconomic status?
- Am I able and willing to recognize and constructively address conflicts that arise based on gender, race, religion, or socioeconomic status?

Adapted from Eisenhower National Clearinghouse for Mathematics and Science Education. (n.d.). *Common bonds: Anti-bias teaching in a diverse society.* Columbus, OH.

that many beginning teachers are frightened at the prospect of teaching in diverse schools, and their expectations for student performance and behavior are often stereotypical and inadequate. **Box 6.3** poses a series of questions you can ask yourself to judge your current capacity to work effectively in a diverse school. In reading Box 6.3, you are prompted to consider the awareness of your own struggle with bias; the country's deeply rooted historical, social, cultural, and political structures; and how these structures impact the teaching of all young people. In encouraging teachers to make a positive difference through culturally responsive and inclusive practices, Timken and Watson (2010) urge teachers to (1) be socioculturally conscious, (2) hold affirming attitudes toward students from diverse backgrounds, (3) embrace the constructivist view of learning, (4) learn about students and their communities, and (5) be an agent of change. As Timken and Watson explain, "Culturally responsive and inclusive teaching is not a separate instructional method to use sporadically . . . It is a frame of mind and a commitment to daily teaching practices that cultivates meaningful, affirming, and equitable learning environments, whereby all students are valued members of the educational community" (p. 148).

Learning Experience 6.2

After reading and considering Box 6.3 we encourage you to engage with an activity commonly referred to as *community mapping*. "Community mapping is a process that promotes increased interaction between the school and the local environs, engaging teachers and students in systematic information gathering about the use of the community in the planning of your teaching and in optimizing the learning of your students" (O'Sullivan, Tannehill, & Hinchion, 2010, p. 58).

How many times have you walked through your community on your way to school or driven down the same streets en route to work? Most of us do one or the other on a daily basis, yet fail to take note of the various types of buildings, assortment of businesses, events on offer to the public, and variety of activities available, all of which make up the community. If we really look, we will see an assortment of indications of the feel of the community that will help us better understand the nature of the community and the types of experiences community members might have. In our busy daily lives filled with family, work, and our own interests we seldom notice other aspects of the community that make it what it is.

Every school resides in a community that is located in a neighborhood, town, or city. In every country, each of these communities has a history, culture, unique geography, special traditions, annual events, public policies, laws, and ethos that guide the daily lives of its people. Treadway (2000) prompts us that, "The relationship between a community and a school should be a two-way street since both have something to offer each other but making that a reality requires that teachers know both what is available and how to make use of that knowledge" (p. 2). With that in mind, conduct community mapping in the neighborhood in which you will be teaching. This community mapping exercise will provide you with the knowledge of what and who are available in your community that might assist you in developing the knowledge, skills, and abilities of your students in a holistic way.

By learning about this community, particularly about its youth outreach and its sport, recreation, and leisure infrastructure, the intention is for you to reflect on what you have learned and how it might impact your understanding of the education of these young people and the ways in which you might link your lessons to opportunities for engagement in sport and physical activity after school. It is anticipated that by doing this you will be able to document the assets and issues of living in this community. In addition, reflect on what you learn about the community and how you can use this information and interactions with people in the community to better connect lessons to the lives of the students you will teach at this site.

Tools you might use for this community mapping include observation, note taking, interviews with community members, discussions with shopkeepers and others who live and work in this community, tourist information brochures, community Internet sites, community maps, and your own photos.

Your specific task: As you collect this information and visual artifacts, create an electronic display of your community and a textual interpretation that tells the community story, implications for student learning, and how it might link to your work with young people in physical education.

Students are often disadvantaged in physical education because of gender, skillfulness, physical appearance, and race. Some of this disadvantage comes from teacher insensitivity or lack of skillfulness, including unequal expectations, differential interaction patterns, and biased selection of activities. Much of it, however, comes from teachers being unaware of, or ignoring, how students treat each other.

Young Peoples' Treatment of Each Other: Caring for Each Other

Everybody who has spent time in physical education classes or on playgrounds observing children and youth in activity understands that students can and do disadvantage and abuse one another, and groups of students are stereotyped and often ostracized from a fair opportunity to participate. The predictable result is student alienation from physical education as a school subject and, subsequently, from a physically active lifestyle. There is a general appreciation that there will be disparities in participation and achievement of students during group work relative to student status. In a study conducted by Brock, Rovegno, and Oliver (2009), economic level, attractiveness, athletic involvement, and personality defined student status on group interactions and decisions. Consequently, this affected whose opinions were acknowledged and which students were silenced. Although the authors qualify that status is specific to the environment and defined by the student culture, it is likely that regardless of environment and school culture there will always be those students who are resigned to never having the required status to be actively involved in the dynamics of group work. It is for these students that we as teachers need to consider how we can best create an environment that enables and encourages equitable interaction and participation.

Student Voice and Choice

Two points for consideration that nicely link our understanding and appreciation between a culturally relevant education and an equity pedagogy are listening to the voices of the students we teach and the co-construction of the physical education curriculum (what Glasby and Macdonald [2004] term a "negotiated curriculum") between teachers and students. Both have the potential to convey to students that "they are legitimate members of the schooling system, and acknowledge that a worthwhile school experience relies on the pupils [students] and teacher informing each others' learning. That is, the teachers' practice of teaching is integrated with and through pupil consultation and subsequent participation" (MacPhail, 2010, p. 229).

In sharing ideas about maximizing participation in physical activities, Stiehl, Morris, and Sinclair (2008) discuss the importance of "change, challenge and choice." That is, providing students with choices among suitable challenges (either offered by the teacher or options generated by the students) will often necessitate changes to an existing activity. Although it may be common practice for the teacher to make most of the decisions about such changes, the authors encourage us to shift the decision making to students, anticipating that this will result in increasing students' interest and involvement as well as gaining a stronger sense of independence and ownership.

An Equity Pedagogy for a Culturally Relevant Education

We propose three profiles related to issues of diversity and bias in teaching: (1) a profile of unacceptable characteristics that result in inequitable, biased learning environments; (2) a profile of acceptable strategies that result in an equitable pedagogy of caring; and (3) a profile of preferred strategies that move beyond a pedagogy of caring to antibias teaching that confronts issues of bias and helps students resolve them within the learning community. An equity pedagogy is defined as "teaching strategies and classroom environments that help students from diverse racial, ethnic, and cultural groups attain the knowledge, skills, and attitudes needed to function effectively within, and help create and perpetuate, a just, humane, and democratic society" (McGee-Banks & Banks,1995, p. 152).

Profile 1: Unacceptable Characteristics That Result in Inequitable, Biased Learning Environments

Using the equity pedagogy definition, identifying the unacceptable teaching profile is fairly easy. In physical education, we find it unacceptable for teachers to create and sustain learning environments within which teachers (1) interact differentially with students based on race, gender, socioeconomic status, or motor skillfulness; (2) communicate differential expectations based on those features; (3) provide more academic feedback to some individuals/groups than others; (4) make gender- or race-stereotyped statements (see **Box 6.4**); (5) let skilled students dominate practice and games; (6) use sexist language in teaching; (7) ignore student gender and cultural differences in choice of activities; (8) ignore and do not intervene in biased interactions among students; and (9) ignore and do not intervene when students harass, intimidate, and/or embarrass one another.

All the characteristics of this profile have been documented from observation of classes in physical education. It is not difficult to change this profile. The teaching skills that need to be instituted are fairly straightforward, sensitive, equitable interaction patterns; that is:

- Thoughtful curricular planning
- Appropriate modeling
- Careful, sensitive monitoring of student behavior
- Intervention strategies to remediate and develop equitable, pro-social behavior and interactions among students

What is more difficult is for teachers to understand that this profile is unacceptable and then make the commitment to see that it gets changed.

BOX 6.4 Avoiding Sexist Language in Teaching and Coaching

Sport has traditionally been male oriented. Many of the common terms in sport are, therefore, male-oriented terms. There are alternatives, and they should be used.

Sexist terms:	*Nonsexist equivalents:*
Guard your man closely	Guard your opponent closely
We don't have the manpower to win	We don't have the depth to win
Second baseman	Second base player
The defenseman	The defense
Three-man teams	Three-person teams
Third man (lacrosse)	Third player
Boys' and girls' push-ups	Extended and knee push-ups
Man-to-man defense	Player-to-player defense
Sportsmanship	Fair play

Learning Experience 6.3

Can you think of any other contributions to add to the sexist terms list in Box 6.4, and appropriate alternatives under nonsexist equivalents? Are you aware of the extent to which you may use sexist terms when you teach and/or coach? What can you do in an attempt to correct inappropriate use?

Profile 2: Acceptable Strategies That Result in an Equitable Pedagogy of Caring

To move from the unacceptable profile to the acceptable profile requires that an equitable pedagogy of caring be developed and sustained. We have already provided the basic description of a caring pedagogy. In this section, we add the application of a caring pedagogy to learning environments of diverse learners. In an important sense, all physical education classes are diverse learning environments because they usually have both boys and girls and they have students at markedly different skill levels. Bias based on gender and skillfulness has been one of the historic inequities of physical education.

A caring pedagogy in a diverse learning environment requires more than good intentions. It requires skills and knowledge that relate diversity issues to pedagogy and subject-matter knowledge (McGee-Banks & Banks, 1995). This would include knowledge about racism, sexism, stereotypes, prejudice, and institutional bias. It also suggests that teachers understand the histories, characteristics, and intragroup differences among major racial and ethnic groups. It is, for example, nearly impossible for teachers to truly respect cultural differences among students and to communicate that respect to their students if they do not have accurate knowledge of those differences and are, instead, gaining knowledge primarily from media stereotypes.

Learning Experience 6.4

Inequity exists at both the individual and institutional levels. Prejudice at either level is unfortunate, and because much power is vested in institutions, inequitable treatment at that level is particularly disabling. A gender inequity at an individual level would entail parents allowing their son, but not their daughter, to play on teams. A gender inequity at an institutional level would entail a school providing twice the support for a boys' team that it does for a girls' team. Can you provide other examples of inequitable treatment at the individual and institutional levels? To what extent do you consider such treatment is intentional?

The teaching skill profile for an equity pedagogy would begin by reversing all of the negative characteristics of the profile previously described. Interactions would be equitable. Expectations would be positive and equitably challenging for all students. Curricular decisions would take differences into account. Modeling, prompting, and feedback would be equitable and appropriate. All students would have equal opportunity to participate, to provide leadership, and to have their voices heard. Skilled students and boys would not dominate participation. Harassment or embarrassment of students by students would be proactively prevented and remediated immediately when it did occur. This is probably the easy part of this shift from unacceptable to acceptable; it can be accomplished by observing and providing feedback about teaching practices and behavior and then monitoring student activity.

This chapter is about developing **learning communities** in physical education and the role of a caring pedagogy within that framework. A major characteristic of learning communities is the common commitment to fairness and caring about one another. A caring pedagogy is meant to establish and sustain a fair learning environment, within which members care about and respect one another. A learning community of diverse learners cannot be built or sustained, however, without the learners themselves coming to grips with their cultural differences and learning to understand and respect classmates who come from backgrounds different from theirs. Students have to feel safe to share their concerns, to disagree with classmates, and to participate in discourse and activities that are intended to build respect and community. A learning community has to be open and challenging, yet also highly supportive, if it is to be a safe learning space (Young, 1998). Most students have had little experience expressing deep concerns about gender, race, ethnicity, and socioeconomic status. Their initial efforts might be halting and clumsy. They might well fear being ridiculed by their classmates. The learning space needs to be "hospitable not to make learning painless but to make the painful things possible" (Palmer, 1993, p. 74).

Profile 3: Preferred Strategies That Move Beyond a Pedagogy of Caring to Antibias Teaching

To move from the acceptable profile to what we believe to be a preferred profile, teachers must be willing to plan for and implement activities that confront inequities and help students develop the knowledge and predispositions to become advocates for equity and fairness throughout their lives. This is not to suggest, however, that within this preferred profile, teachers do not focus on helping students become competent in the subject matter of physical education. The issue is that all students should achieve success, and that cannot happen if the learning environment is inequitable and not culturally relevant to students from different backgrounds. What is added to this main agenda is making the confrontation of bias, particularly as it relates to physical activity and sport, a part of the content that students master, in terms of both knowledge and skills. In the preferred profile, a strong element of **antibias teaching** is added within the learning community. **Box 6.5** asks another series of questions that will allow you to assess the degree to which you engage in antibias teaching.

BOX 6.5 To What Degree Am I Engaged in Antibias Teaching?

- Do my students see me as actively confronting instances of stereotyping, bias, and discrimination when they occur?
- Do I teach and encourage students to understand and respect the feelings and points of view of others who are different than them?
- Do my students understand that I do not judge student performance based on race, gender, or socioeconomic differences?
- Do I plan activities that help students to identify prejudice and discriminatory practices in physical activity and sport?
- Do I help students to develop skills and predispositions to respond appropriately to instances of bias, discrimination, and harassment?
- Do I plan activities that help students to examine and analyze how class, race, and gender in physical activity and sport are represented in the media, school, and local community?

Learning Experience 6.5

As you consider the extent to which you do or do not engage in antibias teaching by responding to the questions in Box 6.5, provide evidence for instances where you respond positively to the questions posed (e.g., in what way do students see you actively confront inappropriate instances?). In instances where you answer no to any of the questions, suggest ways in which you can change your practices to move towards antibias teaching.

We are not suggesting that antibias teaching should take the form of an "in your face" confrontation. Such an approach would effectively eliminate the notion of a safe learning place described earlier. In diverse learning communities, students will understand that they bring differences to the setting. The goal should be to address these disparities in ways that allow for a growing tolerance, respect, and appreciation of diverse perspectives.

Students will exhibit biases in nearly all physical education classes. Evidence indicates that gender bias is nearly always present in physical education (Flintoff & Scraton, 2006; Gard, 2006; Oliver & McCaughtry, 2011; Penney, 2002). Both boys and girls tend to reproduce in class the gender-appropriate roles they have learned in the wider community and from the media. Failure on the part of teachers to address the limitations of these roles serves inadvertently to reinforce them. Teachers who work to provide an equitable learning environment, not only as regards gender but also race, ethnic heritage, and skillfulness, will ensure that all students get equal attention and opportunity to participate and to have their voices heard. This would be a vast improvement over many current conditions, working towards an antibias pedagogy that brings stereotypes in sport and physical activity to the attention of all students and creates the conditions within which these stereotypes can be broken down. This would empower all students to take full advantage of their physical capabilities and to broaden their horizons about what is possible for them in physical activity and sport.

Antibias teaching does not require any new or remarkable teaching skills or strategies. It does require the motivation to attempt it and the perseverance to see it through. How do teachers address these issues? First, they make them part of the content of physical education and willingly give time to address the issues. This, in one sense, is analogous to our argument that the time taken at the beginning of the year to establish class routines and procedures is more than compensated for by increased effectiveness throughout the school year. The difference here is that issues of bias in physical activity and sport are legitimate content issues for physical educators to pursue. Students need time to be made aware of these issues and to process them through discussion and activity.

Teachers also use many different teaching skills to make their antibias teaching effective. They develop and enforce class rules and routines that make it clear that biased behavior is inappropriate. They prompt students in situations where inequities might arise. They utilize antistereotyping comments ("Ron, Glenda is the best setter on your team. You should get the ball to her as often as possible."). They avoid sexist language (see Box 6.4). They use corrective feedback to correct stereotyped or biased comments or actions ("Jake, don't say Tom throws like a girl. Girls can learn to throw as well as boys can. I want you to think about how Tom and the girls feel when that is said."). They use girls as demonstrators as often as boys and not just for activities too often labeled "girls'" activities. They utilize antistereotyping role models (e.g., bulletin boards to include female basketball players and male dancers). They invite antistereotyping guests to class (e.g., girls from the school who have gone on to athletic success). They utilize universal representation in class examples, choices of leaders, and representations on bulletin boards (e.g., in fitness units, they do not always use slim, ultrafit, highly attractive persons with certain body types but rather show that fit persons come in all sizes, shapes, and looks). They consistently reinforce with their students the notion that sustained effort, rather than innate ability, is the key to achievement. They assign antistereotyping tasks within class and as homework (e.g., review how girls are shown in advertisements related to sport products, assess the amount of space or time given to women's sports in the local newspaper or television station, analyze the kinds of sports that African Americans are associated with in television advertisements, analyze the access to and costs of recreational opportunities in various socioeconomic areas of a community). They promote equity through celebrations that emphasize multicultural awareness or the accomplishments of persons who have experienced bias. They shape class discussions around incidents of bias outside of class and gradually help students discuss their feelings about bias in their own lives and within their own class. They develop agreements with students about how class and small-group discussions are conducted (see **Box 6.6**). They use "why are" questions for discussions that reveal institutional bias (e.g., Why are most head coaches white? Why are girls less active during school recess? Why are boys more likely to hog the ball in games?). They select culturally sensitive activities and help extend the students' understanding of activity biases and stereotypes in the wider culture. They group students and assign leadership roles in ways that both ensure equity and allow for advances in the general antibias agenda of their teaching. Oliver's (2010) work focuses on how to understand students (predominantly girls) through collaborating with them to practice strategies for changing body and physical activity inequalities as they see them.

BOX 6.6 Ground Rules for Discussions

If there are any special teaching skills related to antibias teaching, they are most likely to be in conducting class and small-group discussions, simply because discussions are not as commonly used in teaching physical education as they are in classroom subjects. Students will need clear ground rules, practice, and feedback to learn to participate in ways that are consistent with the tenets of a learning community. They are likely to talk over one another, blame one another, and take disagreements personally. Following is one set of ground rules developed for a South Carolina curriculum to fight bigotry:

- Listen patiently and carefully to each student who speaks.
- Express yourself honestly and openly.
- Search for truth from each person's perspective.
- Avoid shaming, belittling, or blaming.
- Maintain each person's confidentiality.

Students need to learn that offensive remarks hurt. They hurt the target of the remark, they eventually hurt the person who makes the remark, and they certainly negatively affect the spirit of the community.

Adapted from Roefs, W. (1998). Better together. *Teaching Tolerance, 7*(2), 34–41.

And, of course, teachers do this using the skills associated with a caring pedagogy, so that students are not threatened but rather feel safe and secure to express themselves both to the teacher and to their classmates, understanding that they will be respected and supported in their efforts to grow and contribute to the learning community. In other words, antibias teaching is forwarded by the application of effective, caring teaching skills.

Finally, the goals of antibias teaching are much easier to reach if the school or, where appropriate, the school district has policies and programs that support such efforts. We have known for some time that schools that have common, consistent behavioral expectations and discipline codes are more effective. We have known for some time that primary schools in which approaches to teaching reading are similar from class to class produce more effective readers. The lesson to be learned from this is that consistency throughout schools and districts results in much stronger outcomes. **Box 6.7** shows how one school district has supported antibias teaching.

Teaching Personal and Social Responsibility

Effective discipline and behavior management are best achieved through a set of proactive strategies, the goal of

BOX 6.7 How District Policy Can Support Antibias Teaching

The Durham School District (North Carolina) approved an antiracism and ethno-cultural equity implementation policy in 1995. The policy set in motion a series of districtwide programs, the major focus of which is the area of curriculum. Among the initiatives are the following:

- Students participate in a 5-day Students Together Against Racism (STAR) program to build student leadership skills and develop plans to combat discrimination and create an environment of social harmony in schools.
- Staff participates in antiracism training and forms antiracism resource teams in schools.
- Antidiscrimination curriculum units are developed at all levels.
- All curricula are reviewed to detect bias and stereotyping.
- An Ethno-cultural Equity and Race Relations department was created to provide in-service education and consult with the antiracism resource teams.
- Antibias employment practices were instituted.
- New teachers are oriented to the program and receive mentoring.

A teacher's efforts to develop and sustain an antibias teaching agenda would be very much enhanced by district policies similar to these. What policies exist in districts/regions in your area?

which is the development and maintenance of appropriate student behavior. All teachers must come to grips with what they believe to be appropriate behavior in physical education classes. This will include behavior in three major categories: (1) interactions between the teacher and students, (2) interactions among students, and (3) interactions with the physical environment (e.g., equipment, facilities). Because context and personal beliefs are important in this area, we do not suggest specific behaviors within these categories. What is important, however, is that teachers build a consensus among their students that the behaviors that are necessary within each category are the right ones for building and maintaining a productive class environment. Only through consensus building can students come to view the behavior norms within a class as "our" norms rather than "her" or "his" norms. When this is done correctly, students and teachers establish what amounts to a social contract that students believe in and help sustain.

Teachers have a much easier time promoting appropriate behavior in their classes if there is a school-wide set of norms for behavior. The likelihood of students feeling that behavior norms are "ours" is very much enhanced by adoption of school-wide behavior norms that all teachers expect and support. Finnicum (1997) argues that physical education teachers should practice *primary prevention*, a concept borrowed from medicine. **Primary prevention** refers to altering the environment to reduce the likelihood that diseases will develop (e.g., creating a safe supply of drinking water in a neighborhood or ensuring that all infants are vaccinated). Secondary prevention refers to detecting the early signs of disease and initiating treatment. The most important kind of primary prevention for physical education teachers is helping children and youth learn how to be responsible for their own behavior and then to act responsibly and helpfully toward their classmates.

The Teaching Personal and Social Responsibility (TPSR) Model

Fortunately, physical education has a well-tested model for achieving the goals of primary prevention—the **Teaching Personal and Social Responsibility** (TPSR) model developed by Don Hellison (2010; Hellison & Walsh, 2002). The model provides a progression of goals through which students move toward becoming fully responsible citizens of the physical education class and extend those behaviors and values outside of class. The goals of TPSR are as follows (Hellison, 2010):[1]

Goal 1: Respect for the rights and feelings of others

- Maintaining self-control
- Respecting everyone's right to be included
- Respecting everyone's right to a peaceful resolution of conflicts

Goal 2: Participation and effort

- Learning what effort means in different situations
- Being willing to try new things
- Developing an optimistic yet realistic sense of personal success

Goal 3: Self-direction

- Staying on task independent of teacher supervision
- Developing a sound knowledge base
- Developing, implementing, and evaluating personal plans
- Learning to work for deferred consequences

[1] Reproduced from Hellison, D. (2010). *Teaching personal and social responsibility through physical activity* (3rd ed.). Champaign, IL: Human Kinetics.

Goal 4: Caring: sensitivity and responsiveness to the well-being of others

- Learning appropriate interpersonal skills
- Helping others without prompting or external rewards
- Contributing to the good of the group
- Being sensitive about other students and expressing that appropriately

Goal 5: Generalizing outcomes: responsibility outside of physical education

- Consideration of the relevance of the four previous goals in a number of settings
- Application of the four other goals in the playground, at school, at home, and in the wider community

Hellison (2010) suggests that respect is the first issue in the learning progression because the class is a community in which the rights of all classmates must be protected. Understanding TPSR as a progression does not mean that you teach respect first, then participation, as if learning about and practicing being respectful is now completed. To the contrary, you must revisit each goal in the progression again and again as you move toward the higher goals.

Many teachers who use the TPSR model rely on turning these goals into a set of levels that provide a simple vocabulary and set of concepts that allow teachers and their students to understand, think about, prompt, and evaluate the level of their personal and social responsibility (Hellison, 2010):[2]

- *Level 0: Irresponsibility.* Students make excuses, blame others, and often deny personal responsibility for what they do and what they fail to do.
- *Level 1: Respect.* Students may not participate well in class activities or show improvement, but they are in sufficient control that they do not interfere with classmates or the teacher; and they maintain this self-control without constant teacher supervision.
- *Level 2: Participation.* Students not only show respect, but also participate fully in class activities.
- *Level 3: Self-direction.* Students not only participate and show respect, but also are able to work without direct supervision and can begin to plan, implement, and evaluate some of their own physical education.
- *Level 4: Caring.* Students not only show respect, participate, and engage in self-directed activities but also support and show concern for classmates and are willing to help others.

The levels provide teachers a shorthand method of communicating with students and an easy system for students to evaluate their own progress. Questions like "What level are you at now, Billy?" or "What do you need to do to move to level 3?" are common. The levels also provide students and teachers a way to learn about what behaviors are examples of each level.

The Enactment of TPSR

The degree to which any teacher has to rely on TPSR as a way of helping young people learn how to treat themselves and others well will differ from school to school and often among classes within the same school. For some teachers, who are confronted with many young people who exhibit level 0 or level 1 behavior frequently, TPSR should become the main goal of the curriculum until most students are at level 3. For teachers in these situations, Hellison (2010) has suggested a range of instructional strategies to teach personal and social responsibility. The two fundamental strategies are "awareness talks" and "experiencing the levels" because the success of this model depends upon all students being fully aware of the levels and learning what the behaviors at the various levels look and feel like.

Teachers who utilize TPSR most often display the levels on large posters so students can see them and refer to them when needed and as constant reminders of the importance of personal and social responsibility.

Awareness talks are brief episodes during which teacher and students discuss levels and various behaviors that are positive and negative examples of a level. These talks can occur at the start of class, at any teachable moment (when an event in class provides an opportunity for learning about the levels), or as a closure during which students reflect on and evaluate their own behavior. One teacher developed a large "target poster" with level 4 as the bulls-eye and the other levels as outer rings of the circle target. When children leave the gymnasium, this teacher has them file past the target and touch the level at which they feel they operated during that class, which is a form of reflection and self-evaluation (Hellison, 2010).

Teachers use various ways to help students experience the levels. Partner tasks require both respect between partners and participation. Self-paced challenges allow for beginning experiences in self-direction. Children learning the concept of personal space and how to maintain it, while moving among classmates who also are in motion, can learn that doing so is an important form of respect. Cooperative learning tasks can help teach respect (Parker & Stiehl, 2010), as can involvement as a team member in a sport season (Siedentop, Hastie, & van der Mars, 2011). Helping spot classmates in a tumbling activity, acting as a retriever for a classmate practicing tennis serves, or fulfilling the role of coach or squad leader can help students experience caring behaviors that are examples of level 4. It also is important that students be taught a specific

[2] Reproduced from Hellison, D. (2010). *Teaching personal and social responsibility through physical activity* (3rd ed.). Champaign, IL: Human Kinetics.

form of conflict resolution. One example students might benefit from is a "talking bench" where they go to talk out their conflict with the contingency that settling the issue is necessary for them to return to activity.

For other teachers, who work with students who have had basic opportunities to learn respect and participate with at least some measure of effort, the TPSR model can be used along with teaching a specific curriculum such as Adventure Education or Sport Education.

Teaching personal and social responsibility may become a significant part of the physical education curriculum for certain classes. Alternatively, it might become an initial unit in the school year for students with whom a teacher has not worked previously. Or it may become embedded in activity units as part of a general classroom management system, thus accounting for only a small part of the overall lesson planning and implementation. However, children and youth do not always grow in personal and social responsibility as an automatic outcome of being involved in sport or fitness activities. To the contrary, such activities have the potential to teach students to be followers or self-directed, to be selfish or caring, to be respectful or abusive of their classmates. The activities themselves tend to be neutral, but they provide the opportunity for students to learn to be one kind of person or another. If you want your students to be personally and socially responsible in the sense described, make sure these values and the behaviors that reflect them are taught effectively and the learning environment is conducive to students understanding, practicing, and improving them.

Once a teacher has developed a caring, culturally relevant, nonbiased environment for the students, potentially through enacting the TPSR model, then students are in a better space to consider how to most effectively contribute to a physical education learning community that encourages them to share similar values and commit to each other's learning, growth, and welfare. The remainder of the chapter engages with the development of a student learning community before unpacking the six characteristics of a learning community. Examples of how to develop learning communities in physical education are then shared.

Defining and Developing a Learning Community

The climate of your classes and your relationships with the students you teach can be characterized by compliance, cooperation, or community. For schools to be effective in meeting their goals, students must comply with rules and procedures. When students comply primarily in order to avoid punishments, the climate of classes is typically not positive, and learning goals are more difficult to achieve. When students actively cooperate in following rules and implementing class procedures, the climate of classes improves markedly, and student performance is likely to improve. The next step would be to build and sustain a learning community within your classes. If you were to successfully develop a learning community, you would likely have students who do the following (Brophy, 2010):

- Are supportive of each other
- Take responsibility for their own actions
- Hold themselves accountable for class success
- Cooperate with one another
- Trust each other
- Feel empowered to make decisions
- Feel positive about the class identity
- Are committed to core values of fairness and caring

Doesn't that sound like the kind of class that would optimize the learning potential of all the students? Doesn't that describe the kind of class you would enjoy teaching? The problem, of course, is that this idyllic state of affairs doesn't just happen. Learning communities have to be developed and then sustained. Many schools are now trying to put in place some of the organizational features that contribute to community building. The challenge to build learning communities has grown out of the belief among an increasing number of educators that children and youth will not only experience positive social growth and develop the values that will help them become productive citizens, but also improve their academic performance and be more likely to become self-directed learners. Having students become self-directed learners means that they must be afforded the opportunity to practice making decisions, and teachers must be willing to not feel that they have to be in control of everything.

Learning Experience 6.6

Reflect back to instances you experienced as a student at school that encouraged you to be a self-directed learner on your own and/or in a group. Share what some of these experiences were. List characteristics of the teaching environment and attributes of the teacher that encouraged such self-directed learning.

It is important to emphasize that learning communities are not necessarily synonymous with working in groups. Both are likely to include individuals with different abilities, interests, and self-esteem, while perhaps allowing personal choices, personal accountability, and decision making. However, students in successful learning communities are supportive, responsible, accountable, cooperative, trusting, empowered, identified with the class, and committed to fairness and caring. Learning communities are more focused on acknowledging and accommodating individual characteristics over a longer period of time than is usually afforded when working in a group.

A learning community exists when students feel valued, supported by their teacher and classmates, connected to one another, and committed to each other's learning, growth, and welfare (Lewis, Schaps, & Watson, 1995; Schaps & Lewis, 1998). Learning communities are not gimmicks, nor are they an educational fad. You cannot just decide one day that learning communities sound like a good thing and expect to develop one the next week. Learning communities have specific characteristics that take time and effort to develop. They are bounded environments that persist over time. It also takes time and effort to sustain learning communities. Members share important common goals, and they cooperate to achieve those goals. They share allegiance to significant symbols and take part together in rituals that emphasize their community. Schools that serve diverse, heterogeneous groups of learners are not easy places within which to develop learning communities, but when they do develop, they can be powerful in their impact on academic and social outcomes.

Six Characteristics of Learning Communities

Boundaries

Communities have boundaries that set them apart. Boundaries can be physical, symbolic, or conceptual. Creating smaller school organizations within a large school is not uncommon in the United States, where class sizes in urban postprimary schools regularly reach 40 to 45. In such instances, a common practice is to split the total school population into smaller "schools" to afford the teachers and students some sense of community. Another system that attempts to create boundaries within which school communities can develop is the *house system*, where schools randomly allocate students to particular "houses" (i.e., groupings of students) for pastoral care (looking after the personal and social well-being of children/youth) as well as encouraging group loyalty through having houses compete with one another at, for example, sporting events. A curriculum that has a clear focus creates a boundary and, pursued to a larger scale, this is one of the features of magnet schools (see www.magnet.edu), where the whole school curriculum is themes based (e.g., where a school prepares students to function in a diverse society), and helps to eliminate, reduce, or prevent longstanding patterns of racial isolation. Indeed, a focused curriculum is a primary feature of school learning communities.

Persistence

A group meant to develop into a community must persist over time, simply because it takes time to develop shared values, pursue common goals, and develop mutual respect and caring. Some postprimary schools are experimenting with having one teacher stay with the same class for several years instead of the class having a different teacher at the start of each school year or changing teachers within the same subject area. In countries with primary physical education specialists, there is a unique opportunity to work with all young children. These are organizational changes that could be accomplished at very little cost and reap many potential benefits as regards the promotion, and subsequent benefits, of learning communities.

Common Goals

Students sharing common goals is different from students sharing similar goals. Common goals exist when success is defined collectively. This is opposite to situations in which some students can succeed only to the extent that others fail. In most schools, academic work is defined individually. In learning communities, educators seek ways to increase the collective pride in, and benefit from, individual successes. Class goals become important. Students applaud and celebrate the successes of classmates because they contribute to the larger, collective goals for the common good of the community.

Learning Experience 6.7

Identify a particular learning outcome or learning goal for school physical education. Consider the way in which the following individuals, working together to contribute to a learning community, could complement each other's strengths by working towards the learning outcome/learning goal:

- A student who has poor movement skills but does not appear inhibited in taking part in physical education
- A student who is physically talented in most physical activities but gets frustrated at their peers' lack of physical ability in particular activities
- A student who has poor language skills and tends to rely, very successfully, on mirroring what their peers do in response to direction from the teacher rather than being prompted by the teacher directly
- An overweight student who has difficulty in undertaking some physical activities due to a limited level of fitness, but who is genuinely interested in helping others

Cooperation

There are numerous ways students can learn about, and eventually engage in, cooperative learning and associated practices. Cooperative learning is widely seen as a solution to many of the problems of instruction in heterogeneous classrooms (Cohen, 1994). Cooperative learning is an instructional model in which students work together in small, structured groups to master the content of the lesson. The teacher's role is to clarify practice goals, ensure tasks are understood, demonstrate appropriate behavior, supply direction, set time limits, state objectives clearly, facilitate learning by monitoring group progress, and provide instruction and guidance in effective group techniques. Students can be performers, recorders, observers, presenters, timers, leaders, and collectors (Hannon & Ratliffe, 2004).

Striving to achieve group goals, participating as peer teachers, successfully filling leadership roles as managers or coaches, and helping with class management are among the most obvious types of cooperative student behaviors we see in physical education classes. In learning communities, teachers express strong expectations of cooperation, take time to show students what cooperation means in specific situations, and celebrate it when it occurs. A cooperative class environment is a building block toward a caring class environment. In learning communities, students eventually grow to care about each other's successes and failures. This goal is more likely to be achieved if students and teachers come to know about each other in ways that extend beyond the curricular focus.

Symbols and Rituals

All communities develop significant symbols and rituals as a means of building and sustaining identity. This is true of ethnic, religious, and sport communities, and it also is true of learning communities within schools. At the school level, educators have always focused on this feature through what is typically called "school spirit." In physical education, classes might adopt a class name and a class uniform. They might also develop a series of ritual celebrations, for example, public performances of what they have learned, within-class tournaments, or special field trips.

Fairness and Caring

Learning communities are built and sustained on qualities of fairness and caring. How many times have you heard a child or youth say, "That's just not fair!"? Of all the growing sensibilities that youngsters have, fairness is among the most important. These elements are also at the heart of educational movements toward breeding good citizenship among students in schools (Ofsted, 2006; Schaps & Lewis, 1998). To be a good class citizen, students have to be committed to a prevailing system of justice within the class. A main focus of the system is learning to care about the rights of classmates as well as their own rights. As discussed earlier in the chapter, the TPSR model provides a progression of goals through which students move toward becoming fully responsible citizens in physical activity and physical education settings. Some strategies for creating a sense of fairness and caring within learning communities include (Schaps & Lewis, 1998):

- A collaboratively developed system of discipline and procedures, as evidenced in a fair play agreement (see **Box 6.8**)

BOX 6.8 A Fair Play Agreement

For the Player

I, ____________________, agree to:

- Always play by the rules
- Respect the officials and their decisions
- Remember that I am playing because I enjoy the sport
- Work at achieving my personal best
- Show appreciation for good plays and good players
- Maintain self-control at all times
- Play fairly at all times

____

Signature

For the Teacher

I, ____________________, agree to:

- Remember that students play for fun
- Encourage my students
- Offer constructive criticism and feedback
- Instruct my students to follow both the letter and the spirit of the rules
- Teach my students that officials are an important component of the game
- Encourage my students to be good sports
- Give every student a chance to play and learn the techniques and strategies
- Remember that my actions speak louder than my words

____

Signature

Modified from Fair Play Canada. (1993). Fair play—It's your call!: A resource manual for coaches (p. 25). Ottawa, Canada: Canadian Centre for Ethics in Sport.

- Regular class meetings to solve problems and develop class norms
- Challenging learning activities that emphasize respectful treatment of classmates
- Opportunities for teachers and students to get to know one another as persons
- Dealing with issues of curricular values, such as fair play or gender bias in sports

Eventually, such practices create a framework and set of expectations for interactions within the class, whether those interactions are part of the student social agenda or related to lesson-designed learning tasks. **Box 6.9** conveys how one school implements a learning community model.

BOX 6.9 A School Learning Community

Schools throughout the world are adopting a learning community model to increase their effectiveness. Manomet School is organized into nine learning communities that have the following attributes:

- Student-centered approach
- Commitment to outcomes by members of the team valuing achievement and showing a commitment to success for all students
- Recognition and reward of worthy achievements
- Spirit of advocacy with regard to students
- Collaborative team policies for behavioral expectations and climate
- Community building among teachers, students, and parents
- Proactive posture in which teams attempt innovations and initiate projects
- Healthy give-and-take that recognizes and celebrates differences

The nine Manomet School communities (55–80 students each) are further divided into "houses" of approximately 18 students, with each house having a teacher leader who acts as a guide, advocate, and friend for the students under his or her care. Within their houses, students express concerns, have their progress monitored, and discuss events related to the learning teams and the larger issues of citizenship and civility. Although the school has a common core curriculum, learning community teams differentiate their curricular foci. Each team has its own name, logo, T-shirt, color, and other features that set it apart. The teams plan a series of specialized activities to build and nurture the sense of community (assemblies, field trips, special dinners, team meetings). Students also represent their houses and learning community teams in clubs and intramurals.

Learning communities in physical education can be enhanced through models-based practice, where the physical education curriculum is theme based. Dependent on the model chosen, each has the capacity, to a lesser or greater extent, to frame a learning community that has *boundaries*, *persists over time*, has *common goals* and *cooperation* toward achievement of these goals, has *symbols and rituals* to build and sustain its identity, and develops a climate of *fairness and caring*. One example is the Health and Wellness framework. The Health and Wellness framework is used throughout the year to frame the physical education curriculum for all students in the third year of postprimary school, between 14 and 15 years of age. Although the focus of the year is on general health-related fitness concepts and aligned components (e.g., cardiovascular and muscular endurance) through an introduction of self-assessments, short-term goal setting, and fitness activities, the curriculum allows for other physical activity areas to be included. The year-group begin the school year with a series of discussions and assessments to establish where they are in regards to health fitness, and the students are asked to set a target for where they would like to be at the end of the school year as regards their health fitness. There are two possible options to subsequently establish a learning community.

The first option is that the year-group divide into teams on the basis of having set similar goals for the end of the year and spend some time considering how they intend to reach their goals, appreciating that they will be expected to supplement their one physical education lesson a week with involvement in physical activity outside of the school curriculum. The team becomes a learning community over time, mapping and accumulating their weekly involvement in physical activity, conscious of attaining their health fitness goals. They share their interest and expertise in particular physical activities with their peers, encouraging individuals to attend physical activity opportunities of which they would otherwise not have been aware, or had no confidence to attend without a peer. In a bid to have the community strive towards the desired goal, it may arise that the more proactive members of the community, as regards increasing their physical activity levels, are required to become facilitators of physical activity for their less active peers. This could entail inviting their less active peers to accompany them when they are physically active and/or to act as motivators for their peers to increase their physical activity levels.

The second option is that the year-group divide into teams that are made up of students who have a wide range of involvement in physical activity and subsequently have identified disparate health fitness goals for the end of year. Each team develops a set of collective goals in a number of areas, including total distances run or walked, a collective bench press goal, and an average recovery rate goal. They discuss how to monitor their performances relative to these goals and begin a series of discussions about the help they could provide each other in reaching the goals. It may evolve that in a bid to achieve the community's accumulated health fitness goals that they assign particular members of the community to work on contributing more to one goal than another. For example, a member who is keen on walking but not bench pressing may be encouraged to focus specifically on contributing to the total distance walked by the team.

Regardless of either option, the teams in which the year-groups are divided remain the same throughout the school year for physical education. The focus on teaching basic fitness vocabulary and introducing related concepts such as cardiovascular fitness remain the focus of the physical education lessons throughout the year, regardless of the physical activity mediums being taught and experienced. The teacher is also required to continually convey and reinforce to students the three primary goals of concepts-based fitness education: (1) students need the opportunity to engage in lifetime physical activities of sufficient intensity and duration necessary to help maximize health benefits, (2) students need to learn why it is important to develop and maintain adequate levels of physical activity and fitness, and (3) students must develop the knowledge base and skills necessary to plan and execute personal activity programs throughout their lives (McConnell, 2010).

Learning Experience 6.8

Each of the following characteristics may have some bearing on an individual's willingness to contribute to a learning community: cognitive ability, culture, fitness level, language, movement skills, physical characteristics, religion, sex, and socioeconomic class. As a teacher, how do you propose to acknowledge some of these differences? How do you propose to acknowledge these differences while at the same time conveying equity in treatment towards all students (i.e., being seen not to favor or penalize any particular student or group of students)?

Physical Education Learning Communities Through a Sport Education Unit

Sport Education is a curriculum and instruction model that encourages students to establish and maintain a physical education learning community through actively promoting all of the six characteristics of learning communities noted earlier in the chapter. Numerous elements of the Sport Education model lend themselves naturally to supporting learning communities. For example, "seasons" extend the length of time in which students work together as a team, "affiliation" encourages students to retain membership for the duration of a season, a "culminating event" allows the team to convey what they have learned throughout the season, and "festivity" encourages the development of teams into learning communities where they identify with a team name and colors as well as publicizing team and individual performances. We share here in what way Sport Education addresses each of the six characteristics of a learning community.

The notion of *persisting teams* popularized by the Sport Education model addresses two characteristics of the learning community. Sport Education teams have names and colors for a uniform that create boundaries as regards differentiating between the members and nonmembers. Teams within a physical education class, as in the Sport Education curriculum model, can become microcommunities if they persist over time. This leads us to considering the characteristic of persistence.

Persisting teams have the potential to evolve into true learning communities, especially if teachers design seasons to last 15 to 24 lessons or teams stay together throughout the entire school year. One postprimary school in Washington (United States) has an Adventure Academy where students spend 2 days a week working as a collective group in physical education, science, and language arts. The assignments and experiences that students have in each subject area are focused around adventure content, with learning tasks and challenges developed collectively throughout the academic year.

The different roles and responsibilities that students are encouraged to take on in Sport Education enhance the cooperation characteristics of the learning community. Within teams, students undertake a number of roles and responsibilities that collectively, through cooperation, increase the likelihood of achieving the set task. For example, if students are working on a gymnastic sequence, cooperation is required among the spotters, the performers, and the judge. If they are working on a particular game, cooperation is required among the manager, the coach, and the players. In both cases the students, regardless of their assigned role, are working towards a common goal, another characteristic of the learning community. Common goals exist when success is defined collectively, in the first instance as a team and then across a class.

Sport Education teams tend to fit the learning community characteristic of symbols and rituals (e.g., rituals could include team name, team chant, uniforms). Siedentop, Hastie, and van der Mars (2011) noted an example of a primary school in Alabama (United States) where students between 7 and 10 years of age joined in an integrative Sport Education season (with art, technology, and life sciences) called the Biome project. The gymnastics season's theme was biodiversity and habitat, with each of the seven participating teams representing different earth ecosystems (e.g., deserts, tropical rainforests, deciduous forests). The students within each class then became team members of one of six teams representing different species within the ecosystem (e.g., birds, mammals, reptiles, fish). Each team had to construct a mascot representing one of the animals and bring it to physical education class each day. The season's competition combined within- and between-class competitions. One way in which the program created rituals was through scheduling within-species lunches; that is, all the birds from each class joined together for lunch.

Another ritual was the season's culminating event, which consisted of a gymnastics meeting at the town's recreation center, during which students had multiple roles. In addition to the traditional noncompetitor roles (e.g., judge, scorekeeper), certain students served as VIP hosts to assist parents attending the event with finding seats and to provide refreshments. This example shows how students learn about communities by all participating in the types of rituals and roles that brings community members together.

As suggested previously in this chapter, a collaboratively developed system of discipline and procedures, as evidenced in a fair play agreement, is a strategy for creating a sense of fairness and caring within learning communities. An example of a fair play agreement drawn up between a class of students and the physical education teacher is provided in Box 6.8. After consultation with their team, the fair play agreement can be signed by the coach/leader of each team within the class, further enforcing the characteristics of boundaries, cooperation, and common goals. A fair play agreement encourages students and the teacher to discuss their respective appropriate and expected behaviors as they conduct themselves within physical education. Agreeing to an appropriate system of discipline and associated procedures encourages students not only to be committed to a prevailing system of justice within the class but also to learn to care about the rights of classmates (and the teacher) as well as their own rights.

CHAPTER SUMMARY

The Sport Education example discussed in this chapter is an effective way of conveying the extent to which the six characteristics of a learning community overlap. Working in teams can actively promote and allow students to experience all six characteristics of a learning community. Working towards common goals is likely to entail cooperation and persistence over time. The onus resides with the physical education teacher to construct a teaching and learning environment that encourages students to work as a learning community. Revisiting the first part of this chapter, this is more likely to be a success if the teacher has developed a caring, culturally relevant, nonbiased environment for their students. Subsequently, the students are potentially in a better space to consider how to most effectively contribute to a physical education learning community that encourages them to share similar values and commit to each other's learning, growth, and welfare.

1. A caring pedagogy invests in the development of students and sustains conditions within which students protect the rights and interests of classmates.
2. Teacher practices such as helping, valuing students, treating students respectfully, being tolerant, encouraging, and supporting are viewed by students as caring.
3. Caring teachers plan challenging and significant activities and help students achieve important outcomes.
4. Students can be disadvantaged in physical education because of attributes such as gender, skillfulness, race, and physical appearance.
5. An equity pedagogy builds class environments that help students from diverse backgrounds achieve outcomes to function well in society and create and sustain a more just and humane society.
6. Unacceptable practices include stereotyping or discriminatory teacher actions and an unwillingness by the teacher to prevent the behavior and/or intervene when students behave in discriminatory ways toward classmates.
7. To become a caring teacher requires skills and knowledge that relate to diversity issues in pedagogy and in the content being taught.
8. Antibias teaching purposefully confronts issues of stereotyping and discrimination and works specifically with students to help them become more tolerant and more willing to be advocates for antibias practices in schools and in the larger community.
9. Students will need to be taught specific communication skills to be able to take part usefully and fairly in antibias discussions within class.
10. The Teaching Personal and Social Responsibility model provides a progression of goals through which students move toward becoming fully responsible citizens of the physical education class and extend those behaviors and values outside of class.
11. Students in successful learning communities are supportive, responsible, accountable, cooperative, trusting, empowered, identified with the class, and committed to fairness and caring.
12. Learning communities have boundaries, persist over time, share common goals, value cooperative practices, identify with community symbols and rituals, and are committed to fairness and caring.
13. Strategies for sustaining fairness and caring include collaboratively developed class procedures and discipline codes, class meetings to solve problems and develop class norms, challenging learning activities emphasizing respect, opportunities to know one another, and willingness to deal with values in the curriculum.

REFERENCES

Bosworth, K. (1995). Caring for others and being cared for: Students talk caring in schools. *Phi Delta Kappan, 76*(9), 686–693.

Brock, S. J., Rovegno, I., & Oliver, K. L. (2009). The influence of student status on student interactions and experiences during a sport education unit. *Physical Education and Sport Pedagogy, 14*(4), 355–375.

Brophy, J. (2010). *Motivating students to learn* (3rd ed.). New York: Routledge.

Chaskin, R., & Mendley-Rauner, D. (1995). Toward a field of caring: An epilogue. *Phi Delta Kappan, 76*(9), 718–719.

Coakley, J. (2008). *Sports in society: Issues and controversies* (10th ed.). New York: McGraw-Hill.

Cohen, E. G. (1994). *Designing groupwork* (2nd ed.). New York: Teachers College Press.

Eisenhower National Clearinghouse for Science and Mathematics Education. (n.d.). *Common bonds: Anti-bias teaching in a diverse society*. Columbus, OH: Author.

Fair Play Canada. (1993). *Fair play: It's your call. A resource manual for coaches.* Ottawa, Canada: Canadian Centre for Ethics in Sport.

Finnicum, P. (1997). Developing discipline policies to prevent problem behaviors. *Teaching Secondary Physical Education, 3*(4), 25–26.

Flintoff, A., & Scraton, S. (2006). Girls and physical education. In D. Kirk, D. Macdonald, & M. O'Sullivan (Eds.), *Handbook of physical education* (pp. 767–783). London: Sage.

Gard, M. (2006). More art than science? Boys, masculinity and physical education research. In D. Kirk, D. Macdonald, and M. O'Sullivan (Eds.), *Handbook of physical education* (pp. 784–795). London: Sage.

Glasby, T., & Macdonald, D. (2004). Negotiating the curriculum: Challenging the social relationships in teaching. In J. Wright, D. Macdonald, & L. Burrows (Eds.), *Critical inquiry and problem solving in physical education* (pp. 133–144). London: Routledge.

Goodman, J., Sutton, V., & Harkavy, I. (1995). The effectiveness of family workshops in a middle school setting: Respect and caring make the difference. *Phi Delta Kappan, 76*(9), 694–700.

Gorard, S., & See, B. H. (2011). How can we enhance enjoyment of secondary school? The student view. *British Educational Research Journal, 37*(4), 671–690.

Hannon, J. C., & Ratliffe, T. (2004). Cooperative learning in physical education: Ideas for teaching health-related fitness. *Strategies: A Journal for Physical and Sport Educators, 17*(5), 29–32.

Hellison, D. (2010). *Teaching personal and social responsibility through physical activity* (3rd ed.). Champaign, IL: Human Kinetics.

Hellison, D., & Walsh, D. (2002). Responsibility-based youth programs evaluation: Investigating the investigations, *Quest, 54*, 292–307.

Larson, A. (2006). Student perception of caring teaching in physical education. *Sport, Education and Society, 11*(4), 337–352.

Larson, A., & Silverman, S. J. (2005). Rationales and practices used by caring physical education teachers. *Sport, Education and Society, 10*(2), 175–193.

Lester, P. M., & Ross, S. D. (Eds.). (2011). *Images that injure: Pictorial stereotypes in the media* (3rd ed.). Westport, CT: Praeger.

Lewis, C., Schaps, E., & Watson, M. (1995). Beyond the pendulum: Creating challenging and caring schools. *Phi Delta Kappan, 76*(7), 547–554.

Lipsitz, J. (1995). Prologue: Why we should care about caring. *Phi Delta Kappan, 76*(9), 665–666.

Lortie, D. (2002). *Schoolteacher: A sociological study* (2nd ed.). Chicago, IL: University of Chicago Press.

MacPhail, A. (2010). Listening to pupils' voices. In R. Bailey (Ed.), *Physical education for learning* (pp. 228–238). London: Continuum.

McConnell, K. (2010). Fitness education. In J. Lund & D. Tannehill (Eds.), *Standards-based physical education curriculum development* (2nd ed., pp. 367–387). Sudbury, MA: Jones and Bartlett.

McGee-Banks, C., & Banks, J. (1995). Equity pedagogy: An essential component of multicultural education. *Theory into Practice, 34*(3), 152–158.

Noddings, N. (1992). *The challenge to care in schools.* New York: Teachers College Press.

Ofsted. (2006). *Towards consensus? Citizenship in secondary schools.* Document reference number: HMI 2666. Manchester, UK: Author.

Oliver, K. L. (2010). The body, physical activity and inequity: Learning to listen *with* girls *through* action. In M. O'Sullivan & A. MacPhail (Eds.), *Young people's voices in physical education and youth sport* (pp. 31–48). London: Routledge.

Oliver, K. L., & McCaughtry, N. (2011). Lessons learned about gender equity and inclusion in physical education. In S. Dagkas & K. Armour (Eds.), *Inclusion and exclusion through youth sport* (pp. 155–171). London: Routledge.

Osler, A. (2005). *Teachers, human rights and diversity.* Stoke on Trent, England: Trentham Books Limited.

O'Sullivan, M., & Kinchin, G. (2010). Cultural studies curriculum in physical activity and sport. In J. Lund & D. Tannehill (Eds.), *Standards-based physical education curriculum development* (2nd ed., pp. 333–365). Sudbury, MA: Jones and Bartlett.

O'Sullivan, M., Tannehill, D., & Hinchion, C. (2010). Teaching as professional inquiry. In R. Bailey (Ed.), *Physical education for learning* (pp. 54–63). London: Continuum.

Palmer, P. (1993). *To know as we are known: Education as a spiritual journey.* New York: HarperCollins.

Parker, M., & Stiehl, J. (2010). Personal and social responsibility. In J. Lund & D. Tannehill (Eds.), *Standards-based physical education curriculum development* (2nd ed., pp. 163–191). Sudbury, MA: Jones and Bartlett.

Penney, D. (Ed.). (2002). *Gender and physical education*. London: Routledge.

Roefs, W. (1998). Better together. *Teaching Tolerance, 7*(2), 34–41.

Schaps, E., & Lewis, C. (1998). Breeding citizenship through community in school. *School Administrator, 55*(5), 22–26.

Siedentop, D., Hastie, P., & van der Mars, H. (2011). *Complete guide to sport education* (2nd ed.). Champaign, IL: Human Kinetics.

Stiehl, J., Morris, G. S. D., & Sinclair, C. (2008). *Teaching physical activity. Change, challenge and choice*. Champaign, IL: Human Kinetics.

Timken, G. L., & Watson, D. (2010). Teaching all kids: Valuing students through culturally responsive and inclusive practice. In J. Lund & D. Tannehill (Eds.), *Standards-based physical education curriculum development* (2nd ed., pp. 123-153). Sudbury, MA: Jones and Bartlett.

Treadway, L. (2000). *Community mapping*. Unpublished manuscript prepared for Contextual Teaching and Learning Project, Ohio State University and U.S. Department of Education.

Wan, G. (2008). Explorations of educational purpose 2. In *The education of diverse student populations: A global perspective*. Rueil-Malmaison, France: Springer.

Wentzel, K. (1997). Student motivation in middle school: The role of perceived pedagogical caring. *Journal of Educational Psychology, 49*(3), 411–419.

Young, L. (1998). Care, community, and context in a teacher education classroom. *Theory into Practice, 37*(2), 105–113.

CHAPTER 7 Preventive Classroom Management

Overall Chapter Outcome

To be knowledgeable about preventive classroom management strategies and how to use them to develop and maintain a positive environment for young people to learn in physical education

Learning Outcomes

The learner will:

- Describe the nature and purpose of preventive management
- Discuss the relationship among management, teaching, and student learning
- Articulate personal expectations for student behavior
- Describe how student expectations for teachers might be sought
- Characterize the nature and purpose of rules and routines in the classroom
- Explain how to effectively teach rules and routines to students and allow them to practice
- Describe how to link the breaking of rules to predetermined consequences
- Clarify their understanding of management time and why it matters in the physical education classroom
- Demonstrate how to use a variety of effective management strategies in the classroom
- Describe how to use the umbrella of active supervision strategies to monitor student behavior

In this chapter we show why sound classroom management is such an important prerequisite for building and implementing quality physical education. However, it bears noting here that the need for teachers to develop these critical class management skills and strategies is based on two key assumptions. First that you understand the need, and have the expectation, for students to learn in physical education. And, second, that you are motivated to develop the necessary skills and strategies to make this possible.

The Nature and Purpose of Preventive Management

Effective class management in physical education does not just happen. Classes that run smoothly, are free from disruptive behavior, are positive environments where students enjoy learning, and optimize the amount of time for instruction and practice are the result of teachers who understand class management and have the skills to develop and sustain a successful managerial task system. Over the past 40 years, researchers have shown conclusively that effective teachers are, first of all, good class managers. Being a good class manager does not make you an effective teacher, but it will provide the opportunity for you to be effective if you care about students and their learning and have the teaching skills and motivation to put them to use consistently.

Effective class management, therefore, is a necessary precondition for effective teaching and learning. There is an old adage that "an ounce of prevention is worth a pound of cure."

BOX 7.1 Key Terms in This Chapter

- *Active supervision:* An umbrella set of strategies that a teacher uses at various times within the lesson, during teacher presentation of tasks, demonstration of skills, student group work, whole class instruction, independent practice, or individual performances. Includes back-to-the-wall, proximity control, with-it-ness, selective ignoring, learning names, overlapping, and pinpointing.
- *FOS principle:* "Focus on the student"; a principle established to encourage the teacher to place the student at the center of all decisions.
- *Managerial episode:* Each managerial task constitutes an episode of time and behavior that begins with some event (most frequently a signal or instruction from the teacher) and ends when the next instructional event or activity begins.
- *Managerial task system:* Establishes the limits for behavior and the positive expectations for students.
- *Managerial time:* The cumulative amount of time students spend in managerial tasks, that is, all the organizational, transitional, and non-subject-matter tasks in a lesson.
- *Momentum:* The smoothness with which the various segments of a lesson flow together. A lesson with momentum has no breaks, no times when activities or transitions slow down the pace.
- *Pace:* The degree to which the lessons move forward at a steady tempo.
- *Preventive class management:* The proactive (rather than reactive) strategies teachers use to develop and maintain a positive, predictable, task-oriented class climate in which minimal time is devoted to managerial tasks and optimal time is therefore available for instructional tasks.
- *Routines:* Part of the framework of an effective and positive management system. Routines specify procedures for performing tasks that are repeated frequently throughout the class.
- *Rules:* Part of the framework of an effective and positive management system. Rules identify appropriate and inappropriate behaviors and the situations within which certain behaviors are acceptable or unacceptable within the class.
- *Teacher's interactive behavior:* Key to good management, this is the result of a teacher's clear, proactive behavior that involves instruction and practice.
- *Transitional task:* The time when students move from one activity to another (e.g., teams changing courts, moving between stations in a fitness lesson, making substitutions in games, changing the demands of a group task in dance, partner balance task in gymnastics).

Nowhere is this truer than in the manner in which teachers manage their students, time, and equipment. Many of the discipline problems that teachers encounter occur because of poor management. That is, in poorly managed classes, students are much more likely to become disruptive. Inadequate or unskilled class management has two negative outcomes. First, it tends to increase discipline problems, and second, it reduces time that can be used for learning and practice.

Preventive class management refers to the proactive (rather than reactive) strategies teachers use to develop and maintain a positive, predictable, task-oriented class climate in which minimal time is devoted to managerial tasks and optimal time is therefore available for instructional tasks. Routines for accomplishing managerial tasks are taught, and students are given sufficient opportunities to practice them. Appropriate ways of behaving during managerial and instructional tasks are also part of the instruction and practice. Students are encouraged to perform managerial tasks well and to behave appropriately, and their efforts to do so are recognized and rewarded. When you visit a class taught by an effective class manager, you see the managerial tasks done smoothly, quickly, and with little attention from the teacher. Unless you were there at the outset of the school year or semester, however, you would not have seen how the teacher employed the organizational and behavioral skills necessary for the system to run so smoothly.

The **managerial task system** establishes the structures through which a physical education class becomes a predictable, smoothly operating system. The managerial task system establishes the limits for behavior and the positive expectations for students. Students know what the managerial tasks are and how and when to perform them. As you will see throughout this chapter, teachers can decide what the specific elements of the managerial system will be and teach the system directly to students, or they can work with the students to develop the system jointly (see **Box 7.2**).

BOX 7.2 The Three Cs: Compliance, Cooperation, and Community

Effective class management and discipline can be achieved in three ways.

- *Compliance*, where teachers organize rules and consequences so that students comply with the class managerial system and behavior rules. Thus, teachers who are sufficiently skilled can establish an effective management system and bring students into compliance with the demands of the system.
- *Cooperation*, which teachers solicit from students by (1) helping them understand how the class managerial system benefits them and (2) bringing them into the decision-making process about how the system is developed and maintained.
- *Community*, where teachers attempt to build a learning community, a shared decision-making community that enables teachers and students to develop and sustain relationships in which self-discipline, responsibility, helping others, and the larger good of the group are emphasized.

There may be some students and some classes where compliance is the best a teacher can achieve. Some students and some classes where cooperation is the best a teacher can achieve; and some teachers who think cooperation is the most appropriate goal to work toward. Other teachers may work with students over an extended period of time and want to develop a learning community. Keep in mind that learning communities cannot always be achieved given the conditions and time constraints under which many physical education teachers work. The key is for you to recognize the differences among the three approaches and to understand the various strategies necessary to achieve them.

Learning Experience 7.1

Reflect on how you might initially set up the rules, routines, and procedures that will guide behavior in the classroom. Describe how you would use compliance, cooperation, or community, or a combination of the three to design the management system.

An effective management system is important because it is necessary to create the time teachers and their students can devote to learning. For teachers for whom student learning is important, time is the most precious commodity. Time spent managing students and responding to disruptive behavior takes away from time for instruction and practice. Remember, teaching is not inherently fun! Constantly having to manage groups of students and discipline misbehaving students is neither fun nor satisfying. Developing an effective class management structure does contribute to making teaching worthwhile, satisfying, and fun. Watching students improve through practice is satisfying.

When considering classroom management, it is crucial to remember safety and the nature of physical education. The mere fact that there are moving bodies in a gym or on an athletic field is conducive to accidents occurring. Keeping students safe is certainly the responsibility of both the teacher and the students, yet it is the teacher who must plan for this aspect of management initially.

Myths and Truths About Management and Teaching

The first myth is that good management and discipline are inherent in good teaching; that is, if you teach well, you will have no management or discipline problems. Choose a good activity and teach it well, as this myth goes, and your students will be well managed and behaved. This is at best simplistic and at worst simply wrong. The truth is that the foundation for good teaching is effective management and discipline. Being a skilled manager does not automatically make you a good teacher, but it creates the time and opportunity for you to be a good teacher. The skills and strategies to become an effective class manager are well known and can be learned and perfected by any teacher who (1) understands their importance and (2) is motivated to employ them.

The second myth is that students will come to physical education with the necessary behaviors to be cooperative learners. There are two reasons why assuming this to be true is dangerous for teachers. Traditionally, teachers have relied on parents to raise their children in such a way that the children come to school with certain behaviors well developed and other behavioral predispositions pretty much in place. We like to call these "school skills." Teachers assume that children have learned to pay attention, to respond to instructions, to try to learn in school classes, to respect each other, and so on. In some schools, for some children and youths, these assumptions may still hold, but, in many schools and for many children and youth, they do not. The truth is that many teachers spend far more time than they want helping children learn basic behaviors to be successful in school and managing and disciplining unruly, sometimes hostile, youth. This is one reason why class management and discipline has been at or near the top of teacher concerns for several decades.

The third myth is that, because children and youth typically enjoy physical activity, they will be enthusiastic about learning in physical education. The fact is that many students come to physical education anxious about being there or determined to do as little as possible. Let's face it: Some students (for diverse reasons) hate physical education! The saddest comment we can make about our profession is that some students have learned to hate physical education by being in poorly managed and poorly taught physical education classes. You should assume that the motivations students bring with them to your classes vary greatly, running the gamut from those who want to avoid physical education as much as they can to those who love it and want as much of it as they can get. Your responsibility is to make physical education work for both of these kinds of students and for all those in between the extremes. Effective class management is foundational to effective teaching no matter what instructional approach is taken. This is true for direct, teacher-controlled instruction, and it is true for wholly learner-centered and learner-controlled instruction. It is true in a classroom in which students are organized in neat rows of desks, and it is also true for the gymnasium and playing fields.

Establishing a Management System

Teacher and Student Expectations of Themselves and Each Other

If we want young people to participate in physical activity now and into their futures, we must focus on their needs and desires. One of our colleagues has penned the term ***FOS principle*** to denote the principle of "focus on the student." In other words, it is our task as teachers not only to design challenging, relevant, and exciting learning experiences to promote student learning and interest but also to set the stage for learning through development of a positive and safe learning environment.

Frequently we observe teachers starting off a new semester/school year by sharing with students the expectations they hold for student behavior. These might include such expectations as students being cooperative, coming to class ready to learn, being willing to try whatever is asked, taking responsibility for their own learning, and consistently providing help to peers. Less often do we observe teachers seeking the viewpoints of students on their expectations for teachers that they perceive as necessary for them to learn, especially in postprimary schools. We suspect that if teachers did seek these insights they might hear such expectations as (1) participating in well-planned, enjoyable lessons developed around content and learning that is relevant, meaningful, and worthwhile to their lives; (2) receiving guidance and feedback to help them improve; and (3) being made to feel valuable and important. We know that a positive, safe, supportive, and enjoyable learning environment is one in which students feel comfortable and able to learn. Setting up a class management system designed to prevent disruption, support student learning, and provide enjoyment of that learning is the first step.

Learning Experience 7.2

Two steps guide this learning experience.

1. Make a list of what you think students expect from their teachers and classes.
2. Begin your next class in the primary or postprimary level by asking your students what they expect from you as a teacher and from the class.

Do students' responses match with what you expected, and what you had planned to deliver?

Behaviour2Learn (see www.behaviour2learn.co.uk) suggests that behavior problems are learned and developed through the relationship students have with themselves, their peers and others, and the curriculum. Key for developing appropriate behaviors is the learning environment that you, as the teacher, create through sharing how you expect students to behave and how it will help them learn, "catching" students being good by praising appropriate behavior, and assisting students in setting realistic personal behavior goals.

An important dimension of teaching is developing relationships with students. A teacher's relationship with students is key to the environment in which learning occurs, the teaching strategies employed by the teacher, the responses and interactions of students, and ultimately the learning that is achieved by students. Teachers can establish a positive relationship with their students by (1) communicating with them, interacting regarding both in and out of school issues; (2) learning more about students' interests and desires; and (3) developing a shared respect between teacher and student. Establishing a positive relationship with students can encourage students to seek learning, value their school experiences, and participate positively in the classroom.

Whether at the primary or postprimary level, teachers and students work together for long periods of time. A level of cooperation that allows both teacher and students to function effectively and without high levels of tension or anxiety must be achieved. The best preventive class management systems are developed as social contracts between teachers and their students. When students are actively brought into the development of the system and understand why the rules, procedures, and routines are important for their class experiences to be successful, they develop an ownership of the system, buying into the system and what it is meant to accomplish. Time spent with students establishing class rules and procedures, and consequences for breaking rules, is time well spent. Teachers should view this as an important learning experience for their students, one in which the student voice is heard and respected. In addition, development of a social contract between teachers and their students is fundamental to learning communities and a caring pedagogy.

Developing Rules and Routines

An effective management system begins with the development of routines and the establishment of class rules for appropriate behavior. Both routines and rules need to be taught, and students need opportunities to practice them with clear, consistent feedback and clear, consistently applied consequences. These routines and rules provide the foundation of the management system in any class.

Routines specify procedures for performing tasks within the class. Any task that is repeated frequently (e.g., taking attendance, stop and start signals) should be made into a routine. A set of routines provides the structure that allows classes to run smoothly, free of delays and disruptions. Routines also relieve the teacher of the need to be a constant traffic cop, directing every management or organizational behavior that occurs in the classroom.

Rules identify appropriate and inappropriate behaviors and the situations within which certain behaviors are acceptable or unacceptable (e.g., talking to a classmate often is acceptable and even encouraged but not when the teacher is trying to explain something to the class). Some rules identify a range of behaviors (e.g., be cooperative) that are situational and can have a range of meanings (e.g., being cooperative in helping put away equipment differs from cooperating with teammates in a game). Other rules are behavior specific (e.g., not running on the pool deck, not picking up equipment until directed are both related to safety).

Research has indicated clearly that teachers who spend time in the early part of the school year—the first several weeks—teaching specific classroom and gymnasium routines not only have an easier time managing and disciplining throughout the school year but also have students who learn more (Burnett, 2002; Brophy & Good, 1986; Marzano, 2003; Siedentop, Doutis, Tsangaridou, Ward, & Rouschenbach, 1994; Todorovich & Curtner-Smith, 2002). Teachers who take time to specifically teach routines such as gaining teacher attention, using equipment, and moving around the available space have fewer problems. Gymnasium routines become part of the content that is taught, which has a high payoff. Primary physical education teachers typically teach routines and rules along with content. They create activities that emphasize certain organizational and behavioral situations that allow teaching of the routines or rules and give students ample opportunity to practice the routines or the behavior specified by the rules. These procedures also provide teachers frequent opportunity to provide feedback, correct errors, and reinforce children who perform the routines well and those who behave in ways specified by the rules. At the postprimary level, teachers more often specify the rules and explain them, along with the consequences of breaking the rules. Often these class rules and procedures are passed out in written form to students as part of class materials and, in some cases, are part of the school procedural guidelines that are given to all students. In some cases, students are asked to take the physical education procedures home and have their parents sign them as an indication that students and parents understand the procedures, rules, and consequences of violations.

Routines and Their Development

Routines should be taught for all procedural aspects of lessons that recur frequently, such as what students should do when they enter the gymnasium and when the teacher gives a signal for attention or the appropriate way to get out and put away equipment. As routines become habitual, they will be used more and less off-task behavior will occur in the situations the routines are designed to address. Routines that are used frequently in physical education are shown in **Table 7.1**. As a teacher, you need to select the routines for the behaviors most frequently conveyed in your own setting. Determine the routines that are necessary to start and then add more as the need arises.

The first series of lessons are critically important in having students practice the many different managerial routines, thus setting the tone of the rest of the school year. Using classroom routines consistently has a profound effect on both student behavior and learning. According to Marzano (2003), the number of disruptions in classes where rules and routines were effectively implemented was considerably lower than the number of disruptions in classes where rules and routines were not taught or reinforced. Routines need to be taught as specifically as one might teach any movement or sport skill. This means explanations, demonstrations, student practice with feedback, and all other elements related to learning are used for teaching routines. For example, most physical education teachers at the primary and postprimary levels teach an attention/quiet routine because they frequently have to stop class activity to provide instructions or feedback or to change the activity. This routine involves a specific teacher signal for gaining the attention of students (a whistle, hand clap, the word *freeze*). The expectation is that students quiet down quickly, place equipment on the floor/ground, and face the teacher. During the first few lessons of the school year, effective teachers will use activities that allow for many stops and starts, just so they can teach these routines.

From the perspective of maximizing students' opportunity for physical activity during physical education lessons, many teachers teach an entry routine that allows for immediate activity. When taught effectively, as a routine, students come to expect to be active when they enter the teaching space. Some teachers teach a fitness-related warm-up for this routine. Others teach a series of stretching activities specific to the physical activity focus of the unit. Those who employ Sport Education have students report to their team court where their team's trainer starts the warm-up. Still others design a task that is posted on the door directing students

TABLE 7.1 Routines Typically Used in Physical Education

Beginning of Class Routines	Use of Materials and Equipment Routines	Transitions and Interruptions Routines	Individual/Group Work Routines	When Teacher Is Teaching Routines	Close of Class Routines
• Students entering class • Taking attendance • Entry activity	• Distributing equipment • Collecting equipment • Space boundaries within lessons • Sharing equipment • When and how to use equipment	• Stop and start signals • Leaving class • Returning to class • Emergency drills • Gathering students for instruction • What to do if a ball or other implement invades space • Transitions between activities • Dispersing students to activity • Unexpected interruptions	• Moving into and out of groups • Expected behavior in groups • Procedure for grouping students • Group roles and responsibilities • Group communication • Relationships within and between groups • Home base	• Student attention • Student participation • Gaining teacher(s) attention • Housekeeping chores	• Closure activity • Lesson closure • Exiting classroom for locker room or next class

to begin to practice specific tasks immediately upon entering the teaching space. You may need to add routines for specific activity units, particularly safety routines for activities that involve equipment, wearing protective goggles in floor hockey, or spotting routines for gymnastics. If you use small-group teaching, leaders or team captains can be given responsibility for routines being performed well.

The following teaching strategies will prove helpful when teaching routines:

- *Explain and show:* Explain the procedure in language that is age specific, and show students what it looks like (this might be done by students themselves).
- *Show correct and incorrect examples:* Show students the incorrect way to do something at the same time you are showing the correct way.
- *Rehearse:* Provide opportunity to practice the procedure. Have a goal for each rehearsal and give immediate feedback (for example, "On the 'go' signal, you have 15 seconds to organize into partners and find a free space in the gym—go!").
- *Expect perfection, reward direction:* Routines can be learned easily and performed consistently, but you must expect perfection and support students as they gradually get better and better. A "That's good, but we can do better" attitude should prevail. If, after some practice, they still fall short, then you can use "positive practice."
- *Use positive models:* When individuals or groups perform the procedure appropriately, point it out to the rest of the class. This both provides support for cooperative students and shows the rest of the students how the procedure looks when it is done well.
- *Provide frequent feedback:* Praise success. Praise improvement. Give behavior-specific feedback rather than general feedback. How you praise will change from primary to postprimary students. In general, students in primary schools will respond favorably when singled out for excellent performance. Once students reach the age of 12, public praise that is delivered by recognizing teams or groups of students is preferable. If you wish to praise an individual student, do it one-on-one while others are practicing.
- *Use activities to practice routines:* Create activities that allow for practice of routines. For example, use an activity in which students have to change partners frequently to practice the attention/quiet routine and the partner routine. As another example, if certain small group activities require a certain number of students, students should be able to get into these groups. This too can be practiced.
- *Periodically check for student understanding:* Ask students to describe the procedure and why it is important to do it well.
- *Prompt, rather than pray:* As students learn a routine, prompt them with the appropriate action rather than standing and praying they remember what to do. For example, if they have 10 seconds to transition to a new formation, after a couple of seconds, put one hand in the air and call out 5, 4, 3, 2, and 1 as you decrease the number of fingers in the air. However, be mindful that this does not become a routine for you. The goal is ultimately for students to come to complete the routine within the set time limit without needing to be prompted.

Learning Experience 7.3

Provide an example of a routine that you might employ at the end of a lesson. Think in terms of lesson closure, where it might take place, how students are grouped, and whether collection of equipment is involved. Remember, a routine is intended to save time and be efficient.

Postprimary teachers are often required to take attendance and report it as soon as class begins. There are multiple effective attendance routines from which teachers can choose. For example, the teacher may choose an attendance routine where students come into the gym, pick up their name/activity card (see **Figure 7.1**) off the floor, hand it to the teacher, and then move to their team space for warm-up. This routine allows the teacher to have personal contact with each student and permits the teacher to know who is in attendance in a time-efficient manner. The sample attendance card also provides a way for the students to maintain a record of some aspect of the lesson (e.g., laps walked, activities achieved). Similarly, team captains can be charged with the responsibility to note team member absences to the teacher.

Another possibility is to employ the initial activity (e.g., team warm-ups/conditioning) as a time for the teacher to quickly determine which students are absent. Notice that this allows the teacher to overlap the managerial task of taking attendance during a time when all students are active. Employing such overlapping skills reflects advanced effectiveness in class management (Doyle, 1986; Kounin, 1970). The key message here is that lining students up standing or sitting along a wall is simply an unacceptable routine because it takes too long (especially with larger class sizes) and takes time away from students being active.

Rules and Their Development

Rules specify behaviors students need to avoid or exhibit to help make classes positive and appropriate environments for all students to learn and grow. Rules help students learn the behaviors and attitudes needed to live cooperatively with

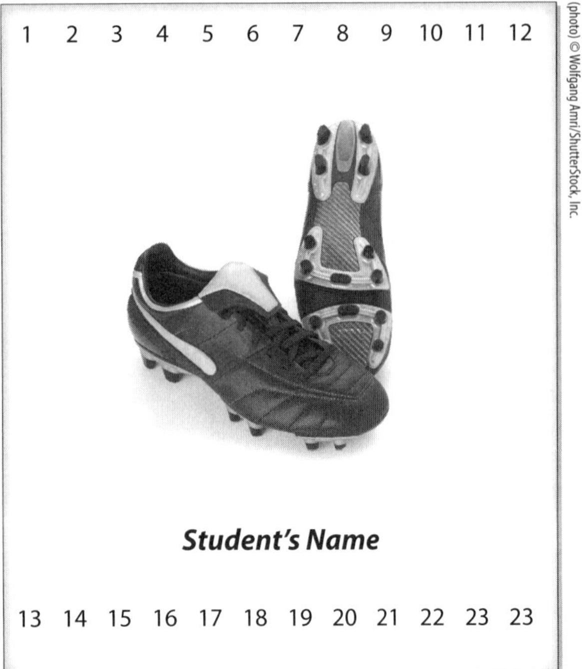

FIGURE 7.1 Sample attendance card.

others in work and in play over a lifetime. Rules can specify both behaviors students should learn and the situations in which they are appropriate or inappropriate (e.g., talking to a classmate is sometimes acceptable, sometimes expected and encouraged, and sometimes inappropriate). The behaviors specified in rules need to be learned and practiced, just as do content skills. Rules tend to differ from routines in that they often specify general categories of behavior that occur in different situations. Rules such as "respect your classmates," "play fairly," and "be cooperative" refer to groups of behaviors that differ from situation to situation but tend to have the same effect. When designing rules, or working with students to select appropriate rules to govern classroom behavior, consider the following categories:

- *Safety:* This involves behavior appropriate to certain kinds of equipment, specific curriculum and instruction models, and behavior related to classmates (e.g., not using a climbing wall without permission and supervision, walking a safe distance behind a peer swinging a golf club, having a spotter when attempting a new street dance jump).
- *Respect others:* This involves behavior related to the teacher and classmates (e.g., encourage others, support peers' efforts, be positive, and avoid hurting anyone physically or emotionally).
- *Respect the learning environment:* This involves behavior related to equipment and the physical space (e.g., keeps the sports hall clean, put away all the equipment after use, care for equipment as if it were your own).
- *Support the learning of others:* This involves behavior related to sharing, supporting, and helping the group (e.g., take responsibility for your role in class, share equipment space, provide peer assistance when needed).
- *Try hard:* This involves behavior such as using time well, staying on task, and making an effort to be on time, be on task, and always try hard.

One method of involving students in the design of rules to guide classroom behavior is to use the full value contract (FVC), which is frequently employed in Adventure Education to set the stage for the classroom to be a safe place for all students to enjoy and be successful. An FVC is an agreement among members of a class whereby they decide on specific behavior guidelines and expectations that will ultimately guide their interactions with one another in class. Throughout the year, students can be reminded of their FVC and brought back to it for discussion, review, and even adding more behaviors as the need arises. **Figure 7.2** displays an FVC designed by an undergraduate student during her teacher education program.

Sometimes rules need to be taught differently than routines. The behaviors that fulfill a class rule such as "respect others" will differ from situation to situation. Therefore, the range of behaviors that comply with the rule—and those that violate it—needs to be taught. When you are developing and teaching rules, the following guidelines will be helpful:

- Rules should be as short and direct as possible.
- Rules should be communicated in language and symbols that are age appropriate.
- No more than four to seven rules should be used because too many rules cannot be effectively written by teachers or remembered by students.
- When possible, state rules positively, but make sure that both positive and negative examples are provided.
- Make sure class rules are consistent with school rules.
- Early in the year (or semester), prompt rules often; give frequent, specific feedback; and consistently acknowledge students who follow rules.

Class rules should be related to consequences. With this in mind, one final bullet point on the design and teaching of rules should be included:

- Develop a hierarchy of consequences (least to most severe), and clearly specify their relationship to rule violations.

One pre-service teacher designed a way for her students to design a FVC using what she labeled a "HANDS-IN" concept.

1. The teacher identifies five significant values or commitments to guide the class in developing their "HANDS-IN" agreement. In this case, the teacher chose

   Safety First **Teamwork** **Commitment** **Be Self-Aware** **Be Honest**

   * The group also can be given the option of choosing their own five values.

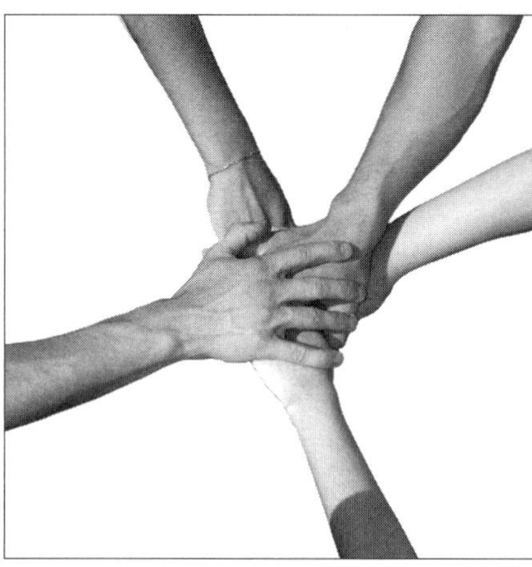

2. Split the pupils into five groups and give each group one of the above values.
3. Each group is given the task of brainstorming key words that represent this value.
4. Have an open discussion among the entire class about what words and attributes each group has identified and suggested.
5. The group selects which words they feel best represent each of the values.
6. Each person should draw and cut out the shape of their hand from their colored piece of paper and write one of the chosen words that represents the value.
7. When this is completed, everyone will post their hand around in a circular fashion.
8. The group has now completed their "HANDS-IN" contract with values and expectations that they feel is most important for a comfortable and effective learning environment.
9. Each member in the group should feel a sense of ownership of the contract. If a member of a group breaks this contract, the visual is there as a reminder for everyone to see.

FIGURE 7.2 A sample full value contract (FVC).

Consequences should be explained to students. Good physical education teachers post both the rules and consequences conspicuously in multiple locations (e.g., the gymnasium, hallways, changing rooms). It is important to keep in mind that rules, to be effective, need to be made clear and then enforced fairly and consistently.

Teachers should prompt compliance with rules often, by pointing out opportunities to behave in ways that fulfill the rule and by publicly acknowledging instances of good examples of behavior as well as instances of student behavior that are not in line with a rule. Students need to be reminded of rules at times other than when a rule violation occurs, for instance, referring to a rule of "working cooperatively" at times other than when there is an argument or inappropriate language being displayed. Asking students about behaviors related to rules is a good way to judge the degree to which they are beginning to understand the rules (for example, asking students about safe and unsafe ways of using equipment).

To move beyond compliance toward cooperation and, eventually, a learning community, students must understand why rules are chosen or jointly developed and why positive or negative consequences are related to following or violating rules. Reasons for rules and consequences, and the relationships among them, do not have to be conveyed through lectures—indeed, that would be ineffective. However, students need to understand why safety is important and why cooperation among learners is essential both for their own development and for the good of the class as a whole. This is best accomplished through giving concrete examples, having students engage in activities that foster the types of behavior you are looking to develop, recognizing positive instances of rule following, and providing lots of specific feedback. Helping students understand why rules are important begins to move the students' perceptions that they are the teacher's rules to a sense that they are their rules.

Almost all teachers develop class rules. Not all, however, teach them effectively; nor do all enforce them consistently. Student perceptions of the fairness of the rules and the consistency and fairness of the application of consequences are fundamentally important to their buying into the managerial system. Teachers should never develop rules they cannot consistently enforce, nor should they specify consequences they cannot consistently deliver.

Managerial Time: What It Is and Why Reduce It

Managerial time refers to the cumulative amount of time students spend in managerial tasks, that is, all the organizational, transitional, and non-subject-matter tasks in a lesson. It is time when no instruction is given, no demonstrations are made, and no practice is done. Therefore, it contains no opportunities for students to accomplish instructional goals. Roll taking, getting equipment out, waiting for an activity to begin, organizing teams, moving from one place to another, and handing out parental consent forms for a field trip are all examples of managerial tasks that contribute to managerial time. We are not suggesting that these tasks are not necessary. However, less-effective teachers consistently spend too much time accomplishing managerial tasks. Research also supports the commonsense notion that disruptive student behavior is more likely to occur during managerial tasks than during instruction or practice tasks. Effectively implementing managerial tasks, therefore, not only reduces managerial time and increases chances for instruction and practice but also reduces the likelihood of disruptive behavior.

An important concept in understanding and reducing managerial time is the managerial task or, as it is sometimes referred to, the **managerial episode**. Each managerial task consists of an episode of time and behavior. Managerial tasks begin with some event (most frequently a signal or instruction from the teacher), and they end when the next instructional event or activity begins. For example, the teacher may blow his or her whistle to gain students' attention (start of managerial task), and then ask students to go to their team court and design an offensive play for moving the disc down the court in Ultimate Frisbee (managerial task ends when teams begin the design of an offensive play).

The total time in all episodes is the managerial time for that lesson. Focusing on managerial tasks allows a specific analysis of where in a lesson and for what purposes managerial time is being accumulated.

The following are examples of managerial tasks:

- Students come from the locker/changing room and await the first signal from the teacher to begin the class (time from the official beginning of the period to the moment when the first instruction is given).
- A teacher blows her whistle and tells the class to assemble on one side of the gym (time from the whistle until the class is assembled and another instruction is given).
- A teacher, having explained a drill, signals students to go to their proper places to begin the drill (time from the dispersion signal to the moment the activity actually begins).
- Inside a gym, a teacher finishes instructions for an activity and sends the class outside to begin the activity (time from signal to leave until the outside activity begins).

Often it is not any one managerial task that wastes a major portion of class time but rather the accumulation of individual episodes that are each a little too long. Many teachers are surprised at the number of managerial tasks in a typical lesson but are pleased to learn that managerial time can be reduced substantially—and often easily.

A particularly important managerial task is the **transitional task**. In any physical education lesson, there are often several instructional tasks, requiring teachers to change from one task to another or from one variation of a task to another (e.g., teams changing courts, moving between stations in a fitness lesson, making substitutions in games, changing the demands of a group task in dance, partner balance task in gymnastics). In any given primary lesson, it is not uncommon to have 15–20 transitional tasks per lesson; in secondary lessons there tend to be fewer transitions, albeit the spaces are larger and the class size is greater, so loss of time often is more dramatic.

Transitions, therefore, account for a large portion of accumulated managerial time. Effective teachers establish routines for all recurring managerial and transitional tasks. When a managerial task system is well established, it not only reduces managerial time and the opportunities for disruptive behavior but also quickens the pace of a lesson and maintains the momentum of that pace throughout the lesson. A quick pace that is maintained throughout the lesson is important to convey to students that they are in a learning environment. A quickly paced, upbeat lesson in which the pace is maintained through a well-established managerial task system probably does more than any other factor to impress upon learners the teacher's intent that they learn and improve. Early research (Kounin, 1970) showed that slowing the pace of the lesson or breaking its momentum with interruptions or other slow-down events tends to increase disruptive behavior and lessen the learning time students acquire. There is no research at this point in time to dispute this notion.

Learning Experience 7.4

Provide an example of a transitional task that might occur in your physical education class. Determine how you might prompt this task to be completed more quickly and thus save time.

The Skills and Strategies Most Important to Preventive Class Management

An effective managerial task system is developed and maintained by using key strategies and some important teaching skills. The primary goal is to develop a system that enables students to do a great deal of self-management, that makes them want to be responsible members of the class, and that allows teachers time to attend to learning-related issues rather than managerial issues.

Starting the Lesson

Managing how you *start the lesson* frequently sets the tone for the entire lesson and those lessons to follow. It sends the message that physical education is important and this is a setting where learning will occur. Younger students often come to the gym ready for activity and eager to become involved. Some older students straggle in and are already trying to avoid participation. For both groups, and for all those in between, the start of lessons is important and should be informative, stimulating, and challenging. A lesson that drags right from the start, because of poor organization and management, is difficult to energize. As you plan each lesson, consider how you might use some of the following points to guide you:

- An entry routine can assist in an effective and smooth-running start to the lesson.
- Start the class on time because promptness establishes the pace and momentum of a class and underscores the importance of what is done in physical education.
- Use a time-saving method for taking attendance such as during the initial activity, with students at home base, by student captains/leaders, or by nonparticipants.
- Provide an initial activity so that when students enter the gym, they have something to do that contributes to lesson outcomes.

Transitions

Effective management of *transitions* is the best place to save overall management time and also is likely to be the best way to decrease chances for disruptive behavior that occurs during dead times in class. Well-managed transitions also send a clear message to students that what happens in physical education is important and requires their attention, cooperation, and enthusiasm. Effectively managing transitions is the surest way to produce what teaching research has described as a "task-oriented climate," so often associated with high learning gains.

The following are management strategies that will result in more effective transitions:

- Develop clear attention, gathering, and dispersal routines. Make sure the students begin the routine on a "go" signal, which is also taught. These are the important keys to moving students around spaces efficiently.
- Always have something for students to do when the transition is completed. This can be either the start of the next activity or specific directions explaining what to do in the new space. Nothing is more detrimental to effective management and discipline than students being asked to wait at the end of transitions.
- Consider having primary children practice a locomotor skill (e.g., skipping, hopping) as they do the transition. This will give them some skill practice during the transition and provide some focus for their movement from place to place.
- Establish a time goal. When establishing expectations for quick transitions, say, for example, "Let's do this in less than 20 seconds," count the time as the transition is being made, and compliment the group when the goal is met. Next time the goal can be reduced slightly until students get the idea of how quickly transitions can be accomplished.
- Use music to manage transitions. With the available technology and software (e.g., see Audacity at www.audacity.sourceforge.net; Garage Band at www.apple.com/ilife/garageband; Seconds Pro, an interval timer for iPhones at https://itunes.apple.com/ie/app/seconds-pro-interval-timer/id363978811?mt=8) that allow you make all kinds of interval music that is really easy to use, teachers can now easily create MP3 files with music that have short blocks of silence inserted. When the music goes silent, it signals that students quickly rotate from one station to the next (such as during a fitness circuit) or switch tasks (e.g., a lifter becomes the spotter and vice versa during a strength conditioning lesson). The expectation is that students are engaged again by the time the music restarts. Effective use of music can be an excellent management strategy. Moreover, students generally enjoy having music playing in the background, and there is some evidence that music can be used as a motivational tool as well (Ward & Dunaway, 1995).

Equipment Transitions

Equipment transitions not only take time but also often create dead time for students not involved in them. Dead time creates opportunities for off-task behavior that can spread and disrupt the smoothness and momentum of the class. There are several ways to avoid this through effectively managing equipment transitions.

- *Have an equipment manager.* If you use teams, consider having an equipment manager as a primary role for each team. That person would organize team members to manage the equipment appropriately.
- *Find different systems for children to exchange equipment.* This could be, for example, month of birth or color of clothing. The point is to keep a smooth flow of students exchanging items. If you use a home base routine that involves numbers or colors, you can use this system for managing equipment exchanges.
- *Organize your equipment storage.* Find ways that facilitate exchange according to whatever system you develop.

Managing Formations

Effective teachers provide many practice opportunities for their students to learn the skills and strategies that are the focus for a lesson. Practice often requires grouping students (scattered, pairs, triads, quads, and the like). Much of the lost management time in lessons can be attributed to students not organizing efficiently for practice formations. The following practices can facilitate efficient organization and management of formations:

- *Teach commonly used formations as routines.* A teacher who uses pairs, triads, and quads frequently should teach them as routines. A teacher should be able to say, "Form practice triangles with players 10 feet apart and each triangle at least 15 feet from the next. Go!" This routine combines a form of a partner routine and the disperse routine.
- *Structure the space for a lesson.* Use cones, hot/poly spots, floor lines, or chalk both inside and outside to delineate practice groupings.
- *Mark the gym floor or paved outdoor space into a grid format.* A grid system is simply a grid of 8- to 10-foot squares. Each square can become a home base. Corners can be used to quickly organize into pairs, triads, or quads. Adjacent squares can be used to organize into larger spaces with more students. When game lines are needed, the grid lines can be used for that purpose also.

For example, as a teacher you could have a class list with each student numbered on the list. At the start of class, ask students to look at the posted colored grid chart (see

	Line 1	Line 2	Line 3	Line 4
Row F	7	15	11	5
Row E	13	8	19	1
Row D	4	20	14	24
Row C	6	22	16	18
Row B	17	9	2	21
Row A	10	3	23	12

FIGURE 7.3 A color grid for grouping students.

Figure 7.3) and find their number, line number, row letter, and color. Once students learn their place with each of these criteria you have a number of different ways to transition students to partners (grid partner is the person next to you; lines 1 and 2 and lines 3 and 4), groups of six (rows A, B, C, D, E, and F, or colors), groups of four (lines 1, 2, 3, 4). Students can easily move from working in their lines to working with their partner to working in a group of five. A couple of teachers were recently introduced to this concept by their student teacher, and after initial skepticism, they have now been converted to its use after seeing how successful it was for young people, with one teacher noting, "Students don't seem to mind being partnered with someone they would not ordinarily pick because it is set by the grid rather than by teacher design."

Momentum and Pace of the Lesson

Momentum refers to the smoothness with which the various segments of a lesson flow together. A lesson with momentum has no breaks and no times when activities or transitions slow down the pace. **Pace** refers to the degree to which the lessons move forward quickly. Kounin (1970) showed that quickly paced lessons that are smooth are clearly associated with more effective teaching and learning.

The following management techniques contribute to the smoothness of lessons:

- Start class on time and with a well-paced activity.
- Manage transitions so that dead time is eliminated.
- Have a procedure for dealing with intrusions. The procedure for dealing with notes from the principal, a public address announcement, a slightly injured student, or a child who begins to cry should allow you to deal with the intrusive event and still keep the class activity going. Some primary school teachers have had success with teaching children a simple cue that tells them the teacher is going to be busy for a few moments and they are to continue their activity and behave responsibly.
- Make your expectations for a smooth, well-paced class clear to your students. Recognize and praise students who try hard and move quickly. Students will soon learn what the norm for the class is to be.
- Show enthusiasm for the lesson, activity, and students. An important teacher behavior for showing enthusiasm is what we call "hustles." Hustles are verbal and nonverbal behaviors that energize students. Interjections such as "let's go," "quickly, quickly," and "hustle!" are cues for students to pick up the pace.

Teacher Interactive Behavior

Good management does not just happen. It is the result of a clear, proactive strategy. It is accomplished through instruction and practice; that is, it is taught and learned. During the teaching and learning phase, the **teacher's interactive behavior** is crucial to success.

- Give explicit instructions, frequent prompts, and regular feedback when establishing the managerial task system.
- Give feedback to individuals and to the class as a whole. Specific feedback, including information on time spent and time saved, is more important than general feedback (such as "good job"/"well done").
- Have high expectations and communicate them frequently at the outset. An expectation is shown through teacher interaction that describes a process or outcome that is to be achieved. Expectations can describe a process ("I expect you to move quickly when you change stations.") or outcomes ("I want you to complete the equipment exchange within 30 seconds.").
- Communicate feedback and expectations. One good way to do this is to post records of managerial performance by students. You can wear a simple wrist chronograph that allows easy measurement and records the times of various managerial episodes. At the outset of the year or semester, this approach can help you set goals and post performance improvements related to those goals.
- Gradually reduce interactions as students become more proficient at management routines. The idea is to have students eventually manage themselves and to have most of the managerial tasks of a lesson become routine. Intermittently, however, continue to praise and recognize students' good behavior and performance.

Safety Guidelines

Both emotional and physical safety are critical to any physical education class and require intentional planning. For students to feel safe the environment must be safe; safety precautions must be planned, and shared with, students. A few ideas that might help guide you in developing safety measures include:

- Develop classroom safety rules and post them in a prominent place for all students to see.
- Revisit safety rules as the year progresses or when some are most essential for a given activity.
- Certain activities such as bouldering/climbing wall, throwing activities in athletics (i.e., track and field), and archery require content-specific safety procedures. It is imperative that you are vigilant in monitoring students' compliance with such safety routines.
- Design emergency systems so students know what to do if a peer is injured. This might involve students knowing to stop activity and sit down, having one student assigned to go immediately to the office for assistance, and having one student designated to collect a first-aid kit and/or ice for injury management.
- Many schools, especially larger ones with expansive outdoor facilities, provide physical educators with two-way radios that help in connecting with emergency medical transport teams. With the prevalence of mobile phones, many teachers carry those with them to use in the event of a medical emergency.

Recognizing Potential Behavior Problems

Regardless of how well the teacher has designed the preventive management system; taught rules, routines, and other management procedures; and allowed students to practice and receive feedback on appropriate behavior, there will still be instances of students being off-task or disruptive. Low-level passive disruption is characterized by a student who is off-task yet not disturbing the learning of peers, whereas high-level active disruption suggests that others are affected by a student's off-task or inappropriate behavior. In other words, the degree of amotivation or disaffection and how a teacher might deal with each differently are central to management in the classroom. There is, however, a set of essential teaching strategies that can assist the teacher in recognizing student behaviors that have the potential to prevent other students from learning. Once the teacher is aware of these behaviors they can be managed before they escalate.

Active Supervision

Active supervision is a crucial teaching strategy that is useful in both the managerial and the instructional task systems. It might be easiest to think of active supervision as an umbrella set of strategies that a teacher uses at various times within the lesson—during teacher presentation of tasks, demonstration of skills, student group work, whole class instruction, independent practice, or individual performances. There is a substantial body of research that supports employing active supervision throughout each lesson (e.g., Hastie & Saunders, 1990; Patterson & van der Mars, 2008; Sariscsany, van der Mars, & Darst, 1995; Schuldheisz & van der Mars, 2001). When these strategies are used in physical education lessons, active supervision is found to

- Maintain a safe learning environment
- Support student learning
- Monitor student progress and success
- Ensure on-task student behavior
- Provide student assistance
- Encourage improvement

The umbrella set of strategies for managing off-task behaviors include back to the wall, proximity control, with-it-ness, selective ignoring, using names, overlapping, and positive pinpointing. Effective use of these will help prevent students' straying off-task, or at least keep it from escalating.

Back to the Wall

The *back to the wall* strategy refers to the teacher being positioned in the gymnasium so that he or she can view at least 90% of the students 90% of the time, thus seeing off-task behavior when it starts rather than after it has taken hold and spread to other students. The idea is to use the gymnasium boundaries or lines on the gym floor to position yourself to allow a view of the entire group. From this position the teacher can scan the entire class while moving in and out among groups of students in an unpredictable manner, interacting and providing feedback along the way. In the diagram of an activity space shown in **Figure 7.4** we have highlighted the danger zone—the area where a teacher would have his or her back to a large number of pupils in the class. If conscious of this zone, teachers can strive to move in a way that allows them to keep their back to the wall and the majority of the class in sight at all times. At all costs, you will want to avoid "piddling in the middle."

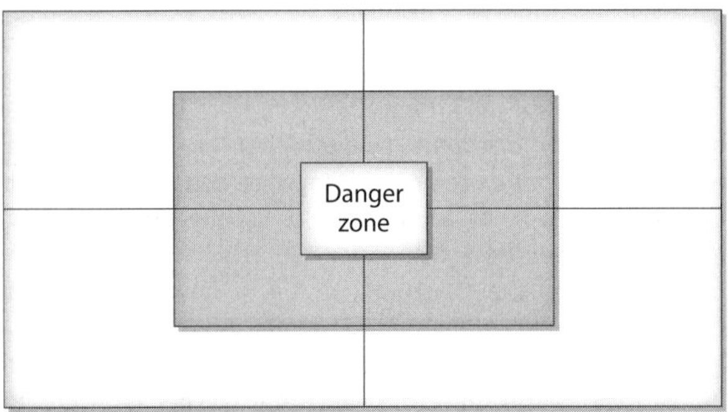

FIGURE 7.4 The danger zone.

A related consideration is the physical arrangement of equipment and location of student groups. You will want to balance the need for having sufficient space between groups to ensure safety, yet not spread out so far that it would hamper your ability to effectively supervise the group and the activity.

Proximity Control

Any of us that have ever misbehaved know that if the teacher or person of authority is near we tend to behave more appropriately, especially if the teacher gives us that serious "don't you dare" teacher look. This is the idea behind the *proximity control* strategy. Move to the problem, give the look, and therefore head off inappropriate behavior and prevent it from escalating. In many cases you need not even say a word.

With-it-ness

As a student, did you ever feel that the teacher had eyes in the back of her head? No matter where the teacher was standing in the class, every time someone started to misbehave the teacher would be right there quickly targeting off-task behavior or using feedback across space to let you know she was aware of what was happening. With-it-ness requires the teacher to know what the class looks like in order to recognize any visual cues that suggest something is not right; what the class sounds like so that a change in noise level might indicate something is amiss; and how the class tends to operate that would highlight behavior patterns that are becoming disruptive. Although disconcerting for the troublesome student, with-it-ness is a benefit to those students who are engaged in the learning experience and get distracted when peers misbehave.

Selective Ignoring

The idea of a teacher choosing her or his battles might be one way to think of *selective ignoring*. In other words, if a student is off-task but not disrupting others, why not ignore the behavior and maintain the momentum of the lesson? In some cases, the teacher may find that selective ignoring can lead to extinction of an unwanted behavior. A student who is not getting the attention desired may stop trying to gain it through this particular behavior (Graham, 2008). A teacher who knows her or his students well may come to recognize that for some students a particular behavior is the norm for them and not intended as a disruption or a way to gain attention from peers or the teacher. When this becomes apparent to the teacher, she or he might assist other students in appreciating the behavior for what it is and ignoring it as well.

Using Names

If teachers are to build positive relationships with their students, help learners to feel valued and worthwhile, and maintain lessons that flow and are not marred by disruptions and poor behavior, learning and using student names frequently are critical. If positioned on one side of the gym when a disruption occurs on the other side, it is more efficient and effective to use feedback across space to a particular student by using his or her name than having to move to the problem because you do not know the student's name. From a positive perspective, using student names to praise behavior, encourage effort, prompt technique, or applaud team play is certainly a strategy to keep students focused on the lesson while promoting appropriate behavior. It also makes it easier for teachers to employ the aforementioned with-it-ness.

Learning Experience 7.5

Learning names is a difficult task. What strategy might you employ to assist you in learning the names of all students you teach at the postprimary level, where class sizes are frequently large?

Overlapping

Consider the following scenario: Thirty students enter your teaching space eager to participate, attendance is due to the office within minutes of the class starting, two boys and one girl need to borrow gear, the initial lesson activity is new today so needs some oversight, and the other physical education class has a substitute today, which often makes things a bit more hectic than usual. A teacher who is able to deal effectively with all of these classroom occurrences is said to be *overlapping* (i.e., doing several things at one time). Maintaining intent while all of these situations are taking place is a learned teaching skill; it does not just happen, it evolves over time. It revolves around strong teacher planning, knowing students well, caring about each of them, effectively running routines, and developing confidence that you can maintain the lesson flow despite any disruptions. Be patient while you develop the ability to overlap a number of events that occur in your physical education classes.

Positive Pinpointing

When students struggle with what an appropriate behavior (or skill in the instructional task system) looks like, a teacher might choose to identify a student or students who are demonstrating the behavior correctly, thus using *positive pinpointing*. Teachers identifying appropriate behavior through positive pinpointing highlights learners, models desired behavior, and reinforces appropriate behavior.

Assessing the Effectiveness of the Managerial Task System

How well does your management system work? The managerial task system should be assessed periodically to make sure it is running as smoothly and efficiently as possible and to identify possible weak components (for example, a particular transition that regularly takes too much time). Monitoring managerial task performance is not difficult and does not need to be time-consuming for the teacher. Managerial task lengths can be easily recorded with a wrist chronograph. You could also tally the number of prompts and interactions you have with students during managerial tasks (the more prompts and interactions, the less students are engaged in self-management). You might also occasionally observe selected students to see how often they have to wait for the next lesson segment to begin or the frequency with which they are off-task during managerial tasks. Not all these observations have to be made in the same lesson; you still have to teach.

As students are actively participating in class activities, there is a series of questions that you want to consider continuously while you are actively supervising their efforts:

- Are students working safely?
- Are students on task?
- Are students working cooperatively?
- How are students interacting among groups?
- Where was I positioned during different parts of class?
- Where did I move as the learning tasks progressed?
- How did I organize the skill practice, and why was it successful or not successful?
- How do I manage students as they participate in lesson tasks?

As you answer these questions and analyze your observation data you may find that managerial tasks are performed quickly, that the next activities begin without student waiting, and that all this gets done without many prompts, desists, or feedback to students. You will then know that you have developed and are maintaining an effective managerial task system.

Learning Experience 7.6

Identify a teacher in your teaching practice setting who has a reputation for providing a positive and well-managed classroom where students take responsibility for their own behavior and learning. Ask the teacher if you may interview him or her and perhaps observe one of his or her lessons to become familiar with the strategies the teacher employs.

CHAPTER SUMMARY

In this chapter we focused on classroom management in physical education, specifically the nature of designing a preventive management system to prevent off-task and inappropriate behavior from occurring. We examined the importance of the teacher–student relationship, working with young people to develop and maintain a positive learning environment, how to develop and teach rules and routines, and the most effective classroom management techniques. Finally, we explored methods of maintaining a productive classroom. Behavior problems are less likely to occur if an effective preventive management plan has been taught and reinforced; however, we know that behavior problems will occur and can be quite distressing for teachers, especially novice teachers.

1. Effective class management is a necessary precondition for effective teaching and learning.
2. Preventive management refers to the proactive strategies used by teachers to develop and maintain a positive, on-task climate.
3. The managerial task system establishes the limits for behavior and the positive expectations for students.
4. Behavior for learning suggests that behavior problems are learned and developed through the relationship students have with themselves, their peers and others, and the curriculum. Key for developing appropriate behaviors is the learning environment, which the teacher is responsible for creating cooperatively with students.
5. Teaching is about relationships. Teaching strategies employed by the teacher, the responses and interactions of students, and ultimately the learning that is achieved by students are all influenced by this relationship.
6. At the foundation of an effective management system is the development, teaching, and monitoring of classroom routines and rules.
7. Rules identify appropriate and inappropriate behaviors and the situations within which certain behaviors are acceptable or unacceptable.
8. Routines are taught for all procedural aspects of lessons that recur frequently.
9. Although they may be taught differently, both routines and rules need to be taught as specifically as a teacher might teach any movement or sport skill.
10. Class rules should be related to consequences so students know the consequences of choosing to violate an agreed-upon rule.
11. Managerial time refers to the cumulative amount of time students spend in managerial tasks when no instruction is given, no demonstrations are made, and no practice is done; that is, organizational, transitional, and non-subject-matter tasks in a lesson.
12. Managerial tasks or episodes begin with some event (most frequently a signal or instruction from the teacher) and end when the next instructional event or activity begins. It is not one managerial task that wastes a great deal of class time but the accumulation of individual episodes.
13. A lesson is typically made up of several transitional tasks such as changing activities, movement of students between stations, or regrouping students for a new activity.
14. An effective managerial task system is developed and maintained by using key strategies and some important teaching skills, such as starting the lesson, transitions, equipment transitions, managing formations, momentum and pace, teacher interactions, and safety guidelines.
15. There is a set of teaching strategies that can assist the teacher in recognizing student behaviors that have the potential to prevent other students from learning.
16. When the umbrella set of strategies known as active supervision is used effectively by the teacher throughout class activities, the result is maintenance of a safe learning environment, support given to student learning, monitoring of student progress and success, on-task student behavior, and students being provided with assistance.
17. The umbrella set of active supervision strategies for managing off-task behaviors includes back to the wall, proximity control, with-it-ness, selective ignoring, using names, overlapping, and positive pinpointing.
18. Teachers should assess their managerial task system periodically to make sure it is running as smoothly and efficiently as possible and to identify areas that need improvement.

REFERENCES

Behaviour2Learn. Home page. Available from www.behaviour2learn.co.uk

Brophy, J., & Good, T. (1986). Teacher behavior and student achievement. In M. C. Wittrock (Ed.), *Handbook of research on teaching* (3rd ed., pp. 328–375). New York: MacMillan.

Burnett, P. (2002). Teacher praise and feedback and students' perceptions of the classroom environment. *Educational Psychology, 22*(1), 5–16.

Doyle, W. (1986). Classroom organization and management. In M. C. Wittrock (Ed.). *Handbook of research on teaching* (3rd ed., pp. 392–431). New York: Macmillan.

Graham, G. (2008). *Teaching children physical education: Becoming a master teacher* (3rd ed.). Champaign, IL: Human Kinetics.

Hardin, C. J. (2008). *Effective classroom management: Models and strategies for today's classrooms* (2nd ed.). Upper Saddle River, NJ: Prentice Hall.

Hastie, P. A., & Saunders, J. E. (1990). A study of monitoring in secondary school physical education. *Journal of Classroom Interaction, 25*, 47–54.

Kounin, J. (1970). *Discipline and group management classrooms.* New York: Holt, Rinehart & Winston.

Marzano, R. J. (2003). *What works in schools: Translating research into action.* Alexandria, VA: Association for Supervision and Curriculum Development (ASCD).

Marzano, R. J., Marzano, J. S., & Pickering, D. J. (2009). *Classroom management that works: Research-based strategies for every teacher.* Alexandria, VA: Association for Supervision and Curriculum Development (ASCD).

Patterson, D., & van der Mars, H. (2008). Distant interactions and their effects on children's physical activity. *Physical Education and Sport Pedagogy, 13*, 277–294.

Sariscsany, M. J., Darst, P. W., & van der Mars, H. (1995). The effects of three teacher supervision patterns on student on-task and skill performance in secondary physical education. *Journal of Teaching in Physical Education, 14*, 179–197.

Schuldheisz, J., & van der Mars, H. (2001). Managing students' physical activity levels through active supervision in middle school physical education. *Journal of Teaching in Physical Education, 21*, 75–90.

Siedentop, S., Doutis, P., Tsangaridou, N., Ward, P., & Rouschenbach, J. (1994). Don't sweat gym: An analysis of curriculum and instruction. *Journal of Teaching in Physical Education, 13*, 375–394.

Todorovich, J. R., & Curtner-Smith, M. D. (2002). Influence of motivational climate in physical education on sixth grade pupils goal orientation. *European Physical Education Review, 8*, 119–138.

Ward, P., & Dunaway, S. (1995). Effects of contingent music on laps run in a high school physical education class. *Physical Educator, 52*(1), 2–7.

CHAPTER 8 Developing Discipline Using Effective Behavior Management

Overall Chapter Outcome

To develop a comprehensive, proactive discipline strategy for a particular developmental level of students that incorporates a specific effort to lead students to being self-directed learners reflecting personal and social responsibility

Learning Outcomes

The learner will:

- Define discipline
- Understand students' perspectives on teachers' use of management/discipline strategies
- Develop a reasoned perspective on the use of punishment and reinforcement as an approach to developing discipline
- Explain why discipline is important
- Explicate the concept of primary prevention
- Explain and apply strategies for changing behavior
- Describe effective praise and related interaction techniques
- Designate and apply reinforcement and punishment techniques for increasing pro-social behavior and decreasing misbehavior, respectively
- Explain the various considerations and recommendations for implementing the various behavior change techniques
- Explain the ultimate goal of a discipline system

When problems arise, the first question to ask should be, "Did I do all I could in using my preventative management approaches effectively?" If you did and you still experience problems with students' behavior, having experience in employing evidence-based **discipline** techniques will help reduce such problems.

Teachers often struggle with issues related to discipline, especially if preventative class management is lacking. Garrahy, Kulinna, and Cothran (2005) found that U.S. elementary school physical educators across varying years of experience and teaching contexts (i.e., urban vs. suburban) mostly depend on the following three strategies for navigating discipline issues with students: (1) trial and error, (2) advice from colleagues, and (3) professional development. Most noted that their teacher education program did little, if anything, to equip them with effective discipline strategies. Teachers increasingly view the parents of students as "accomplices in their child's poor behavior" (p. 59).

Much in line with the dual-directional influence between teachers and students within the ecological framework, there is evidence that students (1) are keenly aware of the management dynamics at play within the class (Cothran & Ennis, 1997) and (2) view teachers as effective managers when they

BOX 8.1 Key Terms in This Chapter

- *Activity reinforcers:* Reinforcers in the form of students' favorite activities or privileges. In primary physical education settings, activities such as jumping rope, shooting baskets, playing soccer, or privileges like getting to be first in line or assisting the teacher with equipment are all potential activity reinforcers.
- *Behavior management:* The formal and planned application of specific and evidence-based techniques based on the behavioral principles of reinforcement and punishment.
- *Consequence:* An event that follows a particular behavior. Consequences may be positive or negative. In physical education environments, they provide the "reasons" for behaving that students need so they can learn new and appropriate forms of behavior.
- *Contingency:* Relationship between the situation or context (also referred to as the *antecedent*), the behavior, and a consequence.
- *Contingency contracts:* In collaboration with the student, the teacher creates a document in which the contingent relationship is explained between the expected student behavior and the delivery of a specified reward (a reinforcer). Also referred to as a *behavior contract.*
- *Differential reinforcement:* The teacher ignores the inappropriate behavior while at the same time reinforcing other more desirable behaviors. There are multiple applications of differential reinforcement, including differential reinforcement of incompatible behavior (DRI), differential reinforcement of alternative behavior (DRA), differential reinforcement of low rates of behavior (DRL), and differential reinforcement of other behavior (DRO).
- *Discipline (as a noun):* As in "This is a class that is disciplined"; a class with few if any instances of inappropriate behavior and ample examples of pro-social behavior among students.
- *Discipline (as a verb):* Application of a consequence deemed negative and negative consequence; implies and focuses on punishment.
- *Group contingency:* The presentation of a reinforcer (i.e., reward) contingent upon the behavior of an individual in a group, a segment of the group, or the group as a whole. Variations of this technique include dependent-, independent-, and interdependent-group contingencies.
- *Positive practice:* The teacher has students engage in an appropriate behavior a specified number of times as a consequence of misbehaving. Although technically a punishment procedure, it does carry with it an educative dimension in that the appropriate behavior is practiced repeatedly. Also referred to as *overcorrection.*
- *Premack principle:* Access to a highly desirable activity is contingent on completing a task that is undesirable and named after David Premack who first coined this contingency. Also referred to as *Grandma's rule.*
- *Prompt:* An extra reminder aimed at ensuring that the behavior occurs. Can be verbal, auditory, tactile, and/or visual. Occurs prior to the occurrence of the behavior. Also called *cues.*
- *Pro-social behavior:* Student behavior that enables achievement of educational and personal growth goals in settings such as physical education lessons.
- *Punishment:* Presentation of a consequence, aimed at reducing or eliminating future instances of the same behavior. If the behavior indeed occurs less frequently it can be said that this consequence was punishing in nature. Conversely, if the behavior persists, it would not be a punishment.
- *Reinforcement:* Application of a positive consequence, aimed at ensuring continued or increased occurrence of that behavior. Applying a negative consequence (also referred to as "punishment") is aimed at reducing or eliminating the inappropriate behavior.
- *Reward cost:* A punishment technique where students lose previously earned points or privileges as a consequence of misbehavior. Also referred to as *response cost.*
- *Social reinforcers:* Verbal and nonverbal forms of attention from the teacher (and/or peers) contingent on the occurrence of desirable behavior/performance.
- *Tangible reinforcers:* Reinforcers that come in the form of stickers, pencils, and the like. Any tangible item can potentially serve as a reinforcer, if it is something that students desire.
- *Time-out:* A frequently used punishment technique aimed at reducing future occurrences of the problem behavior, by removing the student from the class activity for a short period of time as a consequence of misbehaving or breaking a class rule. Technically, time-out is the removal of the chance to earn positive reinforcement.
- *Verbal desist:* A verbal reprimand aimed at having the student cease the unacceptable/inappropriate behavior.

set their expectations for behavior early, are consistent in applying them, and develop positive relationships with students (Cothran, Hodges-Kulinna, & Garrahy, 2003).

Discipline must be considered in the context of the skills and strategies associated with developing a preventive managerial task system. Discipline problems are much less likely to occur when an effective managerial task system is in place. In addition, effective discipline is fundamental to becoming a caring teacher and developing a successful learning community.

We have no illusions about the difficulty of developing and maintaining discipline in today's classes. Some students try to be fully disengaged from physical education. Others seem to enjoy disrupting classes and being rude to teachers. Immature students often make fun of and exclude those who don't fit in. A few students can become physically abusive of others, especially in physical activity settings, where confrontations can occur. In recent years, bullying has emerged as a prevalent phenomenon. To further complicate things, the trend toward the full inclusion of students with disabling conditions has required teachers to further develop and refine their discipline skills to deal effectively with students' disabling behavioral problems. The behavior management strategies introduced in this chapter have been shown to be effective in helping students with disabilities.

Discipline is about developing and maintaining appropriate behavior between teachers and their students and, just as important, among students. This includes, as a basic goal of a discipline program, the absence of certain behaviors that threaten the peaceful, cooperative, productive nature of a class. We define *appropriate behavior* (also referred to as **pro-social behavior**) for students as that which enables the achievement of educational and personal growth goals in an educational setting. Different settings might require other definitions of appropriate behavior. Thus, we will not attempt to define in any specific way what any teacher ought to teach and enforce regarding discipline. But to be productive, all educational settings need high rates of appropriate behavior, no matter how it has been defined. It is insufficient to define appropriate behavior solely by the absence of inappropriate behavior.

The term *discipline* has always been important in teachers' vocabulary. Few in-class aspects of teaching provide more stress than discipline, especially for beginning teachers. School management will often evaluate, at least partially (and sometimes wholly), teachers on their ability to maintain good discipline in classes. Many physical educators will define discipline solely by the management and elimination of inappropriate behavior. To them, discipline means "keeping the troops in line," and the military analogy is not used without reason. For some teachers, maintaining discipline amounts to developing and sustaining a rigid atmosphere in which students avoid misbehavior because of the fear of serious consequences. In some rare instances, in certain school contexts, such an approach may be necessary at the outset as a means of gaining control in out-of-control situations.

We believe that discipline can and should be viewed from the perspective of it being dual-directional in its focus, where it targets both the reduction/elimination of misbehavior and the development of pro-social behavior. Think about it in terms of how we use the term when referring to a good sports team. Good teams are composed of players who are *disciplined* in their preparation and performance. It certainly means more than just the absence of mistakes.

Why Discipline Is Important

Developing discipline in your classes is important for many reasons. First, parents and school management/administrators expect classes to be well managed and well disciplined. Although parents and administrators understand that disruptions sometimes occur and that occasionally some students will become difficult discipline problems, they *expect* that a certified teacher can handle the disruptions and problems effectively, and maintain a focus on learning the subject matter. Teachers invariably rank discipline problems as one of the most important topics for continuing professional development. Beginning teachers across subject matters especially have consistently reported that managing student behavior is a primary concern (e.g., O'Connell Rust, 1994; Olson & Osborne, 1991; Veenman, 1984). O'Sullivan and Dyson (1994) reported that although high school physical educators did not perceive discipline to be a major problem, and worked hard to employ routines and clear and consistent expectations for student behavior, they did see it as distracting from accomplishing instructional goals. Importantly, it appeared that teachers lowered expectations in the instructional task system for compliance within the managerial task system (O'Sullivan & Dyson, 1994).

How teachers manage students' behavior is a main focus of evaluation by school management. More teachers get poor evaluations based on their ability to maintain discipline in their classes than they do for ineffective instructional skills. Nothing produces teacher fatigue and burnout more than having to deal constantly with discipline problems. For your own sanity and well-being, we urge you to learn as much as you can about how to effectively employ both preventive class management and discipline strategies and practice the skills associated with their effective use.

One of the strongest predictors of teacher ineffectiveness is the prevalence of off-task and disruptive behavior in classes. There is conclusive evidence in the teaching research literature that effective teachers are first and foremost good class managers. However, do not misconstrue this to mean that students in a well-managed and effectively disciplined class inherently learn more. There is a difference between creating the conditions for learning to take place and actually facilitating that learning through the design and delivery of meaningful and developmentally appropriate lesson content. Unfortunately, there are many physical education classes in which there is an adequate level of class management and students are well disciplined, but where students meet few, if any, learning goals (i.e., master skills, effectively use tactical moves, reach acceptable physical activity levels). Effective management and discipline create the opportunity for learning to take place, but the teacher must seize that opportunity and employ good instructional strategies, select appropriate content, and monitor student progress if the learning goals are to be realized. Thus, effective management and discipline are necessary preconditions for learning to take place, but they are not sufficient in and of themselves to guarantee learning.

Developing Pro-Social Behavior: Practicing Primary Prevention

Effective discipline is best achieved through a set of proactive strategies, the goal of which is the development and maintenance of appropriate student behavior. All teachers must come to grips with what they believe to be appropriate behavior in physical education classes. This will include behavior in three major categories: (1) interactions between the teacher and students, (2) interactions among students, and (3) interactions with the physical environment (e.g., equipment and facilities). Context and personal beliefs are important in this area, so we do not suggest specific behaviors within these categories. What is important, however, is that teachers build a consensus among their students that the behaviors that are necessary within each category are the right ones for building and maintaining a productive class environment. Only through consensus building can students come to view the behavior norms within a class as "our" norms rather than solely the norms of the teacher. When this is done effectively, students and teachers establish what amounts to a social contract that students believe in and help sustain.

Learning Experience 8.1

What do you see as key examples of student behavior that would fall in the three major categories of behavior listed above?

Teachers have a much easier time promoting appropriate behavior in their classes if there is a school-wide set of behavior norms. The likelihood of students feeling that behavior norms are "ours" is very much enhanced by adoption of school-wide behavior norms that all teachers expect and support. Finnicum (1997) argued that physical education teachers should practice "primary prevention," a concept borrowed from medicine. In that context, primary prevention refers to altering the environment to reduce the likelihood that diseases will develop (for example, creating a safe supply of drinking water in a neighborhood or ensuring that all infants are vaccinated). Secondary prevention refers to detecting the early signs of disease and initiating treatment. Much of what follows in later sections of this chapter is, in this sense, about secondary prevention.

The most important kind of primary prevention for physical educators is to help children and youth learn how to become responsible for their own behavior and then to act responsibly and helpfully toward their classmates. Physical education has a well-tested model for achieving the goals of primary prevention—the Teaching Personal and Social Responsibility (TPSR) model developed by Don Hellison and his colleagues (Hellison, 2011; Hellison et al., 2000). The model provides a progression of goals through which students move toward becoming fully responsible citizens of the physical education class and extend those behaviors and values outside of class. However, if despite employing sound preventative management and building a community of learners, students still persist in inappropriate behavior, then teachers need to address this with specific behavior change interventions.

Teachers have to develop a deliberate plan aimed at supporting and promoting pro-social behavior as well as reducing misbehavior. This plan should include specific information about the desired behavior and the unacceptable behavior of students, along with consequences for both. The plan should be communicated explicitly to students, so they are aware of the consequences. Unfortunately, in many cases, physical educators tend to focus their formal discipline plan solely on the negative consequences in the event that students choose to engage in misbehavior. For example, teachers post the following menu of progressively more negative consequences:

- Quiet warning
- Public warning
- Time-out (self-determined return to activity)
- Time-out (teacher-determined return to activity)
- Time-out for the duration of the class period
- Removal from class and sent to a room (sometimes called a Problem-Solving Room) on campus where the student (while supervised by another adult) is expected to reflect on his or her conduct
- Visit to a school administrator's office
- Phone call home
- In-school lunch period detention
- After school detention
- Suspension from school
- Expulsion from school

This one-sided approach to developing discipline only seeks to reduce inappropriate behavior. There is no guarantee that each of these intended consequences/punishers will actually be effective. For example, being removed from the activity (i.e., time-out) could be something that the student sought in the first place. A phone call to the parents/guardians may not hold much clout if parents have little interest in or concern for how their children conduct themselves. The remainder of this chapter offers an overview of evidence-informed strategies and specific behavior change techniques, including guidelines for implementation and considerations for use.

Changing Behavior

Developing school and classroom discipline is about changing behavior—specifically, changing disruptive behavior to helping behavior or changing rude, abusive interactions to polite, supportive interactions. As we argue, good discipline is not just about eliminating unwanted behavior but also about building and sustaining appropriate behavior (see **Box 8.2**). If teachers employ sound classroom management, coupled with planning and delivering meaningful and appropriate activity experiences that have built-in accountability for pro-social behavior (e.g., Sport Education), then the need to address extreme and/or persistent misbehavior is greatly diminished. Invariably, teachers will meet situations involving misbehavior that require some form of punishment. However, each time a teacher stops or punishes an inappropriate behavior, the opportunity arises to replace it with a more appropriate behavior. Effective teachers do just that. They work on a replacement strategy rather than just an elimination strategy.

We cannot state often enough that building an effective class management system, employing sound instructional techniques, and developing well-designed and meaningful learning tasks will go a long way toward preventing many student behavior problems. Not using managerial routines, spending excessive time in instruction, or using learning tasks where most students are inactive are the perfect recipe for creating more opportunity for disruptive behavior. Although it is easy to then blame students, an honest reflection by the teacher will reveal that such problems are largely self-inflicted.

Well-planned and consistent use of **behavior management** enables teachers to develop classrooms with discipline. Behavior management involves the arrangement of contingencies. A **contingency** is the relationship among the situation or context (also referred to as the antecedent), the behavior, and a consequence. The **consequences** provide the "reasons" for behaving that students need so they can learn new and appropriate forms of behavior (see also **Box 8.3**). These consequences are either positive or negative. Employing a positive consequence (also called **reinforcement**) is aimed at ensuring continued occurrence of the appropriate behavior. Applying a negative consequence (also referred to as punishment) is aimed at reducing or eliminating the inappropriate behavior. As students begin to learn and get better at consistently engaging in appropriate behavior, the consequences can be gradually reduced.

Certain basic strategies apply to every behavior change technique, whether it is learning how to stay on task, respect classmates, follow rules, or use equipment properly. Understanding these strategies and learning how to implement them form the basic foundation of teachers' discipline skills. The following are basic strategies when using specific behavior change techniques:

- *Be specific.* Make sure students know exactly what you want them to stop doing and exactly what you want them to do instead. Specificity helps students learn more quickly, and it also avoids having students believe you do not like them. Particularly when you are using punishment, the goal should be to eliminate the behavior, not make the student feel that he or she is a bad person. The focus should be on what the student(s) did or did not do.
- *Define the change contingency carefully.* The contingency should specify the situation, the behavior, and the consequence. "If you do X in this situation, then

BOX 8.2 Considerations Regarding Punishment/ Negative Consequences

We want to be clear about how we will use the term *punishment* in the context of developing discipline in physical education programs. In many cases, when the general public hear this term used they interpret it as a young child getting spanked. Under no circumstances do we support or promote inflicting any form of physical harm as a means of stopping any type of student misbehavior (including the use of physical activity such as making students or athletes run laps or do push-ups). As we will show, the term *punishment* refers to a general process of applying negative consequences with the goal of reducing future inappropriate behavior. We will provide numerous examples of punishers across different contexts to show how it can come in varied forms.

Historically, education was a place where corporal punishment was not uncommon. Moreover, physical education has a long history of using some form of physical activity as punishment. It is essential that physical educators are keenly aware of the legal ramifications of using such consequences. We encourage you to explore the school (system) policies relative to the use of them. We will emphasize this point more later in this chapter: Under no circumstances should physical educators use either of these consequences!

BOX 8.3 Shouldn't Students Behave Well Without Having to Be Rewarded?

There is no good answer to this question. When teachers use behavior change techniques, they are often criticized by people who assume that students should always behave well just because that is "expected" and the "right thing." That may be good enough for mature adults who behave properly because they have been taught to do so and value the acceptance that society provides for these ways of behaving. It is seldom enough for students who are not very far along to adulthood. No teacher should feel that using specific behavior change techniques is inappropriate.

However, teachers need to use the techniques skillfully and wisely. Far too often, teachers use large consequences (rewards or punishments) where small ones would do nicely. For example, a teacher might send a student to time-out, when a quick one-on-one prompt might have sufficed. Or the teacher might give a student the privilege of coming in before school and shooting baskets, when some well-timed and genuine social reinforcement could have resulted in the same improvement in behavior. An important principle of behavior change programs is referred to as the "principle of least intervention." What it means, quite simply, is that you do as little as possible to get the job done. If you can teach young children to behave appropriately by effectively using social praise and positive feedback, then special privileges or material rewards will be unnecessary. In some extreme cases, privileges and rewards are much more useful because systematic social praise is ineffective or not powerful enough. However, eventually, students should behave well without always being rewarded. It takes practice to learn to use the correct behavior change strategy at the correct time and in the correct way.

Ultimately, we want people to behave in socially acceptable ways for its own sake, and not just to get the reinforcement. Certain critics have called any form of reinforcement a form of bribery. They want students to be "intrinsically motivated." We view it as a process in which students learn to make correct decisions given the options of positive and negative consequences. The learning process in which reinforcement is employed effectively and appropriately, and then fades away gradually, reflects the shift in the decision making when persons decide to act appropriately because it is expected, because others do it, because it is the appropriate thing to do, or because of self-pride. However, in the early stages of learning, students need more immediate, concrete reasons for behaving in appropriate ways.

Y will happen." "If you are not in class at 3 minutes past the hour, then you will receive a detention mark." "Class, if all of you stay on task during our practice drills for the next 10 minutes, then you can pick an activity to end the class for the last 5 minutes."

- *Think small and move gradually.* Behaving better is *learning*. Students learn in small increments. Get them to behave better tomorrow than today, and quite quickly they will be behaving very well. "Reward direction, not perfection" is the best guideline. Avoid trying to change too much at one time. Start with one significant behavior problem, define it and its replacement specifically, provide a consequence, observe the degree of change, and then move on. Typically, students do need more time to learn something new. If you as a teacher believe that students should know what is expected after being told or shown once, you will likely grow impatient and focus mostly on reducing their inappropriate behavior (i.e., the more narrow orientation toward discipline).
- *Start where the student is.* Do not expect miracles of good citizenship from students who have had difficulty behaving. First, get to know your students and what they bring to your class in terms of appropriate and inappropriate behavior. Start with respect and participation; then build gradually on behavior change successes. Continued success at small improvements will allow more ambitious behavior change expectations.
- *Above all, be consistent.* State a fair contingency and follow through on it. Nothing confuses students more, or makes them more distrustful, than teachers who say one thing and do another or who are not consistent in their expectations and treatment of students from one class to the next. Being consistent will help students decide how to behave during class and beyond. That is, we need to get students to the point where once they know how to act appropriately, they choose to do so.

These five strategies underlie behavior change techniques, from decreasing inappropriate behavior to increasing prosocial behavior. Small, specific improvements are achieved by effectively applying contingencies consistently, by using appropriate consequences, and by gradually moving to more complex behavior (e.g., showing care and concern for others, helping out without being asked). As the appropriate behaviors become habit, the immediate contingencies that supported their growth gradually fade.

It is important that you understand that students (just like adults!) misbehave for a reason. Their showing off, acting rude, or remaining off task occurs because they are, in fact, reinforced for doing so. Often the reinforcement may come from getting peer attention, or even inadvertent recognition from the teacher. The task facing most teachers is to develop more appropriate forms of behavior by providing more appropriate reasons for behaving well. Starting in early postprimary years, having students involved in the decision process of what behaviors are desired and unacceptable, and the related consequences for both will help their decision making in how they conduct themselves. In the next sections, we will define the key concepts of reinforcement and punishment that are the basis for specific behavior change techniques aimed at increasing appropriate/pro-social behavior and reducing inappropriate behavior.

Learning Experience 8.2

List 10 student behaviors you see as critical for students to exhibit that would contribute to building a community of learners. Then list 10 student behaviors that would be unacceptable to you and that would detract from building a community of learners. Using the concept of contingency explained earlier, develop a plan of what you would use as possible consequences, and how you might administer the consequences.

Reinforcement: The Use of Positive Consequences

Reinforcement is the process of presenting a positive consequence to each occurrence of behavior, aimed at ensuring that the person will continue to behave in the same way in the future. When a teacher signals "freeze" (the antecedent), students stop quickly (the behavior). This is followed immediately by the teacher's specific praise/feedback (the consequence). When subsequent stops are executed equally quickly, the teacher's praise/feedback serves as reinforcement. Consequences that are highly desirable to individuals are considered powerful reinforcers. For example, physical educators may select activity reinforcers that students identified as desirable. Certain activities (e.g., basketball, aerobics) can be powerful reinforcers, if they are highly desired by students. If the behavior is not sustained, then the consequence technically does not qualify as reinforcement.

Reinforcement is all around us in every aspect of life. Reinforcement comes in countless forms, from getting paid for one's work to getting recognized publicly for accomplishments, getting promoted to a higher position in a company, receiving salary bonuses, receiving a free coffee beverage after purchasing a set number, receiving a free airline ticket upon flying a set number of miles with the same airline, getting car insurance premiums reduced for good driving behavior, and having healthcare premiums reduced for participating in preventative health screenings twice a year.

In sport settings, reinforcement abounds within the activities themselves as well: A tennis player who correctly executes a lob (the behavior) such that the opponent cannot return the shot earns a point (the reinforcer); a soccer player moves across the opponents' goal (the behavior) in a way that draws an opposing defender out of position (the reinforcer), thereby creating space for a teammate to move in and shoot and perhaps score a goal; a closely guarded basketball player who, rather than forcing a shot, passes the ball (behavior) to a teammate who is open and closer to the basket, and takes a higher percentage shot (reinforcer).

Learning Experience 8.3

Beyond the examples listed previously, list five more examples of reinforcement in everyday life and then in sport contexts that you have experienced yourself. What aspect of your behavior was reinforced? What form did the reinforcement take?

Students in primary schools generally wish to please adults (e.g., the teacher). Thus, adult attention (e.g., verbal and nonverbal praise, positive feedback) and privileges such as being made a squad leader, being allowed to assist the teacher with moving equipment, being named captain of a squad, and so on are generally powerful reinforcers. More so perhaps in postprimary schools, inappropriate behavior may be reinforced in certain instances. For example, smiles and quiet laughter from peers may be reinforcing inappropriate behavior by a student.

As we noted in Box 8.3, some forms of reinforcement require minimal effort, whereas others require more extensive planning and oversight. Using reinforcement techniques effectively requires a thorough understanding of which techniques to use, and when and how to use them. Moreover, teachers need to learn about their students' reinforcer preferences. The latter is critical in that not all reinforcers work in the same way for every person. What is reinforcing to some may not be reinforcing to others. Using the previous examples of basketball and aerobics, not all students may like basketball, instead preferring an activity like aerobics.

It is important to remember that verbal and nonverbal praise and feedback are not inherently reinforcing (especially if they are used poorly). The same goes for activities provided as rewards. All such actions by teachers would be examples of reinforcement only if they result in subsequent improved performance on the part of the students.

Techniques for Developing and Sustaining Pro-Social Behavior

The number of interactions that teachers have with their students during a single lesson can be in the hundreds. An interaction occurs whenever teachers convey information to students, such as a one-word prompt ("Careful"), feedback ("Keep that line straighter"), a nonverbal act (a smile or frown), praise ("Thanks for helping with the equipment"), instruction ("I want all partners to watch each other perform and give feedback"), or an expectation ("I expect you all to play this game without arguing"). Few things distinguish the more effective teacher from the less-effective teacher better than the skillfulness in how they interact with students. This section focuses on the use of positive approaches for developing effective classroom management and discipline.

Over four decades of teaching research in physical education has borne out unequivocally that physical educators are far too stingy in their support of appropriate student behavior. Typically, teachers respond negatively or correctively to students when they misbehave. Physical education classes are too full of "be quiet," "pay attention," "listen up," "sh-h," and "that's enough, over there." There is far too little "Thank you, Jack, I really liked your effort today"; "Way to get started quickly, well done"; or "Your group was really focused on having a good practice; I love that." Don't expect to build good behavior and have a warm, nurturing, caring physical education climate without focusing frequently on good behavior and finding multiple ways to recognize and reinforce it. **Box 8.4** shows a few examples of various types of positive interactions teachers can use to motivate and support appropriate behavior.

The hard-liner and stern taskmaster will find little comfort in these pages, at least, not for someone who creates a harsh and punitive class climate and sustains it through an overreliance on punishment and threats of punishment. Decades of research on effective teaching show that the foremost predictor of classes in which students achieve less is a harsh, punitive climate and teachers who too often shame and ridicule students to get them to conform. Students will simply not come to enjoy physical education (and physical activity in general) in such conditions. You do not have to make physical education a warm, fuzzy place in order for students to achieve, but you must at least make it a place in which students are safe from harm, either from yourself as a teacher or from their classmates.

The following strategies for effectively using interaction techniques are essential for helping students learn and grow in physical education, and for developing and sustaining an effective behavior management system. With deliberate practice and good feedback on your performance you can become skillful in their use. The skillfulness that comes from

BOX 8.4 Encouraging Appropriate Behavior Through Positive Interactions

General positive interactions (no specific information content):

Yes!	Good!	Nice job!	Excellent!
Beautiful!	Terrific!	Way to go!	Nice going!
Thanks!	That's the way!	Much better!	Everybody did well!
Great effort!	Outstanding!	Nicely done!	Fantastic!

Specific positive interactions (can be combined with nonverbal acts):

- The Jaguars and Rays teams got their practices started right away. . . . Impressive!
- Thanks for paying attention, Jack!
- Did you all see the way Gabrielle helped David?
- The entire class worked hard during the fitness activities. . . . I'm very proud!
- This group [pointing] was quiet right at the signal!
- Great job freezing quickly—you took only 6 seconds!
- Thanks for helping with the equipment, Justin!

Positive interactions with value content (value content describes why the behavior is important):

- Way to get quiet quickly; now we can begin the game more quickly!
- Thanks, Bill. When you make an effort, the other guys seem to also!
- Ann, you did a great job this week, and I'm sure you had more fun!
- Squad 3 did a great job with the equipment. Now we can start earlier!
- Nice going! When you work that hard during your team practice, it will help you in your games!

Nonverbal positive interactions:

Smiling	Nodding	OK sign	High fives
Clapping hands	Winking	Thumbs up	Applauding

practicing their use is not only in refining the techniques themselves but also in knowing the right technique to use in terms of the situation, such as the kind of students, the setting, and the type of behavior.

- *Clear, specific prompts:* A **prompt** is a teacher interaction that reminds students what is expected of them. When the teacher is developing new behavior (or, indeed, a managerial task system), students should be prompted often. Often, teachers tend to prompt students only after misbehavior has occurred. This is an error in technique because it ties reminders only to misbehaviors. Prompts should also be specific; that is, they should contain specific information about a behavior or the situation in which it should or should not occur. As students grow in their capacity to behave well, prompts can gradually decrease in number.
- *Conveying high, yet realistic, expectations:* Students deserve to be told what is expected of them. Most discipline-expectation interactions will be directed toward process behaviors, such as behaving safely, courteously, and helpfully and staying on task. These should be realistic for the setting and students, yet they should also be optimistic about what students can accomplish. As we share our expectations for student behavior, it might also be appropriate to seek from them what they expect from our behavior. Starting in early years of postprimary schools, actually involving students in deciding on the expectations for general class behavior will help set the tone for creating an environment of shared responsibility and commitment to making the class a positive experience.
- *Frequent and appropriate feedback and praise:* Teachers can provide feedback or praise students individually, in groups, or as a class. As we noted, providing praise effectively is a skill that requires practice. Siedentop and Tannehill (2000) noted the common error committed by teachers who use high rates of the same simple, repetitive statements, such as "Good job" or "Way to go." Praise becomes effective (i.e., reinforcing) only when it reinforces appropriate student behavior. That is, the appropriate behavior increases as a result of praise. Ineffective praise is not a reinforcer if it does not result in improved behavior. **Box 8.5** shows guidelines for delivering effective praise.
- *Effective nonverbal interactions:* We cannot overstress the importance of nonverbal interactions. Students will use nonverbal messages to judge the credibility and genuineness of teachers' verbal interactions. The skillful use of nonverbal interaction starts with ensuring that "your audio matches your video"; that is, your nonverbal and verbal acts are in synch and not contradictory. Experts have suggested that nonverbal interactions are at least as powerful as what is said to students, in that they perceive nonverbal interactions as reflecting the actual feelings and thoughts of the teacher. Galloway (1971) argued that when verbal and nonverbal acts are contradictory, students accept the latter as more valid. Examples of positive nonverbal communication include a sincere smile, thumbs-up sign, muted clapping of the hands, pat on the back, and high fives. The next step is to ensure that you use more positive than negative nonverbal acts. Rolider, Siedentop, and Van Houten (1984) demonstrated persuasively that student perceptions of their teacher's enthusiasm were directly related to the number of times the teacher actually smiled during class.
- *Using public versus private interactions:* Effective teachers know when to communicate approval or disapproval privately to students—a whisper in the ear, a private pat on the back, and a little talk after class. They also understand the power of "conspicuous praise" (Wynne & Ryan, 1997); that is, the public recognition of the good behavior of one student to the

BOX 8.5 Guidelines for Delivering Effective Praise

Effective praise:

- Is delivered immediately and contingently, yet does not intrude on task-related behavior
- Identifies specific aspects of behavior that were done well
- Provides information about why the behavior is important
- Is matched well to the behavior being reinforced
- Is related to standard criteria or previous performance rather than comparison to other students
- Properly attributes success to effort and ability
- Includes expectations for continued success and improvement
- Shows variety, sincerity, and enthusiasm

Major technique errors in delivering praise are:

- Providing only nonspecific, global reactions
- Not providing specific information about the performance
- Comparing too often against peers
- Over- or underexaggerating relative to the performance
- Intruding on task-related behavior
- Being insincere, unenthusiastic, or bland

Adapted from Brophy, J. (1981). Teacher praise: A functional analysis. *Review of Educational Research, 51*, 5–32.

entire class, the names of daily fair players on the bulletin board, and so forth. Asking students who behaved well to write their names on a good behavior poster is another example. Teachers should not assume that public praise and private interactions are only for children. A sincere one-on-one comment of appreciation to a 16-year-old after class, accompanied by a pat on the back, is still a powerful motivator for good behavior.

Another powerful strategy, in both primary and postprimary settings, is the "fill the bucket" activity (see www.bucketfillers101.com). This can be used as part of closures of lessons, where students are invited to fill the bucket of a peer in class by publicly recognizing the specific life skills that the peer demonstrated during the class. Examples of bucket fillers could be helping out someone without being asked, working hard, being supportive, being positive, showing care for a classmate, and so on.

Common types of reinforcers in physical education are social, activity, tangible, and edible reinforcers. **Social reinforcers** are probably the most common and consist of verbal and nonverbal forms of attention from the teacher (and/or peers) contingent on the occurrence of desirable behavior/performance. Adult attention in the form of smiles, thumbs up, and high fives coupled with some form of genuine, credible, and specific praise or feedback is a universally powerful reinforcer. With good practice, this technique is relatively easy to learn and the least burdensome on the teacher.

Activity reinforcers are those activities in which students really enjoy engaging. In primary physical education settings, activities such as jumping rope, shooting baskets, playing soccer, and privileges such as getting to be first in line or assisting the teacher with equipment are all potential activity reinforcers. In postprimary settings, activity reinforcers could include getting time to engage in a choice of a favorite activity such as basketball, volleyball, yoga, or aerobics.

Activity reinforcers are at the center of the **Premack principle** (Premack, 1959). This principle (often referred to as Grandma's rule, as in "Once you complete your homework, you can go play outside") holds that access to a highly desirable activity is contingent on completing a task that is undesirable. Students receiving a set amount of class time (e.g., 8 minutes) to engage in their favorite/highly desirable activity contingent on demonstrating improvement in areas such as attending to teacher instruction, exerting effort during fitness activities, or getting started quickly on a new activity is an example of the Premack principle.

Tangible reinforcers generally come in the form of stickers, pencils, and the like. In essence, any tangible item can potentially serve as a reinforcer if it something that the student desires. In Sport Education, teams earn points for demonstrating fair play and for successful completion of duty team tasks. What makes these potentially powerful reinforcers is that these points are an integral part of how the season competition is structured. That is, they can help teams move up in the league standings.

A final class of reinforcers is edible reinforcers. In many schools, students may get rewarded for their performance by way of some type of food reinforcer, such as a pizza party. Individual teachers may also use certain bits of food, snacks, candy, and soda. Given that a large percentage of students come to school already overweight or obese, and that these types of foods with high fat, sugar, and sodium content are readily available beyond the school environment, we strongly discourage the use of this approach to reinforce certain types of student behavior. There are simply too many other, much more appropriate, reinforcers available.

Punishment: The Use of Negative Consequences

When using *discipline* as a verb, it often implies and focuses on **punishment**: "I had to discipline the student" almost always means that some type of punishment was used. Punishment is a useful and sometimes necessary behavior change technique. It has a technical meaning, which we will describe, and a number of school-based applications that teachers should be familiar with and know how to use effectively. Punishment is composed of a set of valuable techniques within the teacher's total class management and discipline skill repertoire. We use the term *skills* purposefully because, as is the case with reinforcement, punishment techniques have to be used skillfully. There is too much punishment in schools because too few teachers have the skills to develop and maintain pro-social behavior through more positive strategies. Too often, students' behavior is managed largely by way of punishment strategies.

The purpose of punishment is to stop and redirect inappropriate behavior into more useful and productive forms of pro-social behavior. As we explain in **Box 8.6**, punishment should never be used in retribution, to flex your muscles, or to otherwise demonstrate your power. If punishment is the sole or main weapon in the teacher's arsenal of discipline skills, then chances for success are severely limited. Teachers will want to be deliberate in deciding how to apply the negative consequence and what type to use. That is, it should not be an arbitrary choice or one that is used only because it is easy to use or because you are only familiar with using one type of negative consequence.

Remember, the basic purpose of a discipline program is not just to reduce instances of inappropriate behavior but also to redirect students toward pro-social behavior that contributes both to personal growth objectives and to a more positive and productive learning environment. Punishment is the presentation of a consequence with the goal of reducing or eliminating future instances of the same behavior. Its primary objective is to quickly stop the particular behavior. Examples of punishers in everyday life would be getting scolded for being dressed

BOX 8.6 Punishment: The Two-Edged Sword

Classes need rules and standards of conduct. To enforce them, a system of consequences is necessary, and some consequences will be negative in nature. Punishment is a two-edged sword in that it can be used to protect as well as to commit terrible acts against the weak. Some teachers will misuse punishment, and many others do not use appropriate punishment techniques with sufficient skill. Teachers also sometimes use punishment to retaliate personally against a student who has bothered them in some way or when they become frustrated with their ability to get a class to do its work.

When teachers employ punishment to control students, it is fundamentally about power. Power is a basic fact of human life, and some people have more of it than others. Much power is legitimate, such as the power a parent has over a child. Some power, such as the power of a bully on the playground, is illegitimate. The classroom is a prime setting where students learn about power. Teachers have it and legitimately need it. The issue, though, is how they use it. The great potential for misuse of power does not mean that it should be extinguished or surrendered to students. It means, however, that power should be exercised with utmost fairness (Wynne & Ryan, 1997). And, we would add, used skillfully.

We should note that surrendering power to students is quite different from empowering students by helping them learn to make good decisions, lead by example through appropriate behavior, and so on. Developing discipline (defined broadly) is not an either–or proposition relative to "who is in charge." Teachers who are serious about helping students develop their social skills and life skills must create opportunities for students to make good choices, and reinforce those choices.

inappropriately, getting demoted in your job, and getting a monetary fine for violating traffic laws. In the context of sport, negative consequences of athletes' actions in sport also represent examples of punishment. For example, the golfer who hits into the trees is punished by having to search for the ball, having a much more difficult second shot, and likely a higher total score for the round; making a poor pass in soccer close to one's own goal would be punished when it results in a turnover and a score by the opposing team; a person starting out on a strength conditioning regimen who chooses too much weight is punished by the resulting injury that requires time off from exercising; a soccer player who makes a severe tackle from behind receiving a yellow card from the referee; a basketball player who commits the maximum number of personal fouls being ejected from the game; and an ice hockey player who trips an opponent with the hockey stick receiving a 2-minute penalty box stay.

In physical education teaching contexts, punishment can take many forms as well, from something as subtle as a stern stare by the teacher, to being removed from an activity (i.e., time-out), to losing previously earned points or privileges such as being allowed to assist the teacher with equipment cleanup, to more elaborate punishers such as detention. Although the emphasis should be on using reinforcing consequences that will encourage appropriate/productive behaviors, in some instances teachers may need to resort to using certain negative consequences to stop inappropriate behavior in the short term.

A key point to remember is that the effectiveness of the punishment can be determined only by whether it results in fewer occurrences or complete elimination of the inappropriate behavior in the future. If a student persists in the inappropriate behavior following the negative consequence, by definition it does not qualify as punishment. Moreover, what is punishing to one student may not be punishing to another student in the same class. Consider an example during a postprimary soccer lesson. The teacher puts a student who loves to play soccer but who at times taunts and criticizes lesser-skilled classmates, in time-out for a few minutes. Upon returning to the action, the student refrains from engaging in the behavior. Knowing that continuing the behavior would raise the prospect of a second (and perhaps longer) removal from the action likely helped in the decision to refrain from further taunting. In the same class, there is another student who does not like soccer (or physical activity in general). This student also engages in the same inappropriate behavior and is removed using the same consequence. However, upon return, the behavior persists. In this student's case, the time-out strategy is not punishment. In fact, students may deliberately engage in such behavior as a means to avoid having to participate in certain tasks or activities. Thus, teachers must be mindful when deciding about the type and severity of the punishment. And it is equally important for teachers to understand their students' likes, dislikes, and capabilities. Having that understanding allows teachers to be more deliberate and skillful in using negative consequences as a short-term means of stopping unacceptable behavior (at least temporarily).

Some form of punishment may, at times, be needed. However, excessive dependence on it by teachers in the long term makes the physical education experience for students one to be dreaded, and will more likely make physical activity something to be avoided at all cost.

Physical Activity as a Means of Punishment

Using physical activity as a means of stopping inappropriate behavior is the most egregious and unacceptable form of punishment. In the United States, the National Association for Sports and Physical Education (NASPE, 2009) published a formal position statement on the use of physical activity as punishment, indicating that "administering or withdrawing physical activity as punishment is inappropriate and constitutes an unsound education practice" (p. 2). The good news is that between 2000 and 2006, the percentage of U.S. states that prohibit schools from using physical activity as punishment in physical education increased from 2.1% to 16%, and the percentage of states actively discouraging schools from the practice also increased from 25.5% to 56% (Lee, Burgeson, Fulton, & Spain, 2007). However, although the exact occurrence is difficult to track, school staff members are allowed to use physical activity (e.g., running laps, push-ups) to punish students for inappropriate conduct in physical education in almost a third of U.S. schools, and the practice was actively discouraged in less than 10% of schools. The practice likely persists (primarily in postprimary schools) because (1) sport coaches across performance levels continue to model the practice to "motivate" their athletes; (2) teachers were subjected to it when they were students, and saw that "it works" in the short term; and (3) there is an absence of formal policies (with consequences) prohibiting physical activity as punishment, which in essence represents a tacit approval of continued use of this practice.

A second means of using punishment involving physical activity is the withholding of access to physical education class or other physical activity (e.g., recess) for inappropriate behavior in the classroom or for failing to complete assignments in academic subjects. This equally inappropriate approach to punishment is more prevalent in primary schools. Lee et al. (2007) reported that this practice occurs in over 20% of U.S. schools. When physical educators (and coaches) resort to this means of managing student behavior, it actually says less about the athletes, and more about the overall behavior management system that teachers put in place.

Especially in today's context of promoting the importance and value of physical activity, it is inconceivable how physical educators can claim that they are in the business of fostering daily physical activity as a lifestyle for students to embrace, and then to turn around and use physical activity as a means of punishing some other unrelated behavior. Even though it may produce a desired effect in the short term, teachers run the risk of losing credibility with students when sending such conflicting messages.

Techniques for Decreasing/Eliminating Misbehavior

Disruptive or other inappropriate student behavior should be stopped quickly, before it can spread and interfere with the lesson. Even when a good managerial task system is in place, disruptive behavior will sometimes occur. When it does, you will want to have a well-thought-out plan of action, with effective alternatives for dealing with the misbehavior—and then clear and effective consequences for redirecting the student or students into more productive patterns of behavior. In virtually all cases, efforts to reduce inappropriate/unacceptable behavior can and should be accompanied simultaneously by efforts to explicitly redirect students toward pro-social, productive behavior. There are several evidence-informed techniques that teachers can employ in school settings. They include the use of verbal desists, ignoring minor tolerable behavior, differential reinforcement, positive practice, contingency contracting, group contingencies, time-out, and reward cost. The following sections provide an overview along with guidelines and considerations for use.

Verbal Desists

The most common strategy for dealing with misbehavior or disruptions in class is the verbal reprimand—what we refer to as a **verbal desist**. Verbally desisting misbehavior is a useful strategy when it is done skillfully. In studying classroom management, Kounin (1970) showed convincingly that there are specific methods and skills for using desists effectively. Desists must be clear, that is, contain specific information about what the student did wrong. Instead of "stop that," it should be "stop sitting on the basketball." Desists should also have firmness; that is, teachers should follow through on the delivery of the desist so the student knows that what is said is meant. Maintaining eye contact and moving closer to the offender (also called *proximity control*) are examples of firm follow-through. Nonverbal actions can be used as negative consequences, as expressions of disapproval, such as a finger to the lips, standing with hands on hips staring at students, frowns, and so forth. Matching the nonverbal expression with the verbal desist sends a clearer message to students.

Effective desists are also timed appropriately and accurately targeted. A well-timed desist stops the misbehavior immediately after it starts and before it can spread to other students. An accurately targeted desist is directed toward the original offender, not a secondary offender. Effective teachers seldom make timing or targeting errors. When students learn that you time and target your desists appropriately, they know that you know what is going on in the class—what in research is called "with-it-ness" (Kounin, 1970). It will seem to your students that you have eyes in the back of your head. Desists should not be punitive or harsh, and angry desists simply make students uncomfortable and do not improve behavior.

Ignoring Minor Tolerable Behavior

Although disruptive behavior needs to be stopped immediately, there are levels of behavior that might not be wholly appropriate but are tolerable to the teacher. These are typically minor infractions or minor off-task behaviors that do not disrupt the lesson's flow or a teacher's capacity to teach the class. All teachers will have different levels of behavior they are willing to tolerate. What is important is to be consistent from day to day and from student to student about what you will and will not tolerate. Minor tolerable infractions do not warrant verbal desists or punishments.

Differential Reinforcement

In many cases, when teachers try to reduce a problem behavior, they can employ **differential reinforcement**, where the teacher ignores the inappropriate behavior (i.e., no longer reinforces it), while at the same time reinforcing other, more desirable behaviors. There are multiple applications of differential reinforcement. They include differential reinforcement of incompatible (DRI) behavior, differential reinforcement of alternative (DRA) behavior, differential reinforcement of low rates (DRL) of behavior, and differential reinforcement of other (DRO) behavior.

Differential Reinforcement of Incompatible Behavior

With DRI, the teacher reinforces a behavior that a student cannot exhibit at the same time as the problem behavior, and also withholds reinforcement of the problem behavior itself. For example, during a basketball lesson, a student who is supposed to be practicing dribbling persists in intermittently shooting at a basket. The typical reaction of the teacher is often to desist the shooting behavior. Instead, the teacher can reinforce the student's dribbling performance. Similarly, during a class-wide instructional episode, a student cannot be silent and attending while simultaneously talking with a peer. Here the teacher has the opportunity to reinforce the student's silence during instruction. **Table 8.1** includes a list of examples of possible problem behaviors with their incompatible corollaries. **Box 8.7** provides guidelines for using DRI behavior.

BOX 8.7 Guidelines for Effective Use of DRI and DRA

1. Ensure that the behavior to be reinforced is truly an incompatible or alternative positive behavior, and preferably one the student has demonstrated previously (i.e., you know the student can do it).
2. Reinforce the incompatible/alternative behavior immediately and consistently. Especially early on, each time the student demonstrates the appropriate behavior, reinforce each opportunity. For example, a student who frequently interrupts class-wide instruction or fidgets with equipment during those episodes should be reinforced for each instance of demonstrating full attention and leaving the equipment alone, no matter how short the instructional episode might be.
3. At all costs, withhold all reinforcement of the problem behavior. For DRI/DRA to be successful, it is critical that the amount of reinforcement of the incompatible/alternative far outweighs the reinforcement of the problem behavior. Inadvertent reinforcement of the problem behavior may come from the teacher or classmates.

Adapted with permission of Pearson Education, Inc., from Cooper, J. O., Heron, T. E., & Heward, W. L. (2007). *Applied behavior analysis* (2nd ed.). Upper Saddle River, NJ: Pearson/Merrill-Prentice Hall.

Differential Reinforcement of Alternative Behavior

Although similar to DRI, *differential reinforcement of alternative behavior (DRA)* has the teacher reinforce desirable student behaviors that are different from the problem behavior, though not incompatible. In the prior example of the student talking out during class-wide instruction without raising

TABLE 8.1 Examples of Incompatible/Alternative Positive Behaviors

Possible Problem Behavior	Incompatible Positive Behavior
• Being tardy for class	• Being in position for attendance on time
• Talking with classmate during class-wide instruction	• Being quiet and attentive during class-wide instruction
• Fidgeting with equipment during class-wide instruction	• Leaving equipment alone and attending to teacher direction
• Being inactive during episodes of physical activity	• Actively participating in assigned activity
• Using equipment inappropriately (e.g., kicking a volleyball, slamming a racket on the floor)	• Using equipment safely and appropriately
• Cursing	• Refraining from cursing or using more acceptable exclamations (e.g., "darn 'it!", "rats")
• Talking out without raising hand	• Raising hand and waiting until asked to answer a question or speak out
• Practicing techniques other than those assigned by the teacher	• Practicing the task(s) as assigned
• Grabbing, pushing, kicking, etc. of classmates	• Not touching classmates while standing or sitting in close proximity

a hand, the teacher would be employing DRA if she or he reinforced the student's raising of the hand or maintaining eye contact with the demonstration that accompanies the instructions.

Differential Reinforcement of Low Rates of Behavior
The goal of differential reinforcement of low rates of behavior (DRL) is to get the student's inappropriate behavior to a level that the teacher is willing to accept. Thus, the teacher reinforces a lower rate of occurrence of the behavior (as opposed to reinforcing the total absence of the problem behavior, which is introduced later in this chapter). For example, some students may develop a pattern where they are seeking their teacher's attention. This would be especially noticeable during times when they are supposed to be engaging in learning tasks. This attention-seeking behavior may take the form of frequently asking questions, or asking the teacher to watch them do something unrelated to the lesson's activities. As we noted previously, there are instances of inappropriate student behaviors that are minor and/or occur only occasionally. They do not distract the teacher's instructional efforts. However, if the frequency reaches a certain level then DRL would be an effective intervention.

Teachers can choose to use DRL based on how the student did over the course of an entire lesson or break the lesson into short blocks of time. The teacher would set a criterion for how often the student can engage in the misbehavior (e.g., no more than four times per lesson or no more than two times per block of 10 minutes within each lesson). At the end of the lesson, or each block of time, if the student met the criterion the teacher would reinforce the student. **Box 8.8** includes key guidelines for using DRL.

BOX 8.8 Guidelines for Effective Use of DRL

1. Understand the limitations of DRL. One of the downsides of DRL is that it takes some time for the behavior to improve, so if a rapid and substantial improvement is needed, DRL would not be the appropriate intervention choice.
2. Determine the actual frequency of the problem behavior over the course of approximately four lessons. This will provide a baseline of the typical pattern of the problem behavior.
3. Choose a criterion that lies somewhat below the baseline sessions' average. That is, if a student seeks attention from the teacher on average 12 times in a typical lesson, then the performance criterion can be set at 9 times for the next few lessons. As the student improves the criterion can be gradually pushed lower.
4. Be sure to provide feedback to the student throughout the intervention. Keep the student informed as to the progress that he or she is making.

Avoid providing reinforcement if the criterion is not met. Yet do calmly prompt the student to continue his or her effort.

Data from Cooper, J. O., Heron, T. E., & Heward, W. L. (2007). *Applied behavior analysis* (2nd ed.). Upper Saddle River, NJ: Pearson/Merrill-Prentice Hall.

Differential Reinforcement of Other Behavior
A teacher using *differential reinforcement of other behavior (DRO)* would deliver a reinforcer if the student refrains from engaging in the problem behavior for a specified amount of time (e.g., a full lesson or a series of four lessons). Examples of DRO include thanking students for not talking during instructional episodes over the course of a lesson and having a typically misbehaving student earn a point for each gym period during which she or he refrains from arguing with classmates and granting a privilege for every five points earned. DRO is also referred to as *omission training* because the reinforcement is provided contingent on the student refraining from engaging in the behavior. Thus, with differential reinforcement, the teacher's primary focus is on strengthening desirable student behavior.

Positive Practice

With this behavior management technique (also referred to as *overcorrection*), the teacher requires students to engage in an appropriate behavior a specified number of times as a consequence of misbehaving. Although **positive practice** is technically a punishment procedure, it does carry with it an educative dimension in that students practice the appropriate behavior. It is especially effective in terms of improving students' performance in managerial and organizational routines, such as (1) coming to a quick stop upon a teacher's freeze signal, (2) hustling over to gather in one area in the gym during a gather routine, (3) hustling from station to station during a fitness circuit, and (4) returning jump rope equipment quickly, safely, and in a specified manner after use.

The appropriate behavior is always the replacement for what was being done wrong. For example, if students do not execute managerial routines as appropriately or quickly as expected, the teacher can choose to have students practice this routine several times in a row immediately following the occurrence of the problem behavior. **Box 8.9** includes important guidelines for using positive practice.

Teachers should also be aware of the limitations and potential problems associated with positive practice, especially if

BOX 8.9 Guidelines for Effective Use of Positive Practice

When employing positive practice, teachers should be mindful of the following guidelines and considerations:

1. Immediately upon the occurrence of the problem behavior, explain that the behavior is unacceptable and explain why the student(s) must improve.
2. Do so in a calm and unemotional voice. At all costs, avoid criticism and lengthy scolding because it will not increase the effectiveness of the positive practice technique. In fact, it may strain your overall relationship with the students.
3. Provide a brief review of what you expect. This serves as a prompt that reminds students what is expected and acceptable.
4. Let the student(s) practice the correct way of executing the behavior. For example, effective teachers expect students to execute managerial routines such as freezes and forming groups. When students have demonstrated they have learned those routines previously and they then take more time than necessary, positive practice can be employed by having the full class practice that routine immediately (perhaps multiple times if the class shows insufficient progress).
5. Carefully supervise students as they engage in the positive practice activity, and determine if they demonstrate improvement. At this time, do not provide additional reminders about what you expect and avoid providing too much praise or positive feedback.
6. In the subsequent instances where students are to demonstrate the same behavior *do* provide praise/positive feedback.
7. Teachers who find they have to resort to positive practice more frequently on account of students' poor execution of managerial routines should review their overall approach to teaching these routines.

Adapted with permission of Pearson Education, Inc., from Cooper, J. O., Heron, T. E., & Heward, W. L. (2007). *Applied behavior analysis* (2nd ed.). Upper Saddle River, NJ: Pearson/Merrill-Prentice Hall.

it is not used effectively. First, overcorrection does take up valuable class time. Second, it is more labor intensive for teachers because they have to actively monitor the students. Third, for the positive practice sequence to be punishing, it cannot be reinforcing in itself (i.e., students preferring to do the positive practice activity rather than the upcoming learning activity).

Relative to the potential loss of class time, however, if used effectively, it will ensure that in the future students will execute these managerial outlines, which will contribute to the overall pace and momentum of future lessons.

Contingency Contracts

Also called a *behavior contract*, when using a **contingency contract**, a teacher collaborates with a student to create a document in which the contingent relationship is explained between the expected student behavior and the delivery of a specified reward. This particular behavior change technique has been used with great success across many different behaviors (e.g., weight loss, academic performance, athletic skill performance) and settings, including schools.

The key components of a contingency contract are: (1) the task expected, (2) the reward(s), (3) record of performance, (4) specified duration of the contract (e.g., number of lessons or days), and (5) signature spaces for each of the participants. Relative to the task statement it should specify the "what," the "when," and the "how well." That is, the student whose behavior is targeted should be clear about what she or he is expected to do (or avoid), when the task needs to be completed by, and the criteria for successful performance.

One of the attractive features of contingency contracts is that the student actively participates in defining the behaviors, deciding on a reward, establishing the precise contingencies (how much, for how long, and so forth), and evaluating the contract. Importantly, from a learning and development perspective, using contingency contracts is an important step toward starting students on the road to self-management. That is, they get to help make decisions about how they choose to act within the class. Without this, students are more likely to view this process as something that is imposed on them by the teacher. Teachers should not use contingency contracts unless they are willing to negotiate with students on these matters. Specific guidelines for their use are shown in **Box 8.10**.

Learning Experience 8.4

In a school physical education or other physical activity setting (e.g., sport club) where you teach or coach, determine a student or player who has displayed persistent inappropriate behavior for which other planned behavior change techniques have not been successful. Using the steps outlined in Box 8.10, develop and implement a contingency contract. Be sure that the implementation is structured so that you can oversee the student's performance.

BOX 8.10 Guidelines for Effective Use of Contingency Contracts

Using contingency (or behavioral) contracts provide a constructive means of improving student behavior. Teachers should only choose the behavioral contract approach if other planned efforts (e.g., prompts, social reinforcement, time-out) have not resulted in the desired behavior change.

Developing behavioral contracts requires a time investment for both teacher and student(s). We recommend teachers use the following steps to ensure the best chance of success:

1. *Schedule a meeting with the student(s).* Explain why you are proposing the development of a contract, how it would help the student personally, how it would help the class, and how the contract would work. Explain as well that in your role as teacher you will fully participate in developing and implementing the contract.
2. *Decide on one or a few behavior tasks to be addressed.* Ensure that (1) the focus is on positive behaviors, as well as some that the student already has shown success with, and (2) both the teacher and student have a copy of the list of expected tasks/behaviors.
3. *Develop a list of potential rewards.* This would be a list of favorite activities and things/treats. Then decide on what would be a fair reward, ensuring that there is balance between the expected level of performance and the reward. That is, the reward should not be so insignificant that the student views it as not worth the effort, yet also not too extravagant (i.e., too much reward for minimal expectations).
4. *Write the actual agreement/contract.* The actual written contract should specify the expectations for the student(s) (including how well the student is to perform) as well as the settings (e.g., gym, changing room) and the duration (i.e., for how long the student is expected to demonstrate the behavior, such as a week's worth of lessons, or 2 weeks' worth). It may be necessary to specify possible exceptions as well. Furthermore, it should specify when, where, and how much of the reward will be provided. Finally, both the teacher and student(s) sign the agreement. In most cases, having a third, independent party (e.g., a school administrator, parent) sign the contract as well demonstrates that this contract is important and lets this person also ensure that the contract is fair. The contract should have space where the performance of the student can be tracked over the course of the contract. If possible, let the student come in and personally update the record, thus seeing the progress toward earning the reward.
5. *If the problem behavior appears entrenched and difficult to eliminate, consider providing some margin of error.* For example, if the student has been unable to refrain from interrupting the teacher's instructions, an expectation of perfection over the course of three consecutive lessons is likely too high. If and when the student slips up even once on day one of the contract then there would be no more incentive for the student to continue to make an effort. Thus, the first contract may need to include a level of performance that allows some margin of error. Subsequent contracts can include increased levels of performance (i.e., higher expectations) by reducing or fully eliminating the margin of error.
6. *Continue to combine the behavioral contract with other forms of reinforcement.* When the student demonstrates other positive/pro-social behaviors not included in the contract, be sure to recognize these as well.
7. *Closely monitor the student's performance.* This will ensure that the student is indeed improving during the course of the contract period. Furthermore, it will show the student that the teacher is serious about the agreement.

Data from Cooper, J. O., Heron, T. E., & Heward, W. L. (2007). *Applied behavior analysis* (2nd ed.). Upper Saddle River, NJ: Pearson/Merrill-Prentice Hall.

An example of a contingency contract for an individual student is shown in **Figure 8.1**. Examples of problem behaviors where contingency contracting can be used to improve a student's performance include disrupting class peers, class attendance, being tardy for class, and excessive talking during class-wide instructions. Students would have input in terms of the preferred reward(s).

Group Contingencies

The behavior change techniques presented so far have focused on developing pro-social behavior of individual students. However, there are many instances in school environments where teachers can employ contingency management to change the behavior of groups of students (Cooper et al., 2007). A **group contingency** is defined as the presentation of

Contingency Contract

Task		Reward	
Who:		Who:	
What:		What:	
When:		When:	
How well:		How well:	
Student Signature:		Date:	
Teacher Signature:		Date:	
Third-Party Signature:		Date:	

Task Record

M	T	W	TH	F	M	T	W	TH	F

FIGURE 8.1 Sample completed contingency contract.

a reinforcer (i.e., reward) contingent upon the behavior of an individual in a group, a segment of the group, or the group as a whole.

An example would be where over the course of a number of class periods, students can earn a reward contingent on them demonstrating improved performance in some type of general classroom behavior (e.g., refraining from talking during class-wide instructions, improved on-task behavior). Examples of the reward might be access to a highly desirable activity, having music play in the background throughout the class period, extra game time, or minutes toward a full lesson where students get to do choice activities.

Generally, the agreed-upon group contingency is in effect over the course of multiple lessons, where teachers might employ tokens or points that can be gained based on the established contingency. Once the group meets the performance criterion, the token can be exchanged (i.e., cashed in) for the backup reinforcers (e.g., choice activity, game play, free time) (Cooper et al., 2007). For example, the contingency might be where the group can earn 3 minutes of class time toward a choice activity during each of the next four lessons, contingent on all of them being dressed and ready for activity within 4 minutes of the bell signaling the start of the class period. It goes without saying that if the regular learning activities during the unit of work are attractive and enjoyable to the students, they may be more inclined to be ready and prepared for class, thereby negating the need for a group contingency.

There are three categories of group contingencies (Cooper et al., 2007):

1. *Dependent group contingencies* are those where the reward for the entire class group is dependent on an individual student or subset of the whole group meeting the performance criterion on a specified behavior.
2. *Independent group contingencies* are those where only those who meet the performance criterion receive the reinforcer.
3. *Interdependent group contingencies* are those where all members of the group need to meet the performance criterion in order for the group to earn the reward. The interdependent contingency can be implemented in four different ways:
   a. *The group as a whole must meet the criterion.* If, for example, a class has had difficulty remaining attentive during instructional episodes, the contingency might be set up as follows. Students will earn the award if the class as a whole refrains from interrupting the teacher during times when the teacher provides instructional and/or organizational/managerial directions during all but one such episode per class for four class episodes.
   b. *The reinforcer is provided based on a group average.* For example, in a concepts-based physical education program where students frequently have out-of-class homework assignments, the teacher has determined that

few are studying the assigned content. If the teacher wants to ensure that students spend more time studying the material at home for a written culminating exam, he or she could challenge students by offering a reward if the group's average exam score is at least 90%.

c. *One individual student is chosen at random to earn the reinforcer for the group.*

d. *The teacher uses the good behavior game.* A common format for the "Good Behavior Game" is as follows:
   - Depending on class size, divide the class into three or four teams. Each team selects its own name.
   - Emphasize that each team can win, and that they are competing against a criterion, *not* each other!
   - Discuss the specific expectations.
   - Discuss rewards and have students select the final reward.
   - Explain the game. Points are awarded each time a signal sounds. Students should not know when the signal will sound. If all members on a team are working at the time that the signal goes off, the team earns a point. Even if only one member is not "behaving," the team does not receive a point.
   - Use a CD or MP3 file that includes 8 to 10 cues in the form of a loud bell or some other type of sound. Space these sounds at intervals of varying lengths. If at all possible, create multiple versions of the CD/MP3 file, each with differing interval patterns. When the class begins, simply play the MP3 file over the sound system with the volume turned up.
   - Upon each signal, scan the class and determine which teams deserve the point. Praise the teams that are working and let them know that they just earned a point. Explain the reason why certain team(s) did not earn a point.
   - At the end of a class period, total up the points earned by each team, and post the scores.
   - At the end of an agreed upon period (e.g., 4 lessons, 2 weeks), teams that reached the criterion earn their reward.

Given the options available, be sure to choose the most appropriate type of group contingency. For example, if improvement is sought in the behavior of an individual student or a small group, the dependent group contingency would be the appropriate choice. If you want to improve the performance of students differentially (i.e., some you do and some you don't want to reward), the independent group contingency is more appropriate. If your concern is for the performance of the group as a whole, one of the interdependent group contingency choices is appropriate.

With each consecutive game played, teachers can lengthen the game's duration, and/or reduce the number of sounds used per class used to score the teams' performance. Thus, very slowly the game is phased out.

Rationales for Using Group Contingencies

There are several rationales for why teachers should consider the use of group contingencies. They include:

- It can save time during the administration of the consequence (i.e., the reinforcer).
- Often it is impractical to implement contingencies with multiple individual students. For example, if you have a substantial number of students who exhibit disruptive behaviors, it will be difficult to administer a behavior reduction program with each individual student. It will be less burdensome if you can administer one reward to the entire class. Moreover, group-oriented contingencies can be applied across a variety of students, behaviors, and settings.
- Generally, group contingencies are used only if and when less extensive intervention efforts (e.g., ignoring behavior, social reinforcement) have been unsuccessful. Although group contingencies can be aimed at reducing problem behaviors, they still offer a more positive approach in that they target the development of more pro-social behavior.
- When used effectively, group contingencies encourage positive interactions and support among student peers. For example, if an entire class would be rewarded with free time contingent on the performance of an individual student, the prospect of free time would serve to initiate encouragement and support from the class peers toward that individual student. Especially in cases where students with disabilities are the focus of the contingency, typically developing peers can be an excellent support system. This procedure, of providing a reward to a whole group based on the performance of one individual, is called the *hero procedure*. It facilitates positive interaction between students because the whole group will benefit from the performance of the one student who is the target of the contingency. Thus, teachers can capitalize on peer influence or peer monitoring because this type of contingency allows students to act as their own change agents. We should note that if the group contingency is poorly arranged (e.g., an unreasonably high expectation) there is a risk it may place undue peer pressure on a student and have a detrimental effect in the form of scapegoating or, worse, bullying. This harmful outcome must be avoided at all costs by carefully structuring the contingency.

Effective use of group contingencies can produce significant improvements in student performances both in regard to motor skills and fitness development and in relation to managerial and organizational tasks. Examples of student misbehavior where group contingencies would work well include being on time for attendance, hustling when transitioning from the changing room to an outdoor activity venue on the campus, taking attendance in the least amount of time

BOX 8.11 Implementing Group Contingencies: Guidelines and Considerations

Compared to using social reinforcement, group contingencies require careful planning and monitoring by teachers. The following are some guidelines for their implementation:

- *Choose a powerful reward (i.e., reinforcer).* Effective teachers will develop a "reinforcer menu" (based on the preferences noted by students) that lists the preferred rewards.
- *Choose appropriate performance criteria.* The individuals for whom the contingency is applied *must* have the prerequisite skills to perform the expected behavior.
- *Closely monitor both individual student and group performance.* It is very well possible that the performance of the group is improving but that some individual students within the same group are not improving. Some students may even try to sabotage the group contingency, trying to prevent other groups from earning the reward. If that is the case, you will want to arrange a contingency with the individual student in combination with your regular group contingency.
- *Practice the use of group contingencies on a small scale first.* You could use a single class period as a starting point. For example, if student nagging is a persistent and "nagging" problem for you, try the following. At the beginning of class, present the contingency where all students will get 4 minutes of extra game time (or free time, or choice game) if the student group will nag no more than three times. If they nag more often they do not get the reinforcer. The next day you might consider allowing only two nags.
- *Group contingencies are especially effective when used over longer periods of time (e.g., weeks).* Using it one time (e.g., over three to four lessons) will work very well. However, for sustained behavior change, follow the completion of the first contract with additional ones. In doing so, teachers can gradually increase the criterion for earning the reward, and/or gradually reduce the scope/size of the reward.
- *Do not give away the store.* Ensure balance between the behavioral expectation and the contingent reward. That is, avoid extravagant rewards for minimal improvements in students' performance.
- *Combine the use of group-oriented contingencies with other behavior change procedures when appropriate.* That is, continue your use of individual praise that can function as a reinforcer.

Data from Cooper, J. O., Heron, T. E., & Heward, W. L. (2007). *Applied behavior analysis* (2nd ed.). Upper Saddle River, NJ: Pearson/Merrill-Prentice Hall.

possible, dressing for class, starting an initial activity upon entering the gym, not taking excessive time for in-class transitions, reducing nagging/complaining by students, reacting quickly to a signal for attention, waiting to start an activity until the end of the instructions (i.e., waiting for the teacher's "go" signal), and not fidgeting with equipment during instructional episodes.

There is substantial evidence that effectively implemented group contingences can produce substantial improvements in students' behavior/performance when used in primary and postprimary physical education and sport settings (e.g., Hastie, van der Mars, Layne, & Wadsworth, 2012; Hume & Crossman, 1992; Patrick, Ward, & Crouch, 1998; Vidoni, Azevedo, & Eberline, 2012; Vidoni & Ward, 2006, 2009; Ward & Dunaway, 1995). In these studies, teachers reinforced improvements in students' and/or athletes' on-task behavior (e.g., running or swimming laps completed), effort (expressed in heart rates), disruptive behavior, social behavior, fair play behavior, and independent out-of-school physical activity behavior. The contingencies included several types of rewards, including allowing music to be played, providing free time, T-shirts, choice activities, or "mystery reinforcers" (e.g., key chains with different types of sports balls, pins, and pencils). Specific guidelines and considerations for implementing group contingencies are presented in **Box 8.11**.

When using group contingencies, teachers must be mindful of several ethical issues that may surface, depending on how well they are arranged (see **Box 8.12**).

Learning Experience 8.5

When in a school setting where you have observed persistent student misbehavior among multiple students, (1) informally survey the students and determine their favorite activities, and (2) over the course of two or three lessons determine the prevalence of the problem behavior by developing a written log of the students' behavior. What seem to be the most prevalent problem behaviors? Based on the information you gathered, develop a group contingency plan aimed at changing the behavior of the students. Which type of group contingency would be the more appropriate one? Explain why.

BOX 8.12 Using Group Contingencies: Some Ethical Considerations

- Depending on the contingency's setup, it is possible that some students in class may exhibit inappropriate behaviors toward peers who failed to reach the performance criterion, thus resulting in *scapegoating*. Teasing, threatening, and/or ridiculing are examples of scapegoating. Thus, be alert for coercion and covert peer pressure!
- Teachers can avoid the risk of scapegoating by setting appropriate behavior expectations when deciding on the criterion for the group contingency. Performance expectations should be within reach and early on allow a certain margin of error. For example, a group contingency can be set where the entire class receives the reinforcer if 80% of the group is on time and dressed appropriately for class, 90% of the next 10 class periods. Thus, your one or two perennial non-dressing and tardy students may not keep the group as a whole from ultimately receiving the reward.
- Use of a group contingency may be problematic if the contingency to be implemented states that the offender(s) be publicly identified on a chart or poster board. This again could result in scapegoating or bullying. Teachers can prevent this by leaving off students' names from the poster or chart where student progress toward receiving the reward is tracked.

Data from Cooper, J. O., Heron, T. E., & Heward, W. L. (2007). *Applied behavior analysis* (2nd ed.). Upper Saddle River, NJ: Pearson/Merrill-Prentice Hall.

Time-out

One of the most frequently used punishment techniques in schools is some form of **time-out**, where a student is required to sit out from the class activity for a short period of time as a consequence of misbehaving or breaking a class rule. Given its prevalence as a measure of punishment, it deserves extra attention. Technically, time-out is the removal of the chance to earn positive reinforcement intended to reduce future occurrence of the problem behavior. Getting placed in time-out is analogous to the use of the penalty box in ice hockey and rugby, especially in the sense that teachers have a specific place where the offending student goes to spend a specified amount of time.

In physical education/activity settings, if the activity is one in which the student likes to participate, then the student is more likely to see removal from it as punishing. On the other hand, if the student dislikes an activity (e.g., an activity that is perceived as boring, overly difficult, and/or too strenuous), removal from it is unlikely to change future behavior. This highlights the point that the behavior subsequent to the punishment determines whether the consequence was, in fact, punishing.

Generally, a time-out should be of short duration, seldom longer than 3–4 minutes. A timer (such as an egg timer or clock) should be used for the student to time his or her own time-out suspension. Upon the first use of a time-out, teachers may choose to let the student return to action when the student believes she or he is ready to join in the activities. It is helpful if you have the student verbalize to you what he or she did wrong after the time-out period before returning to lesson participation. If the student then engages in inappropriate behavior again, and is placed in time-out again, the teacher gets to decide when the student can return to action. In most cases, the student, while removed from the activity, does remain in the environment. The teacher will need to monitor the student while in time-out, but should refrain from interacting with the student. Moreover, other students in the class should be directed that they are not to interact or make eye contact with any student who is in time-out because those are other possible sources of reinforcement for the student.

Excessive and persistent inappropriate behavior during a lesson may require the student's complete removal from the activity area, coupled with being placed in a room. In some postprimary schools, the behavior management plan may include the use of a separate classroom space that in effect serves as a time-out room, though it may get named something else. In **Box 8.13** we offer specific guidelines to ensure effective implementation of time-out as a behavior change technique.

Employing time-out has several advantages for teachers. First, it can be implemented with relative ease. Second, in regular physical education/activity settings, it is regarded as an acceptable and fair approach to managing students' behavior. Third, whereas other behavior change techniques, such as ignoring the behavior and differential reinforcement, may take longer for behavior change to occur, time-out can bring about quick improvements in students' behavior. And fourth, teachers can combine time-out with differential reinforcement, and maintain a focus on not only reducing the inappropriate behavior but also supporting appropriate behavior.

Reward Cost

Reward cost, also called *response cost*, is a punishment technique where students lose previously earned points or privileges as a consequence of misbehavior. Reward cost is one of the most common forms of punishment in society at large. That is, many rule violations result in the loss of money. For adults, receiving a traffic fine for driving with excessive speed, and having one's automobile insurance premium raised for

BOX 8.13 Guidelines for Effective Use of Time-out

The following are guidelines and considerations for teachers when employing time-out:

- First and foremost, teachers will want to ensure that the activities within lessons are stimulating, attractive, meaningful, and appropriate in difficulty level. This will go a long way toward preventing most inappropriate student behavior. If any of these features are absent, students will be more inclined to avoid participation and choose some type of misbehavior.
- Explain which behaviors will result in being placed in time-out. Students should be aware of the types of behavior that would lead to removal from the class activity.
- Decide on the process used and the length of the time-out. Generally, the time spent in time-out should not exceed 3–4 minutes. However, if the student has previously been in time-out for longer periods, then such short duration time-outs may not be effective.
- As much as possible, remove all possible sources of reinforcement during the time-out period. Especially when students in time-out remain in the environment, peers and friends in the class are potential sources of reinforcement. Provide explicit reminders to the other students that they should refrain from interacting with the student(s) in time-out.
- There may be instances where teachers place two or more students in time-out simultaneously. In that case, ensure that the time-out spaces are located far enough apart so the students cannot talk to each other, which would be a potential source of reinforcement.
- Define the criteria for return to activity. Returning to the class activity should not be based solely on the passage of time. Rather, the student should be monitored to ensure that the problem behavior does not continue during the time-out.
- Be consistent when employing time-out. If students are placed in time-out in some instances of certain misbehaviors but not on other occasions, they will be confused about what the teacher finds acceptable.

Data from Cooper, J. O., Heron, T. E., & Heward, W. L. (2007). *Applied behavior analysis* (2nd ed.). Upper Saddle River, NJ: Pearson/Merrill-Prentice Hall.

having caused a traffic accident are two simple examples of losing a previously earned reinforcer (i.e., money).

In physical education, teachers would need to have an ongoing system in place where students earn points or privileges for performing varying responsibilities and roles in order for reward cost to work. An example of reward cost in physical education/activity settings is "fines" in the form of having points taken away that could be exchanged for minutes of free time. Previously earned privileges such as being first in line or being an equipment manager that are taken away from a student also are examples of reward cost.

In the Sport Education curriculum model, teams earn points for performing several nonplaying roles and demonstrating fair play behavior throughout each lesson. These points directly affect the teams' position in the season's league standings. Thus, there is a built-in accountability system that encourages student fair play behavior and duty team performance. When duty team and/or fair play performance slips over several lessons, teachers can remove some previously earned points (i.e., reward cost), which may result in the team losing ground in the season's competition.

In an outdoor education context, attending a field trip where students get to participate in an all-day hike in a regional mountain range is contingent on earning a minimum number of points during the preparatory class periods that precede the field trip. If during the preceding class periods students falter in some way (e.g., exhibiting unsafe behavior), they lose points.

As is the case with all other punishment techniques, its effectiveness is determined by whether it results in reduced inappropriate behavior. **Box 8.14** provides some guidelines for using reward cost.

Reward cost has several attractive features for use in physical education/activity settings. First, the technique can be implemented with relative ease (assuming teachers employ a type of points/reward system). Second, if used appropriately, reward cost will result in reduced inappropriate behavior relatively quickly. Third, it is easily combined with other reinforcement techniques.

The Ultimate and Long-Term Goal of a Behavior Management System

All teachers are expected to have a discipline plan or system in place for their classes. Well-designed behavior management systems should have the short-term capacity to reduce inappropriate and disruptive behavior quickly and effectively, and then to begin to develop and support appropriate behavior to achieve the goals of a lesson or unit. Behavior management systems also need to be focused on longer-term goals such as student self-control and self-direction.

In the longer term, it is important that schools help students grow as independent decision makers who can weigh the consequences of their own actions and behave responsibly toward adults and their own peers. Students also need to learn to accept the consequences of their actions and not to make excuses or blame others for what was clearly their own misbehavior. Ultimately, they need to learn to behave well without supervision and to persevere in appropriate behavior even in the face of possible negative peer pressure.

BOX 8.14 Guidelines for Effective Use of Reward Cost

The following guidelines and considerations are provided for when teachers choose reward cost as a means of reducing the future occurrence of certain problem behaviors:

- *Ensure that the misbehavior and the fine are stated explicitly.* Students should be provided with a clear explanation as to what the misbehavior is and the fine that results as a consequence.
- *The magnitude of the response cost should fit the severity of the misbehavior.* That is, minor offenses should result in smaller fines, whereas a major offense should result in a larger loss of previously earned privileges/points.
- *If at all possible, apply the fine immediately after the occurrence of the misbehavior.* If this cannot be done immediately, let the student know that you will announce the actual fine at the end of the class period.
- *Have students first build up their bank of reinforcement.* If students have not yet earned a sufficient amount of points or minutes toward time in a choice activity, reward cost is difficult, if not impossible, to implement. Once the amount of points increases, then the impact of reward cost is felt more.
- *Combine reward cost with other reinforcement techniques.* As is the cases with all other punishment techniques, seek out every opportunity to reinforce appropriate behavior (e.g., differential reinforcement of alternative behavior).
- *Consider setting a "bonus reward cost" system.* When students already have a set amount of time allocated for free time for choice activities once a week, or a set amount of time for having music playing in the background, the teacher can offer additional minutes of free time or time with music noncontingently (i.e., the bonus). Any misbehavior would then result in the loss of the bonus minutes.

Teachers should carefully consider the following potential reactions by students when reward cost is applied:

- *Knowledge of the student's history of aggressive or emotional behavior is essential* because certain students may react with strong verbal outbursts upon losing the privilege of points, especially if the reward cost is applied multiple times in a single lesson. This will allow the teacher to decide if reward cost is the appropriate course of action. If such aggressive verbal outbursts occur, try to ignore them as much as possible.
- *Reward cost increases the attention to students' unacceptable behavior.* In itself it is purely a punishment technique. Therefore, it is important that teachers counterbalance the reward cost use with reinforcement techniques aimed at strengthening students' pro-social behavior.
- *Avoid overdependence on reward cost.* Use reward cost only as a last resort and then only for extreme misbehavior.

Data from Cooper, J. O., Heron, T. E., & Heward, W. L. (2007). *Applied behavior analysis* (2nd ed.). Upper Saddle River, NJ: Pearson/Merrill-Prentice Hall.

Students tend to learn these life skills to the extent that (1) teachers effectively teach such content, (2) the school is a place in which there are clear expectations for good behavior, and (3) students get treated fairly and consistently regarding those expectations. If you can develop a discipline system in your physical education classes that is consistent with the school system, yet is specific to your physical activity setting, you will have a better chance to succeed in this important endeavor.

Learning Experience 8.6

- In the school where you are placed for your teaching experience, determine what, if any, school-wide discipline plan is in effect. Next determine the discipline plan in effect within the physical education program. In both cases, place the discipline plan on a continuum from "predominant dependence on punitive consequences" to "predominant dependence on reinforcing consequences," and describe the type of consequences employed. Arrange for time to meet with the physical education teacher and determine his or her personal philosophy on discipline and view on the school's discipline system, including how it was developed, what seems to work well, what does not work well, and what the teacher does or does not like about the school's approach to discipline.
- Describe your own philosophy of discipline. Include your personal experiences that would form the basis of your philosophy on developing discipline.
- Create a specific plan for developing/maintaining discipline in your classes.

TABLE 8.2 A Fair Player System for Developing Effective Discipline

Fair Player	Unfair Player	Nonplayer
• Follows class rules • Respects classmates, teacher, and equipment • Frequently compliments peers • Perseveres • Is helpful in assisting others • Involves classmates • Is appropriately assertive • Actively participates in learning activities • Eagerly fulfills assigned organizational/managerial tasks • Wins and loses games with grace	• Finds ways to cheat • Puts peers down • Hogs ball • Gets frustrated easily and quits • Teases classmates and pouts • Is insensitive to others • Is overly aggressive • Taunts when winning and pouts when losing • Lacks self-control • Requires frequent teacher supervision/attention • Has minimal engagement in learning activity with little energy • Avoids assistance during organizational/managerial activities • Is disrespectful toward classmates, teacher, equipment, and facilities	• Avoids management system • Avoids peers • Hides out during activity • Makes little if any effort toward assigned tasks • Gives "get lost" messages • Requires constant teacher supervision/attention • Lurks on outside of activity • Is nonassertive • Fears failure • Is bored or anxious • Blames others and denies personal responsibility • Gets frustrated and quits on classmates • Teases and pouts • Makes excuses • Cheats

Although we presented the various techniques of reinforcement and punishment separately, teachers can and should use them in combination, again from the perspective of discipline being dual-directional (i.e., simultaneously reducing inappropriate behavior and fostering pro-social behavior). One such approach is shown in **Table 8.2** using the concept of "fair play" as framed by Siedentop, Hastie, and van der Mars (2011). The benefit of this kind of system is that it helps students learn the behaviors that differentiate among a fair player, an unfair player, and a nonplayer. When there are consistent negative *and* positive consequences for students who operate in each of those three categories, then the chance of developing classes full of fair players increases. It is important for teachers to have students who conform to rules and expectations. However, all too often in physical education a system is put in place so that students do conform but are left in a pattern of conformance rather than being helped to grow into more mature, self-directed individuals. To become truly self-directed, students must be weaned gradually and carefully from the normal kinds of behavioral supports that school provides for them as they are learning how to become responsible.

CHAPTER SUMMARY

In practice, preventative management and discipline go hand in hand. If preventative management is used well, and if all students feel safe and valued (and the content presented is exciting and appropriate), then teachers will most likely not need to develop a behavior contract or use group contingencies. However, even under the best of circumstances, there will be instances where students may need extra support in developing discipline in their own behavior. The key is to have a deliberate plan for managing the behavior of students, select the right technique, and employ it appropriately.

In schools where many students come to school without some basic school skills (i.e., following directions, listening during instruction, showing respect toward peers), teachers will need to foreground the development of such skills. This is not likely to be successful without strong preventative management and the development of a strong sense of community of learners.

1. Discipline should be viewed as a means for developing and sustaining appropriate behavior between teachers and students and among students.
2. Discipline is more than merely applying negative consequences for inappropriate student behavior. Indeed, if punishment is the main strategy, then the discipline system is inadequate.
3. Behavior management is important because school management and parents expect orderly learning environments, and teachers find their workplace to be more enjoyable when there is discipline.
4. Well-disciplined classes create conditions in which learning may take place, but the time must be filled with good learning activities.
5. Hellison's TPSR model is a sound approach to help students develop personal and social responsibility within classes and outside them.
6. Basic strategies for changing behavior include being specific, defining contingencies, starting with small chunks of behavior, making gradual changes, being consistent, and starting where the student is.
7. A contingency is the relationship between a behavior and a consequence. The consequence to the behavior can be positive or negative. If it subsequently results in increased frequency of the behavior it served as a

reinforcer. If the frequency of the behavior reduces, or the behavior disappears altogether, the consequence served as a punisher.

8. General strategies for increasing appropriate behavior include clear, specific prompts and rules; high yet realistic expectations; frequent reinforcement; effective nonverbal interaction; and effective public and private communication.
9. Specific techniques for developing and/or sustaining appropriate/pro-social behavior include the use of verbal and nonverbal prompts, social reinforcers (in the form of feedback and praise), tangible reinforcers, and activity reinforcers. The use of edible reinforcers is strongly discouraged.
10. Effective praise requires following known guidelines and avoiding major technique errors (e.g., praising students noncontingently, being general) as well as using a variety of praise techniques.
11. Specific techniques for reducing misbehavior include verbal desists, ignoring tolerable behavior, differential reinforcement of incompatible behavior (DRI), differential reinforcement of alternative behavior (DRA), differential reinforcement of low rates of behavior (DRL), differential reinforcement of other behavior (DRO, also known as omission training), positive practice (also called overcorrection), contingency contracting, group contingencies, time-out, and reward cost.
12. The ultimate goal of a discipline system is to bring students into responsible, mature relationships with their peers, the subject matter, and the school society because this prepares students to generalize those behavioral predispositions beyond the school to the community and the home.

REFERENCES

Brophy, J. (1981). Teacher praise: A functional analysis. *Review of Educational Research, 51*, 5–32.

Cooper, J. O., Heron, T. E., & Heward, W. L. (2007). *Applied behavior analysis* (2nd ed.). Upper Saddle River, NJ: Pearson/Merrill-Prentice Hall.

Cothran, D. J., & Ennis, C. D. (1997). Students' and teachers' perceptions of conflict and power. *Teaching and Teacher Education, 13*, 541–553.

Cothran, D. J., Hodges-Kulinna, P., & Garrahy, D. A. (2003). "This is kind of giving a secret away . . .": Students' perspectives on effective class management. *Teaching and Teacher Education 19*, 435–444.

Finnicum, P. (1997). Developing discipline policies to prevent problem behaviors. *Teaching Secondary Physical Education, 3*(4), 25–26.

Galloway, C. (1971). Teaching is more than words. *Quest, 15*, 67–71.

Garrahy, D. A., Kulinna, P. H., & Cothran D. J. (2005). Voices from the trenches: An exploration of teachers' management knowledge. *Journal of Educational Research, 99*, 56–63.

Hastie, P., van der Mars, H., Layne, T., & Wadsworth, D. (2012). The effects of prompts and a group-oriented contingency on out-of-school physical activity in elementary school-aged students. *Journal of Teaching in Physical Education, 31*, 131–145.

Hellison, D. (2011). *Teaching personal and social responsibility through physical activity* (3rd ed.). Champaign, IL: Human Kinetics.

Hellison, D., Cutforth, N., Kallusky, J., Martinek, T., Parker, M., & Stiehl, J. (2000). *Youth development and physical activity*. Champaign, IL: Human Kinetics.

Hume, K. M., & Crossman, J. (1992). Musical reinforcement of practice behaviors among competitive swimmers. *Journal of Applied Behavior Analysis, 25*, 665–670.

Kounin, J. (1970). *Discipline and group management in classrooms*. New York: Holt, Rinehart & Winston.

Lee, S., Burgeson, C., Fulton, J., & Spain, C. (2007). Physical education and physical activity: Results from the School Health Policies and Programs Study 2006. *Journal of School Health, 77*, 435–463.

National Association for Sport and Physical Education (NASPE). (2009). *Physical activity used as punishment and/or behavior management* [position statement]. Reston, VA: Author.

O'Connell Rust, F. (1994). The first year of teaching: It's not what they expected. *Teaching and Teacher Education, 10*, 205–217.

Olson, M. R., & Osborne, J. W. (1991). Learning to teach: The first year. *Teaching and Teacher Education, 7*, 331–343.

O'Sullivan, M., & Dyson, B. (1994). Rules, routines, and expectations of 11 high school physical education teachers. *Journal of Teaching in Physical Education, 13*, 361–374.

Patrick, C. A., Ward, P., & Crouch, D. W. (1998). Effects of holding students accountable for social behaviors during volleyball games in elementary physical education. *Journal of Teaching in Physical Education, 17*, 143–156.

Premack, D. (1959). Toward empirical behavioral laws: I. Positive reinforcement. *Psychological Review, 66*, 219–233.

Rolider, A., Siedentop, D., & Van Houten, R. (1984). Effects of enthusiasm training on subsequent teacher enthusiasm. *Journal of Teaching in Physical Education, 3*(2), 47–59.

Siedentop, D., Hastie, P. A., & van der Mars, H. (2011). *Complete guide to sport education* (2nd ed.). Champaign. IL: Human Kinetics.

Siedentop, D., & Tannehill, D. (2000). *Developing teaching skills in physical education* (3rd ed.). Mountain View, CA: Mayfield.

Veenman, S. (1984). Perceived problems in beginning teachers. *Review of Educational Research, 54*, 143–178.

Vidoni, C., Azevedo, L., & Eberline, A. (2012). Effects of a group contingency strategy on middle school physical education students' heart rates. *European Physical Education Review, 18, 78*–96.

Vidoni, C., & Ward, P. (2006). Effects of a dependent group-oriented contingency on middle school physical education students' fair play behaviors. *Journal of Behavioral Education, 15*, 81–92.

Vidoni, C., & Ward, P. (2009). Effects of fair play instruction on student social skills during a middle school sport education unit. *Physical Education and Sport Pedagogy, 14*, 285–310.

Ward, P., & Dunaway, S. (1995). Effects of contingent music on laps run in a high school physical education class. *Physical Educator, 52*(1), 2–7.

Wynne, E., & Ryan, K. (1997). *Reclaiming our schools: Teaching character, academics and discipline* (2nd ed.). Upper Saddle River, NJ: Prentice Hall.

SECTION III Designing an Instructionally Aligned Physical Education Program

Introduction

One of the most unfortunate situations to observe in physical education is to see a well-managed class, led by a teacher with good teaching skills, working on content that is boring, insignificant, or developmentally inappropriate for the particular group of students. Designing a meaningful, challenging curriculum is a key element in building a successful physical education program. Translating the intent of that curriculum into units of instruction, then a series of lessons, each of which has an appropriate progression of well-designed learning experiences, is the basic stuff of good planning.

The chapters in this section will help you understand how to align your goals for physical education with choice of curriculum model, instructional models, and teaching strategies as well as the learning experiences and adaptations designed to meet those goals and the assessment to show how well students have achieved the outcomes that define the goals. Although this sounds complex, it is really quite straightforward as you come to understand the idea of instructionally aligned learning and become familiar and skilled at aligning program goals through curriculum design, assessment, and instruction and with the employment of technology to meet the ever-increasing interactive skills of youth.

CHAPTER 9 Curriculum Concepts and Planning Principles

Overall Chapter Outcome

To develop insight into curriculum concepts, principles of curriculum design, and a model for curriculum planning that will encourage the development of a meaningful, worthwhile, and relevant school physical education curriculum

Learning Outcomes

The learner will:

- Define curriculum and its association with program and syllabus
- Explain backward design and instructional alignment as the two main guiding principles of designing and planning curriculum
- Provide examples of common practices in physical education curricula
- Describe the role of curriculum in successful physical education
- Describe objectives and outcomes and examine the relationship between the two
- Engage with international differences in physical education curriculum design
- Specify eight principles of curriculum design
- Explain the different "goods" to which physical education curricula are devoted
- Describe the six-step model for curriculum planning

Before going any further in introducing and discussing curriculum concepts, it is imperative to qualify what we mean by *curriculum* and its relationship to associated terms such as *program* and *syllabus*. **Curriculum** tends to refer to all planned learning for which the school is responsible and all the experiences to which learners are exposed under the guidance of the school (Kelly & Melograno, 2004). These can include school subjects, after-school sport, and extracurricular activities. A school curriculum can contain a set of **objectives** that note instructional intent and **outcomes** that describe what students are expected to achieve across the school curriculum. Along with every other school subject area, all the experiences that students have in physical education while they attend a particular school represent that school's curriculum. Although *curriculum* is commonly used to convey the accumulation of planned learning experiences across the school, it is sometimes used interchangeably with the terms *program* and *syllabus* when a specific school subject lists selected activities and experiences planned to achieve student learning outcomes. It is therefore common for some countries to discuss a physical education curriculum, for others to discuss a physical education program, and for others to refer to a physical education syllabus. Throughout this chapter we favor the use of the term *curriculum*.

Backward Design and Instructional Alignment

It is imperative that the reader understands two concepts, *backward design* and *instructional alignment*, that guide the design and planning of curriculum. Wiggins and McTighe (1998) encourage teachers to plan backwards from the "big ideas" they want students to learn, design assessment tools that will demonstrate students having achieved success, and

BOX 9.1 Key Terms in This Chapter

- *Authentic outcome:* An outcome that requires a performance in a context similar to the one in which the knowledge, skills, and strategies will eventually be used.
- *Backward design:* When curriculum design begins with the exit outcomes and proceeds backwards to ensure that all components are directly related to achieving the outcome.
- *Content standards:* What students should know and be able to do at a particular developmental/grade level.
- *Curriculum:* All planned learning for which the school is responsible and all the experiences to which learners are exposed under the guidance of the school. Curriculum is also used interchangeably with the terms *program* and *syllabus* when a specific school subject, such as physical education, lists selected activities and experiences planned to achieve student-learning outcomes.
- *Curriculum guide:* A formal district/regional document explaining the objectives to be achieved in a subject and the activities thought to contribute to those objectives. Also often referred to as a *curriculum syllabus* or a *graded course of study.*
- *Instructional alignment:* Exists when the objectives/outcomes, activities, instruction, and assessment of a physical education program are matched and compatible.
- *Objectives:* Statements of instructional intent that include situation (condition), task (behavior), and criteria that will guide student learning.
- *Outcomes:* What students are expected to do and know as the result of participating in the program.
- *Outcomes-based curriculum:* A curriculum in which specific outcomes rather than general objectives form the basis of the curriculum.
- *Performance standards:* These tell teachers and students how well the student has to perform to meet the standard. That is, how good is "good enough" for that level.

choose teaching strategies to facilitate students reaching those big ideas. This is commonly referred to as **backward design** and constitutes considering the following:

- What do we want students to know and be able to do as a result of participating in our programs? (curriculum)
- How will we know when they have been successful? (assessment)
- How can we get them there in the most challenging and engaging ways possible? (instruction) (Lund & Tannehill, 2010)

For example, if the goal is to be a fair player during activity, assessment should be to demonstrate fair play in an activity setting and teaching should be learning what it means to be a fair player and practicing it with feedback. If the goal is to be physically active in class daily, assessment should be learners demonstrating daily physical activity and teaching should be providing challenging opportunities for learners to be physically active. Both examples constitute **instructional alignment** where goals, assessment, teaching strategies, and learning experiences are aligned, promoting richer learning for students.

A meaningful and coherent physical education program reflects an alignment among learning goals, assessments that determine if students reach those goals, and the instructional practices that provide students the opportunity to achieve success (Cohen, 1987; Lund & Tannehill, 2005, 2010, 2014). That is, demonstrate alignment between what students are intended to know and be able to do, the opportunities they receive to learn and practice, and how we assess for learning. The first piece of the instructional alignment triad is reflected in goals for student achievement, that is, what it is that students will learn in physical education. The second piece of the triad is assessments that match the learning goal. We must determine what we want students to achieve (goal) and how they might demonstrate success. All learning does not have to be demonstrated in the same way. Just as all students learn differently, so do they demonstrate learning in varying ways. It is up to the teacher to provide opportunities for students to demonstrate their success, their mastery, their competence, and their level of achievement. The final piece of the triad is instruction and how instruction is designed to facilitate learning. It must be done intentionally, thoughtfully, creatively, and in an inviting and individually motivating way.

Common Practices in Physical Education Curricula

Experiences in physical education ought to add up to something significant in the lives of students. Physical education should excite students, engage them enthusiastically in activities they find meaningful, and eventually help them develop lifelong commitments to physically active lifestyles. Sadly, physical education curricula do not always achieve those outcomes. Too many young people move through their school physical education experiences bored, uninterested, and even eventually alienated from the physically active lifestyle that most curricula aim to develop. Too many students wonder where all the excitement is that they see and experience in school sport, in community activity programs, on television, and in fitness centers. In too many school districts/regions, education is planned and delivered with no serious effort to articulate and develop the programs at primary and postprimary levels to achieve significant curriculum objectives.

One major culprit is the continued widespread use of the short-unit, multiactivity curriculum model, what many refer to as a "smorgasbord" curriculum (Taylor & Chiogioji, 1987). Because physical education has many objectives/outcomes, teachers plan the curriculum as a series of short activity units, with a few lessons of isolated, basic skill practice and then a few class periods of a tournament or series of games. Perhaps most alarming is that these same "introductory" units tend to be taught over and over again throughout the physical education curriculum, so that students' physical education experiences are repetitive, uninteresting, and unchallenging. Thus, a student in postprimary physical education might well experience a short volleyball unit in which the first several lessons introduce the serve, forearm pass, set, and spike. These skills are then practiced in drills that often isolate the skills from the context in which they might be used in games. Even so, students seldom get sufficient practice opportunities to become confident about their skills. Then, for several lessons, teams are assigned and games are played. Game play is typically of low quality because students do not have sufficient skills to enjoy the game, having had little opportunity to learn the tactical and strategic elements of volleyball. Many of those students might have had nearly identical volleyball units in primary school, so they leave school with little appreciation for what a great sport volleyball can be and ill equipped to pursue volleyball as a recreational sport in their adult years. Their physical education curriculum has failed them.

Learning Experience 9.1

Reflect on your experience as a student of school physical education at primary and postprimary schools and write down:

- The activity areas to which you were most and least exposed through the physical education curriculum
- The extent to which you experienced the multiactivity program in physical education
- What encouraged or discouraged your participation in school physical education
- The opportunities you were afforded through the physical education curriculum (e.g., team affiliation)
- Your lasting impression of school physical education

Join a group of your peers and share your responses to identify the similarities and differences of school physical education that you have been exposed to.

The Role of Curriculum in Successful Physical Education

Successful physical education, in which most students achieve a large proportion of the objectives/outcomes, is the result of curriculum and instruction coming together in appropriate ways, and is greatly enhanced when facilitative structural arrangements can be put in place. Successful physical education requires the following:

- A meaningful, relevant curriculum that is articulated across ages and school levels
- Effective teaching that helps students become enthused, self-reliant learners
- Organizational arrangements that allow for meaningful engagement and provide sufficient time and support to achieve meaningful outcomes

In the absence of even one of those three components, the program will fall short. A dull curriculum, perceived by students as repetitive, lacking appropriate challenges, and irrelevant, will fail, even when it is taught effectively. An exciting and relevant curriculum can also fail if it is taught ineffectively. A meaningful curriculum that is delivered effectively through appropriate instructional strategies will succeed. Organizational arrangements such as block scheduling (see later in this chapter), persisting groups, learning communities, and links to community programs can all strengthen and invigorate the curriculum.

Learning Experience 9.2

Consider the demographics in the following examples and develop a written outline of what would be a potentially meaningful, exciting, and relevant curriculum that would complement each class:

- A class of twenty-eight 16-year-old boys and girls who attend the school from a wide geographical area and whose physical education exposure has only been hockey due to the interest and expertise of the physical education teacher
- A class of twenty-six 13-year-old boys who wish to play soccer all the time in physical education due to their interest in playing as part of a team and who thrive on exploring how to most effectively play the game.
- A class of twenty-three 14-year-old girls and boys, most of whom live in a disadvantaged area where limited access and support is available to them to be physically active outside of school hours.

This chapter introduces the concepts and language of curriculum and the fundamental principles that guide its development. The chapter also introduces examples of curriculum made by national professional agencies that should form the basis of the curriculum design suggestions made here. This chapter will be most relevant to those who are required to, or want to, (1) develop their own curriculum, (2) adapt what is currently in place, and/or (3) work collectively to develop a physical education curriculum following national guidelines (e.g., the National Association for Sport and Physical Education [NASPE] in the United States, the Department of Education and Skills [DES]/National Council for Curriculum and Assessment [NCCA] in Ireland). The concepts and principles in this chapter will be necessary if you have to start from scratch to build a curriculum. If your program already has a written curriculum in place, this chapter's information will help you determine to what extent your program reflects the three aforementioned criteria for success.

Important Curriculum Terms

To become knowledgeable and skilled in the area of curriculum, you must be able to use the common technical terms. These terms and concepts are employed by teachers and administrators in their everyday work in schools, and a thorough understanding of them is necessary for you to read and apply the professional literature.

Most school districts and many states in the United States have and require a **curriculum guide**, which is a formal district document explaining the objectives to be achieved in a subject and the activities thought to contribute to those objectives. A curriculum guide is also often referred to as a *curriculum syllabus* or a *graded course of study*, and is typically based on the NASPE Content Standards (see **Box 9.2**). Curriculum guides have become very detailed in some districts that have moved toward an **outcomes-based curriculum**, in which specific outcomes rather than general objectives form the basis of the curriculum. This requires more detail in terms of what activities and experiences contribute to the outcomes.

BOX 9.2 NASPE Content Standards

- Standard 1: Demonstrates competency in a variety of motor skills and movement patterns
- Standard 2: Applies knowledge of concepts, principles, strategies, and tactics related to movement and performance
- Standard 3: Demonstrates the knowledge and skills to achieve and maintain a health-enhancing level of physical activity and fitness
- Standard 4: Exhibits responsible personal and social behavior that respects self and others
- Standard 5: Recognizes the value of physical activity for health, enjoyment, challenge, self-expression, and/or social interaction

Reproduced with permission from NASPE. (2004). *Moving into the future: National standards for physical education* (2nd ed.). Reston, VA: NASPE.

BOX 9.3 Differing Presentation of Physical Education Curriculum

Country: Australia

- Curriculum for postprimary physical education: Personal Development, Health and Physical Education (PDHPE) syllabus
- Included in the documentation: aims, objectives, key competencies, and core content

Country: Ireland

- Curriculum for postprimary physical education: Physical Education syllabus
- Included in the documentation: aims, objectives, topics, and learning outcomes

Countries: England, Wales, and Northern Ireland

- Curriculum for postprimary physical education: Physical Education Programs of Study
- Included in the documentation: key concepts, key processes, range and content of activities, and curriculum opportunities

Three examples of how a physical education curriculum is presented in three different countries are noted in **Box 9.3**. In Australia, the documents that denote what is to be taught as Personal Development, Health and Physical Education (PDHPE) in postprimary schools are referred to as a *syllabus*. The syllabus lists the aims, objectives, and key competencies before introducing core content (e.g., better health for individuals and the body in motion).

In Ireland, the physical education document that denotes what is to be taught over the first 3 years of postprimary school (known as the *junior cycle*) is commonly referred to as the physical education *curriculum* or physical education *syllabus*. It lists the aims and objectives of junior cycle physical education before providing topics and learning outcomes for eight areas of study (i.e., adventure activities, aquatics, athletics, dance, invasion games, net and fielding games, gymnastics, and health-related activity).

In England, Wales, and Northern Ireland physical education resides within the National Curriculum framework. The documents denoting what content students are expected to experience in the subject area at particular stages of their schooling are referred to as *programs of study*. Such programs include key concepts (competence, performance, creativity, and healthy, active lifestyles), key processes (e.g., developing skills in physical activity), range and content of activities (e.g., outwitting an opponent in a games situation), and curriculum opportunities (e.g., experience a range of roles within a physical activity).

Considering Objectives

Common to most curricula are *objectives*, which are statements of instructional intent that include situation (condition), task (behavior), and criteria that will guide student learning. Physical educators have traditionally designed objectives in the psychomotor, cognitive, and affective learning domains. Each reflects a different aspect of content to be delivered to students to focus their learning.

- *Psychomotor objectives:* What do you want students to be able to do?
- *Cognitive objectives:* What do you want students to know?
- *Affective objectives:* What do you want students to think or care about?

Objectives are written in terms of teaching intentions and indicate the subject content that the teacher intends to cover. **Box 9.4** notes a selection of objectives from the junior cycle physical education syllabus in Ireland.

BOX 9.4 Examples of Learning Objectives

Through their study of junior cycle physical education students will develop:

- Competence in the performance of a range of activities and the ability to analyze these in the context of technical, physiological, and biomechanical implications for the performer
- The ability to invent, compose, and choreograph physical activity in structured, imaginative ways
- The ability to make decisions relating to physical activity while appreciating consequences in both tactical and moral contexts
- An understanding of the principles, rules, and purpose of different categories of activity, and the criteria for mastery of each
- An understanding of the psychological, sociological, aesthetic, and biological knowledge relevant to physical education
- An appreciation of the value of participation in selected physical activities as a lifelong endeavor
- An understanding of the principles of fairness and tolerance in interaction with others
- The desire and the capacity to acquire a positive sense of self

Reproduced with permission from Department of Education and Skills & National Council for Curriculum and Assessment. (2003). *Junior cycle physical education*. Dublin, Ireland: DES/NCCA, p. 7.

Learning Experience 9.3

Consider the objectives listed in Box 9.4 and share your thoughts on which aspects of student learning they match (i.e., psychomotor, cognitive, affective). Provide a rationale for your reasoning.

Not only do curricula have general objectives in those domains, but unit objectives become more specific, and traditional lesson planning suggests that each lesson should also have identified lesson-specific objectives. This results in three levels of objectives: curriculum, unit of work, and lesson plan. An effective physical education curriculum is one in which the successful teaching of content outlined in the unit objectives (achievable through objectives identified for the related block of lessons attached to each specific unit) increases the likelihood of students successfully achieving the overall objectives of the physical education curriculum and the aligned learning outcomes. **Box 9.5** provides two examples of possible broader physical education curriculum objectives and associated (more specific) objectives related to that main objective that could be delivered through different content areas.

BOX 9.5 Examples of the Relationship Between Curriculum Objectives and Content Objectives

Example 1:

- *Physical education curriculum objective:* Content on how to invent, compose, and choreograph physical activity in structured, imaginative ways
- *Related objective in dance:* Content on how to plan and compose movement in various dance contexts
- *Related objective in gymnastics:* Content on how to select, create, and perform a short sequence based on specific themes

Example 2:

- *Physical education curriculum objective:* Content and learning experiences on the principles of fairness and tolerance in interaction with others
- *Related objective in adventure activities:* Content and learning experiences on how to demonstrate responsible personal and social behavior in adventure activity settings
- *Related objective in games:* Content and learning experiences on how to display an understanding of the dynamics of team efficiency

BOX 9.6 Matching Learning Outcomes with Objectives

Physical education curriculum objective: Content on how to invent, compose, and choreograph physical activity in structured, imaginative ways

- *Related objective in dance:* Content on how to plan and compose movement in various dance contexts
- *Related learning outcome in dance:* Students will plan and compose selected movements in a dance form of their choice
- *Related objective in gymnastics:* Content on how to select, create, and perform a short sequence based on specific themes
- *Related learning outcome in gymnastics:* Students will select, create, and perform a short sequence based on a theme of their choice

Considering Outcomes

Whereas objectives are what the teacher intends to teach, learning *outcomes* are what students are expected to do and know as the result of participating in the activities in a program. Learning outcomes should be defined in ways that show immediately how the outcome would be assessed. That is, the very statement of the learning outcome suggests when it can be known that the outcome has been achieved. Learning outcomes can be viewed as "ends" and curriculum objectives can be viewed as "means" (Lambert, 1996). Learning outcomes must guide the development of objectives because, if they do not, objectives might be achieved, but the desired outcome will not be reached. **Box 9.6** revisits Example 1 in Box 9.5 and matches learning outcomes with the already established curriculum objectives.

Authentic Outcomes and Authentic Assessment

One reform agenda in education has been to stress the importance of **authentic outcomes** (Wiggins, 1993). An outcome is authentic if it requires a performance in a context similar to the one in which the knowledge, skills, and strategies will eventually be used (Siedentop, 1996). Authentic outcomes should thus be evaluated using *authentic assessment* measures, in which the assessment allows students to demonstrate the necessary performance qualities in the appropriate context. For example, authentic outcomes in sport activities would relate to actually performing the sport in a competitive setting, such as a basketball game. In this example, authentic assessment would require information on points scored, shooting percentages, turnovers, rebounds, and the like as well as measures of how successfully a strategy was implemented.

Learning Experience 9.4

Consider the following authentic outcomes and develop an appropriate activity that would allow students to achieve the outcome.

- *Gymnastics:* Students will create and perform a group gymnastic routine that includes locomotion, flight, and balance.
- *Dance:* Students will perform a dance routine that conveys different types/styles of dance.
- *Health-related activity:* Students will create a personal fitness program.

Content and Process Outcomes

In most subjects, primary attention is paid to *content outcomes*, that is, strategically appropriate skills and knowledge that represent what is essential for successful performance in a particular activity. For example, in dance, students would perform dances showing control and sensitivity to the style of dance and to the music. Educators, however, have always believed in the importance of *process outcomes*—those skills and attitudes that manifest themselves in areas such as problem solving, effective communication, teamwork, and fair play. For example, in dance, students would cooperate in groups to discuss, select, and perform dances.

The Contribution of Outcomes to Exit Standards, Content Standards, and Performance Standards

When final outcomes are established for a curriculum, it then becomes necessary to define how the outcomes will be translated to various grade levels for purposes of planning units and lessons. This is done in different ways across countries. In the United States, the final outcomes of a curriculum are defined in terms of *exit standards*. The next important step in curriculum planning is identifying **content standards**, which define what students should know and be able to do at a particular developmental/grade level (NASPE, 2013). The use of content standards as a planning device should be accompanied by **performance standards**, which tell teachers and students how well the student has to perform to meet the standards, that is, how good is "good enough" for that level. Behaviors that indicate progress toward a performance standard are called *performance benchmarks*. Identifying performance standards and benchmarks related to those standards leads quickly and easily to *standards-based assessment*.

In England, Wales, and Northern Ireland, each program of study includes a range of attainment targets to reflect the expectations for students within a particular age range. Level 2 represents expectations for the average 7-year-old, Level

4 for the average 11-year-old, and Level 5–6 for the average 14-year-old. **Box 9.7** lists what constitutes Level 4 and Level 6 in the physical education program of study for England, Wales, and Northern Ireland. This allows the reader to consider the extent to which it would be possible to provide evidence from physical education to determine the level at which a student was achieving.

BOX 9.7 National Curriculum in England, Wales, and Northern Ireland: Levels Specific to Physical Education

Level 4 (11 years of age)

Pupils link skills, techniques, and ideas and apply them accurately and appropriately. When performing, they show precision, control, and fluency. They show that they understand tactics and composition. They compare and comment on skills, techniques, and ideas used in their own and others' work, and use this understanding to improve their performance. They explain and apply basic safety principles when preparing for exercise. They describe how exercise affects their bodies, and why regular, safe activity is good for their health and wellbeing. They work with others to plan and lead simple practices and activities for themselves and others.

Level 6 (14 years of age)

Pupils select and combine skills, techniques, and ideas and use them in a widening range of familiar and unfamiliar physical activities and contexts, performing with consistent precision, control, and fluency. They use imaginative ways to solve problems, overcome challenges, and entertain audiences. When planning their own and others' work, and carrying out their own work, they draw on what they know about strategy, tactics, and composition in response to changing circumstances, and what they know about their own and others' strengths and weaknesses. They analyze and comment on how skills, techniques, and ideas have been used in their own and others' work, and on compositional and other aspects of performance. They suggest ways to improve. They understand how the different components of fitness affect performance and explain how different types of exercise contribute to their fitness and health. They describe their involvement in regular, safe physical activity for the benefit of their health and wellbeing. When leading practices and activities, they apply basic rules, conventions, and/or compositional ideas consistently.

Reproduced with permission from Qualifications and Curriculum Authority. (2007). Physical education: Programme of study for key stage 3 and attainment target.

In the United States, NASPE identifies specific examples of the content standards (see Box 9.2) for grade-level ranges representing K (kindergarten) to 2, 3–5, 6–8, and 9–12. In the previous edition of the content standards, *Moving into the Future: National Standards for Physical Education* (NASPE, 2004), NASPE lists student expectations (reflecting what students should know and be able to do at the end of each grade-level range) and sample performance outcomes (examples of student behavior that demonstrate progress toward achieving the standards for each grade-level range) for each content standard. **Box 9.8** provides an example for grade levels 6–8 (10 to 13 years of age). At this time, equivalent benchmarks to the most recent NASPE content standards are yet to be published.

BOX 9.8 A Specific Example of NASPE Content Standards for Grade Levels 6–8 Using Standard 1

- A physically educated person demonstrates competency in motor skills and movement patterns needed to perform a variety of physical activities.

Student expectations (at the end of grade 8):

- Adolescents are able to participate with skill in a variety of modified sport, dance, gymnastics, and outdoor activities.
- Students achieve mature forms in the basic skills of the more specialized sports, dance, and gymnastics activities.
- They use the skills successfully in modified games or activities of increasing complexity and in combination with other basic skills.
- Students demonstrate use of tactics within sport activities.

Sample performance outcomes (across the 6–8 grade range):

- Serves a volleyball underhand using mature form (e.g., stands with feet apart, watches ball, pulls arm and shifts weight backward, swings arm and shifts weight forward, contacts ball and follows through)
- Performs a variety of simple folk and square dances
- Dribbles a ball while preventing an opponent from stealing the ball
- Places the ball away from an opponent during a tennis rally
- Designs and performs gymnastics (or dance) sequences that combine traveling, rolling, balancing, and weight transfer into smooth, flowing sequences with intentional changes in direction, speed, and flow
- Returns to base position on badminton court following a drop shot
- Uses Fisherman's and Figure 8 knots appropriately for belaying while rock climbing

International Differences in Physical Education Curriculum Design

Curriculum design is usually initiated with the appointment of a committee to do all the preliminary work, including development of an overall district/region/national philosophy and a set of objectives and discussion of which activities best meet the objectives. It is important to be aware that although some countries have decentralized governance for curriculum development to individual regions/states (e.g., Australia), in the United States curriculum development is governed at the school district level. Other countries operate a curriculum design suited to the nation (e.g., Finland, Ireland, New Zealand). Penney (2006) provides an engaging look at physical education curriculum construction and change, providing numerous examples of how curriculum initiatives in physical education vary across countries.

In countries where curriculum development is devolved to individual regions, states, or school districts the curriculum is still guided by a set of national standards/expectations that convey what we want students to know and be able to do. At an individual region, state, or school district level the committee will be composed mostly (and in some cases exclusively) of physical education teachers but might also include a school administrator, a district curriculum director, and a parent. It has become more frequent for curriculum building in schools to involve students, with an assessment of student needs often part of the process. The graded course of study often is broad in scope because it has to allow for sometimes quite divergent points of view of various physical educators within the region/state. Curriculum objectives are defined quite broadly, and there is often a large number of them. The committee then identifies activities appropriate for meeting the objectives, and some effort is made to develop a sequenced primary and postprimary curriculum that adds up to something significant. Subsequently, in some regions/states, the primary school physical education curriculum often differs in objectives and substance from the postprimary school curriculum.

Although the NASPE content standards (see Box 9.2) serve to direct curriculum development in both the United States and other countries such as China and Turkey, there is no national physical education curriculum in the United States. England, Wales, and Northern Ireland share the same national curriculum in which each program of study includes a range of attainment targets to reflect the expectations for students within a particular age range (see Box 9.3). It is unlikely that a national curriculum will be established in countries with a widely varied geographic area (e.g., the United States, where there is huge diversity in climate and economic wealth) and where there is a considerable divide between the public and political perception of the role of school physical education. Even in countries where there is a national curriculum, there is an appreciation that not all students in all places need the same curriculum, and hence the curriculum is sufficiently broad that physical educators can design curricula that are sensitive to local needs and interests and still achieve attainment targets for different ages and abilities of students.

In countries where curriculum development is completed at a national level (e.g., Ireland), there may be a physical education committee representing a number of agencies with a stake in the physical education curriculum. Such agencies can include those representing physical education teachers, teaching unions, parents, teacher education, and those involved in creating and enforcing curriculum documents. In some countries a directive may be delivered from a government department to the agency responsible for the production of curriculum, requesting that a physical education curriculum be considered and produced. The final product is then returned to the associated government department to support the curriculum and decide if the government department is in a position to enable the enactment of the curriculum. Once the curriculum is to be enacted, it falls to individual schools and teachers to interpret the curriculum document in a way that will allow for a meaningful and worthwhile physical education curriculum in the particular school context. The aims and objectives of any curriculum document tend to be sufficiently flexible to allow each school and teacher to accommodate the specific school context (e.g., expertise of the physical education staff, available facilities and equipment) and student characteristics (e.g., previous exposure to physical activities, skill and ability levels, behavioral issues) they are dealing with.

The national movement toward subject matter standards should not lead to a standardized curriculum. Not all students in all places need the same curriculum. The NASPE (2004) framework is sufficiently broad that physical educators can design curricula that are sensitive to local needs and interests and still achieve the exit standards associated with the definition of a physically educated person.

Delivering the Intended Curriculum Design

One of the main problems with curriculum design can be that teachers set out each year to "cover the curriculum." The curriculum is so broad, with so many objectives, that teachers move quickly through short units in their attempts to cover the full curriculum plan for the school year. The result is often that the curriculum has indeed been covered, but very little learning has taken place because there is insufficient time for students to develop mastery in any of the activities. This problematic practice is perhaps somewhat alleviated in instances where a physical education curriculum document is produced for a phase of schooling (e.g., the first 3 years of postprimary school) and recommends that over the 3 years, not in 1 year only, students are exposed to the different activities (Department of Education and Skills & National Council for Curriculum and Assessment, 2003). An example using the

BOX 9.9 Utilizing the NASPE Content Standards to Guide a Phase of Schooling

Teachers might decide that the major focus of the curriculum in grades 4 and 5 (8 to 10 years of age) should be on content standards 3, 4, and 5 (see Box 9.2), which have to do with healthy lifestyles and a respect for differences. For the two school years covering grades 4 and 5, the focus would be on physical activity, fitness, learning about differences, why it is important to respect them, and how respect can be shown in activity settings. The backward design principle (mentioned earlier in the chapter) would be used in a narrow developmental range. This is not to suggest no attention would be paid to other content standards or that there would be no effort to learn skills, no attention to responsible behavior, and the like. They would be attended to, but the main focus for choosing activities, deciding on instructional practices, and optimizing organizational arrangements would be on grade 6 outcomes for standards 3, 4, and 5.

BOX 9.10 Key Features of a Well-Developed Curriculum Guide

- Program philosophy
- Mission statement
- Program time requirements (i.e., length of lessons, lessons per week, weeks per unit of work)
- Curriculum goals (the broad overarching ones)
- Specific curriculum objectives
- Yearly block plan with brief descriptions of individual units
- Master schedule given the available activity spaces (more for postprimary schools where multiple teachers have to work alongside each other in various facilities)
- Unit outcomes (specifying the link with content and performance standards, and the link with the specific curriculum objectives)
- Assessment and grading
- Program and administrative policies
- Facilities and equipment management
- Program evaluation

NASPE content standards to guide a phase of schooling, in this case grades 4 to 5 (8 to 10 years of age), is provided in **Box 9.9**.

Teachers in general have limited options when it comes to curriculum development, finding that they are responsible for either (1) building a new curriculum from the ground up, (2) revising or modifying an existing curriculum, or (3) expanding a current curriculum. In reviewing an existing curriculum guide, teachers should look for a number of features that would allow them to make a judgment about whether the curriculum guide, regardless of whether it is a locally or a nationally developed one, is well-developed and considered. The features are listed in **Box 9.10**.

Learning Experience 9.5

Choose a country and explore the extent to which the physical education curriculum is either constructed regionally/by state or at a national level. Regardless of what level the curriculum is constructed, determine the following:

- Who is involved, and what appear to be the objectives and outcomes?
- Is there an apparent advantage or disadvantage to agreeing on objectives and outcomes at a region/state level rather than at a national level, or vice versa?
- How many of the key features listed in Box 9.10 are evident in the curriculum?

Principles of Curriculum Design

Good curriculum planning can truly guide the instructional activities of physical education. In a very real sense, what you design for in curriculum planning is what you get (ASCD, 1998a). There are eight principles that need to be utilized when planning curricula. These are presented in **Box 9.11** and unpacked in the following paragraph.

BOX 9.11 Principles to Be Utilized When Planning Curricula

1. Develop a clear statement of a limited set of "goods" that physical education should achieve.
2. Acknowledge your beliefs about education and learning.
3. Include students in the construction of the curriculum.
4. Less is more.
5. Use authentic outcomes to improve motivation and learning.
6. Backward design.
7. Plan for and check alignment.
8. Carefully consider the distribution of sequenced experiences.

Develop a Clear Statement of a Limited Set of "Goods" That Physical Education Should Achieve

Curriculum building in physical education inevitably begins with value decisions about what outcomes are most important to achieve, that is, the "good" that a particular curriculum represents. However, there are very different points of view about what constitutes the primary good of physical education. We advocate a limited set of goods. Successful curriculum efforts are the result of a focused vision of a manageable set of goods that leads to a clear focus for outcomes. There are legitimately different visions in our profession about the most important values that physical education should achieve, but it is a critical mistake to start the curriculum-building process by including so many different visions of the good that designing a focused curriculum becomes impossible. Teachers' visions of a curriculum are somewhat determined by their value orientations.

Acknowledge Your Beliefs About Education and Learning

Teachers' reflecting on what they see as the goods of physical education in turn identifies what they value about education and learning, leading to the identification of a "value orientation." Ennis (2003) defines a teacher's *value orientation* as beliefs on what students should learn, how they should learn it, and how it should be assessed. Ennis noted five value orientations, each with a different emphasis on physical education content, the needs and interests of individual learners, and the goals of society. The five orientations are Disciplinary Mastery, Learning Process, Self-Actualization, Social Responsibility and Justice, and Ecological Integration. A short explanation of what is valued in each orientation is available in **Box 9.12**. The Value Orientation Inventory (VOI) is a tool that can be used to ascertain the extent to which a teacher's preferences for several value orientations blend to form their value profile. A teacher's values may reflect a number of the orientations and will inform the physical education curriculum being offered. A teacher may convey different values for different year groups, which could potentially result in students being exposed to the same teacher for a number of years but be involved in different physical education curriculum experiences.

Learning Experience 9.6

Access and download the shortened version of the Value Orientation Inventory. Complete the inventory and return it to your instructor, who will compile the results and report back on where the class, as a whole, has conveyed they reside on the value orientation continuum. Consider the extent to which your preferred value orientation reinforces or challenges what arises as the dominant class value orientation. Provide suggestions on the reasons for the similarities and differences in value orientations across the class.

BOX 9.12 What Is Valued in Specific Value Orientations?

- A *Disciplinary Mastery* value orientation focuses on establishing what knowledge is of most worth and promotes students demonstrating specific performance and knowledge criteria.
- A *Learning Process* value orientation focuses not only on students having the ability to perform and know about performance to be physically educated persons but also that students know how to make decisions and solve problems about being physically active.
- A *Self-Actualization* value orientation uses physical activity as a means to help students develop positive self-esteem and a sense of efficacy, placing the students' needs and interests at the center of the curriculum.
- A *Social Responsibility and Justice* value orientation focuses on teaching students how to cooperate and accept personal responsibility through the medium of physical activity, helping them to develop positive interpersonal relationships in an environment that emphasizes equity and social justice.
- An *Ecological Integration* value orientation promotes the balance among subject matter content, the needs and interests of the individual, and the social setting, helping students understand relationships between the concepts and principles learned in physical education and knowledge learned in other school subjects.

Include Students in the Construction of the Curriculum

By encouraging young people to share how different contexts contribute to their learning about, and involvement in, physical activity, physical education teachers are in a better position to acknowledge and address how physical education and such contexts can most effectively work together to motivate students to choose active lifestyles (MacPhail, 2010). Students can be involved in so many ways in designing the physical education curriculum in partnership with teachers, increasing the extent to which students will engage with a curriculum that they have had some involvement in constructing. This principle is revisited later in the chapter under "The Goods in Physical Education" and "Curricula That Serve Students Equitably."

Less Is More

A clear, limited vision for a physical education curriculum will inevitably lead to reducing the number of outcomes to be achieved, thus allowing more time within the curriculum to achieve them. This, in turn, will lead to longer units of instruction. The curriculum concept of "less is more" has been particularly associated with reform of the postprimary school curriculum (Sizer, 1992) but can apply throughout primary and postprimary opportunities.

Use Authentic Outcomes to Improve Motivation and Learning

Authentic outcomes are contextualized performance capabilities, most often assessed through a final performance or an "exhibition" (Wiggins, 1987). The public performance of a folk dance or a jump rope routine, the performance of a free exercise routine in a gymnastics competition, the individual and collective performances of a floor hockey team in a round-robin tournament, or achievement of the outcomes of a semester-long nutrition and exercise program, are all examples of authentic outcomes. Authentic outcomes provide targets for students. Working toward a final exhibition of what they can do and know can help motivate students to engage in serious learning that is likely to be more fun and valued more.

Backward Design

As discussed at the beginning of the chapter, effective curriculum design begins with the exit outcomes and proceeds backwards to ensure that all components are directly related to achieving the outcome; that is, the practice of looking at the outcomes in order to design curriculum units, performance assessments, and classroom instruction (Wiggins & McTighe, 1998). If, for example, curriculum designers decide they want students to become competent in at least one sport from each of the three categories (invasion, court-divided, and target), that would represent a good. They would then need to define what "competent" means for postprimary students, and start from there to design down to see where they would have to start with beginning learners to reach the desired outcomes. The design down/backward design principle requires that curriculum developers always ask how a proposed curriculum element would contribute to the exit outcome.

Plan for and Check Alignment

As discussed at the beginning of the chapter, alignment exists when the objectives, activities, instruction, and assessment of a physical education program are matched and compatible with the outcomes. If you have skillful, tactical play in volleyball as an outcome, but lessons consist mostly of isolated technique drills and the assessments are a serving test and a wall-volley test, then you have a serious mismatch (i.e., a nonaligned unit). With "skillful, tactical play in volleyball" as a planned outcome, alignment among that, the instruction, and assessment would be established if the following conditions are met: (1) the practice activities are sequenced, developmentally appropriate, and organized around important strategic principles for volleyball; (2) the practice is contextualized (i.e., occurs in authentic conditions as they would be used in game play); and (3) student performance is evaluated by various analyses of actual game play. If your curriculum suggests that developing independent learners is a good, but there is no evidence that students have increasing responsibility and choice, and/or no authentic opportunity to practice taking responsibility, then the curriculum is far from aligned.

Carefully Consider the Distribution of Sequenced Experiences

Many curricula are developed with the assumption that experiences should be sequenced across the primary and postprimary spectrum and that nearly every unit of instruction should include some activities related to the major objectives of the curriculum. Thus, teachers commonly assume that every unit should contribute to the psychomotor, cognitive, and affective domains. They also assume that the best way to help students learn activities such as volleyball, folk dance, or athletics is to provide several units of instruction that are distributed across age levels (for example, volleyball units in primary and postprimary). However, this approach to distribution seldom achieves its intention. Rather than three 6- to 8-day units at those age levels, a 24-day unit at one age level could result in better learning and more enjoyment for the students. **Box 9.13** shares how the NASPE framework is an appropriate tool and guide for considering the scope and sequencing of physical activity units throughout the physical education curriculum.

BOX 9.13 Using NASPE Standards to Consider the Scope and Sequencing of Physical Education Units

Consider NASPE content standards 1 and 2, which deal with competency in movement forms and applying concepts and principles to the development of motor skills, respectively (see Box 9.2). A group of physical educators might decide that standard 1 should be the guiding principle of curriculum in the early years of primary, with perhaps a complementary focus on standard 5 (demonstrating responsible personal and social behavior in activity settings). Thus, the early years of primary would have a clear focus.

Learning Experience 9.7

Read the following two examples, which were responses from two pre-service teachers when asked to consider their beliefs about learning in physical education:

> *Example 1:* In my opinion physical education should be inclusive, enjoyable and mandatory for every member of the class. I feel that I am not too concerned with a student's performance or skills from a technical aspect but rather the fact that they have the base to improve certain skills if they wish to do so. . . . In my class I feel students would be introduced to a large number of topics, some of which are perhaps outside of the mainstream sports so that students can find what interests them and then pursue that rather than being persistent at a topic in which they have no interest. (Courtesy of Shane Hennessy)

> *Example 2:* As a physical educator my aim is to have all students active and participating in the class while developing a better understanding of physical activity. By making learning experiences relevant and meaningful for students I would hope that it would encourage and motivate them to choose active lifestyles outside the PE environment. (Courtesy of Maire O'Regan)

Answer the following:

- Which curriculum planning principles, if any, are reflected in the two student teachers' belief statements?
- Consider the extent to which your values and beliefs on what physical education should "look like" potentially affects students' experiences of physical education.
- Which of the five value orientations described by Ennis (noted in Box 9.12) are reflected in the two belief statements?

The Goods in Physical Education

What goods do students acquire from a physical education program? Is it a lifetime commitment to physical fitness? Is it the ability and desire to participate in recreational sports? Is it the capacity to cooperate with others toward group objectives/outcomes and the ability to provide leadership in groups when and where necessary? Is it a sense of comfort with, and ownership of, their own body and confidence in their ability to control it to perform various physical activities? Is it an aesthetic experience, the appreciation and valuing of the beauty of physical movement activities? Is physical education mostly about learning to be responsible for oneself and helpful to others? All these possible outcomes, and others, have been suggested by various scholars and professionals as representing the primary goods of physical education. Corbin (2002) and Siedentop and van der Mars (2012) wondered whether physical education would stand for anything if we try to be all things to all people, as reflected in the myriad of outcomes that tend to be associated with physical education curricula.

Learning Experience 9.8

Are any primary goods of physical education evident in allowing students to continually participate in what they deem to be the most popular sport (e.g., the continual request in some countries to play soccer) through the school physical education program? If yes, what are they, and how would you determine that these goods are met? If no, how would you envisage reconfiguring the situation to introduce students to the goods of physical education?

Building a Physical Education Curriculum

Building a curriculum begins with making value decisions about what is most important. Value decisions should always be contextualized. That is, the good in physical education is always about a particular group of students, who live in particular circumstances, in specific regions, and at a particular time, when society values some goals more than others. For example, at various points in history society became very concerned about the fitness levels of young people. This is not to suggest that local needs or societal concerns are the primary driving force for curriculum design. Rather, it suggests that value decisions about the vision of a curriculum should not be made without considering these issues. This again reinforces the power of the teacher's value orientation, discussed earlier in the chapter. Values will guide answers to questions such as "What am I trying to contribute to the lives of these students?" and "How do I want their lives to be enriched by having had these experiences?"

Different visions of the good, of course, would lead to diversified curriculum choices and eventually to various programs of experiences, especially when the curriculum design principles described in the previous section are utilized. To achieve the objectives of a curriculum, you must align the outcomes and content standards with the vision.

Involving Students in Defining the Good(s) of the Physical Education Curriculum

There is a point at which students should have an increasing role in helping define the good(s). In postprimary programs, this is most often achieved through an elective curriculum, in which student needs and interests drive both the range of activities offered and student selection from within that range of activities. This is clearly evident in the New

South Wales (Australia) Personal Development, Health and Physical Education syllabus for the final 2 years of schooling. Acknowledging that senior students are likely to have particular areas of interest that they wish to pursue in greater depth, the syllabus offers a significant options component designed to enable students to specialize in chosen areas.

Teachers also have some obligation to help educate younger students to see the difference between an immediate felt need or preference for certain objectives and activities (for example, when many students just want to play soccer in every class throughout the school year) to a more educated sense of what the possibilities are and what their own preferred future might be like in physical education (for example, when students have a better sense of the health and leisure needs and possibilities for their lives).

Being Realistic in What Can Be Achieved Within a Physical Education Curriculum

There has been a growing consensus internationally that not all goods can be achieved in any one program, and that trying to achieve too many objectives results in too little achievement. As Corbin (2002) has argued:

> *While I continue to endorse all the major objectives of physical education, I am convinced that we must narrow our focus if we are to be effective in truly physically educating our students. At all times we should keep all of our objectives in mind; however, our goals are too grandiose. We must narrow our focus and do a few things well, rather than many things not so well. For example, we try to teach every child to perform all of the many sport skills common in the United States. We know we cannot teach every child to play every instrument in the band. Why do we think we can teach every child every sport? At some point we must begin to adopt a strategy that allows us to use our limited time in a more focused way.*[1]

Our first curriculum planning principle discussed previously suggests that a limited, focused set of goods be defined. Too many physical education curricula adopt all of the many goods. In trying to be all things to all students, they frequently fail to achieve anything of substance. The result often is a fragmented program, with a series of short-term experiences where students are repeatedly "exposed" to the same introduction to activities, and leaving teachers working with older students wondering why "these kids still can't play." As Corbin's (2002) quote suggests, given the amount of time allotted to physical education in a school program, choices must be made about which goods are more important than others, for these students, in this place, at this time. If we had 2 hours per day, 5 days per week, for the length of a school year, for all school years, we would have a wider vision for the curriculum and could develop more expansive programs that deliver on a broader range of significant outcomes. To pretend, however, that multiple major objectives can be achieved in the limited time available to most physical education programs is to risk fooling yourself and the public. Programs built around main-theme curriculum models allow for development because the physical educator responsible for them has a vision about what was the primary good to be achieved, selected a curriculum model, and then developed content to achieve that vision and allowed enough time for students to reach significant outcomes.

A Model for Curriculum Planning

The following six-step process for curriculum planning (ASCD, 1998b), when combined with the design principles described previously in the chapter, allows physical educators to create and deliver curricula that achieve significant outcomes and capture the enthusiasm of students, school administrators, and parents. Although the six-step process noted here was shared in 1998, it is still relevant today.

1. *Know the territory.* An effective curriculum plan is specific rather than generic (ASCD, 1998a). A curriculum should always serve a specific group of learners. Physical educators should understand the current performance capabilities of students, the characteristics of the students and the community in which they live, the facilities and administrative characteristics of the school, and the perspectives of the students in the school as well as the parents and caregivers of those students.
2. *Develop a clear program vision.* The "vision thing" is about deciding what limited set of goods the physical education curriculum will achieve. Having completed step 1, the vision will now be for *these* students, in *this* place, and in *this* time. This vision forms the basis for the program's mission statement that would be publicized to students, parents, and school administrators.
3. *Define the objectives and outcomes that fulfill the vision.* We say "outcomes" rather than "goals" because there should be a high degree of specificity about what students will know and be able to do when they complete physical education. Remember that objectives are statements of instructional intent that include situation (condition), task (behavior), and criteria that will guide student learning. Outcomes are what students are expected to do and know as the result of participating in the program.

[1] Reprinted, with permission, from Corbin, C. B. (2002). Physical activity for everyone: What every physical educator should know about promoting lifelong physical activity. *Journal of Teaching in Physical Education, 21*, 138.

4. *Assess how instructional practices and organizational conditions can help or hinder achievement of the outcomes.* There is a variety of instructional practices available to physical education teachers, and their use must be aligned with objectives and assessment practices. For example, the use of small groups to help develop collaborative learning or the utilization of persisting groups to develop teamwork and leadership qualities. Organizational structures such as block scheduling (see **Box 9.14**), the linking of school programs and community opportunities, and longer units of instruction also will affect the potential to achieve outcomes.
5. *Develop the curriculum plan.* The curriculum plan, using the backward design approach mentioned previously, can now be based realistically on the assessment of local conditions, the vision believed to be most salient to those local conditions, a series of outcomes aligned with that vision, and instructional practices and organizational arrangements that assist in achieving the outcomes.
6. *Implement the plan and assess the results.* In order to create a "live" curriculum that continually adjusts and improves, assessment measures need to be agreed upon that will provide evidence of the degree to which the vision is being achieved through significant outcomes. This allows for the best chance that physical educators will, indeed, get what they design.

BOX 9.14 Block Scheduling as a Structural Aid to Curriculum Success

We have emphasized that organizational arrangements can enhance the possibility that a curriculum will be successful in achieving its objectives. One such arrangement is block scheduling, which is increasingly used in postprimary schools. Two configurations are most common. One is the A–B, alternating day model. Classes meet every other day for 90 minutes for an entire school year. The other is the 4 × 4 model. Classes meet every day for 90 minutes for one semester. Although 90 minutes appears to be the norm in block scheduling, class length can range from 80 to 120 minutes.

One study (Shortt & Thayer, 1998–99) found that schools with block-scheduled classes showed marked improvement over those with traditionally organized school days, academic performance of students was better, and there was increased attention to staff development and instructional programs. Administrators reported that block scheduling seems to have a positive impact on lower performing students and on achievement scores for most students. The increases were found for both urban and rural schools.

Bryant and Claxton (1996) surveyed 55 postprimary schools that had moved to block scheduling to assess the effects of the change on physical education. They reported that all comments were positive. Physical educators reported decreased absenteeism, improved student behavior, more teacher collaboration, and more planning time.

Curricula That Serve Students Equitably

Evidence shows that physical education curricula have not served all students equitably. Thus, those who design curricula must think about equity issues. Sometimes curricula are inequitable not as a result of anyone intending that students be served inequitably, but rather because specific issues of equity were not considered during the design phase. The most significant factors in providing an equitable physical education for all young people are the instructional practices and learning environment developed and sustained by the teachers.

It is also important to listen to the voices of the students who we teach and for teachers and students to co-construct the physical education curriculum (what Glasby and Macdonald [2004] term a *negotiated curriculum*). There are now examples available on how students' values and beliefs have informed the development of effective and equitable practices in physical education (O'Sullivan & MacPhail, 2010). Oliver's (2010) work focused on how to understand students (predominantly girls) through collaborating with them to practice strategies for changing body and physical activity inequalities as they see them. This work has more recently been extended into what Oliver and Oesterreich (2012) have termed "student-centered inquiry as curriculum."

Learning Experience 9.9

What mix of preconditions and commitment in a school and a school physical education department would potentially create a collaborative teacher–student relationship that would encourage the co-construction of the physical education curriculum? How would you envisage going about including students in the co-construction of the physical education curriculum? In what way would your approach change with different student age groups?

Relative to the issue of equity, the key question for curriculum designers is: What groups are best and most served by this curriculum? Are males better served than females? Are more-skilled students better served than less-skilled students? Is the curriculum ethnically sensitive? Does it expand the students' capacities to live effectively in an increasingly multicultural world? Does it develop students' critical capacities to know when powerful economic forces in the health, leisure, and fitness industries are manipulating them?

These are not easy questions to answer. What, for example, are the answers to curricular issues that involve gender? We know that girls have been traditionally disadvantaged in physical education, through both instructional arrangements and curricular offerings (Penney, 2002). Not too many years ago girls were offered gymnastics and dance while boys were offered soccer and basketball. We also know that even though activities are less gendered in society than they were a generation ago, many activities are still gendered in physical education. How do curricular designers in physical education deal with that issue? How do they ensure that boys and girls have opportunities to learn activities that may still have a gender association in the larger society? Flintoff and Scraton (2006) provide an interesting historical reflection on the sex-differentiated curriculum, acknowledging that there are no quick fixes to the equity problems that have plagued physical education for some time. The first important step is to raise the questions and keep asking them as a curriculum is being designed or revised.

Learning Experience 9.10

Reflecting on your experiences during school physical education as a student or on a physical education curriculum to which you have had the opportunity to contribute as a pre-service teacher, consider the extent to which the physical education curriculum inadvertently reproduced and/or perpetuated the inequities that exist in the worlds of sport, leisure, health, and fitness. To what extent was physical education responsible for deliberate reproduction?

CHAPTER SUMMARY

To assist the physical education teacher in developing insight into the curriculum design process, this chapter shared the concepts and language of curriculum, fundamental principles of curriculum design, and a model to guide curriculum planning. We have reminded teachers that curriculum development is about change as we move our programs into the future to meet the needs and interests of young people. Our intent has been to assist teachers in designing a physical education curriculum that is meaningful, worthwhile, and relevant to the lives of the students with whom they work. The relationship between learning goals, assessment to measure those goals, and instructional strategies that will allow students to successful reach those goals form the basis of instructional alignment that is introduced and developed throughout this chapter.

1. Although the term *curriculum* is commonly used to convey the accumulation of planned learning experiences across the school, it is sometimes used interchangeably with the terms *program* and *syllabus* when a specific subject lists selected activities planned to achieve student-learning outcomes.
2. Backward design and instructional alignment guide the design and planning of curricula.
3. A successful physical education requires a meaningful, relevant curriculum articulated across grade levels, effective teaching, and organizational structures that allow for meaningful engagements.
4. An objective is a statement of instructional intent that includes situation (condition), task (behavior), and criteria that will guide student learning.
5. An outcome is a description of what a student will know, be able to do, and value as the result of participating in the program. Consideration should be given to both content and process outcomes, addressing the three domains of psychomotor, cognitive, and affective.
6. Principles of curriculum design include (1) a limited set of goods to achieve; (2) acknowledging beliefs about education and learning; (3) including students in the co-construction of the curriculum; (4) determining a finite number of outcomes; (5) ensuring outcomes are authentic; (6) designing down to achieve the objectives; (7) achieving alignment among objectives/outcomes, activities, and assessments; and (8) considering the distribution of activities to optimize effectiveness.
7. Values are important when you are designing curricula and should be used to determine the goods that the curriculum is meant to achieve.
8. To design curricula, teachers should (1) know their students and context, (2) have a clear program vision, (3) define outcomes that represent that vision, (4) assess how instructional and organizational practices help or hinder achievement of those outcomes, (5) design down to alignment, and (6) implement and assess the results.
9. Equity issues of gender, skillfulness, and cultural relevance should be considered when planning curricula.

REFERENCES

ASCD. (1998a). Playing hardball with curriculum. *Education Update, 40*(8), 1.

ASCD. (1998b). Six steps to school improvement. *Education Update, 40*(8), 3.

Bryant, J., & Claxton, D. (1996). Physical education and the four-by-four schedule. *The Physical Educator, 53*, 203–209.

Cohen, S. (1987, Nov.). Instructional alignment: Searching for a magic bullet. *Educational Researcher*, 16–20.

Corbin, C. B. (2002). Physical activity for everyone: What every physical educator should know about promoting lifelong physical activity. *Journal of Teaching in Physical Education, 21*, 128–144.

Department of Education and Skills & National Council for Curriculum and Assessment. (2003). *Junior cycle physical education*. Dublin, Ireland: DES/NCCA.

Ennis, C. D. (2003). Using curriculum to enhance student learning. In S. J. Silverman & C. D. Ennis (Eds.), *Student learning in physical education: Applying research to enhance instruction* (2nd ed., pp. 109–127). Champaign, IL: Human Kinetics.

Flintoff, A., & Scraton, S. (2006). Girls and physical education. In D. Kirk, D. Macdonald, & M. O'Sullivan (Eds.), *The handbook of physical education* (pp. 767–784). London: Sage.

Glasby, T., & Macdonald, D. (2004). Negotiating the curriculum: Challenging the social relationships in teaching. In J. Wright, D. Macdonald, & L. Burrows (Eds.), *Critical inquiry and problem solving in physical education* (pp. 133 144). London: Routledge.

Kelly, L. E., & Melograno, V. J. (2004). *Developing the physical education curriculum*. Champaign, IL: Human Kinetics.

Kovalik, S., & Olsen, K. (1994). *ITI: The model—integrated thematic instruction* (3rd ed.). Kent, WA: S. Kovalik and Associates.

Lambert, L. (1996). Goals and outcomes. In S. Silverman & C. Ennis (Eds.), *Student learning in physical education: Applying research to enhance instruction* (pp. 149–169). Champaign, IL: Human Kinetics.

Lund, J., & Tannehill, D. (2005). *Standards-based physical education curriculum development*. Sudbury, MA: Jones and Bartlett Publishers.

Lund, J., & Tannehill, D. (2010). *Standards-based physical education curriculum development* (2nd ed.). Sudbury, MA: Jones and Bartlett.

Lund, J., & Tannehill, D. (2014). *Standards-based physical education curriculum development* (3rd ed.; forthcoming). Burlington, MA: Jones & Bartlett Learning.

MacPhail, A. (2010). Listening to pupils' voices. In R. Bailey (Ed.), *Physical education for learning* (pp. 228–238). London: Continuum.

National Association for Sport and Physical Education. (2004). *Moving into the future: National standards for physical education* (2nd ed.). St. Louis, MO: Mosby.

National Association for Sport and Physical Education. (2013, April). Annual Board Meeting Minutes. AAHPERD Convention, Charlotte, North Carolina.

Oliver, K. L. (2010). The body, physical activity and inequity: Learning to listen *with* girls *through* action. In M. O'Sullivan & A. MacPhail (Eds.), *Young people's voices in physical education and youth sport* (pp. 31–48). London: Routledge.

Oliver, K. L., & Oesterreich, H. A. (2012). Student-centered inquiry *as* curriculum as a model for field based teacher education. *Journal of Curriculum Studies*, 1–24 (iFirst article).

O'Sullivan, M., & MacPhail, A. (Eds.). (2010). *Young people's voices in physical education and youth sport*. London: Routledge.

Penney, D. (2002). Gendered policies. In D. Penney (Ed.), *Gender and physical education: Contemporary issues and future directions* (pp. 80–100). London: Routledge.

Penney, D. (2006). Curriculum construction and change. In D. Kirk, D. Macdonald, & M. O'Sullivan (Eds.), *The handbook of physical education* (pp. 565–579). London: Sage.

Qualifications and Curriculum Authority. (2007). Physical education. Programme of study for key stage 3 and attainment target. Available from www.teachfind.com/qcda/physical-education-programme-study-key-stage-3-and-attainment-target

Shortt, T., & Thayer, Y. (1998–99). Block scheduling can enhance school climate. *Educational Leadership, 56*(4), 76–81.

Siedentop, D. (1996). Physical education and educational reform. In S. Silverman & C. Ennis (Eds.), *Student learning in physical education: Applying research to enhance instruction* (pp. 247–267). Champaign, IL: Human Kinetics.

Siedentop, D., & van der Mars, H. (2012). *Introduction to physical education, fitness and sport* (8th ed.). London: McGraw-Hill.

Sizer, T. (1992). *Horace's school: Redesigning the American high school*. New York: Houghton Mifflin.

Taylor, J., & Chiogioji, E. (1987). Implications of educational reform on high school programs. *Journal of Physical Education, Recreation, and Dance, 58*(2), 22–23.

Wiggins, G. (1987). Creating a thought-provoking curriculum. *American Educator*, Winter, 10–17.

Wiggins, G. (1993). Assessment: Authenticity, context and validity. *Phi Delta Kappan, 75*(3), 200–214.

Wiggins, G., & McTighe, J. (1998). *Understanding by design*. Alexandria, VA: Association of Supervision and Curriculum Development (ASCD).

CHAPTER 10 Main-Theme Physical Education Curriculum Models

Overall Chapter Outcome

To describe what a physical education program would look like using different main-theme physical education curriculum models and how to design a coherent multimodel physical education program based on varying perspectives of the goods of physical education

Learning Outcomes

The learner will:

- Clarify how the development–refinement cycle has impacted the use of the main-theme physical education curriculum models
- Describe what is meant by a main-theme or focused curriculum
- Explain the extent to which the "goods" of physical education can be enhanced through implementing a main-theme physical education curriculum model
- Delineate the purpose, characteristics, beliefs, and goods for selected main-theme curriculum models: Developmental Physical Education, Adventure Education, Outdoor Education, Sport Education, Tactical Games Approach to Teaching Games, Teaching Personal and Social Responsibility, Social Issues, and Health and Wellness
- Identify the standards/outcomes or syllabus goals that complement or have the most relevance to each curriculum model for the context in which you reside
- Explain the basis for developing a multimodel physical education curriculum
- Demonstrate how a group of teachers might go about designing a multimodel physical education curriculum program for a selected education level

Selecting, planning, and implementing a meaningful curriculum are the most important issues to be addressed by physical education teachers. You should reflect upon and answer some curricular questions related specifically to the children and youth with whom you might work. What is important to learn in physical education? What do you see as the needs for these students? How can we prepare young people for a healthy lifestyle? What do your students view as most important? How does physical activity relate to students' lives outside of school, and what problems do they encounter in accessing activity? What do young people enjoy about physical activity and movement? What will motivate them to take part in your program? What role might students play in designing a meaningful physical education program? What are the current social and cultural problems that will impact teaching and learning? How might a curriculum best facilitate the educational process in this setting?

Several curriculum models have been developed, tested, refined, and further tested in a variety of school settings. The **development–refinement cycle** is no doubt responsible for the success of these curriculum models and their widespread adoption by physical educators seeking to improve

BOX 10.1 Key Terms in This Chapter

- *Adventure Education:* An experiential learning model that provides learners with the opportunity to challenge themselves physically and mentally, work cooperatively as a group to solve problems and overcome risks, and gain respect for, confidence in, and trust in themselves and their peers. Key concepts of the model include full value contract, challenge with choice, experiential learning cycle, and processing/debrief.
- *Concepts-Based Fitness and Wellness:* Focused on the process of physical activity rather than the outcome of students' achieving physical fitness, this model is designed around themes and concepts in three categories (foundational, behavior change, and wellness). These are introduced through a series of classroom-focused concept days that are applied and reinforced through activity days.
- *Cultural studies:* Developed to meet the needs and interests of students from various backgrounds, cultures, socioeconomic levels, and communities. The intent is to develop young people as questioning, curious, and critical participants in sport and physical activity coming to understand how some young people are marginalized by a lack of activity opportunities available in their school and community.
- *Curriculum model:* Focused, theme-based model that reflects a specific set of goods about what is most important in physical education.
- *Development–refinement cycle:* The process by which a curriculum is developed, tested, refined, and further tested in a variety of school settings.
- *Developmental Physical Education:* A set of models designed around the individual learner with the intent of meeting each learner's developmental needs and unique growth patterns within a holistic education emphasizing cognitive, affective, and psychomotor outcomes.
- *Health and Wellness models:* Focused primarily on giving students the knowledge and skills to make independent decisions on physical activity, and the desire to choose to develop and maintain lifetime physical activity as opposed to a sedentary lifestyle.
- *Health-Based Physical Education (HBPE):* Focused on young people valuing a physically active lifestyle and choosing to participate in appropriate activities that promote health and well-being. Key to this model is that it represents a pedagogical model intended to provide guidance to schools.
- *Health Optimizing Physical Education (HOPE):* Designed for young people to gain skills and knowledge for participation in physical activity in order to gain health benefits across the life span. HOPE includes the five components of a comprehensive school physical activity program (CSPAP): quality physical education, school-based physical activity opportunities, school employee wellness and involvement, physical activity in the classroom, and family and community involvement.
- *Instructional model:* Guides the planning, organization, and teaching of knowledge and learning experiences.
- *Main-theme curriculum model:* Characterized by a narrow activity focus that serves as the organizing center for the program, allocates time for students to achieve important outcomes, has a clear sense of a more limited good and arranges sequences of activities to achieve that good.
- *Multimodel curriculum:* An overarching physical education program developed around selected curriculum models at particular points in time that allow significant outcomes at each level and for every child.
- *Outdoor Education:* Uses the natural environment as the context for experientially enjoying the outdoors and gaining understanding and appreciation for the environment; built on three types of learning: physical skills, environmental awareness, and interpersonal growth.
- *Skill theme approach:* Both a curriculum and instructional model with the content of physical education and the pedagogy. Content is organized by skill themes and movement concepts, with children first becoming familiar with movement concepts such as space awareness, effort, and relationships, followed by fundamental movement themes learned first in isolation and then combined with other skills and movement concepts in more complex and variable settings such as games, dance, and other physical activities.
- *Social Issues models:* Initially designed to provide alternative activities that meet the needs and interests of young people by involving them in the curriculum process and inviting them to explore social issues that influence physical activity opportunities, political issues impacting sport, or health themes such as nutrition, obesity, or smoking that impact participation in physical activity.

BOX 10.1 Key Terms in This Chapter (*Continued*)

- *Sport Education:* Intended to provide authentic and rich sport opportunities to all students within the context of physical education, helping them develop as skilled and competent sport participants with the skills and understanding of strategies necessary to participate in sport successfully. Characteristics include seasons, affiliation, formal competition, record keeping, culminating event, and festivity.
- *Student-Centered Inquiry as Curriculum:* Designed to change schools and physical education to facilitate the learning of all young people through engaging students, seeking their input, listening to and responding to their ideas, and inviting them to participate in the design of the curriculum as a means of empowering them to take responsibility for their own learning.
- *Tactical Approach to Teaching Games:* A consolidated, applied and teacher-friendly approach to teaching games that progresses students through three phases: game form (representation or exaggeration), tactical awareness (what to do), and skill execution (how to do it). The model emphasizes questioning students to cause them to think critically to solve tactical problems focused on what you want them to achieve (tactical awareness, skill execution, time, space, risk).
- *Teaching Games for Understanding (TGfU):* Initially designed as an alternative method for teaching games that emphasized students' finding solutions to problems posed to them in game play situations. Now a six-stage model (game play, game appreciation, tactical awareness, making appropriate decisions, skill practice, game play), TGfU places the student at the center of learning in a problem-based context.
- *Teaching Personal and Social Responsibility (TPSR):* Based on the belief that the most important thing we can teach students is helping them take responsibility for their own development and well-being and supporting that of others through shared power and gradually shifting responsibility for their learning from the teacher to the student. TPSR has eight components: core values, assumptions, levels of responsibility, program leader, daily program format, embedding strategies, problem solving, and assessment.

the impact of their programs. These models can be grouped under what we refer to as *main theme* or *focused* curricula. These models tend to have a narrower activity focus than the multiactivity model approach, and they tend to allocate more time to the narrower focus, thus allowing students to achieve important outcomes.

This is not to suggest that these focused curricula are used simply as "recipes" and cannot be altered to meet local needs. They are models, not prescriptions. Physical educators who use them tend to adapt them to their own particular context, which is typically determined by (1) the type and interests of students, (2) the facilities and equipment available, (3) the ethos of the school and community, and (4) the beliefs and values of the teacher. We are also not suggesting that the entire primary through postprimary physical education curriculum should have a singular theme. Quite the contrary, in this chapter we argue that a program can be created by adopting particular models at particular points in the physical education of children and youth, done in a way that allows for significant outcomes at each level, and for every child.

No one program can achieve all the goods in physical education. As you will see in the curricular models described in this chapter, well-designed and thoughtfully developed programs using a coherent curriculum and appropriate instructional models may be able to achieve many of the goods in physical education across the primary and postprimary curriculum. The objectives and outcomes and how they play out will be tempered by the local context in which they exist and the changing conditions that occur within the lives of students. Once you have determined what you believe are the goods in physical education, assessed their relevance to your students, and considered the context of your setting, you are in a position to determine which of the physical education main theme curriculum models you will adopt. Each model attends to a set of specific goods and meets one or more of the outcomes set for student achievement by physical education teacher organizations and/or governing bodies internationally.

Main-Theme Curriculum Models

There is no consensus within the profession on what constitutes the goods to be achieved in physical education. The arguments against the more traditional multiactivity program have resulted from a renewed interest in what we have described as the **main-theme curriculum models**. That is, programs that have a clear sense of a more limited good and arrange sequences of activities to achieve that good.

Main-theme curricular programs develop because the physical educators responsible for them had a vision about what was the primary good to be achieved, considered the context in which they teach, and then developed content to achieve that vision using input and choices from their students. A main theme becomes an organizing center for the program, the central thrust around which content is developed to meet goals. The curriculum model becomes the main theme guiding development of the program. Effective programs stand for something specific and are guided by a main focus that defines their purpose, goals, and intents.

Learning Experience 10.1

What would you suggest should be the main focus for primary and postprimary physical education? Would it be sport, fitness, social issues? Keep in mind that this view might change once you consult your students and review the ethos of the school and beliefs of the community.

Before we discuss the main-theme curriculum models, it is critical to differentiate between a curriculum and an instruction model. The major difference between the two is the content/goods of what is most important in physical education (**curriculum model**) versus how to organize and deliver instruction and learning experiences (**instructional model**). Each is equally important and they build upon each other. To clarify, curriculum models are focused, theme-based, reflect a specific philosophy about what is most important in physical education, and provide a framework that places the student at the center of instructional design. They define a clear focus around the content, and aim toward specific, relevant, and challenging learning outcomes for students. On the other hand, an instructional model will guide delivery of teaching and learning. After a teacher selects the curriculum model to develop and promote the intended learning, the appropriate instructional models to guide the teaching of content must be determined. As noted in Lund and Tannehill (2010), "Metzler (2005) suggests that an instructional model includes a number of strategies, methods, styles, and skills that are used to plan, design, and implement a unit of instruction" (p. 155). In some cases, we see curriculum models described as both curriculum and instruction models. In other cases instruction models are closely linked to a particular curriculum model as the most effective way for students to achieve learning outcomes. For example, the Tactical Approach to Teaching Games is typically taught by teaching through questions, Outdoor Education might be associated with problems-based learning, and Teaching Personal and Social Responsibility employs invitation and choice. Having clarified the difference between the two, it must be recognized that some models are characterized as both a curriculum and an instruction model. We will discuss these as they appear throughout this chapter.

Learning Experience 10.2

Describe the educational accountability movement that exists in your context. How is it being taken on board by local and regional school administrators?

We have chosen to highlight selected physical education curriculum models that are being used internationally. They each have the elements to serve as main-theme curriculum models, with a different notion of good for students in each. Recently we have seen additional physical education curriculum models being introduced with research currently being conducted as the models go through the development–refinement cycle (developed, tested, refined, and further tested in alternative contexts). These newly introduced curriculum models with which we are familiar will be introduced separately or as part of a grouping where they seem to best fit at the moment (e.g., Student-Centered Inquiry as a Social Issues model, Health Opportunities through Physical Education as a Health and Wellness model). There are other curriculum models that we have chosen not to introduce separately because we see them as perhaps being implemented within or alongside another model. For instance, an Interdisciplinary Physical Education curriculum might see science, language arts, and physical education working together to focus on themes and concepts that are the basis of Outdoor Education. Alternatively, a Sport Education dance season might be framed within a history scheme where dance is viewed and mastered from around the world while students gain global historical insights. The curriculum models we have chosen to highlight are as follows:

- Developmental Physical Education models
- Adventure Education
- Outdoor Education
- Sport Education
- Tactical Games Approach to Teaching Games
- Teaching Personal and Social Responsibility
- Social Issues models
- Health and Wellness models

These exemplary models have been developed, promoted, researched, and used successfully in various educational settings at primary and postprimary levels internationally. Each model has a well-defined focus, an underlying philosophy, and a set of assumptions on which it is based as well as specific outcomes and implications for instructional practice. In addition, each model encourages and promotes alignment among intended outcomes, learning experiences, and assessment and has been successfully implemented in different contexts to align with the standards and outcomes of various national bodies (National Association for Sport and Physical Education [NASPE] in the United States, National Council for Curriculum and Assessment [NCCA] in Ireland, Department of Education and Skills in England and Wales, Scottish Government in Scotland). As you read the model descriptions, you will note that we have not identified the NASPE content standards that appear to have the most relevance for each; instead, we ask you to make the match for the context in which you reside. This emphasis does not suggest that these are the only standards addressed by a given model to the exclusion of the others. Rather, we identify the standards that form a major part of the model framework, and learner outcomes will reflect them. We concur with Stiehl and Parker (2010) when they note that, "standards are not designed to stand apart from one another as discrete, unrelated entities. Their strength lies in their integration, just as a child's strength lies in her or his wholeness—the emotional, cognitive, social, spiritual and physical dimensions of self" (pp. 252–253).

Learning Experience 10.3

If you haven't already done so, obtain a copy of the standards/outcomes that have been developed for children and youth to achieve in primary and postprimary physical education in the education system where you study. In cases where these standards/outcomes do not exist, you might refer to the physical education syllabus or another document that highlights the goals that have been set for young people to achieve.

Each main theme curriculum model represents a different vision of how the good in physical education should be conceptualized and developed into a program. As noted earlier, the actual implementation of these models may look quite different when delivered in different settings given the limitations of facilities and teachers' values and beliefs. The perspectives of the students for whom they are designed also need to be given consideration and respect. The idea is to fit the model to the context. There has been a growing consensus internationally, however, that not all goods can be achieved in any one program, and that trying to achieve too many goals results in too little achievement in any area. Although we will introduce the vision and key features of each model and link the expected outcomes to outcomes/standards for student learning, due to space we will not share complete implementation guidelines. Instead we provide a list of what we view as the most useful resources to guide application of each model (see **Box 10.2**).

Developmental Physical Education Models

Pairs of children are striking a ball with a racket across homemade nets. Nets are created with PVC pipes and jump ropes or PVC cross-bars. There are no more than four students at any one net, each with their own space marked. On offense children are practicing striking to different spaces on the court. The defensive player is practicing returning to a center-back court position after every hit. After a bit students retrieve a paper on which notes and drawings were previously made and they begin working on small group projects. Each group's work is slightly different based on their need and interest—some have no net whereas others do. Some groups keep score and others do not. The teacher moves among the children, providing comments, encouragement, and support for individual and partner efforts. These children are working on designing their own games in which they will demonstrate their individual skill in striking with a short-handled racket and their understanding of the concept of space.

Developmental physical education programs are built around the individual learner with the curriculum designed to meet each learner's developmental needs and unique growth patterns. The intent is to provide a holistic education that emphasizes cognitive, affective, and psychomotor outcomes within each individual, while they achieve content-specific goals. As a result of reviewing the work of key scholars and proponents of the leading developmental physical education models (Skill Themes: Graham, Holt/Hale, & Parker, 2013; Movement Education: Rovegno & Bandhouer, 2013; Developmental: Gallahue & Cleland Donnelly, 2003), we have collated a list of the key points that can inform the design and delivery of an effective developmental physical education program for children (see **Box 10.3**).

Developmental models suggest an interactive relationship among the individual, his or her environmental circumstances, and specific objectives of learning tasks with which the learner is engaged. Regardless of choice of developmental model, when done well, it is age related, not age dependent. What, when, and how to teach depends on each individual, rather than being age group appropriate. This implies that physical skills are introduced and developed in a progressive and sequential manner consistent with the individual learner's current developmental level and learning needs. A physical education program based on a developmental curriculum model is designed in a sequential way that allows children to learn skills, achieve success, and improve their

BOX 10.2 Textbook Curriculum Model Resources

General curriculum texts:

- Lund, J., & Tannehill, D. (2010). *Standards-based physical education curriculum development* (2nd ed.). Sudbury, MA: Jones and Bartlett.

Developmental physical education models:

- Gabbard, C., LeBlanc, E., & Lowry, S. (1987). *Physical education for children.* Englewood Cliffs, NJ: Prentice-Hall.
- Gallahue, D. L., & Cleland Donnelly, F. (2003). *Developmental physical education for all children.* Champaign, IL: Human Kinetics.
- Graham, G., Holt/Hale, S. A., & Parker, M. (2013). *Children moving: A reflective approach to teaching physical education* (9th ed.). New York: McGraw-Hill.
- Rovegno, I., & Bandhouer, D. (2013). *Elementary physical education: Curriculum and instruction.* Burlington, MA: Jones & Bartlett Learning.

Adventure education:

- Henton, M. (1996). *Adventure in the classroom: Using adventure to strengthen learning and build a community of life-long learners.* Dubuque, IA: Kendall Hunt.

Outdoor education:

- Gilbertson, K., Bates, T., McLaughlin, T., & Ewert, A. (2006). *Outdoor education: Methods and strategies.* Champaign, IL: Human Kinetics.

Tactical games teaching:

- Mitchell, S. A., Oslin, J. L., & Griffin, L. L. (2003). *Sport foundations for elementary physical education: A tactical games approach.* Champaign, IL: Human Kinetics.
- Mitchell, S., Oslin, J. L., & Griffin, L. L. (2006). *Teaching sport concepts and skills* (2nd ed.). Champaign, IL: Human Kinetics.

Teaching personal and social responsibility:

- Hellison, D. (2011). *Teaching personal and social responsibility through physical activity* (3rd ed.). Champaign, IL: Human Kinetics.
- Hellison, D., Cutforth, N., Kallusky, J., Martinek, T., Parker, M., & Stiehl, J. (2000). *Youth development and physical activity.* Champaign, IL: Human Kinetics.

Sport education:

- Siedentop, D., Hastie, P. A., & van der Mars, H. (2011). *Complete guide to sport education* (2nd ed.). Champaign, IL: Human Kinetics.

Health and wellness models:

- Corbin, C., Le Masurier, G., & Lambdin, D. (2007). *Fitness for life middle school.* Champaign, IL: Human Kinetics.
- Corbin, C., Le Masurier, G., Lambdin, D., & Greiner, M. (2010). *Fitness for life elementary school program package.* Champaign, IL: Human Kinetics.
- Corbin, C., & Lindsey, R. (2007). *Fitness for life* (5th ed.). Champaign, IL: Human Kinetics.

motor performance. A teacher organizing skill progressions developmentally and then challenging a child with appropriately designed tasks using a variety of teaching strategies would reflect a developmental perspective. Although all the developmental models have some differences they also share multiple similarities, which we will explore through the skill theme approach.

Skill Theme Approach

An example drawn from Graham et al. (2013) demonstrates an appropriate developmental progression for striking using the **skill theme approach**. Striking is introduced in the early primary school grades and focuses on the child attempting to make contact with an object using lightweight, short-handled implements. At this point there will be inconsistency, many

BOX 10.3 What We Know About Developmentally Appropriate Physical Education for Children

- Children do not all learn at the same rate, suggesting that physical educators should not expect all children to perform tasks in the same way.
- Children develop motor skill movements and patterns in sequential and, typically, predictable ways, suggesting that physical educators be familiar with basic/common movement sequences.
- Children do not learn at the same time, suggesting that although physical educators might anticipate certain behaviors at a given age, development is age related but not age determined.
- Children develop skills first in isolated environments and then in increasingly more complex environments resembling games, dance, and gymnastics, suggesting that young people gain competence in skill performance before applying them to more complex applications.
- Children develop motor skills and movements by using them more frequently, suggesting that practice is critical.
- Children have less frequent opportunities for informal play in today's societies, suggesting that physical education has a larger role to play in children learning through playful situations.
- Children develop as a result of their interactions with the environment, suggesting that family and friends are critical, as are the opportunities they have to be physical active.

instances of the object being missed, and inefficient skill attempts at striking the object. Appropriate tasks for this level include striking a diversity of objects tossed, dropped, or suspended using different directional strokes with modified lightweight paddles. As students gain in their consistency to strike the object, the teacher designs challenges that require the children to control the object they are striking. These challenges might include striking with varying amounts of force, repeatedly in succession, and in a specific direction or toward an object. Once children are successful with these types of tasks and can contact the object on repeated attempts and direct it in different directions with varying degrees of force, they are ready to move into more complex activities. In this progression, children will use a variety of implements, employ various strokes, and exchange hits with a partner. Success with these tasks indicates the child has developed a mature pattern of striking and has control over both body and implement in stationary and moving situations. The tasks would then move to game-like activities in complex, changing environments.

The skill theme approach is both a curriculum and an instructional model because it describes both the content of physical education and the pedagogy (teaching process). Two major goals of this curriculum are to (1) develop positive attitudes in young people about themselves and physical activity, ultimately resulting in them choosing to be physically active in all stages of their lives, and (2) help children develop their movement competence to allow enjoyment and success in physical activity participation (Graham et al., 2013). The content of the skill theme approach is organized by skill themes and movement concepts rather than by dance, gymnastics, or games. Children begin by becoming familiar with movement concepts such as space awareness (e.g., self-space, pathways), effort (e.g., flow, time, force), and relationships (e.g., of body parts, with others). Skill themes that represent fundamental movements (locomotor, manipulative, nonmanipulative) are then learned, first in isolation and then combined with other skills and movement concepts in more complex and variable settings such as games, dance, and other physical activities. As young people mature they are given the opportunity to apply their knowledge of skills and concepts to a wide range of movement forms that they find enjoyable and have implications for future life choices. These choices are then specialized into developmentally appropriate games, dance, and gymnastics experiences (e.g., small-sided games, inquiry-based teaching, transfer to tactics) and ultimately narrowed with young adults taking charge of their own learning and physical activity experiences as they begin to focus their attention on selected activities.

Learning Experience 10.4

Using your knowledge of basic motor skills, design an appropriate progression for children focused on dribbling using the hands or striking with an implement.

The skill theme approach has four characteristics that combine both the content and the pedagogy of this curriculum and instruction model.

1. *Basic motor skills:* Skill themes are generic, sequenced from basic isolated movements emphasizing key critical elements to more complex tasks combining other skills and movement concepts. The premise is that if children learn the basic motor skills they will be able to apply them to more complex and, ultimately, adult versions of activities.

2. *Developmental levels:* Skill themes use individual students' developmental levels as the benchmark for choice of content, rather than grade level or age. In other words, content and activities are selected by what the children are able to do and may result in children doing different activities or skills than their peers, and even an entire class doing something different than another class of the same age group. In other words, match the task to the ability of the children.
3. *Scope and sequence:* Drawing from motor learning principles, skill themes are visited and revisited at various times across the school year, through massed and distributed practice, rather than being the focus of complete lessons for an extended period of time. In this way, children gain competence and motivation in a particular theme as skill themes are introduced through a lesson segment, revisited for longer lesson portions, and perhaps revisited again for one or two full lessons focused on the skill theme.
4. *Instructional alignment:* In order for children to achieve success in the content being delivered, the teacher must determine what is to be learned, design learning experiences that practice this learning, and finally assess what the children have been practicing. This enables learning to be progressively built on the skills and knowledge being developed by the learner.

Skill themes is a holistic approach to developmental physical education based originally on the early work of Laban (1948) in educational dance. Although the emphasis appears to focus on fundamental skills and movement concepts, it must be emphasized that physical fitness as well as cognitive and affective learning are a major focus of this model. However, rather than any of these components being isolated, the sole focus of a unit, or viewed as a skill theme of their own, each is integrated throughout the lessons in applied ways. For example, while children are participating in a lesson focused on a jumping and landing theme they may be taking part in a series of rope-skipping activities. One of the challenges might be for them to discover, through inquiry-based teaching and learning, which skipping activity makes them the most out of breath and thus has the biggest impact on their cardiovascular output.

Learning Experience 10.5

Given the description of the skill theme approach and the published national standards or outcomes in your country, identify the specific standards that are either a primary emphasis with this model, a secondary emphasis, or, if applicable, not emphasized at all. Provide a rationale for each standard included.

Adventure Education

Standing on the balcony overlooking an adventure lesson, I see two groups of 12–15 students standing side by side with their feet touching the person's feet next to them. Each group is facing in the opposite direction and does not seem to be paying any attention to the other group but are focused on what appears to be their own task. Their arms are wrapped around one another's waists and there is a great deal of chatter and shouts of encouragement as they appear to move as a unit across the space. Apparently their challenge is to work together to get their small group across the hall without losing foot contact. After both groups are successful they come to the center of the hall and stand in a large circle with everyone in the class holding onto a rope. The rope is slowly passed around the group. When the knot gets to each person they share one thing they learned about themselves in terms of cooperation, what allowed their group to be successful, how they felt taking part in this activity, or what or who helped them to be successful.

Experiential learning that provides learners with the opportunity to challenge themselves physically and mentally, work cooperatively as a group to solve problems and overcome risks, and gain respect for, confidence in, and trust in themselves and their peers are key components of **Adventure Education**. They form the basic philosophy of Adventure Education, which is the basis of the model rather than the activities that the teacher uses to achieve them.

Adventure in physical education can provide meaningful and challenging goals toward which students can strive, include problem solving and risk taking in order to achieve those goals, and provide opportunities for experiential learning within a safe environment. Adventure might be viewed as themes-based to allow students to progress toward achieving cooperative and challenge goals, getting acquainted and cooperating, building trust, communicating and collaborating, completing team challenges, problem solving, and performing low-level initiatives. Several concepts key to Adventure Education that set the stage for student interaction and development include the full-value contract (FVC), challenge with choice, experiential learning cycle, and debriefing or processing the experience. We explain each in turn in the following sections.

Full-Value Contract (FVC)

An FVC is an effective way to stimulate learning and assist group members in achieving their goals. The contract is developed by the group highlighting what each member is willing to put into or do during the group experience. The FVC is a way for members of the group to think about their role and behaviors in the group and how those behaviors affect others. As with any contract, the FVC provides the general rules and expectations that will guide group interactions, including such things as cooperation toward achieving group goals, safety guidelines to which all members will adhere, commitment to share feedback with all members, and a willingness to be confronted if not living up to the FVC. Using FVCs is an excellent approach to having students take more ownership and responsibility in the class.

Learning Experience 10.6

When asked to design a method for students to collaboratively design an FVC, one of our preservice teachers suggested the idea of the links on a chain. Each student comes up with a word or phrase they feel is important for everyone to be successful in physical education class. They each write their word/phrase on one of the links on the chain. In doing so they are making a promise to themselves and to each person in the class that they are going to do their best to abide by what they write down. The chain shows that if even one of the links is broken the whole chain suffers. Like in a class, all the words are linked; if one of the phrases or words is not respected or if people don't commit to them, the whole class is weakened. It symbolizes the importance of each aspect of the class and the people in it. The FVC is posted in the gym at every class to remind each person what is expected of them.

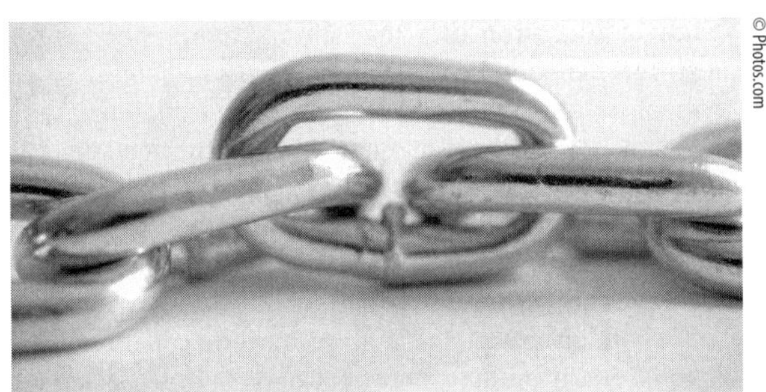

Your task is to select an age level and develop a method for students to collaboratively design an FVC for your own teaching setting.

Challenge by Choice

Based on the idea that not everyone needs to do everything in order to contribute, learn, and be successful, challenge by choice is an invitation for students to participate in a way in which they feel comfortable. It is a chance to try a difficult or frightening challenge in an atmosphere of support and caring, with the understanding that it is ok to back off or play a different role if unable to continue due to a lack of confidence or fear. It is critical to help students recognize that it is the attempt that is important, rather than the result. Challenge by choice does not suggest that a student can opt out of participation; rather, it provides options that might allow him or her to participate more confidently. For example, if you design an activity in which students are asked to hold hands around a circle, a progression of choice to accommodate those who are not comfortable touching each other might be designed. When holding hands is too difficult

- Hold sleeves
- Interlock elbows
- Hold onto a buddy rope (a 12" soft rope with loops for hands on each end)
- Let the students sort out how to stay connected

Experiential Learning Cycle (ELC)

Although experiential learning often is thought of as merely "doing" or being involved, that is only one of the four components of the ELC that is necessary if students are to gain depth and application of learning. The four components of the ELC (as noted in **Figure 10.1**) are (1) activity (the doing in content chosen to meet a learning goal), (2) personal reflection (reviewing what occurred during the activity), (3) abstracting (making connections between ideas and experience), and (4) transfer (application of learning). The ELC may take place several times in a lesson, over a series of lessons, or over time because it is a learning process.

Debriefing/Processing the Experience

Learning in Adventure Education requires processing of the experience to enable learners to make sense of what they gained. In other words, an activity is just an activity until it is processed to help learners create meaning from the experience. Processing encourages and facilitates the learner in making

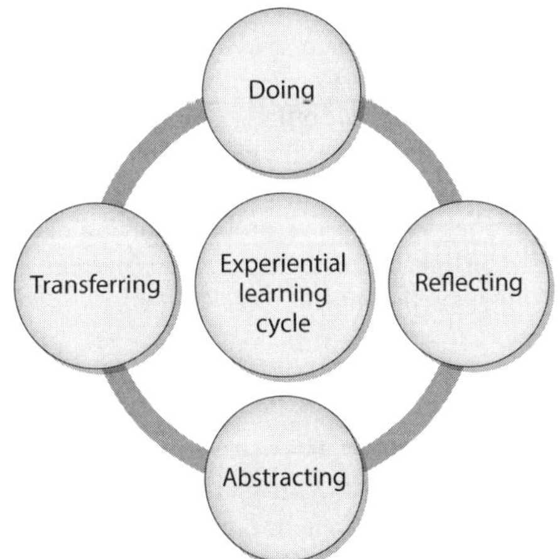

FIGURE 10.1 The experiential learning cycle.
Adapted from Kolb, D. A. (1984). *Experiential learning.* Englewood Cliffs, NJ: Prentice-Hall.

connections between new and previous knowledge, linking concepts and ideas in ways that make them useable, and internalizing new knowledge for future application. Processing can be broken down into a sequence of steps—What? So what? and Now what?—and aligned in the ELC. "What?" takes place during the reflection component of the ELC and asks the learner to identify such things as what they did, how they did it, problems they encountered, and how they felt. When they get to the abstracting component of the cycle, "So what?" causes the learner to analyze and interpret what they identified as occurring when doing the activity, to explain their actions. Finally, the "Now what?" question that takes place during the ELC transfer component prompts the learner to recognize what has been learned and how to apply it to future situations.

An Adventure Education curriculum will look quite different based on the decisions the teacher makes in four categories: (1) the concepts/themes taught (cooperation, communication, trust, problem solving, decision making, team building), (2) the activities selected as the vehicle to achieve these concepts (focused themes-based activities, initiatives, problems to solve, challenges to overcome, cooperative games, individual and group challenges), (3) the format of the program (lengthened class time, weekend experiences), and (4) the instructional models chosen to facilitate student learning and development (cooperative learning, teaching through questions, small group challenges). Regardless of how Adventure Education is delivered, one of the main foci is its experiential approach to learning with physical activity as the means for individual and collective exploration and discovery. The challenges and risks inherent in Adventure programming may produce anxiety and stress. As these challenges are met, self-confidence and self-esteem increase. Many challenges require group effort that brings in the idea of a community of learners, team-building concepts, and group problem solving (see **Box 10.4**).

There are many benefits to a well-developed and delivered Adventure Education program as students learn to cooperate with and depend on each other to solve the problems presented to them. Adventure activities are one way to increase participants' self-esteem, reduce antisocial behavior, promote critical thinking, and improve problem-solving skills. These benefits can be linked directly to numerous outcomes that we hold for student achievement in physical education.

Learning Experience 10.7

Given the description of the Adventure Education model and the published national standards or outcomes in your country, identify the specific standards that are either a primary emphasis with this model, a secondary emphasis, or, if applicable, not emphasized at all. Provide a rationale for each standard included.

Outdoor Education

A weekend orienteering trip to the mountains has been planned. Each small group of skilled orienteers in their final year of postprimary school is responsible for designing a 1.5-mile course for the first-year students experiencing Outdoor Education for the first time. These planners set about studying the map of the territory, interpreting the three-dimensional nature of the symbols on the map—the contour lines that mark the hills and mountains, the blue markings representing either a river or lake, the colored patches that mark the wooded areas of the territory, and the black lines that are actual trails, roads, and power lines. After examining the map for moderately challenging route options that participants might select and maintain that is challenging yet has not too difficult control points, the planners mark these points with a grease pencil on the plastic sleeve into which they have inserted the map. Attempting to keep in mind all they have learned about designing an orienteering course, they attempt to use environmental elevation and water as the control points. As they make each decision, they attempt to ensure variety in the course, select route options that participants might choose, and maintain a course that is challenging yet not too difficult.

Outdoor Education uses the natural environment as the context for experientially helping learners increase their enjoyment of the outdoors and their understanding and appreciation for the environment. In order to achieve this, Outdoor Education is built on three types of learning, (1) physical skills to permit enjoying participation in outdoor activities, (2) environmental awareness related to our natural ecology, and (3) interpersonal growth to allow developing self-confidence and the ability to work collaboratively in a group on an outdoor experience. We will unpack each type of learning in due course. According to Gilbertson et al. (2006), "outdoor education has been described as a place (natural environment), a subject (ecological processes), and a reason (resource stewardship) for learning" (p. 4). Outdoor Education is a holistic experience that, as you will see, is closely linked to Adventure Education—even sharing common components.

Physical Skills

Outdoor activities that make up the Outdoor Education curriculum are those that take place in a natural environment, tend not to involve competition, and typically require a challenge or risk such as fly casting and fishing, hill walking, hiking and backpacking, orienteering with map and compass, or rock climbing. Gaining competence in these types of activities requires learning new and specific skills, gaining expertise and practice in the use of specialized equipment, and maintaining

BOX 10.4 Thread the Rooms

Theme: Problem solving
Target group: Students able to cooperate and communicate
Group size: 9 in a group
Time: 15 minutes
Space: Flat open space large enough for setup as diagrammed
Activity level: Low

Purpose:

To promote problem solving and thinking outside the box. This task also should encourage and reinforce cooperation, teamwork, and communication.

Procedures:

- Set out a grid of cones in the format shown.
- Have one student in each subsquare of the grid (nine students total).
- Set up enough grids for the entire class to participate; each grid of students becomes an adventure team.

The task is to pass a ball so that it enters every student's grid at least once. The conditions are that the ball must stay on the ground, the students must stay in their grid square, and no student can touch the ball more than once. The aim is to complete the task with as few students touching the ball as possible. Here is an example of the ball's route when seven students of the nine touch the ball.

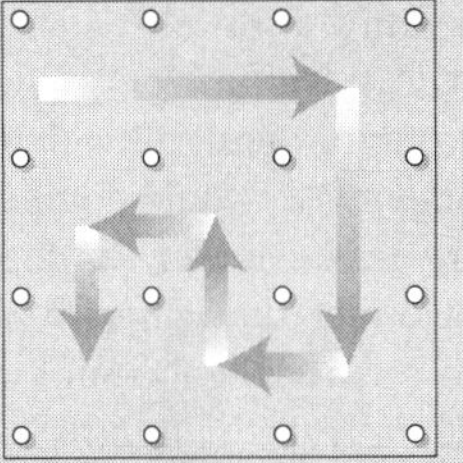

Solution:

With nine students, the actual minimum number of students possibly touching the ball to have it enter each square in the grid is three. However, the students will have to work together and think outside the box to come to this conclusion. We will leave you to determine how this can be achieved.

Debrief:

Each adventure team will debrief the activity. Several members of each team select a question from a hat and the team talks among themselves as they attempt to identify the benefits of the activity for developing their cooperation, teamwork, thinking outside the box, and communication skills. Questions might include

- What skills were challenged in this task?
- What did you find the most difficult part of the task?
- Do you feel you worked well together as a team?
- What was your role as part of the team?
- What hindered team success in this activity?
- How did your team go about solving the task?
- What might have assisted your team to work together more effectively?

the safety of yourself and your peers through knowledgeable application of safety procedures. Whether archery, snowshoeing and skiing, surfing, kayaking and canoeing, mountain biking, anticipating and responding to the weather, or locating a camp site and taking part in camp setup during a camping experience, skill development is crucial. Not all of these outdoor activities can be taught and enjoyed through a school physical education program, but sometimes teachers are surprised by the organizations or groups willing to take part in introducing these activities to young people. After all, surf schools are always looking for new participants for their weekend courses, orienteering clubs often seek new members through schools, and local parks departments count on young people to join summer camps. What better way to access such populations than through working with them in introductory modules in physical education?

Environmental Awareness

Recent warnings of global warming, local and national initiatives to "save the earth," and the worldwide annual Earth Day event have been designed to increase awareness and appreciation of the earth's natural environment. Environmental education and helping young people become aware of our natural settings (e.g., rainforests, flora and fauna), solving environmental problems with which we are faced (e.g., leave no trace, endangered species), and perhaps linking with other subject areas to focus on concepts and principles that overlap (e.g., map reading, conservation, and toxic waste in science) have never been more appropriate. The intent would be for young people to become more knowledgeable about the out-of-doors and gain the necessary skills to make informed decisions and take responsible action within our communities and natural habitat.

Interpersonal Growth

This is where we see the most overlap between Adventure Education and Outdoor Education. As noted previously, a key aspect of Adventure Education is student development of cooperating with others, ability to communicate, working together to solve problems, and building trust with yourself and a group of peers, all which are facilitated in a contrived environment. We would argue that these same interpersonal skills are necessary in Outdoor Education, yet tend to be developed first through adventure programming and then followed up in authentic outdoor settings where the sense of risk is more realistic. In other words, in Outdoor Education, participants encounter real and varied situations about which they must make informed and reasonable decisions on how to respond. These responses will impact nature as well as others, an area that Outdoor Education strives to influence.

The most creative way we have seen Outdoor Education delivered in schools is in Maple Valley, Washington, where the teachers make use of a six-period block schedule to integrate subject areas. The Outdoor Academy integrates physical education, science, and language arts; is theme-based and focused on outdoor recreation (e.g., fly fishing, rock climbing, biking, stewardship); and meets every other day for second-year students (10th grade). Tracy Krause, 2008 NASPE Secondary Teacher of the Year and 2012 National Football League Network Physical Education Teacher of the Year, explains their Outdoor Academy:

> *Our language arts teacher, Jamie Vollrath, uses texts such as* Old Man and the Sea, A River Runs Through It, Into Thin Air, *and* Into the Wild *to teach concepts intended for 10th grade students. Our science teacher, Mike Hanson, uses water quality testing, aquatic invertebrates, evolution, body systems, and the environment to teach experimental design, the 10th grade science focus. The integration occurs when the three of us plan our units together. For example, while I am teaching fly casting and fly tying, Mike is teaching water quality and aquatic insects, and Jamie is teaching* A River Runs Through It. *We are able to take our students into the field several times each month to participate in real science, become environmental stewards (plant trees, trail maintenance), and learn what it means to be conscientious users of public lands.*[1]

Learning Experience 10.8

Investigate your community and identify links that you might make between physical education and Outdoor Education (e.g., an adventure center, parks department program). Describe how you might work cooperatively with this resource to strengthen the outdoor program in your school.

With the wide spectrum of activities that make up Outdoor Education—some that require more social interaction (e.g., hill walking, camping), others a higher degree of fitness (e.g., rock climbing, snowshoeing), and still others more cognitive challenge (e.g., orienteering, fly fishing)—depending on the choice of activities and the purpose for which they are undertaken, Outdoor Education can address numerous learning goals and standards/outcomes.

Learning Experience 10.9

Given the description of the Outdoor Education model and the published national standards or outcomes in your country, identify the specific standards that are either a primary emphasis with this model, a secondary emphasis, or, if applicable, not emphasized at all. Provide a rationale for each standard included.

Sport Education

Students move to their team space in the gymnasium and begin warming up under the direction of their team trainer, who has designed stretches appropriate for the 25-lesson volleyball season in which they are participating. While students are warming up, team managers are reporting attendance to the teacher. As soon as all students are warmed up, they move into skill practice emphasizing the pass, set, and hit in a core drill formation

[1] Reprinted with permission from "Interview with 2008 National Teacher of the Year High School Tracy Krause." © 2013 American Alliance for Health, Physical Education, Recreation and Dance; http://www.aahperd.org/naspe/awards/peAwards/toy/08-T-Krause.cfm.

under the direction of their team captain and with skill feedback from the teacher. After 15 minutes of varied skill practice, the team captains direct their teams to assigned courts for a series of small-sided, three-versus-three volleyball games, which is the first round of games in the season's competitive schedule. Student officials and scorekeepers maintain the pace of the games to ensure that the first round is completed by the close of class. Prior to class dismissal, the duty team compiles the scores and records them on the publicity board while the team equipment managers collect the volleyballs. Members of each team select the member whom they feel displayed the most team effort for the day and that individual's name is put on the fair play board.

In this scenario, students are actively engaged in the sport as it is actually played, working on skills in a realistic game-play situation, taking charge of various aspects of warm-up, practice, and game activities, and all under the direction of their selected team leaders. Students are interested and involved in their own sport experience, so their efforts toward improvement have a focus.

Sport Education defines the content of physical education as sport and provides direction on how sport can be introduced to all students within the context of physical education. Based on the assumption that sport derives from play and is an integral part of many international cultures, within this model, sport is defined as "playful competition" (Siedentop, 1980). Sport Education is a curriculum model designed to provide students with an authentic, in-depth, and educationally rich sport experience within physical education. It is intended to move isolated skill practice through drills out of the curriculum and into sequential, progressive, and realistic game-like situations in which students learn to organize and manage their own sport experience. The primary objective is the development of skilled and competent sport participants through which learners have the opportunity to develop the skills and understanding of strategies necessary to participate in sport successfully throughout life. Although content may be similar in some instances, Sport Education, when used well and with appropriate instructional models employed, does not fit into a multiactivity format of short units of instruction.

Sport Education evolved from the perspective that physical education was not teaching sport in ways that allowed students to experience an authentic sport experience. A major focus of this model is to help students become skilled sportspersons and provide opportunities for them to take responsibility for their own sport and physical education experiences. Six features characterize Sport Education and distinguish it from more traditional forms of physical education: seasons, affiliation, formal competition, record keeping, culminating event, and festivity. Although these features are typically seen and experienced in after-school and organized sport, they are less frequently a part of physical education in schools in a more traditional curriculum. We think they should be, and describe our understanding of each feature and its application to physical education in the following sections.

Seasons

Sport is organized into seasons lasting longer than the typical physical education units (primary 10–12 lessons, postprimary 18–20 lessons). These longer seasons include both practice and competition built into every season to enable students to gain skill and competence in all aspects of the game. Within these seasons, activities tend to be modified into small-sided games that allow all students to be successful and have more opportunities to participate.

Affiliation

Students are members of equal ability teams and maintain membership in that team throughout an entire season. All students learn multiple roles within the team, therefore taking responsibility for aspects of planning and running the season. All members are first and foremost team players. In addition, all team members must learn to play what are called *duty team* roles that function on competition days and might include referee and scorekeeper. Ideally, as both the teacher and students become comfortable in a Sport Education season, every student might have responsibility for a nonplaying role in addition to his or her main role as player. These nonplaying roles might include such roles as coach, captain, trainer, publicist, equipment manager, and any other that might assist the teacher and teams in overseeing functioning of the season. Finally, depending on the sport or activity that is the focus of the season, specialist roles might be required such as choreographer for a dance troupe, starter in athletics, line judges in net games, and safety officer in weight training.

Formal Competition

As noted previously, a season includes both practice and competition, and these competitions themselves will tend to be progressive, perhaps singles competition followed by pairs competition in badminton, 2 v 2, 4 v 4, and 6 v 6 Ultimate Frisbee competition, and perhaps levels of difficulty in gymnastics competition. Regardless of which type of progression is designed for the season, it is posted and followed just as would be done in authentic sport. This formalized competition schedule makes practice sessions and roles more meaningful as players and teams begin to see their progress throughout competition.

Record Keeping

Maintaining a record of performance is key to Sport Education because it allows individual students to recognize their progress and teams to be acknowledged for strong performances, and might serve as a tool for individual and team goal setting. In addition to serving to inform players on their performance, records are also a method for determining team standings across the season. Sport Education encourages season standing to be determined using a point system that recognizes fair play, teamwork, role performance, and other aspects of sport beyond the win/loss record, and these types of data can be recorded and publicized as well.

Culminating Event

Typically sport seasons end in some type of culminating event, whether it is the Ryder Cup in golf, Wimbledon in tennis, the Heineken Cup in Irish rugby, or the biggest culminating event of all, the Olympic Games. In Sport Education, the emphasis on the culminating event is intended to recognize all participants, involve play by all, and provide opportunities for success in all aspects of the season. Part of this culminating event should include an awards ceremony to recognize team standing, skill performance, teamwork, and aspects of the season that were successful and important.

Festivity

Sport is festive. Teams are prepared, excited, and committed; fans come to observe and cheer on their favorite team; sport venues are filled with banners, flags, and slogans; and fans are decked out in colorful team attire. This is a huge aspect of sport that is included in a school Sport Education season, and helps young people to learn that sport isn't just about the winners but is about the enjoyment of taking part, improving, and being successful.

During a Sport Education season the roles of the teacher, students, and community change within the framework of physical education. Siedentop, Hastie, and van der Mars (2011) described the teacher's role as that of being an "instructional engineer" sharing responsibility with learners as they begin to take responsibility for their sport experience. The balance of teacher–student roles shift (see **Figure 10.2**) when taught through a student-centered Sport Education season (right) rather than a more traditional approach (left).

As the teacher facilitates learning, provides and shares instruction with students, works with students to manage the environment, and assesses student achievement, the learners become skilled at assuming responsibility and leadership, working as a cooperative team, and learning with and from one another. They become decision makers and problem solvers holding each other accountable for fair play and teamwork.

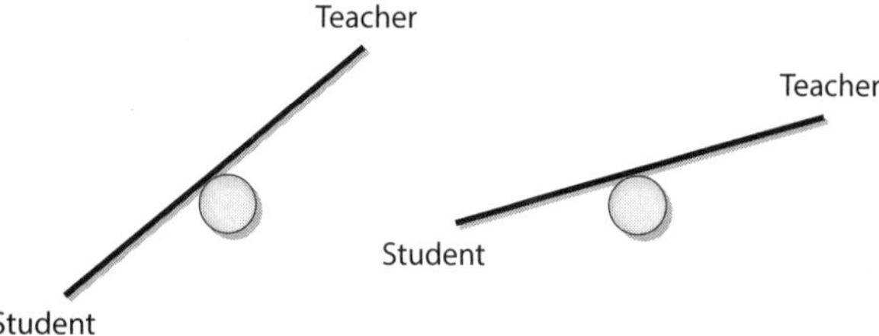

FIGURE 10.2 The changing roles of teacher and student.

Learning Experience 10.10

Begin to outline the design of a Sport Education season to be delivered to your students.

1. Context for season
   a. Age group or class
   b. Sport
2. Teams
   a. Number of teams and team size
   b. Team selection process
   c. Strategies to build team affiliation
3. Roles
   a. Determine and define roles
   b. Student role selection/assignment
   c. Strategies for teaching roles
4. Festivity
   a. Awards, recognition, rituals, and traditions
5. Season design
   a. Length of season
   b. Competitive schedule
   c. Culminating event
6. Record keeping
   a. Scoring
   b. Statistics
7. Extra touches
   a. Newsletter
   b. Handbook
8. Facilities and equipment
   a. Include everything from pencils to stopwatches to referee jerseys

With its focus on demonstrating motor skill competence, being physically active, and taking responsibility for their personal and social behavior, a well-designed and delivered Sport Education season should facilitate all students achieving specific standards and learning goals.

Learning Experience 10.11

Given the description of the Sport Education model and the published national standards or outcomes in your country, identify the specific standards that are either a primary emphasis with this model, a secondary emphasis, or, if applicable, not emphasized at all. Provide a rationale for each standard included.

Tactical Games Approach to Teaching Games

A number of years ago, while observing a postprimary school physical education class, I was surprised to see boys and girls spread out on the field in a number of 4 v 4 games, maintaining possession of the ball and providing support to the ball carrier rather than seeing a clump of players moving down the field all surrounding the ball like a large amoeba. During a short interval, players grouped around the teacher, who was questioning them on the goal of the game, what was necessary for them to be successful, why particular skills or movements would assist them in improving, and if they knew how to perform the skills/movements identified. Although the students indicated short, crisp passes were necessary, they admitted that they were not great at performing them. With that the teacher set the students up into a skill practice task, demonstrated how and what to do with critical points on passing and receiving emphasized, and then started practice providing feedback as students progressed. This skill practice did not last an extended period of time, but was directed by specific goals for achievement. When the teacher put the children back into the same game, they carried on with what appeared to be improved performance. In questioning the teacher, she indicated that this was the Tactical Approach to Teaching Games, and although her students "were not yet better players, they had more fun because they knew what to do and when to do it."

Games teaching constitutes a huge portion of most physical education programs, yet often games are not taught in realistic and challenging ways. They tend to focus on winning, favor the elite performer, and leave many less skilled young people standing to the side with no notion of how to play the game. Although many teachers teach both game skills and tactics, they often teach them in isolated ways that do not help players understand what to do, when to do it, why it will help, and how to do it effectively. At least one of the authors of this book was guilty of this when teaching middle school physical education a number of years ago. Not knowing games well, students in the classes learned skills in isolation and practiced through a multitude of drills (not necessarily game-like), and then finally played in a tournament, with the teacher assuming they would know how it all fit together. In hindsight, they really did not learn how to play the game, thus their enjoyment was limited.

The **Tactical Approach to Teaching Games** evolved from the early work of Bunker and Thorpe (1982) on **Teaching Games for Understanding (TGfU)** and Ellis (1983) and Almond's (1986) games classification system. Bunker and Thorpe (1982) identified several problems associated with skill-based games teaching, including a lack of student motivation for skill practice and their inability to perform skills or make appropriate decisions during game play. As a result, they designed TGfU as an alternative method for teaching games, which emphasized students' finding solutions to problems posed to them in game play situations. TGfU is a six-stage model that places the student at the center of learning in a problem-based context.

1. *Game play:* The lesson begins with a game that is modified and/or exaggerated to set students up with tactical problems. The modifications and exaggerations developed are a result of the developmental level of the students, space and equipment available, and number of players.
2. *Game appreciation:* As students play the game they come to understand that their responses are based on the restrictions placed on them through the modifications and exaggerations.
3. *Tactical awareness:* If a well-designed game, it should represent the same problems, principles, and skills of the parent form of the game, with students becoming aware that by making appropriate decisions and using selected tactics, they can successfully play the game.
4. *Making appropriate decisions:* Typically students need help in making appropriate decisions (e.g., "Do I shoot, pass, or dribble?"). This can be achieved by the teacher asking questions that cause the students to think about what to do and how to do it.
5. *Skill practice:* Once students recognize how the skills are used in the game, they are likely to understand that they need to practice the specific skills or movements, and be willing to take part in well-designed skill practice tasks to allow them to improve performance.
6. *Game play:* Putting students back into a game allows them to see how much they have improved as a result of this cognitive and psychomotor development process.

As Mitchell, Oslin, and Griffin (2003) worked with TGfU they developed the Tactical Games model, which is a consolidated, more applied, and teacher-friendly approach (see **Figure 10.3**). They advocate for development of tactical frameworks (tactical breakdown for different game forms with tactical problems and solutions) and identification of game complexity levels (appropriate developmental sequencing of content). As students are helped to make sense of tactical problems and associated decisions, Tactical Games teaching emphasizes the importance of questioning if students are going to think critically to solve tactical problems. They suggest building questions by what you want the students to achieve. For example, if you are working toward

- *Tactical awareness*, ask, "What do you . . . ?"
- *Skill execution*, ask, "How do you . . . ?"
- *Time*, ask, "When is the best time . . . ?"
- *Space*, ask, "Where is/can . . . ?"
- *Risk* or *exploration*, ask, "What choices . . . ?"

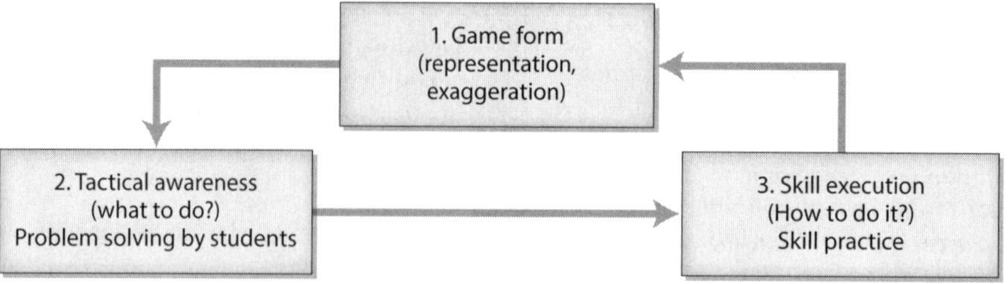

FIGURE 10.3 The Tactical Games model.
Adapted with permission from Mitchell, S., Oslin, J. L., & Griffin, L. L. (2006). *Teaching sport concepts and skills: A tactical games approach* (2nd ed., Figure 1-2). Champaign, IL: Human Kinetics.

It is hoped that this tactical focus will assist students in carrying their understanding over to other similar games. For instance, whether pickleball, badminton, table tennis, or tennis, net games have more similarities than they have differences (e.g., goal of game, striking an object with an implement, court divided, tactical problems). By using a tactical approach, teachers can design progressive, developmentally appropriate lessons that help students learn and apply tactics and skills across a range of similar games.

Learning Experience 10.12

To help you understand the idea of transfer of skills and tactics from one game to other like games, select one of the game categories (invasion, net/wall, striking/fielding, target) and identify the similarities between games in this category.

Mitchell, Oslin, and Griffin (2003) designed a planning framework to guide lesson design within the instructional component of the Tactical Games approach that has proven useful for teachers in delivering the approach.

- Tactical problem
- Lesson focus
- Objectives
  1. *Game:* Conditions/goal/questions
  2. *Practice task:* Goals/cues/extension
  3. *Game*: Conditions/goal
  4. *Closure*

Although the Tactical Games approach focuses on games, the learning outcomes that students strive to achieve go beyond game performance to include understanding strategies and tactics applied to game play, As students gain skill and knowledge in game play, they will enjoy participating in games activity for the enjoyment and challenge.

Learning Experience 10.13

Given the description of the Tactical Approach to Teaching Games model and the published national standards or outcomes in your country, identify the specific standards that are either a primary emphasis with this model, a secondary emphasis, or, if applicable, not emphasized at all. Provide a rationale for each standard included.

Teaching Personal and Social Responsibility

When arriving to the athletics fields, it appears there is a range of activities taking place, all related to disc sports and/or events. One group of youth is engaged in a high-level 7 v 7 competitive game of ultimate, another appears to be challenging themselves in various individual technical disc field events (maximum time aloft, throw, run and catch, and throw for distance), and a third group is playing a five-hole game of disc golf in pairs. A student who is challenging himself in the throw for distance event explains that they have been given the choice of which activity they want to take part in depending on how much effort they want to exert. He indicates he does not much care for team games and tends to get frustrated and angry, so prefers to focus on what he can do on his own. One of his classmates involved in the competitive game seems to thrive on the teamwork component and spends a great deal of time interacting with, and encouraging, her peers. The teacher appears to move among the groups, talking to many of the students informally, challenging others, and in a couple of instances merely watching quietly; she seems to make decisions based on what the students need. As the class comes to an end, the teacher brings the class in and they all sit in a circle. Discussion revolves around how class went today and whether students met the teamwork goals they had set for themselves. One student indicates the barriers he ran into in his interactions while another acknowledges a peer who helped her through a difficult game decision.

Hellison's **Teaching Personal and Social Responsibility (TPSR)** model can be used as a means of practicing primary prevention by helping students learn how to be responsible for their own behavior and to act responsibly toward their classmates. Hellison's notion of responsibility levels goals for students to achieve in their development as responsible individuals both in and outside of the classroom. Although Hellison acknowledges that teachers, faced with frequent behaviors that impact both teaching and learning, often use the responsibility levels to manage the classroom rather than teach responsibility, he reminds us that behaviors are only one aspect of responsibility, with attitudes, values, and beliefs forming the basis for displayed behaviors.

Hellison tells a story of how the TPSR model came to be what he calls a "theory-in-practice" because it continues to develop and evolve through practice. In coming to understand TPSR, the first question with which we are challenged is, "What's worth doing in physical education?" (Hellison, 2011). As we have seen throughout this chapter, teachers have many views of the goods of physical education, which differ greatly and can include wanting students to enjoy being active, competent in sport and games, adventurous and willing to take risks in the outdoors, or even maintaining a level of fitness. Hellison (2011) concluded that for him, "helping my students to take more responsibility for their own development and well-being and for supporting the well-being of others was perhaps the best contribution I could make" (p. 6). He suggests this requires sharing power with young people, allowing them to take responsibility for their own experiences and gradually shifting decision making to them.

In this section, we discuss TPSR as a curriculum model highlighting what Hellison refers to as a flexible framework "of basic values, ideas and implementation strategies" that make up the model. The TPSR framework is composed of eight critical components that Hellison (2011) describes as follows:

- *Core values* place the children first and focus on helping them be the best they can be across all aspects of their lives (i.e., emotional, social, cognitive, and physical).
- *Assumptions* around which TPSR is based include recognition that teaching personal and social development must be intentional, programs need to be directed and include a limited set of specific goals, and that TPSR needs to be embedded into the content through effective teaching strategies.
- *Levels of responsibility* focus young people on personal and social responsibility content for which they are accountable and must take responsibility. These levels/goals are displayed in a progression for teaching and learning. Although these levels/goals tend to be built one upon the other, Hellison reminds us that not all students will progress in the same fashion or at the same pace. **Table 10.1** displays the levels of responsibility and the components for which students must take responsibility.
- A program leader in the physical education class is the teacher who designs and teaches the program. *Program leader responsibilities* include the five themes of empowerment (shift of responsibility to the student), self-reflection (What's worth doing? Is it working? What's possible?), embedding (TPSR levels and strategies integrated with the content), transfer (responsibility beyond the gym and into students' lives), and our relationship with young people (relationships matter and must be about the individual). Hellison suggests although the levels are the responsibility of the students, these themes are the responsibility of the teacher/program leader as they guide daily implementation of TPSR.

TABLE 10.1 Components of the Levels of Responsibility

Levels	Components
Level I Respecting the rights and feelings of others	1. Self-control 2. Right to peaceful conflict resolution 3. Right to be included and to have cooperative peers
Level II Effort and cooperation	1. Self-motivation 2. Exploration of effort and new tasks 3. Getting along with others
Level III Self-direction	1. On-task independence 2. Goal-setting progression 3. Courage to resist peer pressure
Level IV Helping others and leadership	1. Caring and compassion 2. Sensitivity and responsiveness 3. Inner strength
Level V Transfer outside the gym	1. Trying these ideas in other areas of life 2. Being a positive role model for others, especially younger children

Reproduced from Masser, L. (1990). Teaching for affective learning in physical education. *Journal of Physical Education, Recreation and Dance, 61*, 7. Reprinted by permission of the publisher (Taylor & Francis Ltd., http://www.tandf.co.uk/journals).

TABLE 10.2 Daily Program Format

Feature	What It Looks Like
Relational time	Initially referred to as *counseling time*, teacher interactions can take place before, during, or after class and include a friendly chat or just checking in with a student on how he or she is feeling.
Awareness talk	Conducted with the entire class as a way to introduce the idea of taking responsibility. Teaching the levels of responsibility becomes part of the awareness talks and may occur gradually and ultimately involve students sharing their understanding of the levels.
Physical activity plan	The majority of the lesson should involve the integration of TPSR with the activity focus and learning experiences designed for the students.
Group meeting	Held toward the end of the lesson, the group meeting is intended for students to share their insights on how the lesson went and how they and their peers did, bring up problems they encountered, and discuss what the teacher did or didn't do.
Self-reflection time	This is the time at the close of the lesson when students assess their own behavior, how they helped or hindered others, achievement of their responsibilities, and how they might transfer their learning to other aspects of their life.

- *Daily program format* (see **Table 10.2**) is designed to guide every class session and involves five teaching strategies, each of which addresses one of the themes (empowerment, self-reflection, embedding, transfer, and relationship with young people) already described.
- *Suggested embedding strategies* require the teacher to know the lesson content and TPSR content, the pedagogy involved with individual activities and those that promote TPSR, and how to design learning experiences that integrate the two in worthwhile and appropriate ways. This is a huge aspect of teaching TPSR and perhaps the most difficult to gain the skill and experience needed to do so effectively. It seems teachers are often able to interact on various levels with different students (relational time), teach the responsibility levels (awareness talks), and even lead students in reflecting on how responsible they were in class (self-reflection time), yet are less able to integrate affective behaviors (cooperating, caring, respecting) into a physical education lesson. For example, if a teacher is attempting to motivate students (Level II) to participate in a fitness circuit, TPSR suggests providing young people with choices. At a teachers' workshop in Ireland, Hellison challenged us to complete 10 push-ups, or "as many as you can," using either full push-up position or modified, and in an aerobic activity to choose a distance and pace to complete a run. The scenario you read at the start of the TPSR section is an example of Level III—on-task independence. Students are invited to take part in one of three activities designed by the teacher based on their own self-identified needs, interests, and abilities.

One way to begin might be to define the affective personal and/or social behavior so you can teach it. In other words, Level I identifies students having cooperative peers, but what does a cooperative peer look like, what do they do to make them cooperative, and how can a student recognize cooperation in another person? If we define cooperation as teamwork, sharing common goals, praising, encouraging, and assisting others, then we are able to design learning experiences in which students are better able to develop these skills rather than just hearing us say, "Come on, let's cooperate." For example, a team might be asked to choose a team name to identify themselves for a basketball season they are starting. Once in the season, the team is charged with setting a team goal for the day's lesson and determining how they might support one another in achieving it. As members of a team with which they can identify, the idea of building team status in the class might serve to reinforce the idea of cooperating to achieve success.

Learning Experience 10.14

Try this planning strategy. Select a personal or social behavior that you would like to teach (e.g., sharing, listening, trusting). Define that behavior in terms of what it would look like. Then design a learning experience in an activity of your choice that would allow students to develop this behavior.

- *Problem solving* and how to deal with students who do not want to participate, or who choose not to take responsibility for their own behavior or the treatment of others, is something that all teachers must be prepared to encounter. Reflection in action is basically when a teacher assesses a situation as it occurs and makes an on-the-spot decision on how to respond.

TPSR proposes what has become known as a *solutions bank* that is filled with "if–then" ideas. For example, if Jamie gets angry while participating in a group activity and pushes another student, solutions might include putting him in a time-out away from his peers, possibly spending some quality relational time with him, asking him to give an apology to his peer, or maybe Jamie would suggest that when he is starting to get upset, he just give you a high sign and remove himself from interaction with others until he calms down.

- *Assessment* of TPSR and its implementation in physical education needs to reflect and measure the core values and TPSR themes. This may be done through formal and informal student and teacher lesson evaluations. For example, a class might be striving to reduce the number of conflicts that occur during their invasion games unit because competition and frustration tend to foster arguments. Time is spent during various lessons learning and practicing different ways to handle disagreements (negotiation, sitting out of class, self-officiating, or making new rules). The teacher and students keep a public record of the number of conflicts that occur each day, how they are resolved, and what steps might be taken to maintain the progress being made. Group meetings and reflection time are perhaps the most useful and immediate methods for having students assess their personal and social responsibility; however, more formal types of assessment might include student reflection on behavior or assessment rubrics developed for specific situations. One of the most important consequences of students assessing themselves is the empowerment it provides for them, especially if the teacher acknowledges and uses their input.

Learning Experience 10.15

Given the description of the Teaching Personal and Social Responsibility model and the published national standards or outcomes in your country, identify the specific standards that are either a primary emphasis with this model, a secondary emphasis, or, if applicable, not emphasized at all. Provide a rationale for each standard included.

Social Issues Models

When walking out of a sports store last week, I was approached by a young man asking if I had a moment to chat with him about a cultural studies project he was doing in his physical education class. He shared that he and his peers had been invited to help the teacher develop the physical education curriculum for their final year of postprimary school. As a first step, they were conducting a community mapping assignment focused on examining in detail the town's youth outreach and its sport, recreation, and leisure infrastructure. They were collecting information to identify the physical activity opportunities available to young people, assess how much these physical activity settings are accessed and used by young people, critique facilities for physical activity in and beyond the school (e.g., safety, attractiveness, gender, age, special needs, accessibility, cost), and understand how and why young people might become engaged in physical activity during and after school hours. He and his peers were speaking to young people, senior citizens, store owners, youth organizations, and any members of the community willing to share their perspectives. By gaining insight about this aspect of the community, it was hoped that these young people might better appreciate what is available to them when they leave school, influence their teachers' planning for a positive physical education experience, facilitate links between school physical education and the activity outlets in the community and advocate for the improvement of physical activity facilities and opportunities for youth in the local community.

Traditional physical education tends to be based on a sporting model focused on games teaching with the outcome being teachers, students, and the public considering sport and physical education as one entity. We have come to recognize that an overemphasis on sport may suit some students well, yet on the other hand it may cause some young people to choose not to take part in physical education, find their needs and interests overlooked or ignored, shy away from physical activity they associate with sport, or even not find access to the sport/activity of their choice outside of school (Ennis, 2003; Lawson, 1998). As Tannehill (2007) noted, "We need to do things differently, move away from curricula that mirror only what has been done in the past, and build programmes that reflect the desires and needs of young people so that they might persist in their efforts to develop physically active lifestyles." Suggestions proposed by numerous researchers who have worked with youth (e.g., Enright & O'Sullivan, 2010b; Oliver, Hamzeh, & McCaughtry, 2009) encourage providing alternative activities that meet the needs and interests of young people, offering students an element of choice in activities and effort, consulting youth on what types of activity appeal to them, and inviting students to be involved in the design of the physical education program.

Cultural Studies

The **Cultural Studies** curriculum model, as initially proposed by Kinchin and O'Sullivan (1999), was an attempt to meet the needs and interests of children and youth from various backgrounds, cultures, socioeconomic levels, and communities and is an example of a **Social Issues model**. The intent is to develop young people as questioning, curious, and critical participants in sport and physical activity in today's society. Through reflecting on their own experiences in physical activity and sport, students are encouraged to consider how these fit with their personal needs and interests and how some individuals are marginalized by activity opportunities available in their school and community. They are prompted to consider sport and physical activity beyond their communities, both nationally and internationally, and to uncover the cultural and social influences that impact physical activity and sport, such as provision and accessibility, and the positive and negative outcomes of sport and physical activity to individual and community well-being. There are many directions that can be explored within the cultural studies curriculum model, from social issues that influence physical activity opportunities to political issues impacting sport, or from health themes such as obesity to the influence of drugs on athletic performance.

The Cultural Studies curriculum model allows students the opportunity to be physically active in a selected movement form or sport while also exploring the issues related to the sport or physical activity from various perspectives. Cultural Studies intends to help young people make meaningful connections between what happens in physical education and aspects of their lives beyond the classroom including family, friends, and others in the community. For example, during a dance unit, the physical education teacher at a postprimary school and her students decided to coteach a "dance across the generations" theme unit. On the first day of class, students watched the YouTube video, MrVeedeoMan (see www.youtube.com/watch?v = dSLduZTInTA?), which is a fun presentation of dance over the last 50 years. Students worked as a dance troupe to discover the types of music and dances that their family had been involved with over the past few generations, from older siblings to parents and from aunts and uncles to grandparents. Troupes interviewed family members, filmed video clips of family members dancing, and developed their own routine to reflect these dance moves. During class, the students took part in teacher-designed lessons to focus on rhythm and various dance concepts, troupe- or individually led practice of specific dance steps, and viewing of numerous student-resourced YouTube or video dance displays. A final event allowed dance troupes to display their artifacts and demonstrate their routines, with students sharing insights they had gained about dance and their own family histories.

The Cultural Studies curriculum model continues to evolve as do the settings where it is being developed and studied. In the United States, Kinchin (1998) and Kinchin & O'Sullivan (1999) began by examining the perceptions of students participating in a cultural studies unit focused on gender, the body, and media influences in sport. Their next step was a study of student and teacher reactions to a social inquiry unit in sport applied in postprimary physical education (O'Sullivan, Kinchin, Kellum, Dunaway, & Dixon, 1996). Influenced by this work and that of Oliver and colleagues, discussed in the next section, Enright and O'Sullivan (2010a) used participatory action research as a pedagogy to help a group of postprimary girls in Ireland design, coordinate, and evaluate a student-led physical activity club in an after school program in an Irish secondary school. Recently, the National Council for Curriculum and Assessment in Ireland has included cultural studies, renamed Contemporary Issues in Physical Education, as one of the five curriculum models framing teaching and learning in physical education for all students in their final 3 years of postprimary school (see www.ncca.ie/en/Consultations/Senior_Cycle_Physical_Education/LCPE_Framework.pdf).

Student-Centered Inquiry as Curriculum

Over the past number of years, Kim Oliver and her colleagues have focused on learning to listen and respond to young people using inquiry-based approaches (Oliver & Hamzeh, 2010; Oliver, Hamzeh, & McCaughtry, 2009; Oliver & Lalik, 2004a, 2004b). As a culmination of this work, Oliver and Oesterreich (2011) have introduced **Student-Centered Inquiry as Curriculum** as a way to change schools and physical education to facilitate the learning of all young people. They suggest that this change must involve engaging the students, seeking student input, listening to and responding to student ideas, inviting students to participate in the design of the curriculum to meet their individual needs and interests, and ultimately empowering students to invest in, and take responsibility for, their own learning. Oliver et al. (2010) advise that if preservice and practicing teachers are to understand how to use inquiry as a means of listening to student voices, then teacher educators must become skilled at using inquiry in their education programs and demonstrating it in applied ways in our classrooms. In other words, they suggest that the teacher education curriculum needs to redesign itself to reflect student-centered inquiry as well. From Oliver et al.'s (2010) perspective, this redesign of teacher education includes recognizing that teacher education need not be university-based and should reflect such changes as (1) a flexible syllabus should be open to change yet with enough structure to support preservice teachers; (2) physical education might be more significant to young people if taught, and learned, through concepts- or themes-based approaches rather than content-based; and (3) pedagogical issues, such as classroom management strategies, might best be taught as they occur in the classroom with young people.

Student-Centered Inquiry as Curriculum suggests that preservice teachers' learning be student centered while helping young people to be aware of physical activity opportunities available to them. Oliver et al. (2010) support the idea that preservice teachers be actively engaged with teaching young people while they themselves are learning, suggesting that the two go hand-in-hand. In order for this to occur, an environment that allows for growth among preservice teachers and youth in schools is critical. It must reflect respect, caring, and understanding among and between all involved in the teaching and learning setting.

There are four phases in the cyclical process of Student-Centered Inquiry as Curriculum: planning, responding to students, listening to respond, and analyzing responses. In order for student-centered inquiry as curriculum to work, the cyclical process must take place with teacher educators and preservice teacher at the same time it is taking place with preservice teacher and students. This allows inquiry to take place in two cycles simultaneously to impact the learning of teacher educator, preservice teacher, and student. Oliver et al. (2010) emphasize that by living a Student-Centered Curriculum as Inquiry model, and implementing it with students in a physical education setting, preservice teachers learn to be student-centered teachers.

Learning Experience 10.16

A World Café is a collaborative dialogue that draws together the collective ideas, knowledge, and perspectives of a group, shares the outcomes of discussion in an interactive forum, and develops creative insights and solutions to challenging problems. The room is set up like a café with four or five people at each table.

Discussion rounds of 15–20 minutes focused on one topic take place, with notes being kept on large poster paper. Move and share takes place after each discussion round. One person remains at the table to share what happened with the next group while the other members separate to different tables. Discussion continues and deepens with each new round until everyone has moved to each table. Finally, after all rounds are completed, groups come together for a large discussion to share their insights and ideas.

Set up a World Café with your teaching peers. Focus on social issues related to physical education, physical activity, and sport. Attempt to identify issues that might serve as the focus of a Cultural Studies or Student-Centered Inquiry unit.

Adapted from www.rainmaker-coaching.co.uk/worldcafeknowledgecafe

Kinchin and O'Sullivan (2010) note that, "there is little to no 'curricular space' for consideration of the role of sport and physical activity in students' lives, or how individual, community and societal factors enhance or inhibit personal and sustained commitments to lifelong healthy lifestyles" (p. 345).

Learning Experience 10.17

Given the description of the cultural studies model and the published national standards or outcomes in your country, identify the specific standards that are either a primary emphasis with this model, a secondary emphasis, or, if applicable, not emphasized at all. Provide a rationale for each standard included.

Health and Wellness Models

It is Monday morning and students come to physical education prepared to self-assess their progress on developing cardiovascular fitness in a physical activity of their choice. Each student has set a personal goal and determined their training heart rate zone necessary to reach that goal. Students enter the gymnasium from the changing rooms and pick up their heart rate monitors from the rack, get them on and secure, and begin to warm up in various activity groups. Those who have selected jogging head outdoors while the step aerobics group begins low-level stepping. The inline skaters move to their workout area while the basketball players begin activity. They warm up until their heart rates reach their self-determined training zone and they then attempt to maintain this level for 20 minutes. Warm down is done as a group as students interact and talk about how they felt during activity. Students download the information from their monitors to the class computer; note on their own physical activity cards how many minutes they spent below, at, or above their training zone; and make notes in their physical activity journal. They will take time to reflect on their performance and how well they are working toward achieving their goals.

Historically, physical fitness has been regarded by some as the major goal of physical education. In the United States, part of this was an outgrowth of poor youth fitness for the purpose of military readiness. Physical education thus became a prime vehicle to improve youth fitness. As exercise physiology evolved as an exercise science subdiscipline, this goal was coupled with an emphasis on strenuous activity that adhered to frequency, intensity, and duration guidelines. Such physical education classes tended to either focus on one or two aspects of fitness in a single session, which were often said to be overly strenuous and boring, resulting in young people being disheartened, or involved merely an introductory fitness segment (i.e., calisthenics) that did little more than warm young people up for activity. More recently, our conceptions of fitness education have changed and, as a result, so have the outcomes we expect from what was known as fitness education. Today, physical education programs are focused primarily on giving students the knowledge and skills to make independent decisions on physical activity choices and the desire to choose regular participation over a sedentary lifestyle. Corbin, Pangrazi, and Welk (1994) provided an excellent summary contrasting these two fundamentally different "exercise prescription model" and "lifetime physical activity model" perspectives.

> *Although programs using continuous high intensity (high heart rate) activity are not physiologically harmful to children, they are not the most appropriate for children. It is possible, given what we know about effort/benefit ratios and developmental needs of children that such activity can decrease rather than increase motivation for future activity.*[2]

The main goal of this more recent curricular focus is to provide young people with the skills and knowledge that will prepare them to develop and maintain lifetime physical activity. Lack of physical activity, rather than poor physical fitness, has been identified as a cardiovascular risk factor, hence, the health-related focus. A lack of physical activity in combination with poor eating habits has resulted in a high number of children and youth being overweight or obese. With this in mind, physical activity initiatives have been developed internationally and are being implemented with the goal of educating the public on the importance of physical activity and to get people moving. In the United States there are numerous initiatives sponsored by the President's Council on Physical Fitness (see www.fitness.gov), the National Physical Activity Plan (see www.physicalactivityplan.org), the Active Schools Acceleration Project (see www.activeschoolsasap.org/about/asap), and the Let's Move Active Schools program (see www.letsmoveschools.org), to name a few. In other countries similar schemes are being implemented, such as Active School Flag (see www.activeschoolflag.ie) and Get Ireland Active (see www.getirelandactive.ie) in Ireland, the Physical Education and Sport Strategy for Young People in the United Kingdom (see www.education.gov.uk/publications/standard/Physicaleducation/Page1), and the Active Schools program in both Scotland and New Zealand.

In response to the consequences of inadequate physical activity and poor eating behavior, the Centers for Disease Control and Prevention (CDC) in the United States published a set of evidence-based guidelines that reflect research conducted between 1996 and 2009, combine healthy eating and physical activity, and target primary and postprimary schools (see **Box 10.5**). Recognizing that all guidelines might not be appropriate for every school, the CDC encourages schools to assess the needs of the school and available resources in determining which are most feasible for their context.

BOX 10.5 School Health Guidelines to Promote Healthy Eating and Physical Activity

- Guideline 1: Use a coordinated approach to develop, implement, and evaluate healthy eating and physical activity policies and practices
- Guideline 2: Establish school environments that support healthy eating and physical activity
- Guideline 3: Provide a quality school meal program and ensure that students have only appealing, healthy food and beverage choices offered outside of the school meal program
- Guideline 4: Implement a comprehensive physical activity program with quality physical education as the cornerstone
- Guideline 5: Implement health education that provides students with the knowledge, attitudes, skills, and experiences needed for lifelong healthy eating and physical activity
- Guideline 6: Provide students with health, mental health, and social services to address healthy eating, physical activity and related chronic disease prevention
- Guideline 7: Partner with families and community members in the development and implementation of healthy eating and physical activity policies, practices and programs
- Guideline 8: Provide a school employee wellness program that includes healthy eating and physical activity services for all school staff members
- Guideline 9: Employ qualified persons, and provide professional development opportunities for physical education, health education, nutrition services, and health, mental health, and social services staff members as well as staff members who supervise recess, cafeteria time, and out-of-school-time programs

Reproduced from Centers for Disease Control and Prevention. (2011). School health guidelines to promote healthy eating and physical activity. *Morbidity and Mortality Weekly Report, 60*(RR–5), 1–76. Available from www.cdc.gov/mmwr/pdf/rr/rr6005.pdf

Concepts-Based Fitness and Wellness

Physical education should do more than merely provide students with opportunities to be physically active and develop

[2] Reproduced from Corbin, C. B., Pangrasi, R. P., & Welk, G. L. (1994). Toward an understanding of appropriate physical activity levels for youth. *President's Council on Physical Fitness and Sport Research Digest, 1*(8).

a level of personal fitness. Its educative responsibility is to also provide students with the knowledge and skills to make positive, independent decisions and physical activity choices. As McConnell (2010) noted, in **Concepts-Based Fitness and Wellness** the teacher's focus should be on the process of physical activity rather than the outcome of students achieving physical fitness. In other words, it is critical to help young people gain the knowledge and skills needed to develop and sustain a physically active lifestyle over the lifespan. With the limited time students have in physical education, it is not possible for them to be physically active at a moderate to high level and also learn the concepts and principles that guide them in developing physical activity habits. This suggests that the onus is on physical education to motivate and educate young people to make informed and positive physical activity choices outside of the school day. Young people must ultimately take responsibility for their own physical activity lifestyle, daily physical activity habits, and choices that impact their well-being. Corbin and Lindsey (2007) provided a description of this progression as students take responsibility for their own activity choices as the "stairway to fitness" (see **Figure 10.4**), which helps to focus learners on making appropriate physical activity decisions.

In order to teach young people the knowledge and skills necessary to choose an active lifestyle, concepts-based fitness and wellness education is designed around themes or concepts from one of three categories, *foundational* (setting of physical activity goals, self-assessment, components of health-related fitness), *behavior change* (time management, social support), and *wellness concepts* (relaxation techniques, nutrition). Themes and concepts are introduced and

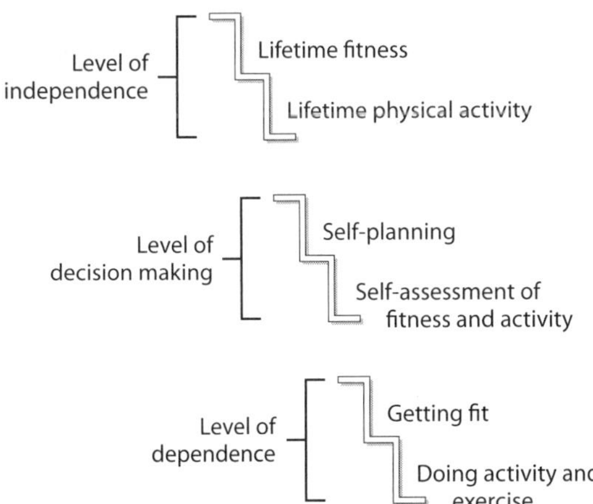

FIGURE 10.4 The stairway to lifetime fitness.
Adapted with permission from Corbin, C., & Lindsey, R. (2007). *Fitness for life* (updated 5th ed.), p. 14. Champaign, IL: Human Kinetics.

developed through a series of classroom-focused concepts days that are applied and reinforced through activity days. Activity days typically involve activity-based lab sessions focused on lifetime activities and sports. Students make personal choices on which they will take part in and self-assess the various concepts being explored. Corbin and Lindsey's (2007) Fitness for Life uses a concept-based model and is one of the most well-known and frequently used curricula in this area. This particular model now also includes versions for use with primary and early postprimary students (Corbin, Le Masurier, & Lambdin, 2007; Corbin, Le Masurier, Lambdin, & Greiner, 2010).

Health Optimizing Physical Education (HOPE)

Health Optimizing Physical Education (HOPE) includes the five components of a Comprehensive School Physical Activity Program (CSPAP) (see www.aahperd.org/naspe/publications/teachingTools/cspa.cfm). CSPAPs, as outlined by NASPE (2011), include (1) quality physical education, (2) school-based physical activity opportunities throughout the day (i.e., before, during, and after the school day), (3) school employee wellness and involvement, (4) physical activity in the classroom, and (5) family and community involvement. Metzler, McKenzie, van der Mars, Barrett, and Ellis (2013) indicated the primary goal for HOPE is for "learners to acquire knowledge and skills for lifelong participation in physical activity for optimal health benefits" (p. 24). In order to achieve this goal with the amount of time young people spend in school, Sallis and colleagues (2012) suggested that school physical education is the most likely setting for youth to be prepared for an active lifestyle while also enjoying a sufficient amount of physical activity during in-school hours. Stensel, Gorley, and Biddle (2008) argued that physical education is a setting where children and youth have the opportunity to participate in physical activity, time to practice basic motor skills, and the ability to gain competence in more advanced movement forms through guided practice by a qualified teacher, which leads to increased interest in physical activity and ultimately improves all aspects of fitness (physical, mental, emotional, and social). An additional point worth noting relates to the relationship of physical education and physical activity with academic performance, especially in light of efforts to improve academic performance of children and youth. A comprehensive review of the evidence surrounding this relationship indicates that time in physical education and physical activity can affect academic behavior and achievement positively (Centers for Disease Control and Prevention, 2010). In a similar review, Trost and van der Mars (2009) concluded that,

- Decreasing (or eliminating) the time allotted for physical education in favor of traditional academic subjects does not lead to improved academic performance.

- Increasing the number of minutes students spend per week in physical education will not impede their academic achievement.
- Increasing the amount of time students spend in physical education may make small positive contributions to academic achievement, particularly for girls. (p. 60)

The HOPE curriculum is based on a social-ecological model (SEM) (Lox, Martin Ginis, & Petruzzello, 2010) that suggests behavior develops as it is influenced by supportive interrelated environments (public policy, social, physical, individual surrounding contexts) in which we live. This implies the need for family and community interactions to focus on providing young people with physical activity opportunities, for teachers to work toward improving nutrition and physical activity policy in the school, and for educators to design physical education and after-school programs to educate youth about physical activity and healthy living. HOPE can be viewed at two levels, interpersonal and organizational, as a means to build and maintain these multiple supportive environments that impact young people's access to and decisions about physical activity and healthy choices.

HOPE intends to develop students' psychomotor and behavioral self-management skills as well as physical fitness by creating and providing physical activity opportunities for them throughout the day, in and outside the school physical education setting. HOPE is designed in strands as opposed to content units, with each strand identifying learning outcomes, different learners, learning activities, and assessments. **Table 10.3** provides an overview to guide design of a HOPE-based curriculum from the planning, implementation, and assessment levels. It is worth remembering that when designing a HOPE program, the primary goal of helping learners *acquire knowledge and skills for lifelong participation in physical activity for optimal health benefits* must be kept in mind. It will also become obvious that without the support and collaboration of parents, teachers, administrators, community professionals, and organizations it will be difficult to design and implement an effective HOPE program. The environment where HOPE is implemented will determine the content (high rates of physical activity, nutritional considerations), learners (students, parents, administrators, community), time (before, during, after school), place (school, home, community), and type of instruction (activity, discussion, group problem solving). An excellent example of a program to promote physical activity among children and youth is being implemented at Meadowview Elementary in Farmington, Minnesota (see www.activeschoolsasap.org/featured-schools/meadowview-elementary). The teacher, Joe McCarthy, has developed a culture of physical activity by designing and implementing three programs that supplement school physical education and provide different opportunities for students—the Jammin' Minute (an exercise program delivered to every class by a fifth-grade student to start the school day), the Running Club (designed to increase physical activity for students during recess), and the Century Club (encourages students to be active outside of school time).

Learning Experience 10.18

Using Table 10.3 to guide you, choose a learning outcome for one of the strands, and design a learning experience for each different population of learners listed and SEM level.

Health-Based Physical Education (HBPE)

Similar to the HOPE initiative, **Health-Based Physical Education (HBPE)** focuses on "pupils valuing a physically active life, so that they learn to value and practice appropriate physical activities that enhance health and wellbeing for the rest of their lives" (Haerens, Kirk, Cardon, & De Bourdeaudhuij, 2011, p. 3). HBPE is proposed by the authors as a pedagogical model and is based on the work of Jewett et al.'s (1995) curriculum models and Metzler's (2005) instructional models. HBPE was developed with the intent of providing guidance to schools on how to design their own HBPE programs to meet a specific context.

HBPE intends for students to experience physical education guided by learning outcomes that will result in physical activity participation that extends across a lifetime by drawing from the research base on transfer of learning and long-term behavioral change. Haerens et al. (2011) suggest that although HBPE is intended for use by teachers and schools, there are what they refer to as nonnegotiable aspects of the model that cannot be overlooked—key learning outcomes (value and enjoy physical activity), assumptions about learning and teaching (self-actualization and social reconstruction), and the domain priorities (affective, cognitive, and motor). They have called for a series of research-focused meetings where researchers and practitioners work towards the development of an HBPE model for physical education aimed at promoting a lifetime of physical activity (Haerens et al., 2011).

In all the **Health and Wellness models** described in this section, students are expected to choose a physically active lifestyle, apply movement concepts to their participation in physical activity, gain a level of physical fitness, and enjoy movement. For example, if students use the stairway to fitness (see Figure 10.4), they select the types of activities that fit their individual health and wellness goals, determine how to maintain their physical activity efforts, and record personal development and progress.

TABLE 10.3 HOPE Planning, Implementing, and Assessing Framework: Program Strands

Strand	Learning Outcomes	Examples of Units, Learning Activities, and Events	Learners	SEM Level
Before/during/after school extended physical activity programming	Promote high rates of moderate to vigorous physical activity (MVPA) and health-related knowledge to supplement scheduled PE program	• After-school dance • Lunch disc activities • Before-school walking club • Drop-in time in gym	• Primary and postprimary students	• Individual
Sport, games, dance, and other movement forms	To learn sport, games, dance, and other movement forms as a source of lifelong participation in physical activity	• Skill themes • Invasion and/or net games • Individual sports • Low-level initiative challenges • Outdoor programming • International dance	• Primary and postprimary students	• Individual
Family/home education	To teach parents, guardians, and other family members to promote physical activity, better diet, etc. at home and in the community	• School open house display • Parent organization presentation • How to read FITNESSGRAM • Healthy cooking courses • Behavior change strategies • School website • Accessing community resources	• Parents, guardians, other family members, and caregivers	• Individual • Interpersonal • Organizational • Policy
Health-related fitness	To promote weekly moderate to vigorous physical activity (MVPA) according to national standards To promote individual achievement of "Healthy Fitness Zone" on standardized measures	• High MVPA units • Designing a personal physical activity plan • Family physical activity strategies for home • Knowledge of health-related fitness	• Primary and postprimary students	• Individual

(*continues*)

TABLE 10.3 HOPE Planning, Implementing, and Assessing Framework: Program Strands (*Continued*)

Strand	Learning Outcomes	Examples of Units, Learning Activities, and Events	Learners	SEM Level
Diet and nutrition for physical activity	To learn and demonstrate knowledge of diet and nutrition that enhances physical activity	• Diet and nutrition for physical activity class • Parent health seminars • Analysis of school nutrition program • Consultations with school food staff	• Primary and postprimary students • Parents/guardians • School food staff • School administrators	• Individual • Interpersonal • Organizational • Community • Policy
Physical activity literacy • Consumerism • Technology • Advocacy	To acquire knowledge and appreciation that can increase and enhance participation in and enjoyment of physical activity	• School health fair • Guest speakers from the physical activity business community • Guest speakers from community advocacy organizations • Seminar on finding web resources for physical activity • Seminar on buying physical activity equipment and clothing	• Primary and postprimary students • Parents/guardians • Other teachers • School food staff • School administration • Community organizations	• Individual • Interpersonal • Organizational • Community
Integration of HOPE across all school subjects (includes recess)	To increase non-physical education teachers', administrators', and school staff's knowledge of and support for children's physical activity and improved dietary habits	• Integrated content units across the school curriculum • Classroom activity breaks (e.g., Take10!) • Seminar on promoting high physical activity at recess • Workshop on recess socialization	• Primary and postprimary students • PE teachers • Other teachers • School administration	• Individual • Interpersonal • Organizational

Modified from Metzler, M., McKenzie, T., van der Mars, H., Barrett, S., & Ellis, B. (2013). A comprehensive school physical activity program called HOPE (health optimizing physical education). Part 1: Establishing the need and describing the curriculum model. *Journal of Physical Education, Recreation, and Dance, 84*(4), 41–47. Reprinted by permission of the publisher (Taylor & Francis Ltd., http://www.tandf.co.uk/journals).

Learning Experience 10.19

Given the description of the Health and Wellness model and the published national standards or outcomes in your country, identify the specific standards that are either a primary emphasis with this model, a secondary emphasis, or, if applicable, not emphasized at all. Provide a rationale for each standard included.

Designing a Coherent Primary and/or Postprimary Multimodel Curriculum

Individual teachers, or groups of teachers within one building, may select from these curriculum models and provide a successful and effective physical education program for their students. However, if children and youth are to leave our programs after postprimary school as physically educated individuals, then all programs in which they participate must have a distinct focus, and be exciting, challenging, relevant to their needs, and designed to achieve the "physically educated" goal. Each of the curriculum models we described meets one or more of the NASPE K–12 content standards. None alone meets all the standards. This suggests that a coherent primary/postprimary **multimodel curriculum** might be designed to achieve all the standards and build upon the skills, knowledge, attitudes, and behaviors outlined within them.

Teachers can design a multimodel curriculum that reflects their perspective on where each standard is best emphasized to meet the varying needs and interests of their diverse populations. It takes communication among teachers in a school at a particular level (primary or postprimary) and/or within a school district across the entire program to achieve this outcome. How do we make it work? What steps do we need to take? Once teachers at each level have determined the goods of physical education, the NASPE content standards (in the United States) or learning outcomes/goals (in other contexts) become the next step. As a group, teachers can reflect on what these standards/outcomes might look like at the primary and postprimary levels. Where should the emphasis be placed? Which are most appropriate for each level of learners? What is important or of interest to youth at each level? Once teachers come to some type of collective agreement, they are beginning to describe the criteria that will guide program development at each level and allow selection of a curriculum model(s) to achieve its success. **Table 10.4** shows two examples of what a group of teachers

TABLE 10.4 Standards by Level

Example 1		
Primary priorities	Standard 2	Applies knowledge of concepts, principles, strategies, and tactics related to movement and performance
Postprimary (middle) school priorities	Standards 1 and 5	Demonstrates competency in a variety of motor skills and movement patterns and recognizes the value of physical activity for health, enjoyment, challenge, self-expression, and/or social interaction
Postprimary (high school) priorities	Standards 3 and 4	Demonstrates the knowledge and skills to achieve and maintain a health-enhancing level of physical activity and fitness and exhibits responsible personal and social behavior that respects self and others
Example 2		
Primary priorities, K–3	Standard 2	Applies knowledge of concepts, principles, strategies, and tactics related to movement and performance
Primary priorities, 4–5	Standards 3 and 5	Demonstrates the knowledge and skills to achieve and maintain a health-enhancing level of physical activity and fitness and recognizes the value of physical activity for health, enjoyment, challenge, self-expression, and/or social interaction
Postprimary (middle) school priorities, 6–8	Standards 3 and 5	Demonstrates the knowledge and skills to achieve and maintain a health-enhancing level of physical activity and fitness and recognizes the value of physical activity for health, enjoyment, challenge, self-expression, and/or social interaction
Postprimary (high school) priorities, 9–10	Standards 3 and 4	Demonstrates the knowledge and skills to achieve and maintain a health-enhancing level of physical activity and fitness and exhibits responsible personal and social behavior that respects self and others
Postprimary (high school) priorities, 11–12	Standards 1 and 5	Demonstrates competency in a variety of motor skills and movement patterns and recognizes the value of physical activity for health, enjoyment, challenge, self-expression, and/or social interaction

might develop as a result of combining their collective perspectives on the importance of the new NASPE standards across a primary and postprimary program. Clearly, the physical education programs teaching toward these priorities will be quite different as the teachers interpret and unpack the standards (Lund & Tannehill, 2010) to meet the needs and interests of their students, the views of the community, and the facilities and equipment to which they have access. Every group of teachers attempting to develop a coherent curriculum could develop an equally varied, yet important, set of outcomes across or within each level.

Learning Experience 10.20

Reflect on your views on the standards that guide physical education, and prioritize them for the age level you teach.

Once a teacher, or group of teachers, has determined their interpretation of a physically educated person and outlined which standards will be the focus at each level, they are ready to select the most appropriate curriculum model(s) to achieve these goals. Which curriculum model would be a best fit for NASPE's new standard 3? The goal of participating regularly in physical activity might be achieved through a Concepts-Based Fitness and Wellness curriculum, the main goal of which is to prepare children and youth for a lifetime of physical activity. This would include the knowledge, concepts, attitudes, and skills necessary to make appropriate activity choices and monitor participation in them. Alternatively, standard 3 could be met through a well-designed and challenging Sport Education season, Teaching Personal and Social Responsibility, or the Tactical Approach to Teaching Games.

Suppose you determine that an important set of outcomes for exiting the early years of postprimary (middle) school physical education is that students will be able to think critically, develop problem-solving strategies, demonstrate respect and support for their peers, and accept physical activity challenges. Which curriculum model might provide the most appropriate means to achieve such goals? Adventure Education, with its focus on personal and group challenges, problem solving, and risk taking, could meet these outcomes.

Choice of a curriculum model provides a framework within which content decisions can be made and learning outcomes identified. Two curriculum models may be selected within one program, with students choosing the one that meets their interests and needs. Teachers may also blend three models to deliver physical education at one level. These might be mixed and matched as a means of meeting a set of goals that the students and teacher have identified as important. Each curriculum model has a place in physical education, yet is designed to allow students to achieve very different types of outcomes.

There must be alignment among our beliefs about the goods of physical education, the curriculum model we select to achieve these goods, and the match between the two. For example, if you have determined that achieving and maintaining a level of physical fitness is most critical and then select Adventure Education as your curriculum model, you would not have much alignment between beliefs and practice. But if your focus is on providing children and youth opportunities to explore the relationship among physical activity, themselves, and the larger community within which they live and select the Cultural Studies curriculum model to facilitate this, you would have a strong alignment. If your intent is helping students to become competent, skilled, and self-motivated sport participants able to manage and direct their own sport experience and you attempt to achieve this through a multiactivity program, you would again not have achieved alignment between beliefs and practice. Had you chosen Sport Education to achieve this, you would have chosen well. It is clear to see how using this framework to guide planning could result in a multimodel curriculum being developed and implemented at a school or district level.

Physical education today is faced with a dilemma, the response to which will both promote and enhance our content in primary and postprimary education or lead to its demise. Recycling our old curricula that have been used repeatedly in the past will not help us solve the problems encountered by children and youth as they negotiate our programs. Teachers need to examine the context in which they teach, come to know and understand the students who live within that setting, and determine issues of greater significance that will impact these contemporary youth. Our task is to use our knowledge and expertise to guide the delivery of physical education content while leaving open options for youth to play a role in curricular decisions.

A multimodel curriculum need not be restricted to schools and be under the sole and direct supervision of physical educators. There are countless resources and personnel in the community who are skilled, knowledgeable, and interested in working with children and youth in physical activity settings. Utilize those resources without giving up quality programming. Schools and community can work together to deliver physical education, in some cases more effectively and thoroughly, and often in a more exciting way than when either does it in isolation. Physical activity offerings not typically included in a physical education curriculum (e.g., canoeing, taekwondo, cycling) can become part of a cooperatively taught module or an off-campus program designed to meet an elective for interested students. Providing physical activity options outside the school day allows students to participate for extended periods, and access physical activity beyond the school setting, often when they are physically more alert. When developing class schedules, think beyond physical education remaining within the traditional 8-hour day and examine options that might also work, such as evenings, weekends, or even weeks during school holidays. For example, students in physical education at Sisters High School in the northwestern United States actually get to apply the outdoor adventure skills they learned in a prerequisite course when they travel to Nepal to deliver critical medical and other supplies to local citizens who live in a very remote region of the Himalayas.

CHAPTER SUMMARY

Students' voices can be solicited on the issues discussed in this chapter as well as about activity choices that best suit their personal needs and interests. These kinds of modifications broaden the scope of what we have typically seen in physical education and can be fit nicely into the goals of the curriculum models described previously. It takes creativity, a willingness to do things differently, and communication between teachers and students and teachers and facilitators available in the community.

1. Main-theme curriculum models are focused, theme-based, reflect a specific philosophy about a physical education program, provide a clear focus around the content, and aim toward specific, relevant, and challenging learning outcomes for students.
2. Through the development–refinement cycle, main-theme curriculum models are developed, tested, refined, and further tested in a variety of school settings.
3. Effective teachers who use the main-theme curricula tend to adapt them to the needs of their particular context (students, facilities and equipment, school/community ethos, and teacher beliefs and values).
4. Developmental curriculum models suggest that what, when, and how to teach depends on each individual, and is age related as opposed to age dependent. Thus, physical skills are introduced and developed in a progressive and sequential manner consistent with each individual learner.
5. Skills themes is a holistic approach that emphasizes fundamental skills and movement concepts integrated with cognitive and affective learning goals throughout lessons in applied ways.
6. Adventure Education provides opportunities for experiential learning, individual physical and mental challenges, cooperation, and problem solving while students gain confidence in, and trust in, themselves and their peers.
7. To help learners to enjoy the outdoors and understand and appreciate the environment, Outdoor Education aims toward prioritizing three types of learning: physical skills, environmental awareness, and interpersonal growth.
8. Sport Education is designed as an authentic and educationally rich sport experience within physical education where students learn to organize and manage their own sport experience. It intends to provide sequential, progressive, and realistic game-like situations with students developing into skilled and competent sport participants.
9. The Tactical Approach to Teaching Games is focused on teaching both game skills and tactics in an integrated way so that students will learn to understand what to do, when to do it, why it will help, and how to do it effectively.
10. The main goal of the Teaching Personal and Social Responsibility model is to assist young people in taking responsibility for their own development and well-being and for supporting that of others through sharing power with students so they might take responsibility for their own experiences and gradually shifting decision making from the teacher to students.
11. Cultural Studies is designed to develop young people as questioning, curious, and critical participants in sport and physical activity through reflecting on their own experiences in relation to what is happening in society and how some individuals may be marginalized by a lack of activity opportunities available in their school and community.
12. Student-Centered Inquiry as Curriculum encourages seeking student input, listening to and responding to their ideas, and engaging them in designing the physical education curriculum to meet their individual needs and interests, and ultimately for them to take responsibility for their own learning.
13. Health and Wellness curriculum models are focused on giving students the knowledge and skills to make independent decisions on physical activity choices and the desire to choose participation over a sedentary lifestyle.
14. A coherent multimodel curriculum involves matching the various curriculum models across the curriculum based on determining the value placed on physical education, choosing the important content standards at each level, and then selecting the curriculum model to match these beliefs.

REFERENCES

Almond, L. (1986). Reflecting on themes: A games classification. In R. Thorpe, D. Bunker, & L. Almond (Eds.), *Rethinking games teaching* (pp. 71–72). Loughborough, UK: University of Technology.

Bunker, D., & Thorpe, R. (1982). A model for the teaching of games in secondary schools. *Bulletin of Physical Education, 18*(1), 5–8.

Centers for Disease Control and Prevention. (2010). *The association between school-based physical activity, including physical education, and academic performance.* Atlanta, GA: Department of Health and Human Services.

Centers for Disease Control and Prevention. (2011). School health guidelines to promote healthy eating and physical activity. *Morbidity and Mortality Weekly Report, 60*(5). Atlanta: Author. Available from www.cdc.gov/mmwr/pdf/rr/rr6005.pdf

Corbin, C., Le Masurier, G., & Lambdin, D. (2007). *Fitness for life middle school.* Champaign, IL: Human Kinetics.

Corbin, C., Le Masurier, G., Lambdin, D., & Greiner, M. (2010). *Fitness for life elementary school program package.* Champaign, IL: Human Kinetics.

Corbin, C. B., & Lindsey, R. (2007). *Fitness for life teacher's edition* (5th ed.). Champaign, IL: Human Kinetics.

Corbin, C. B., Pangrazi, R. P., & Welk, C. J. (1994). Toward an understanding of appropriate physical activity for children. *President's Council on Physical Fitness: Research Digest, 1*(8), 1–8. Washington, DC: President's Council on Physical Fitness.

Ellis, M. (1983). *Similarities and differences in games: A system for classification.* Paper presented at the AISEP Conference, Rome, Italy.

Ennis, C. A. (2003). Using curriculum to enhance student learning. In S. J. Silverman & C. A. Ennis (Eds.), *Student learning in physical education: Applying research to enhance instruction* (2nd ed., pp. 109–127). Champaign, IL: Human Kinetics.

Enright, E., & O'Sullivan, M. (2010a). Can I do it in my pajamas? Negotiating a physical education curriculum with teenage girls. *European Physical Education Review, 16*(3), 203–223.

Enright, E., & O'Sullivan, M. (2010b). Carving a new order of experience *with* young people in physical education: Participatory Action Research as a pedagogy of possibility. In M. O'Sullivan & A. MacPhail (Eds.), *Young people's voices in physical education and youth sport* (pp. 264–285). London, UK: Routledge.

Gallahue, D. L., & Cleland Donnelly, F. (2003). *Developmental physical education for all children.* Champaign, IL: Human Kinetics.

Gilbertson, K., Bates, T., McLaughlin, T., & Ewert, A. (2006). *Outdoor education: Methods and strategies.* Champaign, IL: Human Kinetics.

Graham, G., Holt/Hale, S. A., & Parker, M. (2013). *Children moving: A reflective approach to teaching physical education* (9th ed.). New York: McGraw-Hill.

Haerens, L., Kirk, D., Cardon, G., & De Bourdeaudhuij, I. (2011). Toward the development of a pedagogical model for health-based physical education, *Quest, 63,* 321–338.

Hellison, D. (2011). *Teaching personal and social responsibility through physical activity* (3rd ed.). Champaign, IL: Human Kinetics.

Jewett, A. E., Bain, L. L., & Ennis, C. D. (1995). *The curriculum process in physical education.* Boston, MA: Brown and Benchmark.

Kinchin, G., & O'Sullivan, M. (1999). Making physical education meaningful for high school students. *Journal of Physical Education, Recreation and Dance, 70*(1), 40–44, 54.

Kinchin, G., & O'Sullivan, M. (2010). Cultural studies curriculum in physical activity and sport. In J. Lund & D. Tannehill (Eds.), *Standards-based physical education curriculum development* (2nd ed., pp. 333–365). Sudbury, MA: Jones and Bartlett.

Kinchin, G. D. (1998). Secondary students' responses to issues of gender in sport and physical activity. *Journal of Sport Pedagogy, 4*(1), 29–42.

Laban, R. (1948). *Modern educational dance.* London: MacDonald & Evans.

Lawson, H. S. (1998). Rejuvenating, reconstituting, and transforming physical education to meet the needs of vulnerable children, youth and families. *Journal of Teaching in Physical Education, 18,* 2–25.

Lox, C. L., Martin Ginis, K. A., & Petruzzello, S. J. (2010). *The psychology of exercise: Integrating theory and practice* (3rd ed.). Scottsdale, AZ: Holcomb Hathaway.

Lund, J., & Tannehill, D. (2010). *Standards-based physical education curriculum development* (2nd ed.). Sudbury, MA: Jones and Bartlett.

McConnell, K. (2010). Fitness education. In J. Lund & D. Tannehill (Eds.), *Standards-based physical education curriculum development* (2nd ed., pp. 367–387). Sudbury, MA: Jones and Bartlett.

Metzler, M. (2005). *Instructional models for physical education* (2nd ed.). Scottsdale, AZ: Holcomb Hathaway.

Metzler, M. (2010). *Instructional models for physical education* (3rd ed.). Scottsdale, AZ: Holcomb Hathaway.

Metzler, M., McKenzie, T., van der Mars, H., Barrett, S., & Ellis, B. (2013). A comprehensive school physical activity program called HOPE—Health optimizing physical education. Part 1: Establishing the need and describing the curriculum model. *Journal of Physical Education, Recreation, and Dance. 84*(4), 23–34.

Mitchell, S. A., Oslin, J. L., & Griffin, L. L. (2003). *Sport foundations for elementary physical education: A tactical games approach.* Champaign, IL: Human Kinetics.

National Association for Sport and Physical Education. (n.d.). 2008 national teacher of the year high school. Available from www.aahperd.org/naspe/awards/peAwards/toy/08-T-Krause.cfm

National Association for Sport and Physical Education. (2011). Overview of a comprehensive school physical activity program. Available from www.aahperd.org/letsmoveinschool/about/overview.cfm

Oliver, K. L., Archuleta, J., Blazer, C., De La Cruz, K., Martinez, D., McConnell, J., et al. (2010, March). Student-centered and inquiry-based physical education teacher education. Paper presented at the American Alliance of Health, Physical Education, Recreation and Dance Conference, Indianapolis, IN.

Oliver, K. L., & Hamzeh, M. (2010). "The boys won't let us play": 5th grade *mestizas* publicly challenge physical activity discourse at school. *Research Quarterly for Exercise and Sport, 81,* 39–51.

Oliver, K. L., Hamzeh, M., & McCaughtry, N. (2009). "Girly girls *can* play games/*Las niñas pueden jugar tambien*": Co-creating a curriculum of possibilities with 5th grade girls. *Journal of Teaching in Physical Education, 28,* 90–110.

Oliver, K. L., & Lalik, R. (2004a). "The beauty walk, this ain't my topic": Learning about critical inquiry with adolescent girls. *Journal of Curriculum Studies, 36,* 555–586.

Oliver, K. L., & Lalik, R. (2004b). Critical inquiry on the body in girls' physical education classes: A critical poststructural analysis. *Journal of Teaching in Physical Education, 23,* 162–195.

Oliver, K. L., & Oesterreich, H. A. (2011, Feb.). Student-centered inquiry as curriculum. Paper presented at the Association for Teacher Education, Orlando, FL.

O'Sullivan, M., Kinchin, G., Kellum, S., Dunaway, S., & Dixon, S. (1996). Thinking differently about high school physical education. Paper presented at the AAHPERD National Convention, Atlanta, GA.

Pratt, D. (1994). *Curriculum planning: A handbook for professionals*. Toronto: Harcourt Brace.

Rovegno, I., & Bandhouer, D. (2013). *Elementary physical education: Curriculum and instruction*. Burlington, MA: Jones & Bartlett Learning.

Sallis, J. F., McKenzie, T. L., Beets, M. W., Beighle, A., H., Erwin, H., & Lee, S. (2012). Physical education's role in public health: Steps forward and backward over 20 years and HOPE for the future. *Research Quarterly for Exercise and Sport, 83*(2), 125–135.

Siedentop, D. (1980). *Physical education: Introductory analysis* (3rd ed.). Dubuque, IA: Wm. C. Brown.

Siedentop, D., Hastie, P. A., & van der Mars, H. (2004). *Complete guide to sport education* (2nd ed.). Champaign, IL: Human Kinetics.

Siedentop, D., Hastie, P. A., & van der Mars, H. (2011). *Complete guide to sport education* (3rd ed.). Champaign, IL: Human Kinetics.

Stensel, D., Gorley, T., & Biddle, S. J. H. (2008). Youth health outcomes. In A. Smith & S. Biddle (Eds.), *Youth physical activity and sedentary behavior: Challenges and solutions* (pp. 31–58). Champaign, IL: Human Kinetics.

Stiehl, J., & Parker, M. (2010). Outdoor education. In J. Lund & D. Tannehill (Eds.), *Standards-based physical education curriculum development* (2nd ed., pp. 247–269). Sudbury, MA: Jones and Bartlett.

Tannehill, D. (2007, Oct.). Involving teachers in the design of a coherent physical education curriculum. Paper presented at the Physical Education Association of Ireland (PEAI) Annual Conference, Limerick, Ireland.

Trost, S., & van der Mars, H. (2009). Why we should not cut PE. *Educational Leadership, 67*, 60–65.

CHAPTER 11 Assessment Considerations for Promoting Meaningful Learning in Physical Education

Overall Chapter Outcome

To share different definitions and types of assessment that can be used to inform the design of authentic, meaningful, and relevant assessment tools in physical education

Learning Outcomes

The learner will:

- Explain the sequential considerations of the why, what, when, who, and how of assessment
- Differentiate between assessment and grading
- Explain assessment *for* learning
- Explain how learning experiences and assessment can be the same
- Differentiate between formal and informal assessment
- Differentiate between norm-referenced and criterion-referenced assessment
- Distinguish between formative and summative assessment
- Describe alternative assessment and differentiate between an authentic assessment and a performance assessment
- Explain the roles of teacher assessment, self-assessment, and peer assessment
- Provide examples of how a grading system can match the outcomes of a program

For many years the field of physical education has been able to ignore assessment and has not been held accountable for collecting evidence on student learning in physical education. However, this is changing due to a growing interest in the physical education literature and practice regarding the necessity of enhancing student learning through appropriate, relevant, and worthwhile assessment (Chan, Hay, & Tinning, 2011; Georgakis & Wilson, 2012; Hay & Penney, 2009, 2013; Rink, 2007). Our concern is that prospective and qualified physical education teachers need to be better positioned and skilled to understand and practice effective assessment and to know how to manage the assessment data collected.

In discussing assessment in physical education, Carroll (1994) encourages us to think about five questions: Why assess? Who is going to assess? What will be assessed? When will it be assessed? and How will it be assessed? All five questions are somewhat inter-related; this chapter provides more insight into the first three questions. As a brief overview of what each of Carroll's (1994) key questions of assessment relate to:

- *Why assess?* This is addressed in understanding and appreciating the differences between formative and summative assessment and norm-referenced and criterion-referenced assessment. Both paired concepts are discussed in this chapter.

BOX 11.1 Key Terms in This Chapter

- *Alternative assessment:* An umbrella term for all assessments requiring students to generate a response. Different from a one-time, formal assessment.
- *Assessment:* A variety of tasks and settings where students are given opportunities to demonstrate their knowledge, skill, understanding, and application of content in a context that allows continued learning and growth.
- *Assessment "for" learning:* Occurs at the site of learning, shares learning goals and success criteria, supports learning through feedback, fosters self-assessment and independence, and leads to improved learning.
- *Authentic assessment:* Reflects real life, is performed in a realistic setting, and mirrors what students do outside of school.
- *Criterion-referenced assessment:* Relates performance to a given standard, allowing the teacher and student to document how well a student is mastering certain skills.
- *Formal assessments:* Tend to be standardized and controlled types of assessment.
- *Formative assessment:* Intended to provide feedback to impact the ongoing instructional process, demonstrating that learning is taking place.
- *Grades:* Report a student's performance by attaching a mark to indicate the level of performance. The grade is generally calculated by averaging the results of several different assessment measures that occur throughout a grading period.
- *Informal assessments:* Tend to be less-structured assessments that are integrated into the learning process.
- *Norm-referenced assessment:* Arises when the teacher and/or student compares performances within a group; common when conducting the more traditional forms of assessment such as skill tests and fitness tests.
- *Performance assessment:* Requires students to create something using problem solving, critical thinking, application skills, reflection, or other learned skills to demonstrate learning.
- *Summative assessment:* Provides a final judgment on learning, determining whether learning has or has not happened.
- *Traditional assessment:* Tends to refer to the use of motor skills and fitness as a form of assessment where the main goal is to train students' physical abilities and performance.

- *Who is going to assess?* This involves the teacher, student, both teacher and student, or an external moderator. The potential role of each is discussed in this chapter.
- *What will be assessed?* This is addressed throughout the chapter and can include an infinite number of possibilities including analysis, attitude, behavior, knowledge, practical performance, quality, skills, and tactics. This is further related to the discussion on formal and informal assessment.
- *When will it be assessed?* This includes considering assessing in a teaching and learning situation (discussed in this chapter under "Alternative Assessment"), postlesson, or in lessons other than physical education. In considering when to assess, the assessment can be continuous, periodic, or terminal.
- *How will it be assessed?* This includes a selection of traditional assessments (e.g., skill tests, written tests, fitness tests) and performance assessments (e.g., portfolio, projects, game play, journals).

Learning Experience 11.1

Reflect back on your experience of school physical education as a student and your exposure to assessment in physical education. In instances where you can remember assessment being part of your physical education experience, consider why the assessment was being carried out, who conducted the assessment, where the assessment took place, when you were assessed, and how you were assessed. If you cannot remember assessment being carried out, can you identify possible instances where it could have complemented your physical education experiences? Use the prompts in **Box 11.2** to aid your thinking to be like that of an assessor.

BOX 11.2 A Guide to Thinking Like an Assessor

Focus on determining whether students have really grasped a concept or topic.

- Tell students what they need to learn and why it is important.
- Teach students what you told them they needed to learn and make it applicable and challenging.
- Test students on what you have taught them and they have practiced.

This chapter intends to share with the reader not only the way(s) in which assessment determines what students should know and be able to do (Lund & Tannehill, 2010) but also the ways in which assessment is about gathering, interpreting, and using information about the processes and outcomes of learning. In backward design there are three stages: (1) plan your results, (2) develop assessments, and (3) plan instruction. Designing appropriate and worthwhile assessments is the essence of backward design and instructional alignment, encouraging us to measure what we value and value and act on what we measure. Assessments should match what you want students to know and achieve and what they were taught and practiced.

Learning Experience 11.2

Consider the following two assessment scenarios for the stated learning outcome and determine which of the two is more appropriate, relevant, and meaningful as a measure of the learning. On what grounds do you make the decision?

Learning outcome: For learners to be able to participate successfully in a game of doubles tennis

Scenario: Students undertake a 6-week unit of tennis, meeting once every week for 60 minutes. Throughout the unit students are given the opportunity to progress from singles to doubles matches; are introduced to the skills of the serve, forehand, and backhand; and, when relevant, tennis rules and protocols are introduced and reinforced.

- *Assessment 1*: At the close of the tennis unit, a true/false and multiple-choice examination on rules and protocols is administered, followed by a series of skills tests on key skills necessary for game play, including the serve, backhand, and forehand.
- *Assessment 2*: Several times throughout the tennis unit, students work with a partner to assess and record their success on a set of skills (serve, forehand, backhand) when performed in singles and doubles matches. Once per week, when students are playing in a tennis match, the duty team keeps records of their skill at playing (game tactics), interacting appropriately with their partner (verbal support and encouragement), selecting and performing game tactics (game statistics), following the rules governing tennis (violations tally), and enjoying the competition whether they win or lose (verbal comments and demeanor). Finally, students maintain a progress journal highlighting aspects of the game they are performing well and areas that need improvement. They set goals for their performance in an attempt to improve their weaknesses and maintain their strengths.

If you selected the second assessment as being more appropriate, you are correct. This more authentic assessment provides a holistic picture of students in a real-life situation, as opposed to only a glimpse of what they can do in an isolated and controlled setting. The second scenario provides the learners with feedback to improve performance while allowing them to see where they stand in relation to the goal of playing successfully in a tennis match.

Assessment and Grading

When you hear the term *assessment* do you think of grades? They are, in fact, related, yet quite different. Grades are a reality of schools. **Grades** report a student's performance by attaching a mark to indicate the level of performance. The grade is generally calculated by averaging the results of several different assessment measures that occur throughout a grading period (e.g., homework, quizzes, and projects). Grades are intended to communicate to students how they are doing relative to course expectations and serve as a motivator for future effort, to inform parents of how their child is performing in a course, and to provide a yardstick for school management to examine program effectiveness. Although the intent of grading is appropriate, most of those involved with the grading process (teachers, students, and parents) are not satisfied with how grades are used, especially in physical education. In physical education, grades are generally not based on a series of performance measures that spans an extended period of time, but rather tend to reflect one-shot assessments that occur at the close of a unit of instruction. Teachers tend to grade students using a variety of variables other than skill performance or knowledge. Sometimes physical education teachers are prohibited from grading on performance or pass/fail is the standard. Most frequently, students are graded on participation, attitude, behavior, and attendance (Lund, 1992). In other words, physical education teachers tend not to grade on learning or performance. Teachers not only do not grade on learning but also typically do not assess students in physical education in any substantive way. Several reasons have been noted to explain why physical education lacks a culture of assessment (Lund & Veal, 2008). Explanations for this critical shortcoming range from physical educators reporting feeling ill-prepared to conduct sound assessment of student learning, to poorly designed skills tests that lack validity, to the subject of physical education not being on par with classroom subjects for which there are state or national exams annually. It has also been suggested that preservice teachers need to be adequately trained to conduct meaningful and appropriate assessment that can be incorporated into physical education lessons (Goc Karp & Woods, 2008).

Assessment refers to a variety of tasks and settings where students are given opportunities to demonstrate their knowledge, skill, understanding, and application of content in a context that allows continued learning and growth. Although assessment and grading tend to go hand-in-hand and are frequently considered synonymous, you can see that they are not. To overcome this perception of sameness, we must learn to view and use assessment for purposes other than testing and evaluation. Teachers must be taught that well-designed and thought-out assessments throughout a unit of work can improve the quality of teaching and increase the amount of learning that occurs on a daily/weekly basis. Assessment can serve as a tool to track students' performance progress and allow them to take responsibility for their own learning and improvement. Tracking and regularly monitoring student progress results in greater motivation and achievement.

The Changing Philosophy of Assessment

Assessment is now conceived of as being more fully integrated into the teaching/learning process and providing documentation of student learning and achievement. This move emphasizes meaningful learning outcomes and performance-based assessments that are significant, reflect real-life situations, and involve students in worthwhile and relevant tasks.

The stronger the link between assessment and learning outcomes, the higher student achievement will be. This suggests that stating goals, providing learning experiences that allow students to progress toward those goals, and holding students accountable for achieving those goals by integrating assessment throughout the teaching/learning process will be most effective. Does this mean that you should teach toward the assessment? If it is a good assessment that is relevant and directly measures the learning goal, then yes. For instance, if the intended outcome were for students to be able to design and perform a tumbling routine to music, then having them select the music to match their choice of tumbling elements would be appropriate. Allowing students adequate time to practice their developing stunts to music during mock performances would increase mastery and integration of the skills. Finally, having a class performance of tumbling routines as the culminating event would match the intended outcome and would directly measure what they have learned and practiced. In another scenario, the learning outcome might be for students to recognize their feelings of anger or frustration in physical activity settings and to control/manage those emotions in a constructive way. We might select an assessment that allows them to reflect upon their feelings, identify them, and keep a journal of what brought those feelings on and how they handled the situation. This requires that students learn how to recognize their personal feelings and the behaviors and actions that reflect them, and to develop a habit of noting, in a daily journal, occurrences of these instances and how they react to them. Reinforcing the concepts of big picture goal (BPG) and big picture assessment (BPA), **Box 11.3** denotes matching big picture goals and assessments that support teaching towards the assessment because the assessments presented are relevant and directly measure the success (or not) of the big picture goal.

Does this suggest that the learning experiences and assessment tasks are the same? Yes, but not exclusively. Students need to have opportunities to practice what you want them to learn and what will be assessed (what is commonly referred to as "instructional alignment"), yet practice of other innovative tasks can also be beneficial to and facilitate learning. In addition to practicing the final assessment in the previous example, students might be involved with such activities as developing a feelings collage that represents what they feel, learning to note the amount of frustration or anger they are experiencing on a feelings thermometer, or developing a

BOX 11.3 Instances Where Teaching Towards the Assessment Is Good Practice

BPG:	*BPA:*
In small groups students will design and perform a dance and share a rationale and history of the dance form.	Students design and perform a dance in small groups and describe the rationale and history of that dance form.
Students will design a personal physical activity program that will incorporate nutrition and physical activity.	Students design a personal physical activity program that will enable them to assess and monitor their physical activity levels.
Students will demonstrate responsibility for their own safety and the safety of others, through a group gymnastics performance.	During a group performance, students demonstrate responsibility to ensure self and peer safety throughout the performance.

series of flash cards that provide them with alternative solutions for handling their feelings. Practicing the complement of assessments allows a consistent accountability system to monitor student progress with interventions to improve student learning built into the process. The more realistic the performance assessment, the more students will be motivated to perform, and the result will be more learning, improvement, and success. All of this reinforces the current push toward assessment as an integral part of the teaching/learning process and what is now commonly referred as *assessment "for" learning* (Black et al., 2003; Carless, 2005). A number of studies report the enactment of assessment "for" learning in the physical education context (Casbon & Spackman, 2005; Hay, 2006; MacPhail & Halbert, 2010). Assessment "as" learning is a phrase that also refers to the active involvement of students in their own learning (Gibbons & Kankkonen, 2011).

Learning Experience 11.3

In small groups, provide additional examples to those in Box 11.3 that denote when teaching to the assessment is good practice.

Assessment "for" Learning

Assessment "of" learning tends to encompass assessment that is remote from the site of learning, measures achievement, is based on marks/grades, and is typically practiced through formal examinations. **Assessment "for" learning** occurs at the site of learning, shares learning goals and success criteria, supports learning through feedback, fosters self-assessment and independence, and leads to improved learning (Black et al., 2003).

The key principles of assessment "for" learning are (1) sharing the learning intention, (2) sharing the criteria for success, and (3) providing feedback based on the criteria for success. This involves students assessing their own learning and teaching being adjusted to take account of the outcome of assessment "for" learning. In sharing the learning intention, the teacher needs to make the learning intention clear to students in language they can understand, using a variety of methods, and involving students in decision making (e.g., how will we go about doing/learning this?). In sharing the criteria for success, teachers need to ensure that the students know the criteria against which their work will be measured, involve students in articulating those criteria, and when assessing work, sticking to the predetermined criteria. In offering feedback, teachers should (1) provide feedback on the learning task rather than on the individual, (2) suggest to students what they are aiming for (i.e., what is the bigger picture), (3) encourage students to judge their own work by how much they have learned and the progress they have made, (4) help students to understand where they are in relation to learning goals and how to make further progress, and (5) encourage collaboration among learners.

A study following the use of assessment "for" learning in physical education (MacPhail & Halbert, 2010) found that students appreciated the learning intention being shared with them, feedback, the associated assessment instruments, the structure of lessons, and the focus on learning. There was, however, some concern among the students regarding the introduction of written work within physical education. Teachers in the same study who had agreed to pursue an assessment "for" learning approach reported appreciating the benefits of (1) effective planning, (2) students experiencing ownership of their own learning, (3) the associated assessment instruments, and (4) the professional development that had resulted from being involved in assessment "for" learning. Some teachers commented on the increased investment of time that was necessary to familiarize themselves with the associated planning and preparation.

Assessment Defined

Assessment involves collecting, describing, and quantifying information about performance. In physical education, we typically see teachers assessing students on fitness tests, isolating skills in contrived settings, or awarding points subjectively for effort, dress, and participation. Fitness and skill tests tend to fail to produce information on what children might be learning in and through physical education.

The focus on assessment that authenticates student achievement demands that teachers be able to show what students are learning in physical education (Lund, 1992). This goes beyond identifying the content covered in class and requires that we be able to demonstrate (1) what students have learned, (2) what they can do, (3) how they have changed, (4) how they can share their knowledge and skills, (5) what real-life applications they can implement, and (6) how their physical activity choices reflect their status as independent learners. How can all of this be evidenced? Assessing student data to demonstrate such learning outcomes requires ongoing or continuous assessment, a focus on various types of learning outcomes, viewing assessments as learning tools, utilizing both formal and informal assessment measures, and selecting a multitude of assessment tactics and strategies.

Formal and Informal Assessment

There is a spectrum of ways to assess student performance that includes both formal and informal means. These may be viewed on a continuum from standardized and controlled assessment (formal) on one end to less-structured assessments that are integrated into the learning process (informal) on the other end (see **Figure 11.1**).

Formal assessments tend to be removed from real life and are contrived. These types of assessments may measure

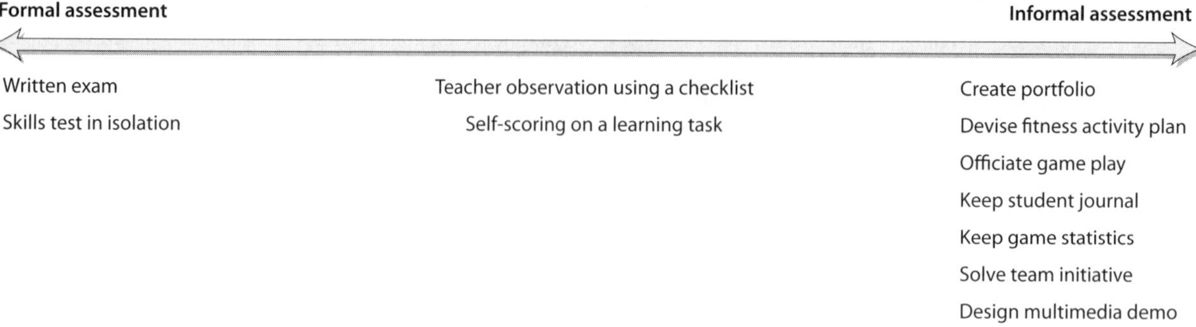

FIGURE 11.1 The assessment continuum.

student performance, but that performance cannot be generalized to other situations. We frequently see the set in volleyball assessed by the number of times a student can set the ball against the wall above a 6-foot line. Although this may demonstrate how many times the student can set the ball in this fashion, it certainly does not indicate how well the student will perform receiving a pass from a teammate and setting it to the hitter in a game of volleyball. Another student in volleyball may score well on a rules test but, when officiating a game, have difficulty recognizing violations or identifying the consequences for committing them. However, there will be instances where a formal assessment is not decontextualized from the learning outcome and is deemed to be the most relevant and authentic assessment to the identified learning outcome. For example, if the learning outcome focuses on students observing and analyzing a skill performance for correct technical elements, a formal and authentic assessment would be for the students to analyze a video performance—their own or their peers'.

Informal assessment is a means of using assessment as a learning experience to promote growth. Using our volleyball example, it would be possible to have our duty team in Sport Education keeping game statistics on the number of sets attempted as well as successful and unsuccessful sets for all students. This would provide information on what students are able to do in a game setting. As for learning and demonstrating knowledge of rules, we could have students involved in a 3 v 3 game and, when a foul occurs, stop the game and have the teacher ask students to identify the foul and the consequence. This allows students to experience the foul and its consequence in a realistic game and provides an environment in which questioning and discussion can take place for clarification.

A common difference between formal and informal assessment is whether the teacher ends up with a record (hard copy or electronic) of student learning. This record of performance can be used for a host of purposes such as to (1) track student progress, (2) provide student feedback, (3) determine the appropriateness of the manner in which a unit of work is structured, (4) provide an indication of student learning for grading purposes, and (5) conduct a program evaluation.

Learning Experience 11.4

Consider instances in which you, as a teacher of physical education, are more likely to favor either formal or informal assessment. Are there instances in physical education that lend themselves to introducing both formal and informal assessment?

Formative and Summative Assessment

Two other terms that are related to formal and informal types of assessment measures are formative and summative. Both have their place in assessment, but there is a clear distinction between assessment that is intended to provide feedback to impact the ongoing instructional process (formative) and assessment that provides a final judgment on learning (summative). One demonstrates that learning is taking place (formative), and the other determines whether it has or has not happened (summative). It is the timing of the assessment that tends to distinguish between summative and formative, with summative assessments tending to arise when teachers traditionally (if at all) develop a record of performance only at the end of a unit of work (e.g., written tests, skill tests).

Formative assessments can be both formal and informal. A formative assessment in a dance unit may be formal in that peer-observation sheets are distributed among the students for them to comment on a peer's performance of a particular dance element. An informal assessment could arise when, in watching the class work together in groups, the teacher draws attention to one group to illustrate and re-emphasize a particular dance component that is the focus of the lesson. Although there is room for both formal and informal assessments contributing to formative assessments, we contend that best practice is to increase the number of relevant formal assessments throughout the learning progress of students. This increases the recording of evidence of progress in students' learning and encourages both students and teachers to consider assessment as an integral part of the teaching and learning process.

Formative assessment is used to provide continuous, ongoing information and feedback to both students and the teacher about progress toward learning goals. These types of assessments allow teachers to identify students who are struggling or experiencing learning difficulties so that they might provide them with guidance to overcome these problems. Such assessments also allow the teacher to identify the more-able students who may require further challenges to increase their learning. Formative assessments suggest adjustments in instructional processes, help learners improve performance, tend to be informal in nature, and may also act as a learning experience or step in the learning process. The formative assessments themselves might be identical to those used in the summative measure of student learning, yet in the first instance, they provide students with practice and feedback on their progress rather than judging them as correct or incorrect. That is, a summative assessment can be an accumulation of (formal) formative assessments that have been completed throughout a unit. When assessment is used in this ongoing and continuous manner, it is directly linked to instruction and tends to motivate learners to want to improve and achieve. Formative assessment in this light seeks information to improve instruction and thus influence student learning. In summary, formative assessment serves four key purposes:

1. Provides feedback to both student and teacher to monitor learning and identify learning difficulties
2. Informs revision of teaching practice through assessment information
3. Allows learners to assess their own performance, maintain a record of their progress, and identify their own weaknesses
4. Assists in the assigning of a final grade on completion of a unit

Summative assessment occurs at the end of an instructional sequence, tends to be formal in nature, and is intended to provide an evaluation of student learning for grading or comparative purposes. In other words, summative assessment determines exit success and how well students achieved the intended learning outcomes. In line with the current emphasis on student learning as an outcome of education, summative assessment is perhaps more critical than it has been previously. This importance suggests, however, that summative assessments be adequate measures of the intended outcomes so they truly reflect learning. This certainly increases the accountability of teachers being able to facilitate and provide evidence from a range of assessments that appropriately and accurately record student performance, not only in their capacity to participate in physical activities but also in demonstrating their theoretical knowledge. **Box 11.4** notes the school physical education examination options across a number of countries and the associated assessments that are to be utilized to provide evidence of student learning.

Learning Experience 11.5

Revisit the three BPGs and associated BPAs noted in Box 11.3. For each, pair with a classmate to consider a formal assessment, an informal assessment, a formative assessment, and a summative assessment. Join up with another pairing and discuss the similarities and differences between your choices for each type of assessment, considering whether all potential assessments would be worthwhile and relevant.

Traditional Assessment

Traditional assessment in physical education (e.g., fitness tests) has been, and continues to be in some contexts, popular. As stated previously, fitness and skills tests tend to fail to produce information on what children might be learning in and through physical education. The prevalence of motor skills and fitness as a form of assessment is a reflection of a kind of physical education whose main goal is to train students' physical abilities and performance, what Tinning (1997) calls "discourses of performance" in physical education. Such discourses have been reported to have negative effects on students, and in some instances even alienate students from physical education, particularly those who are physically less able than their more-able peers. It has been suggested that an emphasis on health-related physical fitness tests rather than a sole focus on the physical fitness aspect would provide a more relevant and appropriate experience for students, in the hope that they would be encouraged to exercise/be physically active more regularly (Keating et al., 2009). Contemporary interest in health-related physical education programs is not to be confused with a revival of personal fitness testing. Rather, such programs use formative and authentic assessment strategies to engage students in understanding the goals of particular types of activity and how they can become responsible for incorporating physical activity into their daily lifestyles.

Alternative Assessment

There is a growing interest in assessment practices that are closer to teaching practice, and along with this movement, a set of assessment terms has evolved. These terms might be considered a means of viewing assessment differently and

BOX 11.4 Assessments Attached to Examination in School Physical Education

Physical Education Senior Syllabus (Australia)

A verification folio is required, which is a collection of student responses to assessment instruments on which the level of achievement is based. A student's verification folio for physical education must contain (1) six assessment instruments, three of which are physical responses and three that relate to each of the focus areas (i.e., learning physical skills, processes and effects of training and exercise, and equity and access to exercise, sport, and physical activity in Australian society), and (2) a student profile that is a summary of the student's performance on those tasks included in the folio.

A-Level Physical Education (England and Wales)

1. Two written papers consisting of three sections each: (a) Applied anatomy and physiology; (b) acquiring, developing, and performing movement skills; (c) contemporary studies in physical education and sport; (d) exercise and sport physiology; (e) psychology of sport performance; and (f) Olympic games: a global perspective.
2. Coursework where students follow a minimum of two physical activities and produce a written action plan and evaluate and appreciate a live performance in one of their chosen activities.

(Proposed) Leaving Certificate Physical Education (Ireland)

1. Personal performance project in which students are required to complete an action research project on one of three selected physical activities.
2. Written examination to examine (a) knowledge and understanding of the theoretical factors that affect participation and performance in physical activity and the relationships between them, (b) learners' concept and process knowledge in relation to the personal performance project, (c) learners' engagement with a case study designed to require learners to apply their learning in a particular physical activity scenario, and (d) clarity and coherence in management of ideas and answers.

Higher Grade Physical Education (Scotland)

1. Performance in which a student is required to develop their performance within a minimum of two physical activities.
2. Analysis and development of performance in which students are required to observe and reflect upon their performance and then consider and apply key concepts from three of four areas of analysis: (a) performance appreciation, (b) preparation of the body, (c) skills and techniques, and (d) structures, strategies, and composition.

thus allowing us to link it more closely to learning. It is necessary to understand this assessment language in order to design and implement an effective assessment model.

Alternative assessment might be considered the umbrella term for all assessments that are different from the one-shot formal tools traditionally used in the past (Hopple, 2005). López-Pastor and colleagues (2012) overview the alternative assessment approaches in order to provide a conceptual framework for assessment and a language for alternative assessment for physical educators. Alternative assessments require students to generate a response rather than choose from a set of responses. Ideally, alternative assessment involves students in actively solving realistic problems through application of new information, prior knowledge, and relevant skills. The development of the Game Performance Assessment Instrument (GPAI) for assessing learning in games (Oslin, Mitchell, & Griffin, 1998) can be regarded as an alternative to sport skill tests because it is more consistent with assessing learning within game contexts than in assessing isolated skills. These alternative assessments might then be considered either as *authentic assessments* or *performance assessments*, depending upon what the student is asked to do.

An **authentic assessment** reflects real life, is performed in a realistic setting, and mirrors what students do outside of school (Mintah, 2003). This might include submitting a scorecard to demonstrate competence on the golf course, monitoring and recording the percentage of time spent within a training heart rate zone on a 30-minute jog using a heart rate monitor, or the entire class keeping daily training logs of their physical activity record.

A **performance assessment** requires students to create something using problem solving, critical thinking, application skills, reflection, or other learned skills to demonstrate learning (Lund & Tannehill, 2010). A student could design an orienteering course for his peers to navigate. Another student might maintain a portfolio documenting her scores on successively complex gymnastics routines over the postprimary years. Other students might consult, collaborate on, and successfully complete a group initiatives project. In each case, (1) tasks can be individual, with partners, or even in groups; (2) assessment can reflect psychomotor, cognitive, or affective types of learning; (3) scoring may be determined by the student or peers or be designed by the teacher; and (4) feedback may be inherent in the task, self-imposed, or provided externally by peers or the teacher.

It is possible that authentic and performance assessments can be done in the same assessment. For example, the assessment of a gymnastic routine in a gymnastics unit is authentic in that it is performed in a realistic setting and is also a performance assessment in that it requires students to create something that demonstrates learning. Another example of an authentic and performance assessment is the use of the GPAI in a games unit where, in the context of a game, students are not only performing in a realistic setting but also being assessed on the extent to which they can accurately observe and articulate their learning of what constitutes effective decision making and skill execution in the game.

In line with the notion of assessment being ongoing, cumulative, and learning oriented, it must reflect formative, informal practices as outlined by alternative types of assessment. Whether you are selecting authentic or performance assessments because we know that assessment and learning are closely related, assessment practices must mirror the learning process. If, as has been suggested, students only learn what will be assessed, then building assessment into the learning process should increase the amount of learning that occurs.

Grading

Early in the chapter, we suggested that grading was a requirement of most schools and that physical education teachers tend to grade students based on participation, attitude, attendance, and behavior. If, however, grades are intended to communicate to students how they are doing relative to course expectations and serve as a motivator for future participation, then they must be based on learning outcomes and performance that demonstrates that learning. In other words, grades should not be based on misbehavior, presence in class, or participation. These are managerial issues that can be attended to through a well-designed preventive management system and consistent use of effective discipline strategies. This is not to say that participation should not be a part of the grading system. If our intent is for students to become physically active throughout their lives, then participation is critical. When participation is identified as one aspect of the grading system, it must be defined, specified, associated with specific outcomes, and measured in meaningful ways. Kovar and Ermler (1991) provide ideas on how to build participation into the teaching/learning process and thus give it a meaningful outcome for students:

- Stating clear participation expectations
- Having no uniform requirements for participation (except decent attire that allows the student to participate)
- Allowing students to choose activities within the class
- Soliciting student input on activities included in the curriculum
- Contracting for certain grades
- Introducing new activities frequently
- Practicing old skills in new ways to stimulate interest

If grades are going to be meaningful and useful to students, the criteria behind them must be explicit and shared with learners before instruction begins. This will allow them to understand the expectations and provide them with the opportunity to set their goals toward achieving them.

The grading system must match program outcomes. This suggests that teachers identify the learning outcome categories to be included in the grading system, determine how they will be weighted, and define the criteria that will form the basis for each portion of the grade. We have already indicated the importance of selecting assessment strategies that measure what students are expected to learn and reflect an accurate picture of their progress.

Every grading system will look different. Each is based on a specific set of learning outcomes and expectations. **Table 11.1**

TABLE 11.1 Sport Education Grading System

Learning Outcomes	Weighting	Criteria	Measurement
Competent sportsperson	40%	• Sufficient skill performance • Strategy execution • Knowledgeable games player	• GPAI • Skill checklists/rating scales • Game statistics
Literate sportsperson	25%	• Demonstrates responsibility in team roles • Team player	• Officiating rules • Role assessments
Enthusiastic sportsperson	25%	• Fair player • Active participant • Optional activity	• Journals • Participation log
Independent learner	10%	• Responsibility for own progress	• Goal setting and maintenance log

provides an example of grading systems specific to the Sport Education curriculum and instructional model. This is not to say that Sport Education is always graded in this fashion. The teacher and students will have a voice in determining what will best meet their needs and the direction they are moving within this model.

Table 11.2 breaks Adventure Education learning outcomes down using the new National Association for Sport and Physical Education (NASPE) physical education content standards. Weighting is determined according to the emphasis of the curriculum and instructional model, and criteria are identified based on the teacher's interpretation of how those would play out in the program. Assessments are then selected to reach those criteria and outcomes. This is an example of a **criterion-referenced assessment**, which relates performance to a given standard, allowing the teacher and student to document how well a student is mastering certain skills. This acknowledges the extent to which a student can complete a learning experience and provides criteria by which the student can strive for a better fulfillment of what is expected (Redelius & Hay, 2012). This is in contrast to a **norm-referenced assessment**, when the teacher and/or student compares performances within a group, and is common when conducting the more traditional forms of assessment such as skill tests and fitness tests. This results in students' performance being assessed in comparison to their peers and does not necessarily acknowledge the extent to which a student has improved his or her performance.

Learning Experience 11.6

- *Task 1*: On an 8 1/2- by 11-inch sheet of paper, draw a cat on a mat. As a group decide who has drawn the best cat on the mat.
- *Task 2*: Now on another piece of paper draw another cat on a mat. This time, the cat is to have hair, two eyes, two ears, a nose, a mouth, a tail, a collar, four legs, whiskers, and be sitting on a mat. For each of the named features score 1 point and mark your drawing out of a score of 10.

Discuss which task is norm-referencing and which is criterion-referencing.

Learning Experience 11.7

Consider in what way a physical education teacher could incorporate formative and authentic assessments when introducing students to fitness and skill tests, focusing primarily on criterion-referenced assessment.

TABLE 11.2 Adventure Education Learning Outcomes

Standard	Emphasis	Criteria	Assessment
1. Demonstrates competency in many forms and proficiency in a few movement forms	10%	• Safely participates in adventure activities • Demonstrates adequate skill to be successful in tasks	• Safety checklist • Skill performance rubric
2. Applies movement concepts and principles to the learning and development of motor skills	10%	• Applies skills in adventure environment	• Support skill rating scale • Application of concepts checklist
3. Exhibits a physically active lifestyle	10%	• Actively participates in tasks	• Teacher and self-assessment profiles
4. Achieves and maintains a health-enhancing level of physical fitness	10%	• Fit enough to successfully complete adventure tasks	• Fitness progress on tasks to match needs of activities
5. Demonstrates responsible personal and social behavior in physical activity settings	20%	• Demonstrates cooperative, responsible, and caring behavior to peers	• Peer assessment • Self-assessment • Journal • Solving team initiatives
6. Demonstrates understanding of and respect for differences among people in physical activity settings	20%	• Shows respect for all peers • Provides support to each group member • Seeks to involve everyone in tasks	• Social behavior rubric • Interactive activities checklists
7. Understands that physical activity provides opportunities for enjoyment, challenge, self-expression, and social interaction	20%	• Accepts challenges, thinks critically, problem solves, and displays enthusiasm in interactions with peers and the tasks	• Problem-solving rubric • Activity profile and log

Who Is Going to Assess?

When we focus on who conducts assessment, we can consider a number of connotations: (1) the student can self-assess, (2) the student can be involved in peer assessment, (3) the teacher can assess, and (4) the teacher and student can assess together. Carroll (1994) draws attention to a number of traits that will influence both teachers' and students' stance towards assessment in physical education. For teachers he notes that their biography, knowledge of aims and objectives, knowledge of students, and general attitude towards physical education will all come into play. For students he notes that their biography, knowledge of teacher's requirements, attitude to physical education, and knowledge of aims and objectives will affect their engagement with assessment. When both the teacher and student are involved in the same assessment, this can be completed separately or through negotiation. If helping students take responsibility for their own learning and their own physical activity experience is a program goal, then allowing them to take part in their own assessment would be important. Using a contract system for grading would be an appropriate strategy. It requires students to set personal goals, determine how to achieve them, and design the criteria to which they will be held accountable for success. Determining the expectations for each step along the way and identifying what reflects a grade at each step are up to the student. How to measure progress toward their goals can be determined either exclusively by the students or in conjunction with the teacher. Contract grading sets the stage for the learner to interact with the teacher in determining appropriate goals and how to measure them. It gives teachers the opportunity to encourage students to analyze their own performances and determine how they might improve.

Figure 11.2 is a fitness contract developed by a 15-year-old postprimary student who wants to feel better, improve his best mile time of 14 minutes, and increase the distance he can run comfortably three times per week. Regardless of the grading system you select, accurate records of student performance must be kept. A comprehensive system of maintaining these records can be created either manually or through the use of a computer program. Avery (2012) suggests that schools implement web-based assessment of students' physical education achievement, encouraging online assessment to be used by teachers, parents, and administrators. Several grading programs are available for the teacher to maintain student grades using computer software. The Easy Grade Pro program (see www.easygradepro.com) provides a variety of ways for the teacher to keep a record of student progress and design ways to improve performance. Software is available for both PCs and Mac computers as well as iPads and iPhones. Physical education software is discussed further by Castelli and Holland Fiorentino (2008).

Goal: Over the course of the term, I will improve my mile time to under 12 minutes, be able to increase my running distance to 3 miles, and enjoy participating in running activities.

I, ____________________, will fulfill the following contract to earn an A in the fitness component (three times per week):

- Warm up and warm down as part of my activity each day
- Walk/run the cross-country circuit three times per week during class
- Increase my running distance each day until I can run the entire 3-mile course
- Monitor my workouts each day using the heart rate monitor and maintain my heart rate in my training zone (60–80% of my maximum) for the running portion of my workout
- Set short-term goals for every 2 weeks to guide me through my workouts, for example:

  End of week 2: Continuous run without stopping or walking
  End of week 4: Reduce 30 seconds from mile run time
  End of week 6: Reduce 15 seconds from mile run time

- Maintain a log of my time running versus walking, 3-mile running times, weekly 1-mile time, and heart rate above, below, and within training heart rate zone
- Maintain a journal of how I am feeling each week, relating how I feel to the improvement (or lack of improvement) I am making each week

FIGURE 11.2 Sample fitness contract.

CHAPTER SUMMARY

This chapter has shared the ways assessment determines what students should know and be able to do in physical education as well as the ways assessment gathers, interprets, and uses information about the processes and outcomes of student learning. The three stages of backward design, (1) planning results, (2) developing assessments, and (3) planning instruction, have been clarified. The key to backward design and instructional alignment of learning is designing appropriate and worthwhile assessments that encourage teaches to measure what we value while valuing and acting on what we measure. Assessments should match what you want students to know and achieve and what they were taught and practiced.

1. In discussing assessment in physical education we are encouraged to consider five interrelated questions: (1) Why assess? (2) Who is going to assess? (3) What will be assessed? (4) When will it be assessed? and (5) How will it be assessed?
2. Assessment allows students to demonstrate their knowledge, skill, understanding, and application of content in a context that allows continued learning and growth.

3. Grades are intended to communicate to students how they are doing relative to course expectations, motivate them for future effort, inform parents of how their child is performing, and provide a yardstick for the administration to examine program effectiveness.
4. There are numerous instances where teaching towards the assessment is good practice.
5. Assessment "for" learning places assessment as an integral part of the teaching/learning process and documents student learning and achievement.
6. Learning experiences and assessment are the same to the extent that they allow learners the opportunity to practice what you want them to learn and what will be assessed.
7. Formal assessment tends to be removed from real life and is contrived whereas informal assessment is a means of using assessment as a learning experience to promote growth.
8. There is a clear distinction between assessment that is intended to provide feedback to impact the ongoing instructional process (formative) and assessment that provides a final judgment on learning (summative). One demonstrates that learning is taking place (formative), and the other determines whether it has or has not happened (summative).
9. Alternative assessment is an umbrella term for all assessments that differ from the traditional one-time formal tools traditionally used in the past. Ideally, it involves students in actively solving realistic problems through application of new information, prior knowledge, and relevant skills.
10. Authentic assessment is performed in a realistic setting and mirrors what students do outside of school. Performance assessment encourages students to create something using problem solving, critical thinking, application skills, reflection, or other learned skills.
11. If grades are going to be meaningful and useful to students, the criteria behind them must be explicit and shared with learners before instruction begins.
12. Criterion-referenced assessment relates performance to a given standard, allowing the teacher and student to document how well a student is mastering certain skills.
13. Norm-referenced assessment is when the teacher and/or student compares performances within a group, and is common when conducting the more traditional forms of assessment such as skill tests and fitness tests.
14. Assessment can be conducted by students self-assessing, students peer assessing, the teacher assessing students, and the teacher and student assessing together.

REFERENCES

Avery, M. (2012). Web-based assessment of physical education standards. *Journal of Physical Education, Recreation and Dance, 83*(5), 27–29.

Black, P., Harrison, C., Lee, C., Marshall, B., & Wiliam, D. (2003). *Assessment for learning: Putting it into practice.* Berkshire, UK: Open University Press.

Carless, D. (2005). Prospects for the implementation of assessment for learning. *Assessment in Education, 12*(1), 39–54.

Carroll, B. (1994). *Assessment in physical education. A teacher's guide to the issues.* London: Falmer Press.

Casbon, C., & Spackman, L. S. (2005). *Assessment for learning in physical education.* Leeds, UK: BAALPE.

Castelli, D. M., & Holland Fiorentino, L. H. (2008). *Physical education technology playbook.* Champaign, IL: Human Kinetics.

Chan, K., Hay, P., & Tinning, R. (2011). Understanding the peadagogical discourse of assessment in physical education. *Asia-Pacific Journal of Health, Sport and Physical Education, 2*(1), 3–18.

Georgakis, S., & Wilson, R. (2012). Australian physical education and school sport: An exploration into contemporary assessment. *Asian Journal of Exercise and Sports Sciences, 9*(1), 37–52.

Gibbons, S. L., & Kankkonen, B. (2011). Assessment as learning in physical education: Making assessment meaningful for secondary school students. *Physical and Health Education Journal, 76*(4), 6–13.

Goc Karp, G., & Woods, M. L. (2008). Preservice teachers' perceptions about assessment and its implementation. *Journal of Teaching in Physical Education, 27*(3), 327–346.

Hay, P., & Penney, D. (2009). Proposing conditions for assessment efficacy in physical education. *European Physical Education Review, 15*(3), 389–405.

Hay, P., & Penney, D. (2013). *Assessment in physical education. A sociocultural perspective.* Oxon, UK: Routledge.

Hay, P. J. (2006). Assessment for learning in physical education. In D. Kirk, D. MacDonald, & M. O'Sullivan (Eds.), *The handbook of physical education* (pp. 312–325). London: Sage.

Hopple, C. J. (2005). *Elementary physical education teaching and assessment. A practical guide.* Champaign, IL: Human Kinetics.

Keating, X., Harrinson, L., Chen, L., Xiang, P., Lambdia, D., Davenhover, B., et al. (2009). An analysis of research on student health-related fitness knowledge in K–16 programs. *Journal of Teaching in Physical Education, 28*(3), 333–349.

Kovar, S., & Ermler, K. (1991). Grading: Do you have a hidden agenda? *Strategies, 4*(5), 12–14, 24.

López-Pastor, V. M., Kirk, D., Lorente-Catalán, E., MacPhail, A., & Macdonald, D. (2012). Alternative assessment in physical education: A review of international literature. *Sport, Education and Society, 18*(1), 57–77.

Lund, J. (1992). Assessment and accountability in secondary physical education. *Quest, 44*(3), 352–360.

Lund, J., & Tannehill, D. (2010). *Standards-based physical education curriculum development* (2nd ed.). Sudbury, MA: Jones and Bartlett.

Lund, J., & Veal, M. L. (2008). Measuring pupil learning—How do student teachers assess within instructional models? *Journal of Teaching in Physical Education, 27*, 487–511.

MacPhail, A., & Halbert, J. (2010). "We had to do intelligent thinking during recent PE": Students' and teachers' experiences of assessment for learning in post-primary physical education. *Assessment in Education, 17*(1), 23–39.

Mintah, J. K. (2003). Authentic assessment in physical education: Prevalence of use and perceived impact on students' self-concept, motivation, and skill achievement. *Measurement in Physical Education and Exercise Science, 7*(3), 161–174.

Oslin, J. L., Mitchell. S. A., & Griffin, L. L. (1998). The game performance assessment instrument (GAPI): Development and preliminary validation. *Journal of Teaching in Physical Education, 17*(2), 231–243.

Redelius, K., & Hay, P. (2012). Students' views on criterion-referenced assessment and grading in Swedish physical education. *Physical Education and Sport Pedagogy, 27*(2), 211–216.

Rink, J. (2007). Editorial: PE teaching: It's ALL about outcomes. *p.e.links4u newsletter, 9*(7). Available from www.pelinks4u.org/archives/070107.htm.

Tinning, R. (1997). Performance and participation discourses in human movement: Towards a socially critical physical education. In J. M. Fernandez-Balboa (Ed.), *Critical postmodernism in human movement, physical education, and sport* (pp. 99–121). New York: SUNY Press.

Wiggins, G., & McTighe, J. (1998). *Understanding by design*. Alexandria, VA: ASCD.

CHAPTER 12 Appropriate Assessment Instruments in Physical Education

Overall Chapter Outcome

To encourage the design and implementation of appropriate assessment instruments/assessment tools that match meaningful outcomes identified to guide student learning and share examples of potential assessment instruments/assessment tools

Learning Outcomes

The learner will:

- Explain guiding principles in matching the assessment task to meaningful outcomes identified to guide student learning
- Identify and describe a variety of assessment measures and when they would most appropriately be used
- Discuss the possibilities of assessing through observation, including checklists, rating scales, and peer assessment
- Demonstrate how portfolios, journals, and event tasks play a role in assessment in physical education
- Consider the appropriate use of written tasks and skill tests as a form of assessing in physical education
- Explain how and why self-assessment and peer assessment are central to assessment in physical education and provide tools that encourage both
- Explain an authentic way to assess game play through the Game Performance Assessment Instrument
- Compile and use scoring rubrics/guides to establish scoring criteria
- Articulate the extent to which the chosen assessment is reliable and consistent
- Demonstrate ways in which to remember to assess

Critical to good assessment is carefully matching the assessment task to the meaningful outcomes you identified to guide student learning. The learning experiences or student assignments can be numerous and varied, as long as the choices closely reflect the intended outcomes and provide learners the opportunity to demonstrate their progress toward achievement of those outcomes. Herman, Aschbacher, and Winters (1992) provide six questions to guide development of effective assessment tasks that we have applied to a fitness example.

1. *Does the learning experience match specific instructional intentions?* If you want students to assess their levels of fitness, determine their specific fitness needs, and design a fitness prescription to guide their fitness activity program, then having them do exactly that as the assessment task would be appropriate.
2. *Does the learning experience adequately represent the content and skills you expect students to attain?* You need to determine exactly what it is you want students to be able to do and what content, knowledge, and skills it will require. In the previous example, students need to decide which fitness tests to use, evaluate their own levels of fitness based on test results and determine their needs for improvement, and be able to use fitness concepts to design an appropriate fitness prescription.

BOX 12.1 Key Terms in This Chapter

- *Assessment steps:* Encourage students to engage with a challenge and determine what they would like to be able to do related to this challenge before considering how they could best pursue these goals on a week-by-week basis.
- *Assessment wheel:* Encourages the student to record, reflect on, and map learning related to the big picture goal and to assess progress towards this goal.
- *Checklist:* A list of statements, dimensions, characteristics, or behaviors that are basically scored as yes or no, based on an observer's judgment of whether the dimension is present or absent.
- *Event task:* Simulates real life; allows multiple solutions and responses; is important, relevant, and current in an attempt to stimulate student interest; and can be completed in a single time frame.
- *Journals:* Allow students to reflect on and share their thoughts, feelings, impressions, perceptions, and attitudes about their performance, an event, an assignment, or other learning experiences.
- *Observation:* Likely to be the most frequent assessment measure, in which a teacher provides feedback, manages the classroom, and informs teaching practice. Students can also be encouraged to observe and assess a peer's performance.
- *Peer assessment:* Where students observe, make appropriate judgments, and record or provide feedback to their peers.
- *Portfolio:* A collection of student work that documents the student's effort, progress, and achievement toward a goal or goals.
- *Rating scale:* Indicates the degree or quality of the criterion to be met.
- *Scoring criteria:* Included in a scoring rubric/guide to judge a performance or product.
- *Scoring rubric:* Defines the criteria by which a performance or product is judged. Sometimes referred to as a scoring guide.
- *Self-assessment:* When students are given the opportunity to assess and modify their own performance, acknowledging that students first need to be taught how to do this.
- *Skills tests:* When designed in an authentic way, can determine performance level and provide feedback to learners.
- *Student log*: A record of performance on specific behaviors or criteria over a given period.

3. *Does the learning experience enable students to demonstrate their progress and capabilities?* This requires you to determine whether the learning experience is fair relative to expectations for prior knowledge and opportunities for students to have learned and practiced necessary skills. Critical to the previous example would be whether students have been taught relevant fitness tests and concepts related to improving components of fitness. Depending upon your intent, you could ensure that all content has been taught or provide resources to challenge students to problem solve on their own.
4. *Does the assessment use authentic, real-world learning experiences?* We know that realistic learning experiences tend to motivate learners to achieve and also provide possibilities for transfer outside of the classroom to real-world settings. If we expect young people to maintain a health-enhancing level of physical fitness, then their ability to assess and monitor their own behavior is relevant and meaningful.
5. *Does the learning experience lend itself to an interdisciplinary approach?* Frequently, realistic learning experiences cross over subject boundaries and require students to apply knowledge and skills from other domains. Fitness prescription includes determining target heart rate training range, which requires the calculation of percentages and other mathematical functions and thus asks the student to apply content from another subject area.
6. *Can the learning experience be structured to provide measures of several goals?* Most programs identify goals for learners that come from the motor/physical, cognitive, and affective domains, as discussed previously. Some learning experiences might assess students in two of these areas. During fitness testing, students may be required to interact with a partner or small group to successfully complete the selected tests. This would measure affective skills of collaboration, teamwork, and cooperation.

Alternative forms of assessment that include realistic and performance-based approaches are an ideal way to conduct continuous, formative assessment throughout the learning process. These approaches allow alignment of outcomes, instruction, and assessment, yet place new demands on both the students and the teacher. Students must take responsibility for demonstrating their learning, and the teacher must design realistic assessments to allow this to occur. Alternative assessments are established by determining meaningful outcomes prior to beginning instruction and then teaching toward and assessing the desired learning. The learning experiences should also provide a meaningful and continuous picture of student progress, rather than pieces of discrete information.

In the same way that some content remains unspecified until the learners themselves interpret it, the same is often true of assessment. Not all knowledge, skills, behaviors, values, attitudes, or changes students make can be quantified and measured. As Kirk (1993, p. 252) indicated, "What students say, what they write, the adaptations and changes they make to their actions over time, are all appropriate and relevant evidence of learning."

We need to ask, "What must my students demonstrate to show they have a grasp of the content?" and "What will successful student understanding look like?" This again suggests that the final assessments and scoring criteria be thoughtfully developed and then become the focus of instruction and student learning experiences. We also might ask, "Are there ways that students can demonstrate their skill and knowledge that are unique to them and their own personal style and ways of learning, or must all students show what they know in the same way?"

In recent years, physical educators have learned numerous methods to monitor student progress, retention, understanding, and physical performance that we demonstrate through the various curriculum and instruction models. Each of the physical education curriculum and instruction models provides abundant opportunities for authentic assessment to measure progress toward meaningful outcomes. But the teacher need not be the only one who assesses student performance. If assessment is designed as continuous and formative and to serve a variety of purposes, then the teacher, the student, or even a peer can play a role in the assessment process. We describe a variety of assessment tasks and link them to meaningful outcomes to clarify assessment tasks appropriate for use within the various models. The remainder of the chapter focuses on a variety of assessment measures and when they would most appropriately be used in physical education.

Observation

You have heard the old saying that "teachers have eyes in the back of their head." This suggests that teachers know what is going on in their classrooms ("with-it-ness"), which students are having difficulty, who is successful, and when an event results in student off-task behavior. Experienced teachers frequently use **observation** in their classes (1) as a means to provide feedback, (2) to manage the classroom, (3) to inform teaching practice, and (4) as a tool for students to assess a peer's performance. As teachers become comfortable using observation, they are often able to convert their informal observations into criteria that they can then formalize and record using a checklist or **rating scale**. These tools ease the collection of information on student progress.

Learning Experience 12.1

Consider the extent to which physical education teachers use observations as a means to provide feedback, to manage the classroom, and to inform teaching practice. Provide examples for each and a reason why observation tends to be the favored form of assessment for physical education teachers.

An observation tool can be used as a momentary time sample (see **Figure 12.1**). In this instance the teacher has chosen five students who they intend to observe at six particular instances throughout the class to ascertain if they are active (denoted by *A*) or inactive (denoted by *IA*). The tool can be made sufficiently small for the teacher to keep it in a pocket while teaching and pull it out to complete at various points throughout the class, denoting if the student is active or inactive by circling *A* or *IA*, respectively. Or, if teachers have a device such as an iPad they could employ a similar version of this form in spreadsheet format.

In using the momentary time sampling tool, a teacher may note that one particular student tends to be inactive throughout the class. If this occurs, the teacher can then focus on that student over a number of subsequent lessons to determine patterns in his or her participation (see **Figure 12.2**), providing evidence on lack of participation before talking with the student in question. It is important that focusing on one individual's participation is not at the detriment of the teacher providing meaningful and worthwhile physical education experiences for all other students in the class.

Changing the focus of Figure 12.1 from active and inactive to communicative (denoted by *C*) and uncommunicative (denoted by *UC*) or cooperative (denoted by *C*) or uncooperative (denoted by *UC*) (see **Figure 12.3**) provides a teacher

	1	2	3	4	5	6
Thomas	A IA	A IA	A IA	A IA	A IA	A IA
Fiona	A IA	A IA	A IA	A IA	A IA	A IA
Therese	A IA	A IA	A IA	A IA	A IA	A IA
Aoife	A IA	A IA	A IA	A IA	A IA	A IA
Robert	A IA	A IA	A IA	A IA	A IA	A IA

FIGURE 12.1 Momentary time sampling for involvement in physical activity.

	Activity	How long?	Enjoyment
Session 1			
Session 2			
Session 3			
Session 4			

FIGURE 12.2 Participation log.

	1	2	3	4	5	6
Thomas	C UC	C UC	C UC	C UC	C UC	C UC
Fiona	C UC	C UC	C UC	C UC	C UC	C UC
Therese	C UC	C UC	C UC	C UC	C UC	C UC
Aoife	C UC	C UC	C UC	C UC	C UC	C UC
Robert	C UC	C UC	C UC	C UC	C UC	C UC

FIGURE 12.3 Momentary time sampling for communication or cooperation.

observation tool that could be used to assess the extent to which students are achieving a learning outcome related to Outdoor Education, such as "Students will work together to achieve the goals of the overnight trip," and the associated elements of communication and cooperation.

Learning Experience 12.2

How could you ensure that the collection of data on a select number of students throughout a class would not be detrimental to the experiences of other students in the same class?

Additional examples of observation tools include how to document minutes of student moderate to vigorous physical activity during physical education (Surapiboonchai et al., 2012), assessing personal and social responsibility within a physical education class (Wright & Craig, 2011), measuring motor skills in physical education classes (Ericsson, 2007), and the use of teacher and student observation checklists in primary school physical education (Connor, Mulcahy, Ní Chróinin, & Murtagh, 2011).

Checklist

A **checklist** is a list of statements, dimensions, characteristics, or behaviors that are basically scored as yes or no, based on an observer's judgment of whether the dimension is present or absent. A checklist may be used for process types of behavior (e.g., followed correct sequence of steps) or, more typically, as a product measure (e.g., critical elements performed). Whether process (sequence) or product (outcome) criteria are used to measure performance, the teacher, peer, or other observer determines whether the criteria were exhibited. A checklist makes criteria for performance public and allows students to clarify what they are expected to do and even to play a role in their own learning. A checklist, however, provides only limited information on whether a specific criterion was demonstrated and nothing about the quality of the performance.

The checklist shown in **Figure 12.4** allows the student, teacher, or peer to indicate whether the appropriate steps were taken in resolving a conflict situation in class. It does

	Situation 1			**Situation 2**		
	Self	Teacher	Peer	Self	Teacher	Peer
A. Ask "What's the problem?"						
B. Brainstorm possible solutions						
C. Choose the best solution						
D. Do it!						

FIGURE 12.4 Conflict resolution strategies checklist.

	First putt		Second putt		Third putt	
	Yes	No	Yes	No	Yes	No
Balanced						
Square blade						
Comfortable grip						
Still body						
Eyes over ball						
Smooth, even stroke						

FIGURE 12.5 Putting critical element checklist.

not provide information about the tone of voice or nonverbal mannerisms that might instigate problems. If students are unable to resolve their own problems in class after consulting the conflict resolution strategies checklist, but the teacher finds that all the steps are being followed, then additional information is needed. This might be obtained by collecting anecdotal notes of what behaviors and language characterize the interactions during the process.

Checklists also can move the focus away from process and turn it toward outcome (e.g., were the elements present or not present in the performance?). **Figure 12.5** shows such a checklist for putting in a golf unit. Checklists that are too complex and cumbersome may actually decrease the amount of accurate information that can be obtained, especially if they are being used for peer assessment or a student viewing his or her own performance on video.

A checklist could be used to assess two outcomes related to Outdoor Education, "Students will select appropriate clothing to suit the weather on an overnight trip" (see **Figure 12.6**) and "Students will participate in an overnight trip following 'leave no trace' concepts" (see **Figure 12.7**).

	Yes	No		Yes	No
Socks (5–6 pairs)			Rain pants		
Walking shoes			Sweats		
Comfortable camp shoes			Long johns		
T-shirt/tank top			Long-sleeve shirt		
Hoodie/fleece jumper			Turtleneck		
Gloves/mittens			Scarf		
Wind breaker			Warm hat		
Rain jacket			Underwear		

FIGURE 12.6 Equipment checklist.

Items to check off	Completed	Not completed
Fire is out and ashes are gone		
Tent is put away properly		
All garbage has been thrown away		
Personal items are packed and ready to go		
All hiking/climbing equipment is put away		
Food items have been packed or thrown away properly		

FIGURE 12.7 Clean site checklist.

Learning Experience 12.3

In a small group, consider an appropriate checklist for two learning outcomes related to Outdoor Education, "Students will work together to achieve the goals of an overnight trip" and "Students will successfully participate in hiking and orienteering." Share the ways in which the suggested checklist for each learning outcome is appropriate. Is it possible to have multiple appropriate checklists for one learning outcome?

Other examples of checklists include a checklist for physical education teachers to promote the physical activity and fitness level in the physical education program (Hill & Turner, 2007) and an observation checklist of the developmental stages of components for repetitive hopping (Nonis, Parker, & Larkin, 2004).

Peer Assessment Observation

We frequently see formal and informal **peer assessment/** observation experiences used in physical education as part of peer tutoring, to keep a record of the number of appropriate skill attempts, to provide feedback on students following a routine, or to indicate if critical features have all been included. Peer observation/assessment is a central part of peer tutoring (also referred to as *peer-assisted learning*). Peer tutoring has a rich empirical base in terms of its effectiveness in bringing about student learning in education, special education, and physical education (Greenwood, Maheady, & Carta, 1991; Ward & Lee, 2005). Peer tutoring can be used in a variety of ways. For example, it might be used where just two students are paired, with one partner trained to assist the other to complete a learning task. Class-wide peer tutoring (CWPT) is an approach in which the entire student group is placed in pairs and the roles of tutors are reciprocal in nature (Johnson & Ward, 2001). A third version of peer tutoring is called *peer-mediated accountability* (PMA). PMA is much like CWPT but with one critical difference. In the case of PMA, the tutee is provided knowledge of the result of the practice but no feedback on the technical execution. PMA has been shown to be highly effective in increasing the amount of practice that students get during the lesson compared to traditional lessons (Ward & Lee, 2005). Notice that peer tutoring is an excellent means of ensuring that more students are getting feedback on their performance than any one teacher could ever provide to groups of individual students. One of the most attractive features of peer assessment is that both the performer and the observer learn during a peer-directed task; that is, the observer needs to be focused in his or her assessment, and this can be of help once he or she practices the skill.

If this type of assessment is going to be effective, students must know the criteria and what they look like when performed appropriately. In addition, students need to be taught how to observe, how to make appropriate judgments, and how to record or provide feedback to their peers. It is also imperative that students understand that their assessment of a peer is intended to provide feedback to improve performance. Teacher modeling of assessment is an appropriate place to begin training students to gauge performance.

Following this, they can gain practice observing and collecting data by counting a partner's appropriate skill attempts, timing some aspect of the performance, measuring the distance of an event, and then moving on to using a basic checklist and rating scale as previously described. **Figure 12.8** shows a complex checklist that requires the peer to observe a series of motor skills in a routine and make judgments on skill inclusion as they progress through the sequence.

The "stars"		Top notch	
Acknowledge the judge		Acknowledge the judge	
Body wave		Straight body stretch	
Step forward into a lunge (hold 3 counts)		One-leg balance (hold 3 counts)	
Forward roll to stand		Step into lunge (hold 3 counts)	
On incline mat			
On flat mat			
Arabesque (hold 3 counts)		Down into body sweep	
Chasse		Back walkover	
Pivot on half-turn on balls of feet		Pivot one half-turn on balls of feet	
Cartwheel to one-leg balance (hold 3 counts)		Back roll to stand	
Straight jump		Jump one half-turn	
Backward roll to stand (hold 3 counts)		Handstand (hold 3 counts)	
Stand stretch to end		Forward roll to stand stretch to end	
Acknowledge the judge		Acknowledge the judge	

FIGURE 12.8 Gymnastics compulsory routine partner checklist.

Student name	Legal	Ace	Short	Long
Player 1				
Player 2				
Player 3				
Player 4				

FIGURE 12.9 Sport Education badminton game statistics.

Students can be taught to play a more critical role in assessing performance in realistic settings. They can be taught how to serve as statisticians and maintain the official game/match statistics that serve as performance feedback to the teacher and that make up the formal record of game performance. A simple set of statistics might be kept on students' performances on the badminton smash in either singles or doubles play, as shown in the form in **Figure 12.9**.

Learning Experience 12.4

How would you teach students how to observe, how to make appropriate judgments, and how to record or provide feedback to their peers in preparing them to conduct peer assessment?

A more complete yet complex set of statistics can also be kept accurately by students once they have gained more experience. The examples in **Figure 12.10** can be used to keep one set of data (serve) on one student or that same set of data on all students. Once they become adept at maintaining this one set of data, students can move on to collecting two sets of data (serve and serve receive). This same procedure is followed for attack and set and finally the complete set of game statistics (serve, serve receive, attack, and setting) for all students using the combined statistics score sheet. This set of score sheets can be modified depending on students' ages and abilities. They can also be adapted to whatever skills and combination of skills students are using in game play. This needs to be taught, modeled, and practiced until students feel comfortable collecting game statistics and until their peers feel that the data collected are accurate and reflect their performances.

Portfolio

A **portfolio** is a collection of student work that documents the student's effort, progress, and achievement toward a goal or goals. A portfolio is a powerful tool that allows learners to take responsibility for demonstrating, monitoring, and displaying their own learning. Portfolios allow students to celebrate what they can do and to display evidence that demonstrates their success. In order to select materials to reflect their progress, students must examine their work, reflect on what it presents, and assess it relative to the portfolio goal. This self-selection, reflection, and assessment process makes portfolio development an instructional tool.

A portfolio is not, however, an assessment until several issues have been considered and negotiated: (1) an assessment purpose is determined, (2) how and what to select for inclusion are defined, (3) decisions on how they may select portfolio materials and when they may be selected are articulated, and (4) criteria for assessing either the entire collection of materials or the individual aspects of it are identified (Herman, Aschbacher, & Winters, 1992). These issues are essential for designing a portfolio task, and student involvement in them is critical if students are to take ownership of their own learning and achievement. Perhaps most crucial are decisions related to what is to be included as samples of student work and then the criteria that will define and measure that body of work. Several questions that the teacher needs to consider relate to whether progress toward a goal or improvement will be assessed and, if so, how they will be measured. If the portfolio includes a variety of materials, how will these materials be weighted in the overall assessment? Issues related to how the portfolio can be assessed are included later in this chapter. **Box 12.2** includes two portfolio assignments that could become assessments. The second was designed and implemented by a group of postprimary schoolteachers who have revised their entire curriculum to meet the needs of their changing youth population. The two goals included in Box 12.2 (of the six identified in the Moscow High School curriculum) also are the goals for the portfolio assignment.

Portfolios may take a variety of formats and utilize numerous tools. Electronic portfolios allow collection, organization,

Serve and serve receive

Serve					**Serve and receive**			
Player	Ace	Legal serve	Illegal serve	Service %	Settable pass	Legal pass	Illegal pass	Receiving %

Serve

- \+ Serve results directly in point scored, opponent unable to make legal play on ball
- 0 Serve is legal and playable by an opponent
- – Illegal serve, out of bounds, in net, or foot fault

Serve and receive

- \+ Pass goes directly to setter and is dealt
- 0 Pass is legal and playable by opponent or teammate
- – Illegal pass, out of bounds, or unplayable

Attack and set

Set					**Attack**			
Player	Assist	Legal set	Illegal set	Set %	Kill	Legal attack	Illegal attack	Attack %

Set

- \+ Set results directly in point scored by a kill set
- 0 Legal set playable by opponent or teammate
- – Illegal set, out of bounds, in net, or foot fault

Attack

- \+ Attack results directly in point scored, opponent unable to make legal play on ball
- 0 Attack is legal and playable by an opponent
- – Illegal attack, out of bounds, in net, or foot fault

Complete game statistics

	Serve				Serve receive				Attack				Set			
Player	A	LS	IS	S%	SP	LP	IP	R%	K	LA	IA	A%	A	LS	IS	S%

This statistics sheet requires the statistician to use the same scoring conventions as on the individual statistics sheets.

FIGURE 12.10 Forms for data collection.

BOX 12.2 Sample Portfolio Assignments

Adventure trust-building portfolio:

- *Goal:* To become a group member who has learned to trust and is willing to actively participate as a member of the group.
- *Portfolio purpose:* After each group activity, prepare a summary report that describes the activity: (1) what happened; (2) the role you played in that activity; (3) reactions, support, or other behaviors of your peers; and (4) how these influenced your ability to trust and feel safe in the activity. At the close of the adventure experience, you will review your summary reports, reflect upon the growth you displayed developing trust and the behaviors of your peers that facilitated this growth, and share your perceptions on this process.
- *Portfolio evidence:* Summary report including what happened, your role, interactions with others, influences on your trusting, and perceptions on the trust-building process.

Moscow High School wellness portfolio:

- *Goal 1:* Students will interpret and analyze effects of a variety of influences on their emotional health.
- *Goal 2:* Students will recognize the relationship between proper nutrition, fitness, and optimum wellness.

Portfolio evidence:

- Write journal entries to communicate stress inventory results, identify consequences related to level, identify situations that result in stress-level increases, and identify alternative responses for these situations.
- Role-play effective nonviolent strategies in potentially volatile situations, and provide a written reflection concerning personal growth as an outcome of this activity.
- Develop a personal fitness prescription that will address strengths and weaknesses in your personal fitness level, and monitor your progress toward reaching fitness goals.
- Develop and incorporate fitness and nutrition strategies for improving overall health.

Adapted from Karla Harman, Moscow High School, 1999.

and storage of a variety of types of information into an electronic file. Information may represent digital pictures, scoring rubrics/guides from different assignments, digitized video segments, text, graphics, scanned photographs, and physical activity or fitness scores. More appropriate from our perspective are the programs that allow students to create their own electronic portfolio. There are numerous electronic portfolios designed for the teacher and student to collect, store, and even revise student work. How electronic portfolios are set up and arranged in each setting depends on the hardware and software available, how time is apportioned, and the teacher's skill and comfort in teaching the necessary technology know-how to students and arranging the environment to support this type of work.

Reflection is another skill that students need to be taught to help them take responsibility for their own learning and allow them to make sense of their progress. Reflection is the process of thoughtfully examining a situation, experience, the learning process, or personal feelings and attempting to make sense of them (i.e., What do they mean? What are their implications? How might I have behaved differently?). In addition to portfolios, several other assessment tools (e.g., journals, self-assessments) require the learner to reflect on some aspect of performance in order to respond thoughtfully.

Learning Experience 12.5

Consider how you could use a portfolio to map your own development as a teacher. What types of evidence could you include that would convey your (1) philosophy on teaching, (2) student learning, (3) materials used in class, (4) feedback from students and parents, (5) professional development, and (6) level of planning?

Melograno (2000) suggests an eight-step process that can aid physical education teachers in designing portfolio systems appropriate for physical education programs. The eight steps are (1) determine general and specific purposes; (2) decide the type(s) of portfolios to be used; (3) establish an organizing framework; (4) identify construction, storage, and management options; (5) establish a process for selecting items;

(6) determine reflection and self-assessment techniques; (7) plan conference strategies; and (8) develop evaluation criteria and procedures.

Journals

Journals allow students to reflect upon and share their thoughts, feelings, impressions, perceptions, and attitudes about their performance, an event, an assignment, or other learning experiences. A journal serves as a means of describing a situation, reacting to that situation, reflecting upon your actions, and using those reflections to learn and to grow. In this sense, the journal becomes a useful learning tool that can begin to demonstrate patterns, themes, and relationships that either facilitate or inhibit development. Journal writing may be (1) conducted in class as a unit/season experience, (2) linked to a specific aspect of instruction through a homework assignment, (3) become a habit for students to develop as part of activity participation, and/or (4) be a means of helping students examine their beliefs and attitudes toward a specific topic.

Journals can take a variety of formats and intents. They might be as open as "What were your feelings about . . . ?" They may seek a response to a set of specific questions, or they may be an ongoing set of reflections on an issue or experience. To help develop a sense of confidence in movement settings, students might be asked to keep a weekly journal throughout the year in which they write about their performance in each activity and identify where they felt successful and why. In another instance, students might be striving toward a series of fitness goals and maintain a journal noting their progress toward them, barriers they encountered, and their feelings about goal achievement. In each case, journal writing involves reflection; that is, going back and recapturing thoughts, feelings, and events and interpreting what they mean personally. Student journals have been utilized to convey how postprimary students demonstrated support for and resistance to implementation of a physical education curricular initiative (Kinchin & O'Sullivan, 2003) and to explore how adolescent girls articulate their embodiment and navigate their embodied identities within the physical education context (Fisette, 2011).

Journal entries generally are not viewed as right or wrong and may include both positive and negative instances. Because journals reflect personal feelings, thoughts, and perceptions, they typically are not graded for their content. They may provide a record of student views on success and failure and information on how students process experiences. Journals can, however, be assessed for completion or by using a set of criteria that guided the journal writing itself. Care must be taken in scoring the student journal because it may tend to stifle reflection, honesty, and the sharing of personal feelings and perceptions. **Box 12.3** conveys a journal program that could be used to encourage students to reflect on and record their daily class activities.

Event Tasks

Event tasks (1) simulate real life; (2) allow for multiple solutions and responses; (3) are important, relevant, and current in an attempt to stimulate student interest; and (4) can be completed in a single time frame. Examples of event tasks include (1) the culminating event for a gymnastics season; (2) successfully getting your entire team through a complex outdoor group initiative; (3) organizing, implementing, and monitoring a wellness fair for the community; and (4) students designing a game that would use concepts of striking, speed, and accuracy. Although an event task can be performed in a single instructional time period, planning may take time out of class or over an extended period. An individual student or a group may perform an event task. Well-designed event tasks reflect critical learning outcomes, provide opportunities for learners to apply knowledge and skill to a meaningful task, and allow learners to demonstrate a level of achievement. **Box 12.4** lists some event tasks across various curriculum models for several year groups.

Two event tasks that could be used as formative assessments to assess learning outcomes related to Outdoor Education are noted in **Box 12.5** and **Box 12.6**.

Learning Experience 12.6

In a small group, consider an appropriate event task for two other learning outcomes related to Outdoor Education. Students will work together to achieve the goals of an overnight trip and will successfully participate in hiking and orienteering. Share the ways in which the suggested event task for each learning outcome is appropriate. Is it possible to have multiple appropriate event tasks for one learning outcome?

Written Tests

Probably the most typical form of assessment for cognitive concepts and general knowledge used in physical education is the written test. It is generally true/false, multiple choice, and perhaps short answer. Typically, we see children and youth studying (or carrying around) a handout covering the rules, procedures, and etiquette that guide a sport or activity. Before play begins, students are tested on how well they know this information that will allow them to participate successfully. Despite our reluctance to encourage the use of written tests, they need not be ineffective if designed in an applied manner that challenges students to critically think about the question (problem) in order to solve it. For instance, providing students

BOX 12.3 Sample Journal Assignments

Cooperation as an integrative theme:

- *Theme:* Cooperation is a theme identified by an entire postprimary school as a necessary social skill that students need to master to function effectively throughout life.
- *Journal task:* Students will reflect upon how cooperation is used throughout life and from the perspective of different content areas. As students identify situations where cooperation is critical, they will describe it and discuss how and why it is critical and how well they feel they cooperate in each situation.

Floor hockey:

- *Goal:* Student journals were used to determine the students' ability to reflect upon their experiences during the Sport Education floor hockey season.
- Prompts:
  - *Entry 1:* We have learned about fair play today. Why is fair play important? Who needs to play fair during game play? How does fair play help while participating in a game? How can you encourage fair play in others?
  - *Entry 2:* Read the attached article and respond to it. Try to organize some thoughts and ideas that tie in with the things we have talked about in class the last couple of days.
  - *Entry 3:* This article talks about Tracy winning the Little League Good Sport Award. Tracy says she tries to "spark her teammates" and "cheer them up." What can you say about being a good sport? Try to come up with some ideas to expand on this topic.
  - *Entry 4:* Describe the importance of teamwork while playing offense and while playing defense. Are there similarities or differences between offensive and defensive teamwork?
  - *Entry 5:* We have captains and managers on each team. These people fill in the roles of the team leaders. What things does a team member look for in a leader? Is it possible for other team members to also be leaders? Explain and expand on this subject.
  - *Entry 6:* The Reds have not had a captain since 1988. Why do you think they went this long without one? Think about what we have worked on in class, and respond to the following questions: Why does a team need a captain? Why are captains important in our class? Is it possible for a team to go without a captain? What would be the consequences of our teams not having captains? Explain and expand on your thoughts.
  - *Entry 7:* Respond to the following statement: "Winning isn't everything, it's the only thing."
  - *Entry 8:* What would you tell a teammate who is making negative remarks? He might say, "I hate this game. I'm going to quit" or "I hate my team. No one passes me the puck."
  - *Entry 9:* We started this season talking about fair play. As the season nears the end, do you think your team is still concerned with fair play? If not, what can you do to help your team remember to play fair? If your team is still playing fair, how did you help your team continue to play fair? Explain.
  - *Entry 10:* Is the team player who scores goals and assists (scoring statistics) always the best (most valuable) player or the fairest player on the team? Explain.
  - *Entry 11:* Is fair play important as the season goes along? In other words, was fair play more important at the beginning of the season and now is winning more important at the end? Can winning and fair play be important to your team at the same time? Explain.

Adapted from Tom Gilbert, 1997, Trinity School.

BOX 12.4 Event Tasks

Sport Education, Acro-sport, Partner Task

The culminating event for the season is a partner competition performed to music. Your task is to design a 90-second routine with a partner to music of your choice. The routine must include four different balance stunts, two locomotor and two nonlocomotor actions, two inversions, and weight transfers.

Fitness and Wellness Education Fun Run, Group Task

Organize and implement a fun run for faculty and students. To be included are a prerun meal, training workshop, maps to guide the runners, applications and run information, awards, and publicity.

Developmental Physical Education, Individual Task

Role-play examples of physical activity situations that might reflect hurt, anger, frustration, defensiveness, unethical behavior, or other emotions detrimental to performance or fair play. Students will then lead a discussion with the class to identify alternative types of behaviors to overcome these harmful ones.

The Culture of Sport, Personal Sport Culture, Individual Task

Students demonstrate their understanding of their personal sport culture by developing a biography of their sport and leisure involvement and the nature of those experiences. The individual experiences are presented as part of a "gallery walk" in which students display oral and pictorial perspectives of their lives in and views of sport and leisure activities (Kellum, Dixon, O'Sullivan, Kinchin, & Roberts, 1992).

Fitness and Wellness Education, Group Task

Students select a daily morning health message prompting students, teachers, and administrators about some aspect of health and wellness and arrange delivery of it throughout the school. For instance, they might provide guidance related to nutrition and sound eating habits or be more specific about daily needs for physical activity.

Fitness and Wellness Education, Partner Task

Students work in pairs to make life-size drawings of themselves participating in a favorite fitness activity. One student demonstrates an activity on a large piece of paper while the partner traces that activity. Students then display their activities and talk about which health- or fitness-related concepts are most critical to it.

Individual Task

Students demonstrate an activity they enjoy and identify the muscle groups used to perform it.

BOX 12.5 Event Task to Assess Students' Understanding of "Leave No Trace" Concepts

Learning outcome: Students will participate in an overnight camping trip following "leave no trace" concepts.

1. With your small group, read the following scenario: Students set off for the hike into the hills for their camping trip with their gear and equipment packed so that they have easy access to water, compasses, and maps. Although they are not completely sure of the route, they feel comfortable that the map will direct them adequately. Two of the boys in the group snack on trail mix as they walk, storing their wrappers in a plastic bag on the side pocket of their packs. As the students traverse the route they attempt to choose a path that does not have a lot of vegetation because they do not want to trample the greenery along the way. A few of the hikers find the flowers and trees lovely and pick a bouquet to put in their tent on arrival at the campsite. When they do arrive at the area in which they will set up camp, the students begin to examine the area for the best place to put up their tents. One group chooses a place that sits just above the river so they will have easy access for the morning kayaking. As the campers prepare for dinner they are disappointed by the postings indicating that campfires are prohibited due to fire safety, but they have enough supplies that this will not impact their meals. After taking part in skits, singing, and telling ghost stories, the campers move to their tents to sleep for the weekend activities.
2. Determine if the participants are following the leave no trace principles. In what way are they following the leave no trace principles? If they are not, be able to share with the class what they were doing incorrectly.
3. The class will assess your analysis of the scenario.

with a game scenario to analyze allows them to demonstrate their knowledge of the rules and procedures governing an activity. **Box 12.7** provides an archery example used in a physical education class at Beechcroft High School that demonstrates this well (also see **Figure 12.11**).

Written tests are often a means of assessing whether students understand critical elements or performance cues that impact performance or know necessary safety procedures. Although this knowledge can be assessed most effectively in

BOX 12.6 Event Task to Assess Students' Appropriate Choice of Clothing

Learning outcome: Students will select appropriate clothing to suit the weather on an overnight trip.

1. With your team, select clothing for the 1-day trip.
2. Navigate the five-control-point orienteering course that notes particular weather conditions at each control point.
3. When arriving at each control point, dress your hiker for the weather.
4. Note your clothing decisions on the task card.
5. Final debrief of decisions will guide where learning is still needed.

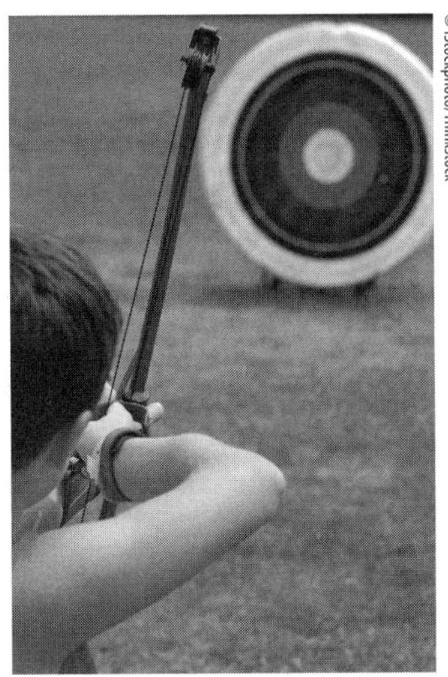

FIGURE 12.11 An archery exam.

BOX 12.7 Archery Exam

1. Sally has just come outside to shoot. She reaches for a bow, immediately picks it up and checks it, then checks her arrows. After giving the command to check equipment, the teacher calls for bows up. Sally shoots her three arrows and hits the following: one in the blue, one in the black, and the final arrow splits the red and the yellow. After shooting her third arrow, Sally puts down her bow and begins playing around with her friends. They chase each other, hit each other, and wrestle. Once given the command to retrieve, Sally gets her arrows and returns to her line twirling them.
   - What did Sally score on each individual arrow? Total score?
   - What safety rules did Sally violate?
2. Bill has three arrows to shoot. On his first arrow, he hits the white. On the second arrow, he picks up the arrow, places it under the bow, places his three fingers on the string, draws, aims, and hits the blue, but it bounces off. On his third arrow, Bill places the arrow on the bow, places his three fingers on the string, aims, and releases. He hits the black. Bill is so excited that he runs out to get his arrows once the command is given to retrieve.
   - What did Bill score for each individual arrow? Total score?
   - What shooting steps did Bill perform incorrectly or forget to do?
   - What safety rules did Bill violate?
3. Tonya arrived late to class with a new hairstyle, new shoes, new gold hoop earrings, and a brand new Nike shirt with her name airbrushed on it. After going through the proper shooting steps, Tonya hit the target three times. One arrow hit the white, one hit the blue, and her final arrow hit the bulls-eye. She was so excited she ran out in her new shoes and stood by her target. When she arrived there, she noticed the arrow in the white only had two feathers. Tonya had just completed her best round of archery.
   - What was the score for each individual arrow? Total score?
   - What safety rules did Tonya violate?
4. Edward has four arrows to shoot. He hits the yellow, which bounces off, white, red, and his final arrow misses a passing squirrel. Once given the command to retrieve, Edward yanks his arrows from the target and returns to his line with the arrows in his back pocket.
   - What did Edward score for each individual arrow? Total score?
   - What safety rules did Edward violate?

Adapted from Mary Henninger, Beechcroft High School Archery Exam.

a realistic setting, there are ways of designing written tests to achieve this in a problem-solving and applied fashion. For example,

Jim is taking part in a climbing unit in his fifth-grade class. These two questions from his written exam relate to his knowledge of communication when climbing or belaying a climber.

1. *Outline the set of commands that are used to initiate the backup belay. Explain what each command means.*

____

____

____

____

2. *What is the meaning of these commands?*

Tension ______________________

Slack ______________________

Falling ______________________

Slowdown ______________________

Another example of how to gain an understanding of what students have learned about concepts introduced is to use an in-class assessment or a homework assignment.

Skills Tests

Skills tests tend to be isolated and do not reflect performance in a realistic setting. However, when designed to assess performance in an authentic way, they may be useful to determine performance level and provide feedback to learners. The Davis Bowling Skills Test (Davis, 1994) is an effective example of a skills test that also serves as a learning experience and can be used in an ongoing fashion. Students bowl one game of 10 frames using two balls per frame unless they score a strike. The goal is to score 20 points (two points per frame) on the skills test. Points are awarded only for the following:

- Hitting the headpin on the first ball
- Making a strike on the first ball
- Making a spare on the second ball

An open frame does not score points. One frame may serve as the entire skills test or be combined with a series of frames, with the entire set of scores, or the average score used to reflect performance. **Figure 12.12** shows a sample score sheet.

First trial:		**Date:**		**Total score:**
Student name:			**Class:**	
Frame	#1 pin	Strike	Spare	Total
1				
2				
3				
4				
5				
6				
7				
8				
9				
10				

FIGURE 12.12 Sample bowling score sheet.

Learning Experience 12.7

Consider a test for a particular skill (e.g., dribbling, kicking, throwing, catching, underhand serve, overhead serve) and determine how best to conduct the skill in a realistic setting. For example, if you choose the skill of dribbling, you may look to identify an authentic skill setting within a modified game of hockey or soccer. If you choose underhand serve, you may look to consider an authentic game situation for badminton or volleyball.

Although collecting and summarizing game statistics provide a measure of individual and group game performance, other instruments provide a more complete picture of skill and tactical performance during game play. If the intent of teaching games is to improve game performance, then assessing game performance should include all aspects of game play in the context in which the game is actually played. This is quite different from the typical isolated skills tests we see administered in contrived, controlled, non-game-like settings in school physical education.

We have selected the Game Performance Assessment Instrument (GPAI) (Oslin, Mitchell, & Griffin, 1998) to demonstrate an appropriate alternative to the more traditional skills tests. GPAI was designed to allow teachers to observe and code performance behaviors that demonstrate ability to perform effectively in games. These behaviors span different kinds of games and were determined in consultation with teachers' knowledge in a variety of games. The components of game performance include the following:

- *Base:* Appropriate return of performer to a home recovery position between skill attempts
- *Adjust:* Movement of performer, either offensively or defensively, as required by the flow of the game
- *Decision making:* Making appropriate choices about what to do with the ball (or projectile) during a game
- *Skill execution:* Efficient performance of selected skills
- *Support:* Off-the-ball movement to a position to receive a pass
- *Cover:* Providing defensive support for a player making a play on the ball or moving to the ball (or projectile)
- *Guard/mark:* Defending an opponent who may or may not have the ball (or projectile)

Not all components apply to all games, and some components are more critical to one game than another. GPAI allows for assessing all components of game play or selecting those that fit most closely with the game, purposes of instruction, and students working at different levels. This instrument uses a tally system to code appropriate and/or efficient as well as inappropriate and/or inefficient performances. Coding all four would provide the most complete picture of performance. **Figure 12.13** demonstrates how you

Scoring Criteria:

Decision made

- Player attempts to pass to an open teammate
- Player attempts to score at the end zone

Skill execution

- Reception-control of pass and set up of the Frisbee
- Passing-ball reaches target

Support

- The player appeared to attempt to support the Frisbee carrier by being in/moving to an appropriate position to receive the pass

	Decision made		Skill execution		Support	
Student	A	IA	E	IE	A	IA

FIGURE 12.13 Form for coding in ultimate Frisbee.
Key: IA, inappropriate; IE, inefficient; A, appropriate; E, efficient.

might code one student in ultimate Frisbee when the focus has been on maintaining possession and scoring.

Once data have been collected, they can be grouped for each component of game performance and overall game involvement. Performance measures can be computed using the totals of the different game components and inserted into the following formulas:

- Game involvement = total appropriate decisions + number of inappropriate decisions + number of efficient skill executions + number of inefficient skill executions + number of supporting movements
- Decision-making index (DMI) = number of appropriate decisions made + number of inappropriate decisions made
- Skill execution index (SEI) = number of efficient skill executions + number of inefficient skill executions
- Support index (SI) = number of appropriate supporting movements + number of inappropriate supporting movements
- Game performance = [DMI + SEI + SI]/3

Self-Assessment

If our intent is to make assessment an educative process to improve student performance, then students must be able to assess and modify their own performance. Because students do not have access to teachers at all times during the day, during summer vacations, or when they graduate from school, their ability to take charge of their own performance is critical. Students should not expect to achieve success the first time they attempt to perform a new task, so being able to assess and make corrections is crucial for them. Students must be taught the key learning experiences to achieve this self-assessment goal (i.e., the standards, the criteria, the know-how) and be given opportunities to practice assessing performance in such a way that they can make appropriate and necessary adjustments to be successful.

Student **self-assessment** can take a variety of forms. The intent of all self-assessment for students is to critically analyze aspects of their performance for comparison to their own goals, teacher-designed criteria, or peer performance standards. Self-assessment requires the student to reflect on performance, learn to compare what a performance feels like (kinesthetic knowledge) to what it should look like, and be able to analyze correct versus incorrect performance. Self-assessment can be as simple as recording the number of successful attempts on a checklist, ranking performance in comparison to progress toward target goals, or measuring and maintaining records of a personal fitness or activity profile.

The assessment wheel and assessment steps are two self-assessments that arose as part of an assessment for learning study conducted in Ireland where students were to take greater responsibility for what is learned and how it is represented (MacPhail & Halbert, 2010).

Assessment Wheel

The **assessment wheel** is a simple form of student self-assessment that does not depend solely on language to communicate student understanding. It encourages the student to record, reflect on, and map their learning related to the big picture goal and to assess their progress towards this goal. It also identifies any learning gaps that may exist and encourages students to plan for the next phase of their learning as well as providing a context for feedback (i.e., inform discussion between student and teacher). The wheel can be used to track progress and at the end of a unit of work can be used as a means of documenting student learning.

Figure 12.14 shows an assessment wheel that has been completed by a student in response to the extent to which they believe they are practicing the essential components to successfully achieve the noted big picture goal/challenge (e.g., "plan, organize, and take part in a class athletics meeting"). The student has twice assessed themselves throughout the 6-week athletics unit, and their assessment wheel conveys that they believe they are most proficient in throwing and jumping (by shading out to the circle edge of the respective components) and are clearly less proficient in working in groups and measuring and recording. Although the assessment wheel is predominantly designed as a self-assessment, a teacher can communicate at which level they believe the student is operating at for each criterion by adding a solid black line to each of the circle segments. The solid black line in Figure 12.14 denotes that the teacher believes that the student is underestimating their performance related to working in groups, overestimates their implementation of safe practice, and agrees with the student's assessment of all other criteria. Room also is allowed for the student and teacher to independently comment on the experience of the big picture goal/challenge.

Learning Experience 12.8

Prepare an assessment wheel related to the following Outdoor Education assessment: "Students will cooperatively and successfully complete an overnight trip at an outdoor center and participate successfully in a day hike and orienteering event."

Assessment Steps

The **assessment steps** (see **Figure 12.15**) encourage students to engage with the big picture goal/challenge and determine what they would like to be able to do related to this challenge. Once they have identified this, they then need to consider how they could best pursue these goals on a week-by-week basis (each step in Figure 12.15 matches with each week of a physical education unit). The assessment steps can result in students within a class noting significantly different

Name: John Peterson
Class: St. Harold's
Date: 2/16/2014

Measure record
Working in
Officials
Analyze
Throw efficiently
Implement safe practices
Run efficiently
Jump efficiently

Challenge
Plan, organize and take part in a class athletics competition.

Student Comment
I enjoyed most of the athletics. The throwing was the easiest, but I didn't enjoy being in a group competition. The teacher is too fussy about safety and it's difficult to remember the rules.

Teacher Comment
John has contributed well to the work of the class, especially in learning correct techniques and helping other students. His attention to safety practices must improve; he should take time to observe others who are more aware of safe practices.

1 – I haven't started this yet
2 – I can do this sometimes but I find it hard
3 – I can perform this at a reasonable level most of the time
4 – I can perform at a high level always

FIGURE 12.14 Assessment wheel.
Modified from Dr. Ann MacPhail. (2007). Assessment in Junior Cycle Physical Education: Final Evaluation Report (Appendix 2).

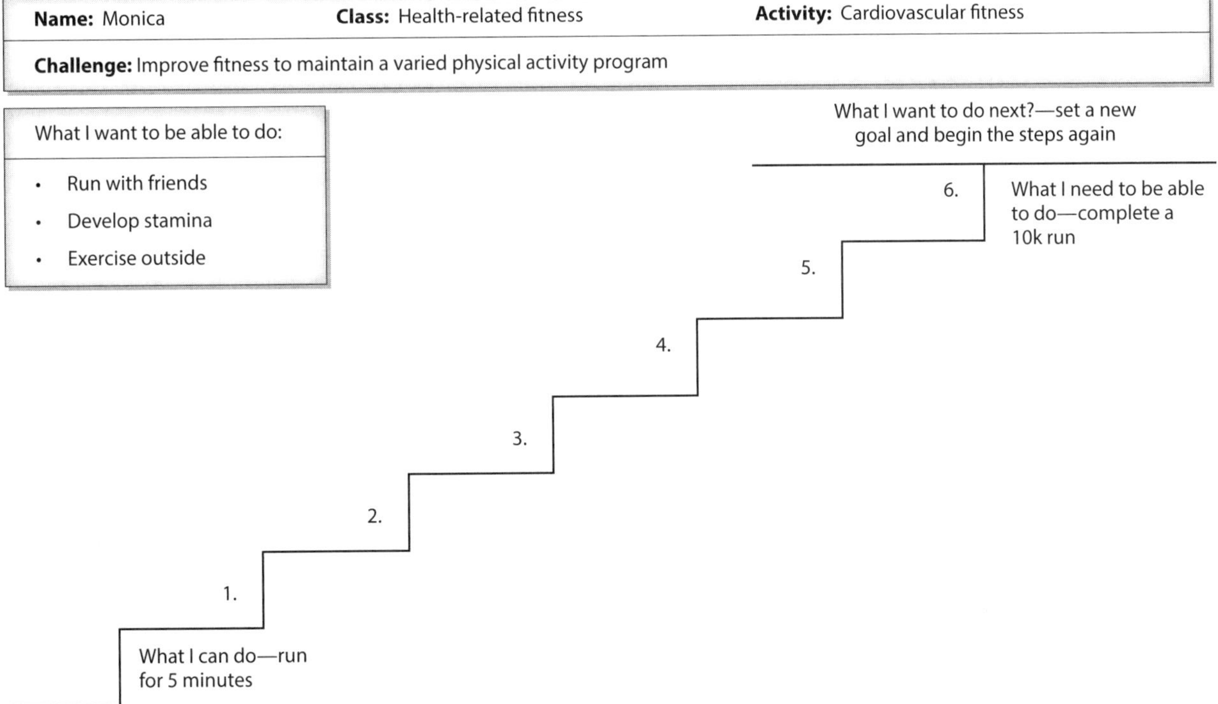

Name: Monica
Class: Health-related fitness
Activity: Cardiovascular fitness
Challenge: Improve fitness to maintain a varied physical activity program
What I want to be able to do:
• Run with friends
• Develop stamina
• Exercise outside
What I want to do next?—set a new goal and begin the steps again
6.
What I need to be able to do—complete a 10k run
5.
4.
3.
2.
1.
What I can do—run for 5 minutes

FIGURE 12.15 Assessment steps.
Modified from Dr. Ann MacPhail. (2007). Assessment in Junior Cycle Physical Education: Final Evaluation Report (Appendix 2).

ways in which to reach the stated big picture goal/challenge. This is likely to result in the teacher having to accommodate numerous learning experiences on a weekly basis, encouraging and facilitating self-directed learning.

Jambor and Weeks (1995) offered a video technique to help students take responsibility for improving their own performance. Interpersonal Process Recall (IPR) is most useful for students who understand what a motor skill should look like, have had some practice assessing their own performance, and are willing to interact with the teacher and peers on their performance. This technique puts students in the role of directing the viewing of their video and leading the analysis and discussion. The teacher becomes the facilitator, asking questions, seeking clarity, and prompting analysis of different movements. As students view the video, they may choose to stop it for discussion at any point to highlight what they see, how they felt, or what they consider significant or critical to them. The teacher's role during this discussion is to help the students delve more deeply into what they are viewing, their reactions to it, and the possibilities for changing a performance. Students must be allowed to work through this process with guidance rather than being told what is wrong and how to correct it. The collaborative nature of the interactions is intended to prevent students from getting defensive about their performance and to encourage them to identify errors themselves.

A **student log** is a record of performance on specific behaviors or criteria over a given period. A student log can be maintained by an individual (fitness or weight training log), partners (win/loss record in badminton), or the entire class (mileage record toward the goal of running across the country). Logs can be simple (activity performed) to complex (time of day, weight training exercises, frequency, intensity, and feelings about the workout) and utilize technology or the more traditional forms of documenting.

To use a log like that in **Figure 12.16**, students conduct a personal fitness assessment, identify fitness needs, establish short-term and long-term goals, select activities to meet those goals, design a weekly fitness plan, and develop the log to monitor progress. As they begin to participate in this fitness plan, they maintain a daily log of their progress.

These logs can be maintained on computers in the classroom using spreadsheet software. If only one computer is available, individual students or the leader of a group of students can enter the data at the close of every class session. Raw data can be turned into a graph to reflect either individual or group work and posted (e.g., minutes of exercise with heart rate [HR] within training range). Students could be required to maintain an activity log that allows them to record and assess their participation level using the following rating scale (last column in Figure 12.16):

1. Not much effort (no improvement on test scores)
2. Participated some of the time
3. Participated most of the time
4. Participated the entire hour

Learning Experience 12.9

Describe the benefits of using peer and self-assessment in addition to teacher observation/assessment. Are there instances in physical education where it is imperative that all three types of assessment are utilized? Are there instances in physical education where one type of assessment would be more appropriate than all three?

Establishing Scoring Criteria: Using Scoring Rubrics/Guides

Scoring criteria are the key to turning assessment tasks into true assessments, rather than just a series of learning

Date	Fitness activity	Minutes	Resting HR	Exercise HR	Resting HR	Laps	Notebook	Rating scale

FIGURE 12.16 Woodward High School activity log.

experiences or tasks that students perform. A scoring rubric/guide defines the criteria by which a performance or product is judged. Essentially, it consists of levels of performance (criteria) and a list of characteristics describing performance at each level. Scoring rubrics/guides can be used to judge performance for many assessment strategies, including portfolios, journals, group projects, and some event tasks.

Figure 12.17 offers an example of a generic four-level racket games (e.g., badminton, tennis, pickleball) scoring rubric/guide (see also Siedentop, Hastie, & van der Mars, 2011; van der Mars & Harvey, 2010). Given the target learning outcomes for a unit or season, teachers can select one or more game performance indicators and determine students' performance levels as they progress throughout the unit and across years. The tool allows teachers to select from an array of substantive learning outcomes including (1) techniques, (2) tactics, (3) knowledge of game rules, and (4) fair play behavior.

Select the term that best matches the player's performance for the observed indicator(s).				
How points generally are scored		Generally Fewer Unforced errors More winners ⟷		Generally More Forced errors Fewer winners
Game play performance indicators	**Exceeds**	**Meets**	**Developing**	**Struggles**
Technique: serving	Potent: Uses serve as an attacking weapon, with variance in placement and speed.	Reliable: More consistent and firm but without varying of placement and/or speed.	Passive: Simply gets the ball/shuttle in play but often with a lob-like trajectory.	Inconsistent: Serve is put in play only sometimes.
Technique: shot execution	Unpredictable: Employs variety of shots (e.g., lobs; fore/backhand, drops, smashes, clears) and aims to move opponent out of position.	Emerging: Hits shots with more consistency but still tends to favor some; shots are hit more flat, leaving opponent with less time to react.	Loopy and arched: Shots are mostly lobbed to the opponent with little deliberate change of speed and direction.	Inconsistent: Shots only sometimes result in maintaining rally; points scored are mostly a result of unforced errors.
Tactics: shot selection	Widely varied: Uses wide variety of shots at the right time; takes advantage of game situations and shots reflect consideration of opponent's and own court position and with good precision.	Varied: Starts to vary shots at the right time; shots reflect consideration of opponent's and own court position but while using a variety of shots, the precision still lacks consistency.	Two shots: Keeps ball/shuttle in play but offers opponent easy return opportunities; uses/favors a couple of shots but precision still lacking.	One shot: Favors mostly one shot (e.g., forehand) regardless of game situation; shots are sometimes wild, and very inconsistent; and still focused mostly on cooperative rallying.
Tactics: ball/shuttle placement	To open spaces: Hits ball/shuttle consistently to deep/short corners either short or long; uses angles depending on opponent's court position; and recognizes opponent's strengths and weaknesses.	Some active placement: Places the ball/shuttle to uncovered spaces when it is hit directly to him/her; hits ball/shuttle more toward the corners (away from opponent) but without looking to land it near the lines; and works the opponent either short or long, using the angles depending on opponent's court position.	Returns to opponent: Returns the ball/shuttle in most cases but with little placement and/or consideration of opponent's position; struggles to place ball/shuttle when on the move.	Survival focus: Aims to simply get the ball/shuttle back over the net; no concern for a specific spot on the court; and may even struggle to get the ball/shuttle over, so may need "no barrier" net to play the game and larger racquet and/or other modifications to play a game.

(*continues*)

FIGURE 12.17 Racquet games scoring rubric/guide.

Reproduced with permission from D. Siedentop, P. A. Hasite, & H. van der Mars, 2011. *Complete guide to sport education*, 2nd ed. (Champaign, IL: Human Kinetics), 168–170.

Select the term that best matches the player's performance for the observed indicator(s).				
How points generally are scored		Generally Fewer Unforced errors More winners ←→		Generally More Forced errors Fewer winners
Game play performance indicators	**Exceeds**	**Meets**	**Developing**	**Struggles**
Tactics: ball/shuttle placement	To open spaces: Hits ball/shuttle consistently to deep/short corners either short or long; uses angles depending on opponent's court position; and recognizes opponent's strengths and weaknesses.	Some active placement: Places the ball/shuttle to uncovered spaces when it is hit directly to him/her; hits ball/shuttle more toward the corners (away from opponent) but without looking to land it near the lines; and works the opponent either short or long, using the angles depending on opponent's court position.	Returns to opponent: Returns the ball/shuttle in most cases but with little placement and/or consideration of opponent's position; struggles to place ball/shuttle when on the move.	Survival focus: Aims to simply get the ball/shuttle back over the net; no concern for a specific spot on the court; and may even struggle to get the ball/shuttle over, so may need "no barrier" net to play the game and larger racquet and/or other modifications to play a game.
Tactics: decision making	Plays smart: Effectively uses information about opponent's moves and shots to select own movement and shot selection.	Controlled: Uses a shot if it is the appropriate one but not as if it has been planned for and set up; considers opponent's shot selection, placement, and court movement to a limited extent.	Reactive: Reactive shots rather than planned ones; shows hesitation and/or late reaction on where and when to move and what shot to employ.	Does not use: Focuses mostly on just making contact; uses limited types of shots.
Tactics: court coverage movement (recovery to base position)	Fluid moves: In control of base position; plans movements a play ahead to be where the opponent will return to the ball/shuttle; consistently incorporates movement to the shot and returns to base position after execution of each shot; and uses fluid/effective footwork to get to and play strokes even when off-balance.	Strokes and moves: Recovers back to base position after most shots, attempting not to be stranded; incorporates movement into the shot, returning to base position after each shot; uses fluid and effective footwork to play the next stroke even when off-balance; some control of central court position but at times, court movement is less fluid.	Reacts to ball/shuttle: Court position is determined by the shot making of the opponent, rather than a planned one; struggles to return to base position after playing effective shots from opponent; leaves open space for their opponent to play the ball into; recovery from shots is delayed due to being off-balance; and the limited footwork tends to be clumsy.	Static: Player does not respond to the placement of the ball/shuttle; no concept of base position or it is incorrect, thus, starting play out of position and losing before they start; and player is rooted to one place on the court and strikes the ball/shuttle from there when possible.

FIGURE 12.17 Racquet games scoring rubric/guide. (*Continued*)

Select the term that best matches the player's performance for the observed indicator(s).				
How points generally are scored		Generally Fewer Unforced errors More winners ⟷		Generally More Forced errors Fewer winners
Game play performance indicators	**Exceeds**	**Meets**	**Developing**	**Struggles**
Tactics: anticipation skills	Consistent: Consistently anticipates opponent's next shot by watching racquet head, body position, court movement, and placement of the ball/shuttle from their own shot.	Some anticipation: Tries to anticipate opponent's next play but not early/quick enough to gain an advantage moving to the ball/ shuttle to catch opponent out of position with next shot; shots are thus still somewhat more defensive in nature.	Sporadic: Sporadic anticipation of opponent's next play; little advantage gained and cannot catch opponent out of position with their next shot; and shots are taken later and are defensive in nature.	Little to no anticipation: Reacts to all plays by opponent; constantly on the defensive; and primarily concerned with how to hit shots (i.e., judging the correct pace with which to hit shot).
Knowledge of game rules as player	Rule violations are absent from play, such as: Double-hits, keeping score, diagonal serving, foot faults, and hitting a ball that clearly is heading out of bounds. Requires no reminders.	Rule violations occur rarely, such as: Double-hits, keeping score, diagonal serving, foot faults, and hitting a ball that clearly is heading out of bounds. Requires no reminders.	Aware of rules but still fails to execute, such as: Double-hits, keeping score, diagonal serving, foot faults, and hitting a ball that clearly is heading out of bounds. Requires few reminders.	Lacks awareness of rules—violations occur frequently, such as: Double-hits, keeping score, diagonal serving, foot faults, and hitting a ball that clearly is heading out of bounds. Frequent reminders needed.
Fair play behavior	Model: Shows respect to classmates, teacher, equipment, and facilities; works productively and effectively with teammates; eagerly fulfills assigned nonplaying roles; shows perseverance and appropriate assertiveness; when needed, resolves conflict quickly and effectively; wins and loses with grace; and consistently attends class, is on time, and is prepared.	Fair play: Is in control of self, and needs little teacher supervision; shows respect to classmates, teacher, equipment, and facilities; when needed, resolves conflict quickly and effectively; participates in most team and class activities; fulfills assigned team role(s); rarely misses class; and few, if any, tardies.	Little: Minimal control of self and needing frequent teacher supervision; not participating fully; may interrupt others; reluctant to try their best; tries to hide out from the activities; taunts others (including teammates, officials, and others); blames others, and denies personal responsibility; gets frustrated and quits on teammates; teases and pouts; makes excuses; misses several classes; and tardy at times.	None: No control of self and needing constant teacher supervision; no appreciable participation; interrupting others; makes few, if any, attempts at participation; hides out from activities; taunts others (including teammates, officials, and others); easily overreacts and creates conflicts; blames others, and denies personal responsibility; gets frustrated and quits on teammates; teases and pouts; makes excuses; and misses class regularly and/or is frequently tardy.

FIGURE 12.17 Racquet games scoring rubric/guide. (*Continued*)

An Example of Assessing Within a Specific Program: The Comprehensive School Physical Activity Program

In terms of assessing the impact of a Comprehensive School Physical Activity Program (CSPAP), one can look at the degree to which a school maximizes its caloric footprint. Simply put, if a school increases access to and opportunity for health-optimizing physical activity for more students (and adults) over the course of a single school day, week, or school year, as a school it increases the number of calories that are expended. There are several observable indicators that a CSPAP can use to demonstrate that it is directly impacting a school's caloric footprint. Some are specific to one CSPAP component whereas others reflect impact on multiple components. They include:

- *The number of students who choose to enroll in physical education beyond the requirements:* This indicator directly reflects the extent to which students who have completed their required physical education courses return for additional opportunities. One example of this metric is what happened at Sheldon High School in Eugene, Oregon, several years ago. One of its teachers, Nanci McChesney, introduced yoga courses as part of the physical education curriculum. Students at that school are required to take physical education classes for 1 year only. Before too long students had to be put on waiting lists to enroll in these courses, and many of them are repeating courses beyond the required coursework.
- *The number of physical venues that are accessible, usable, and supervised for students before school, during recess, at lunch time, and after school:* U.S. postprimary schools generally have expansive built-in physical activity facilities. McKenzie, Marshall, Sallis, and Conway (2000) noted that the odds of students seeking out physical activity beyond physical education improve when three prerequisite conditions are met. First, they must have access to facilities. Second, equipment must be provided. Third, there has to be oversight by adults.
- *The number of students who actually visit their school's activity venues and engage in health-optimizing (i.e., moderate to vigorous) physical activity.*
- *The number of teachers, support staff, and community members who make use of the available activity venues at a school campus over the course of a week.*
- *The physical activity levels of adults utilizing the school's physical activity venues during nonschool hours.*

These indicators provide the kind of evidence that can be used to demonstrate how a school is moving toward creating an activity-friendly environment for all.

A **scoring rubric**/guide is first and foremost an assessment tool that teachers and students can use to gauge the level and quality of student performance formally and informally throughout the learning process. However, the use of a scoring rubric/guide also can help enhance and focus instruction so teachers can facilitate students' learning. When assigning a task (e.g., a game, a dance performance, a report), teachers want to ensure that they communicate clearly to students the activity's specific goals and what the teacher will look (criteria) for in the performance. A well-developed scoring rubric/guide (1) conveys to students what the intended level of task performance looks like and (2) makes levels of development (i.e., learning) public. Thus their use promotes good performance by showing that quality work is achievable and expected. Importantly, because the scoring rubrics/guides contain specific criteria for guiding and evaluating performance, they also form the basis and provide the language and dimensions for immediate, focused, useful, and informative feedback.

Scoring rubrics/guides should be prepared and shared before instruction begins so that both students and teacher know expectations and so that the students can use the rubric to guide and assess their own work (Arter & McTighe, 2001; Lund, 2000). There are two key steps for designing a scoring rubric/guide:

1. Identify the performance task.
2. Define all criteria at the highest level, and then break those levels down into a four-point scoring rubric/guide. Design level 3 to reflect a performance that would be considered acceptable. Level 4 then would represent students demonstrating above the accepted level of performance for the task. Each criterion must be teachable and represent a key attribute of the performance being assessed.

When first employing scoring rubrics/guides, physical educators may wish to limit it to include three levels of performance to ease the process of incorporating their formal and formative use throughout daily instruction. We strongly suggest obtaining copies of sample scoring rubrics/guides that others have used in physical education to serve as a framework to development of scoring rubrics/guides or to be adapted for specific needs (Birky, 2012; Burt, Schroeder, & Hurley, 2008). As scoring rubrics/guides are developed, they can be compared to samples of student work to see if the established criteria are appropriate. If not, teachers can make revisions and try again. The key is that the scoring rubric/guide (1) must capture what is worth assessing and (2) reflect quality performance. Woods and Anderson (2002) provide an example of students designing and implementing an evaluation scoring rubric in an aerobics unit, explaining that input from a rubric students designed in small groups was used to design a single rubric that the class agreed upon

Task Goal: To work as a collaborative team to successfully solve the presented problem.				
Performance Indicators	Performance Level 4	Performance Level 3	Performance Level 2	Performance Level 1
Works toward achievement of group goals	Actively helps identify group goals and works hard to meet them	Communicates commitment to the group goals and effectively carries out assigned roles	Communicates a commitment to the group goals but does not carry out assigned roles	Does not work toward group goals or works actively against them
Demonstrates effective interpersonal skills	Actively promotes effective group interaction and the expression of ideas and opinions in a way that is sensitive to the feelings and knowledge base of others	Participates in group interaction without prompting, expresses ideas and opinions in a way that is sensitive to the feelings and knowledge base of others	Participates in group interaction with prompting or expresses ideas and opinions without considering the feelings and knowledge base of others	Does not participate in group interaction, even with prompting, or expresses ideas and opinions in a way that is insensitive to the feelings and knowledge base of others
Contributes to group maintenance	Actively helps the group identify changes or modifications necessary in the group process and works toward carrying out those changes	Helps identify change or modifications necessary in the group process and works toward carrying out those changes	When prompted, helps identify changes or modification necessary in the group process or is only minimally involved in carrying out those changes	Does not attempt to identify changes or modifications necessary in the group process, even when prompted, or refuses to work toward carrying out those changes

FIGURE 12.18 Sample scoring rubric/guide.
Adapted from Marzano, R. J., Pickerington, D., & McTighe, J. (1993). *Assessing student outcomes: Performance assessment using the dimensions of learning model.* Alexandria, VA: ASCD.

and applied. **Figure 12.18** shows a sample scoring rubric/guide designed for use in assessing team-building experiences in preparation for a high ropes initiative.

Learning Experience 12.10

Design a scoring rubric/guide to assess the extent to which students have achieved the Outdoor Education assessment, "Students will cooperatively and successfully complete an overnight trip at an outdoor center and participate successfully in a day hike and orienteering event." Define all criteria related to the assessment and then decide the highest level of accomplishment for each criterion before breaking levels down to complete a four-point scoring rubric/guide for each criterion.

Reliability and Consistency

Physical educators are deemed to be knowledgeable and expert in the content they teach. That implies that they know what is important to teach and assess. Moreover, it implies that they know how to effectively observe and judge the quality of student performance. Physical educators are expected to make professional judgments about their students' progress in learning. Whether you are using alternative assessment to provide feedback to learners, to inform the instructional process, or to reflect a student's progress, the measure must be reliable and consistent. This basically suggests that a teacher would score a student's performance the same way on successive trials, or that if two similarly experienced people are scoring the same performance, each would give the same score. This becomes a bit problematic with alternative assessment due to its reliance on teacher judgment. Assessment must be equitable to all students. Thus, teachers must be knowledgeable about content, design/employ assessments that fairly and appropriately match the learning goal, select scoring criteria that adequately represent the performance to be judged, and make judgments as consistently as possible. There are no hard and fast rules to govern measuring the reliability of alternative assessment, yet the purpose for which results are used is important. It would be unfair to base a student's grade on assessments that do not measure what they are intended to measure or on information obtained in an unfair or unreliable manner.

Practicing Formal Assessment of Student Learning in Physical Education

Earlier we noted the lack of a culture of assessment in physical education. Importantly, the historic lack of accountability across school, district, state/province, and national levels is the primary reason why physical education has been allowed to largely ignore the task of formal assessment of substantive learning outcomes. However, today's environment in education is likely to require physical education to make this a much more central part of daily teaching. Carroll (1994) introduced five key questions: Why assess? Who will assess? What to assess? When to assess? and How to assess? In an effort to show how formal formative assessment can be a more manageable task for physical educators, we now turn to the issue of *remembering to assess*.

Remembering to Assess

The problem of remembering to assess is important, because physical educators typically rarely engage in formal formative assessment of student learning. Thus, it is a skill that requires deliberate practice on the part of teachers. In a paper, van der Mars, Timken, and McNamee (2008) demonstrated the effectiveness of prompting in assisting experienced physical educators to engage in such assessment. They employed a "Motivaider" prompting device (see www.habitchange.com).

Motivaiders are small prompting devices that remind users to engage in a behavior. The device is a countdown timer worn on a waistband or belt that vibrates for 3 to 5 seconds at the end of each interval. Prompting has been used in a variety of settings and has been shown to successfully change people's behavior. For example, van der Mars, Timken, and McNamee (2008) used the device with a 90-second interval to help remind experienced secondary school physical educators to collect formal assessment data on students' moderate to vigorous activity levels and game play indicators. The teachers reported that it took only a couple of class periods to get used to being reminded to formally assess selected target students. It is essential that the assessment teaching function become habitual rather than an afterthought. By selecting few outcomes, embedding your assessment in lessons throughout the season, and focusing on a small group of students in each lesson, you will be in a better position to determine and document your students' learning.

CHAPTER SUMMARY

Once physical educators become familiar with and confident in introducing effective assessments into their lessons, they can then begin to consider how best to use the outcomes of such assessments to convey to parents and guardians how effectively their child is learning in physical education (Claxton, 2009; Pantanowitz, Lidor, Nemet, & Eliakim, 2011; Wilkinson & Schneck, 2003). This would entail teachers considering the purpose and timing of such reporting to parents. It is likely the purpose would be to provide information about a child's learning, progress, and achievement that can then be used to support further learning. The principles of effective reporting, what to include in the report, and how best to present information in plain language would also need to be considered by the teacher.

1. An assessment is good to the extent that it matches the intended outcome and learning experiences. A series of assessment design questions allows determining whether the intended outcome is relevant and meaningful and the learning experiences are aligned with it.
2. Teachers become skilled at observing student performance and are often able to convert their observations to checklists and rating scales in an attempt to obtain written data of what occurred.
3. Peers can learn from assessing one another and, when trained, are able to provide useful feedback using rating scales and checklists or by maintaining game statistics.
4. A portfolio is a useful form of self-assessment that puts the responsibility on the students to demonstrate their learning. It documents a student's effort, progress, and achievement toward a goal(s) and involves student reflection on personal growth and progress.
5. A journal allows students to reflect upon and share their thoughts, feelings, impressions, perceptions, and attitude about their performance, an event, an assignment, or other learning experiences. A log is simply a record of performance on a specific behavior or criterion.
6. Well-designed event tasks reflect critical learning outcomes, provide opportunities for learners to apply knowledge and skill to a meaningful task, and allow learners to demonstrate a level of achievement.
7. Written tests can be designed so that the student must think critically about a problem in order to solve it, and may thus strengthen the physical response in the more realistic setting.
8. When skills tests are designed to assess performance in an authentic way, they may be a useful learning experience to determine performance level and provide feedback to learners.
9. If assessment is to be truly an educative process, then self-assessment is a critical component in which students must be trained to assess and modify their own performance. The assessment wheel and assessment steps are two self-assessments that allow students to record their own development.
10. Maintaining game statistics or assessing game performance is necessary if a teacher really wants students to be able to play a game, rather than perform skills in isolated situations.

11. A scoring rubric/guide defines the criteria by which a performance or product is judged and can be used for a number of assessment measures: portfolios, journals, activity logs, group projects, event tasks, or individual routines.
12. A series of steps to guide teachers in developing scoring rubrics/guides to meet their assessment needs has been identified. To be meaningful, grades must be designed to match the physical education program with the criteria shared with learners prior to the onset of instruction.
13. To address the issues of the chosen assessment being reliable and consistent, teachers must be knowledgeable about content, design/employ assessments that fairly and appropriately match the learning goal, select scoring criteria that adequately represent the performance to be judged, and make judgments as consistently as possible.
14. Formative assessment of learning has not typically been part of physical educators' repertoire of teaching skills. To start building it into regular lessons on an ongoing basis, the recommended strategies are to (1) select few outcomes, (2) spread assessment over the entire unit/season, (3) target a small number of students per lesson, and (4) consider using a prompting device to ensure that teachers remember to do formative-formal assessment.
15. Formative assessment can be extended to consider how best to use the outcomes of such assessment to convey to parents and guardians how effectively their child is learning in physical education.

REFERENCES

Arter, J., & McTighe, J. (2001). *Scoring rubrics in the classroom: Using performance criteria for assessing and improving student learning*. Thousand Oaks, CA: Corwin Press.

Birky, B. (2012). Rubrics: A good solution for assessment. *Strategies, 25*(7), 19–21.

Burt, T. L., Schroeder, C., & Hurley, K. S. (2008). Stretching the rubric. *Illinois Journal for Health, Physical Education, Recreation, and Dance, 62*, 15–20.

Carroll, B. (1994). *Assessment in physical education. A teacher's guide to the issues.* London: Falmer Press.

Claxton, D. B. (2009). Data for principals, parents, and other stakeholders in physical education: Statistical assessment made easy with Excel. *Strategies, 22*(5), 20–24.

Connor, A. O., Mulcahy, C., Ní Chróinin, D., & Murtagh, E. (2011). Assessment tools in primary physical education: Enhancing teaching and learning. *Physical Education Matters, 6*(1), xviii.

Davis, K. (1994). North Carolina children and youth fitness study. *Journal of Physical Education, Recreation and Dance, 65*(8), 65–72.

Ericsson, I. (2007). MUGI observation checklist: An alternative to measuring motor skills in physical education classes. *Asian Journal of Exercise and Sports Science, 4*(1), 1–7.

Fisette, J. L. (2011). Incidences of student support for the resistance to a curricular innovation in high school physical education. *Physical Education and Sport Pedagogy, 16*(2), 179–197.

Greenwood, C. R., Maheady, L., & Carta, J. J. (1991). Peer tutoring programs in the regular education classroom. In G. Stoner, M. R. Shinn, & H. M. Walker (Eds.), *Interventions for achievement and behavior problems* (pp. 179–200). Washington, DC: National Association for Psychologists.

Herman, J., Aschbacher, P., & Winters, L. (1992). *A practical guide to alternative assessment*. Alexandria, VA: ASCD.

Hill, G.M., & Turner, B. (2007). A checklist to promote physical activity and fitness in K–12 physical education programs. *Journal of Physical Education, Recreation and Dance, 78*(9), 14–20.

Jambor, E., & Weeks, E. (1995). Videotape feedback: Make it more effective. *Journal of Physical Education, Recreation and Dance, 66*(2), 48–50.

Johnson, M., & Ward, P. (2001). Effects of classwide peer tutoring on correct performance of striking skills in 3rd grade physical education. *Journal of Teaching in Physical Education, 20*(3), 247–263.

Kellum, S., Dixon, S., O'Sullivan, M., Kinchin, G., & Roberts, M. (1992). High school physical education comes alive at your school: A unit on the culture of sport for your students. Paper presented at the American Alliance for Health, Physical Education, Recreation and Dance, Atlanta, GA.

Kinchin, G. D., & O'Sullivan, M. (2003). Incidences of student support for and resistance to a curricular innovation in high school physical education. *Journal of Teaching in Physical Education, 22*(3), 245–260.

Kirk, D. (1993). Curriculum work in physical education: Beyond the objectives approach. *Journal of Teaching in Physical Education, 12*(3), 244–265.

Lund, J. L. (2000). *Creating rubrics for physical education.* Reston, VA: National Association for Sport and Physical Education.

MacPhail, A., & Halbert, J. (2010). "We had to do intelligent thinking during recent PE": Students' and teachers' experiences of assessment for learning in post-primary physical education. *Assessment in Education, 17*(1), 23–39.

Marzano, R. J., Pickerington, D., & McTighe, J. (1993). *Assessing student outcomes: Performance assessment using the dimensions of learning model.* Alexandria, VA: ASCD.

McKenzie, T. L., Marshall, S. J., Sallis, J. F., & Conway, T. L. (2000). Leisure-time physical activity in school environments: An observational study using SOPLAY. *Preventive Medicine, 30*, 70–77.

Melograno, V. J. (2000). Designing a portfolio system for K–12 physical education: A step-by-step process. *Measurement in Physical Education and Exercise Science, 4*(2), 97–115.

Nonis, K. P., Parker, H. E., & Larkin, D. (2004). The development of hopping: An observation checklist for educators. *Journal of Physical Education and Recreation, 10*(1), 8–18.

Oslin, J., Mitchell, S., & Griffin, L. (1998). Game performance assessment instrument (GPAI): Development and preliminary validation. *Journal of Teaching in Physical Education, 17*(2), 231–243.

Pantanowitz, M., Lidor, R., Nemet, D., & Eliakim, A. (2011). The use of homework assignments in physical education among high school students. *Journal of Research in Health, Physical Education, Recreation, Sport and Dance, 6*(1), 48–53.

Siedentop, D., Hastie, P., & van der Mars, H. (2011). *Complete guide to sport education* (2nd ed.). Champaign, IL: Human Kinetics.

Surapiboonchai, K., Furney, S. R., Reardon, R. F., Eldridge, J., & Murray, T. D. (2012). SAM: A tool for measurement of moderate to vigorous physical activity (MVPA) in school physical education. *International Journal of Exercise Science, 5*(2), 127–135.

van der Mars, H., & Harvey, S. (2010). Teaching and assessing racquet games using "Play Practice"—Part 2. *Journal of Physical Education, Recreation, and Dance, 81*(5), 35–43, 56.

van der Mars, H., Timken, G. L., & McNamee, J. (2008, April). Coaching physical education teachers to integrate formal assessment into their daily instruction. Paper presented at the AAHPERD National Convention, Dallas-Fort Worth, TX.

Ward, P., & Lee, M. (2005). Peer-assisted learning in physical education: A review of theory and research. *Journal of Teaching in Physical Education, 24*, 205–225.

Wiggins, G., & McTighe, J. (1998). *Understanding by design*. Alexandria, VA: Association for Supervision and Curriculum Development.

Wilkinson, C., & Schneck, H. (2003). The effects of a school physical education and health website on parental knowledge of the program. *Physical Educator, 60*(3), 162–168.

Woods, M. L., & Anderson, D. (2002). Students designing and applying evaluation rubrics in an aerobics unit. *Physical Educator, 59*(1), 38–56.

Wright, P. M., & Craig, M. W. (2011). Tool for Assessing Responsibility-Based Education (TARE): Instrument development, content validity, and inter-rater reliability. *Measurement in Physical Education and Exercise Science, 15*(3), 204–219.

CHAPTER 13 Developing Effective Teaching Practices

Overall Chapter Outcome

To become aware of what teachers do to make a difference in student learning and gain the skills and knowledge to begin that process in your own practice

Learning Outcomes

The learner will:

- Describe the characteristics of a professional physical educator
- Distinguish learning students and active teachers
- Explain how to design physically and emotionally safe learning environments
- Explain how to design a challenging and meaningful learning environment
- Describe how to use the 10 instructional principles
- Describe what it means for lessons to be an arrangement of tasks
- Describe how to communicate learning tasks effectively through both the teacher and the environment
- Articulate how to choose content to match a curriculum model
- Describe developing progressions of instructional tasks
- Explain developing tasks for tactical awareness in games teaching
- Describe how alignment fits into teaching progressions
- Depict how to modify task complexity
- Differentiate between closed and open skills
- Describe how to assess teaching and explore the tools to do so

Our three goals in writing this text are (1) to help you better understand how to be a better teacher in physical education settings, (2) to help you improve your teaching skills, and (3) to motivate you to want to become an effective, engaged, and **professional physical educator**. Of these three goals, the desire to become an effective teacher and to stay engaged with continuing professional development is the foundation upon which your future success is built. As Larry Locke noted in 1975, it isn't *bad* teaching that plagues physical education so much as it is *non*teaching. For example, you may have seen or even participated in physical education classes that could best be characterized as "supervised recreation." The teacher may have had the skills to be effective but wasn't motivated to use them. You have observed teaching from a student's view most of your life. Sometimes teaching looks simple, but that is an illusion. Effective teaching is complex. To teach several classes well each day, 5 days a week, for the length of a school year is difficult and requires both skills and the motivation to persevere in using and improving them.

Learning to teach effectively is like learning to be good in sport or any other movement form. If you want to get better, you have to know a lot about the skills and strategies of the sport, practice frequently under good conditions, and get help in the form of instruction, supervision, and feedback

BOX 13.1 Key Terms in This Chapter

- *Active teacher:* Believes that he or she can make a difference with students, develops a management system that helps students stay on task, plans and implements an instructional program that is action oriented, motivates students and holds them accountable for performance, and does so within a class climate that is supportive and respectful.
- *Check for understanding:* Questions and/or strategies used to determine if students understood and retained directions and instructions.
- *Effective task communication:* When tasks are communicated in such a way that students will attend to and comprehend the information the teacher presents and that information is sufficient for students to initially do the task as described.
- *Extending–refining cycle:* Rink's model for developing progressive instructional tasks. It consists of the informing task (initial task), refining tasks (to improve quality), extending tasks (to make the task more difficult), and applying tasks (to employ skill/strategy in authentic ways).
- *Instructional alignment:* When there is a match among the intended outcomes, instructional processes, and assessment.
- *Learning student:* Is cooperative, eager to learn, enthusiastic about the opportunity to learn more, and responsible for his or her own behavior; enjoys learning and practices purposefully to improve, and is helpful to peers who are similarly engaged in learning.
- *Plenty of perfect practice:* Practice that is pertinent (appropriate for the abilities, interests, and experiences of students), purposeful (lessons are kept on task in a climate that is both safe and challenging), progressive (skills and strategies are organized in ways that lead to sequential, significant learning), paced (activities are sequenced, difficult enough to be challenging yet allow successful practice), and participatory (students are constantly active and learning is equitable for all students).
- *Professional physical educator:* Intends for students to learn, plans for and monitors student enjoyment and progress, manages students to decrease disruptions and increase learning time, organizes learning experiences to match student abilities, and is motivated to be competent and caring.
- *Progressions:* Learning tasks that move students from less complex and less sophisticated tasks to more difficult and complicated tasks.

from those who know more than you do. Once you gain skills in doing a sport, you must have sufficient motivation to continually maintain and improve those skills, especially when the techniques and strategies of the sport evolve. So it is with becoming an effective, engaged teacher, that is, a professional physical educator.

Effective physical educators intend the students in their classes to learn and to enjoy doing the activities they are learning. To accomplish this, effective teachers manage students well to decrease disruptions and increase time for learning. An effective physical educator could do this by helping students take responsibility for their own learning and behavior. Effective physical educators then organize learning time with activities matched to student abilities so that an optimal amount of learning takes place. The assumption is clear: Effectiveness in teaching physical education should be judged by the quality and quantity of student learning. This starts with the intention to have students be different in some positive way (e.g., more skilled, take responsibility for their own learning) as a result of participating in and learning in your class.

This text is written with the assumption that you want to be that kind of a teacher—competent, qualified, and caring. If you have the motivation to become an effective teacher and persevere in that quest during your first several years of teaching, you can achieve a level of effectiveness that will mark you as a competent professional physical educator. Effective teachers orchestrate a repertoire of teaching skills to meet the ever-changing demands of the learning situation. Few things are more enjoyable than watching a motivated, skilled physical educator working with a group of students who are obviously learning and enjoying the learning. You can be that kind of teacher.

Research on teaching has shown clearly that teachers can make a difference. Who your teachers are and what they do in class will affect how much you learn, how you feel about the subject, and how you feel about yourself as a learner. Teachers can, on occasion, also touch the lives of students, influencing them in profound ways. We cannot forget, however, that the primary purpose of schooling is to help students learn and grow in ways that eventually lead to productive work, leisure, and citizenship. The main role of teachers in achieving that primary purpose is in developing and sustaining an effective instructional system (Wiggins, 1989). Through this role, physical education teachers provide an equitable, quality education for all students.

Learning Experience 13.1

Consider why you chose to become a physical education teacher. What and/or who motivates you? What and/or who do you want to influence? What are the benefits you expect to gain for students, yourself, and society?

Teaching and Learning

What is at the heart of effective teaching and learning? Educational psychologists, whether from a behavioral or cognitive perspective, seem to agree that for students to get better at anything they have to engage in sustained, deliberate practice. We know a lot about the conditions that define what psychologists call "deliberate practice" or "perfect practice." Physical education teachers can arrange the conditions for deliberate practice using a variety of instructional models and teaching strategies, meaningful curriculum choices, and facilitative organizational features. It is the quality and quantity of student involvement that reveals the effectiveness of an instructional task system.

Teaching becomes more enjoyable when students are enthusiastically engaged in learning. We begin here by focusing on a learning student. We will then turn to our explanation of an active teacher. We do that because we want to emphasize that it is *what students do* that is at the heart of understanding effective teaching. The quickest and surest way to assess the degree to which a physical education teacher is effective is by watching closely what students do in class. You cannot assess teacher effectiveness by focusing on what the teacher is doing. Indeed, a casual observer can get fooled by focusing solely on the actions of the teacher and ignoring the more important focus on the actions of students.

The Learning Student

In physical education, the **learning student** has these characteristics:

- Is cooperative
- Is eager to learn and enthusiastic about the opportunity to learn more
- Is responsible for his or her own behavior
- Enjoys learning and practices purposefully to improve
- Is helpful to peers who are similarly engaged in learning

Students who exhibit these characteristics are a pleasure to work with, and they also continually stretch a teacher because they want to know and do more. But how do young people become learning students? Students can acquire these characteristics over time through the influence of effective teachers. Assuredly, home backgrounds and community expectations play a role here as well. The bulk of evidence, however, suggests that the influence of teachers, over time, is crucial in helping young people become learners in the sense we have used the term here.

Students learn most of what they know, and can do, through **plenty of perfect practice** (see **Box 13.2**). Repeated practice is necessary for achieving the mastery students need to use skills, tactics, and knowledge in applied settings. This is true for learning fractions in mathematics, and it is true for learning the front walkover in gymnastics or the forearm pass in volleyball, mastering the weak-side help defense in basketball, skillfully orienting a compass when navigating an orienteering event, or making appropriate decisions when communicating with a teammate. Repeated, successful, relevant practice leads to accuracy and speed, two of the necessary components of skill performance and decision making. To be used in applied settings, such as games, skills and tactical knowledge need to reach the level of "automaticity" (Bloom, 1984), where they can be used quickly and accurately in response to the changing demands of the setting. If we want students to build lifelong habits of participation and physical activity, this is the level of performance that physical education needs to achieve for it to be successful as a school subject.

BOX 13.2 Plenty of Perfect Practice

A physical education teacher education program in Adelaide, South Australia, once used the phrase "plenty of perfect practice" as its main guidance for effective teaching. Plenty of perfect practice is realized when student learning experiences can be described as follows:

- *Pertinent:* Lessons are appropriate for the abilities, interests, and experiences of students.
- *Purposeful:* Lessons are kept on task in a climate that is both safe and challenging.
- *Progressive:* Skills and strategies are organized in ways that lead to sequential, significant learning.
- *Paced:* Activities are difficult enough to be challenging yet allow successful practice, and the sequence of activities is smooth and has brisk momentum.
- *Participatory:* Students are constantly active and learning is equitable for all students.

The notion of plenty of perfect practice is thoroughly consistent with both teacher effectiveness research and learning theory. It provides a simple, convenient reminder of what is important in planning for, and implementing, effective learning in physical education.

The learning student is increasingly able to take responsibility for his or her own learning. The goal is to help students become *independent* learners. We don't know as much as we need to know about how to develop such learners. What is most obvious is that young people cannot become independent learners unless they are gradually required to work cooperatively and make decisions, are given informative feedback on their efforts, and are held accountable.

The learning student in physical education learns the knowledge, skills, and strategies that will enable him or her to achieve a physically active, healthy lifestyle. In the United States, the National Association for Sport and Physical Education (NASPE) suggests a variety of attributes for a physically educated person (see www.naspe.org). These attributes are stated as outcomes, which means they represent what students should know and be able to do as a result of their experiences in physical education. Reviewing these outcomes will let you see just how difficult effective teaching in physical education is and that to contribute in some important degree to the achievement of those outcomes your students must take on the characteristics of a learning student.

Learning students, through the process of becoming physically educated, will learn important lessons about themselves. They will learn to see themselves as capable learners. They will learn to see themselves as physically competent and active. They will learn that school and educational experiences in general are helpful and supportive. They will learn that, to get better at something, it is useful to have an effective teacher. These lessons help to shape a lifetime learner.

Learning Experience 13.2

Ask a teacher if you might sit in and observe his or her physical education class. Identify three students to observe—one who is highly skilled, one who is moderately skilled, and one who is low skilled. Take turns observing them as the lesson unfolds, noting what they do, how they respond to tasks, and how they interact with peers. Discuss your findings with a peer and link the discussion to what we know about learning students.

The Active Teacher

An **active teacher** is one who believes that he or she can make a difference with students, develops a management system that helps students stay on task, plans and implements an instructional program that is action oriented, motivates students and holds them accountable for performance, and does so within a class climate that is supportive and respectful. We choose the label of *active teacher* to emphasize the difference between the effective physical educator and the stereotype of the teacher who just "throws out the ball," who doesn't seem to care much about students other than keeping them from being too disruptive.

Active teachers keep students consistently engaged and help them to become better learners. Active teachers frequently use whole-group instruction and well-organized small-group instruction. When students are assigned tasks, the teacher supervises the work carefully. In the classes of active teachers, students are seldom passive. They respond frequently. The pace of instruction and practice is brisk, yet within the students' abilities and developmental levels. Eventually, students receive the message of this approach to teaching, and they learn to work independently and cooperatively with a sense of purpose. In **Box 13.3** we provide summaries of the major findings of research on teacher effectiveness that describe the important strategies used by active teachers. Although this research was conducted and reported throughout the 1980s, it has yet to be contradicted and so provides us with important insights and guidance. This research has shown that these characteristics of active teachers are particularly useful and relevant to teaching (1) young children, (2) less-skilled students, (3) students from educationally disadvantaged backgrounds, (4) beginners at any age level, and (5) well-structured activities in which learning needs to build sequentially. Students who most physical education teachers teach fall into one or more of these categories. Highly skilled, eager, and bright students can also learn from teachers who have these characteristics, but, of course, they tend to learn no matter what methods teachers use.

Teachers teach; students learn. Although teachers can learn *from* students, teachers cannot learn *for* the students. Students learn through their involvement with the content and they get better through purposeful practice. What teachers can do is influence the kind of work students do and the intensity and duration of their engagement with the learning tasks. This involvement, on a lesson-by-lesson basis, is the key to understanding effective teaching. This is true whether the student engagement is related to motor skill, tactical, cognitive, or social objectives. It is also true whether the instructional model is direct or indirect, group, small group, or individualized.

If you want to improve your students' motor skills, fitness, knowledge, social skills, or attitudes, influence the quality and quantity of their involvement with content in class (and out of class, too). In attempting to influence the nature of their involvement, always remember that how students react to instructional tasks, through modifications, will influence the potential for learning. This is why we advocate for teachers to strive to develop a learning climate that is characterized by cooperation and, where possible, over time to build a learning community.

BOX 13.3 Summaries of Active Teachers Teaching Strategies

- *Belief in their own efficacy:* Active teachers believe that students can learn and that they have the skills to help them learn.
- *Time, opportunity to learn, and content covered:* Active teachers allocate as much time as possible to content coverage and provide all students with sufficient opportunities to learn.
- *Expectations and roles:* Active teachers communicate high, realistic expectations to their students and develop a clear, work-oriented class climate. Teacher and student roles are carefully defined, with students being given adequate instruction and time to learn their roles.
- *Class management and student engagement:* Active teachers establish class routines early in the school year, and manage by using these well-established structures. Rules are clear and consistently related to equally clear consequences. The purpose of effective management is to create maximum time for learning the subject matter.
- *Meaningful tasks and high success:* Active teachers design instructional tasks that are meaningful for students and lead to authentic outcomes. Tasks are challenging but also allow students to experience success.
- *Pacing and momentum:* Active teachers create and sustain a brisk pace for class activities and prevent events from disrupting the momentum of this pace. The result is a climate of energy and purposefulness.
- *Appropriate guidance:* Active teachers communicate content with clear, brief demonstrations and explanations, followed by sufficient guided practice, with frequent feedback and checking for understanding, to allow students to benefit from independent practice.
- *Active supervision:* When guided practice shows that students understand the tasks and have eliminated major technical errors, they are shifted to independent practice, which is actively supervised by the teacher, who monitors progress and maintains a task-oriented practice session.
- *Accountability:* Active teachers hold students accountable for appropriate participation in practice, for task completion, and for performance outcomes.
- *Clarity, enthusiasm, and equitable support:* Active teachers communicate clearly, are enthusiastic about their subject matter and their students' achievements, and are supportive of all learners in their efforts to learn and improve.
- *Building from student understanding:* Active teachers begin by assessing what their students understand about the activities and their meanings, and then use this information in planning and implementing lessons. They frequently solicit input, with the result that students feel they have a say in class life.

Learning Experience 13.3

Based on the data you collected on the three students in the previous learning experience, describe how you, as an active teacher, might provide support and feedback to each of the students in an attempt to help them become learning students motivated to participate and learn in your class.

Designing Physically and Emotionally Safe Learning Environments

A major responsibility of every physical education teacher is to provide a safe learning environment for students. Safety should be considered when planning, but it is in the implementation of a lesson that safety must be foremost. Participation in physical activity comes with inherent risks—risks that challenge students' notion of feeling safe (e.g., conscious of a dangerous situation such as running on a wet pool deck), risks that could cause injury (e.g., accidents during activity may result in physical harm), and risks that come with specific types of activities (e.g., physical contact in basketball or rugby). Student safety is the responsibility of the teacher, acknowledging that students also need to be taught and held somewhat responsible for their own safety and the safety of others. Whether considering the managerial or the instructional task system, safety is critical. Students must be taught in a safely engineered environment, taught about safety procedures and practices, and helped to feel safe (emotionally and physically) in this setting.

From a managerial perspective, safety can be planned for in advance of implementation by assessing risks and ensuring that all precautions have been taken into consideration and applied—facilities are clean and risk free, equipment is in good working order, and equipment and people are arranged in the safest way possible. Whenever a potentially hazardous activity is being undertaken, the teacher should emphasize *clearly* the *rules* that have been established with regards to the hazard. These rules should be described and prompted often, and students should be held accountable for obeying them. To do less is to risk both student injury and a legal action. This is not to suggest that activities involving risk should not be used in the physical education program. Quite the contrary, one goal of the program should be to help students learn to take some risks and want to participate in activities that may involve an element of risk. Many sport and outdoor activities have risks and the potential for physical injury. What needs to be emphasized are the rules regarding safety in terms of the specific activity and the space within which it is practiced and played.

Drawing on the work of the European Education Consultants, Kelly (1997) suggests a risk assessment scale that physical education teachers employ as they prepare for teaching (see **Table 13.1**), recording their findings and making appropriate safety adjustments. Once the teacher is confident that all safety precautions have been taken to ensure a safe environment, he or she should develop, teach, post, and review gymnasium/activity space safety rules and procedures. Designing a preventive management plan and developing a contingency management plan will be useful in facilitating students' choice of behaviors and actions that might pose risk to themselves and peers.

When planning for instruction, students' physical and emotional safety should be the teacher's first priority. Students must be taught how to safely perform a learning task, spot a peer who is performing a risky skill, wear necessary safety equipment, and work with a peer/buddy when undertaking tasks that involve risk. From a teaching perspective, teachers must consider all decisions that will allow them to build safety into the learning experiences they design for student participation and learning. These considerations must include designing appropriate progressions, choosing safe content, grouping students for learning, ensuring students have the prerequisite skills necessary to participate, and that lessons include the teaching of task safety precautions and performance guidelines.

TABLE 13.1 Risk Assessment Scale

Scale	Risk	Risk Defined
1	Not likely	No risk identified; chance or a one-off might result in an accident
2	Possible	Likelihood of an accident occurring is low
3	Quite possible	Accident may happen if additional substantive factors occur
4	Likely	Accident is likely due to normal circumstances that might occur
5	Very likely	Unless factors change, an accident will happen

Students not only need to *behave* safely, but they also need to *feel* safe about what they are doing. This means they should feel comfortable about their participation, and should be willing to participate fully. They will have emotional safety to the degree that their efforts are supported and are not met with ridicule and negative comment. Students will also feel comfortable, and tend to behave safely too, if they have experienced an appropriate progression to shape their skills and if they have a background of related successes. If they have experienced the proper progressions, they will be challenged by current tasks and feel able and willing to perform them safely.

Learning Experience 13.4

You are designing an Ultimate Frisbee unit for your third-year postprimary students. The class of 30 students meets for the first class of the day, when the weather tends to be a bit damp. Activity will take place on the outdoor sport fields and each student will have their own disc to begin activity. Review your plans for the unit, consider the students whom you are teaching and the facilities and equipment to be used, and identify five recommendations to reduce the risks your students might encounter. Discuss your list of recommendations with a peer and share a rationale for their inclusion.

Regardless of whether an accident occurs during the managerial or the instructional task system, procedures must be in place with which both the teacher and the students are familiar. Every school has a safety policy and guidelines to guide these procedures, and these should be accessed, reviewed, and posted in the gymnasium. Steps for the teacher to take if, and when, an accident occurs include (1) appraise the situation, (2) protect students not involved in the accident, (3) attend to the accident and injured person(s), and (4) inform the appropriate persons (administration and/or emergency services). Although these steps appear straightforward, the teacher responding immediately and students knowing their roles thoroughly are paramount.

Learning Experience 13.5

Access the safety guidelines that impact your teaching and the safety of your students in the context in which you teach. This might include local and national guidelines, procedures published by the physical education association, safety policies of the school, and specific practices of the physical education department. Make a list of the key aspects you would teach to your students to prepare them for an accident, should it occur in your classroom.

Finally, the teacher must be constantly alert to unsafe student behavior. Students are not mature adults. Often, in the excitement of an activity, they do not behave in fully mature ways. Teachers need to be aware of student behavior that jeopardizes the student's own safety or the safety of others. Unsafe behavior should be desisted immediately, and specific feedback should be given as to why the behavior is unsafe. Active supervision (noted previously and discussed later in this chapter) is the best strategy to help teachers keep in close contact with what their students are doing.

Ensuring a Challenging and Meaningful Learning Environment

What makes a lesson challenging and meaningful to students? There are several important answers to that question. First, curricular choices and curricular design are important for a successful physical education. Curricular choices are always contextual. That is, they are for a particular group of students in a particular setting. Curricular planning should allow for a sufficient amount of time in units for students to achieve significant progress toward meaningful unit goals, which should be defined in authentic terms.

Curricular choices should take into account the cultural relevance of activities to the students' lives and help extend students' perspectives of what activities might be relevant to their lives. This is tricky territory. It takes tremendously skillful teaching, and the development of a cooperative spirit in classes, for teachers to satisfy what students perceive to be their immediate interests, yet also help them extend those interests. This certainly cannot be accomplished without a class climate in which student voices are heard and open discussion and trust define relationships.

A challenging learning environment will develop when unit goals are authentic and when teachers design tasks (or work cooperatively with students to design tasks) that continually provide challenge but also allow for success. Because not all students will have the same skills or background in any activity, provision of challenging tasks that allow for success must include a variation of task difficulty within tasks. The inclusion model allows students to select from a range of difficulty levels within a basic task framework, thus helping to ensure that all students are challenged and can be successful. When students are consistently challenged by meaningful tasks and successfully accomplish them, their learning is positively affected, their interest in the activity is strengthened, and their motivation to persist in getting better is increased.

Teachers are able to design more meaningful instructional tasks when they take the time to find out what a particular activity or skill means to students at the outset of a unit. Teachers make a mistake when they assume that activities and skills mean the same things to students as they do to the teachers who design them. What do students think is the purpose of volleyball? What does it mean to them to strike a ball with their forearms? What does it mean to them to be able to hit the ball with their forearms and direct it toward a target? We know that students construct meaning from their involvement with an activity, that they build meaning on existing knowledge. We also know that, if the knowledge they start with is inaccurate or incomplete, the meanings students construct are likely to be inaccurate and incomplete (Resnick & Williams-Hall, 1998). Thus, teachers must take the time to assess what meanings and understandings students bring to a particular content and then work to ensure that their knowledge and understandings are accurate as they use instructional tasks to build on that base.

The physical education learning environment should also be intellectually challenging. There is no reason to dumb down physical education. There are nuances to skill development and tactical play. There are aesthetic dimensions to sports and dance. There is a wealth of health-related information and meaning to exercise. Students should be encouraged to ask questions, to seek answers. They should be encouraged to explore the ideas that grow from engagement in physical activity. They should be encouraged to express themselves and their reactions to developing arm strength or playing a zone defense. Teachers who find ways to let students know that they value expression, questioning, and the interplay of ideas contribute to a climate of openness in which student voices are respected and improve the intellectual climate of the class.

Learning Experience 13.6

Reflect back on your experiences in physical education. Identify the factors that made physical education a challenging, meaningful, and exciting environment in which to participate. At the same time, identify which factors made physical education boring, repetitive, or not worth your energy to pursue. How would you intend to establish such factors for students you will be teaching in your physical education class? How would you intend to address the factors students share with you?

Ten Instructional Principles

Yellon (1996) proposes 10 instructional principles to aid the teacher in understanding how best to teach, how to design new and refine existing instruction, and how to provide a language for both the teacher and the student to guide the teaching and learning process. Briefly, the 10 principles are:

1. Teaching should be *meaningful*, relevant, and authentic to the learner and related to past experiences, current contexts, and future aspirations. This suggests interacting

with, listening to, and integrating students' desires into the curriculum.

2. Effective teaching is built on and linked to students' *prerequisite* knowledge and skills, which ultimately will result in differentiated learning tasks to meet the needs and interests of all students.
3. In order for students to learn most effectively, the environment must reflect *open communication* where learners are valued, guided, and supported in achieving goals that are shared through transparent means in a trusting relationship.
4. *Prioritizing essential content to be learned* is a first step in designing effective instruction. Define the learning goal, identify what that learning will look like when the student is successful, clarify the steps/procedures necessary for achievement of the goal, and plan instruction to achieve these targets.
5. Not all students learn in the same way through identical pedagogies. Developing and using *learning aids* is a means of assisting all learners to be successful. They stimulate recall, guide practice, emphasize key points, and vary support for learning.
6. Whether through your actions (e.g., voice, lesson pace, movement), choice of learning experiences (e.g., cases, student-designed tasks), selection of teaching strategies (e.g., questions, challenges), or variety in content delivery (e.g., demonstrations, student exploration) it is critical to gain and maintain the learners' attention through *novel pedagogies*.
7. *Modeling* of mental, interpersonal, and physical skills is critical to effective instruction and should include the learner being told what to attend to in a demonstration, repeating the key points of the demonstration, and following the directions while they attempt the skill.
8. *Active appropriate practice* suggests that learners practice a skill or a task in an authentic way, progressing into more in-depth and "real life" applications as they gain mastery.
9. *Encouraging conditions and consequences* are essential if students are to enjoy learning and choose to continue the learning process. This requires the learning context to be emotionally and physically safe, built on accurate and specific feedback to promote learning, and couched in feelings of value and respect.
10. Yellon (1996) calls *consistency of all instructional elements* the secret of instructional design and states that, "there are certain components we need in an effective piece of instruction, and each component has to be consistent with the others."

Lessons as Arrangement of Tasks

Lessons should be viewed as an arrangement of tasks. This is a useful way to view lessons because it focuses on what students do in the lesson. Every lesson has managerial and instructional tasks, and teachers should never forget that students always have social tasks to accomplish. Students will enter the gymnasium or need to move to an outdoor space (entry tasks, initial activity tasks, transition tasks). They will have to be informed as to what content will be practiced for the lesson (informing, refining, extending, and applying instructional tasks explained later in this chapter). They may have to organize differently for different instructional tasks (transitional tasks, equipment replacement tasks). At some point, they may have to gather and disperse to receive instruction and return to practice. The lesson will eventually culminate in closure, and students will move to their classrooms or changing/locker room. How all these tasks are implemented determines the success or failure of the lesson from an instructional point of view.

Students engage in instructional tasks regardless of the instructional model utilized. What does differ in various instructional models, and in a sense defines their categories, is how tasks are *mediated* in the teaching/learning process. The two primary categories are (1) models in which teachers mediate instruction and (2) models in which students mediate instruction. Teachers can mediate tasks directly, as in group-oriented active teaching models, or indirectly through a task or station teaching model or self-instructional models. Many teachers are experimenting with instructional models in which much of the instruction is mediated by students, as in peer or reciprocal models, small-group instruction, Sport Education teams, a cooperative learning format, or problems-based learning. What is important here is to understand that our focus for viewing a lesson as a series of tasks requires you to think first about what students will do in that lesson. This focus helps you see the degree to which you are facilitating the purposeful practice that will lead to important student outcomes.

Table 13.2 contains the main elements of a typical physical education lesson, showing the tasks students would perform and the important instructional functions that the fulfillment of those tasks contributes to an effective lesson. The lesson shown assumes a direct, teacher-mediated model consistent with what we have called active teaching. Some instructional functions get repeated throughout the lesson.

Table 13.3 provides a similar analysis of the main elements of a lesson, showing the tasks students would perform and the important instructional functions that the fulfillment of those tasks contributes in Sport Education, where many of the instructional and managerial tasks are mediated by students. The instructional functions are similar to the teacher-mediated example, but, in Sport Education, most of the actual instructing and managing is done by students with the help and guidance of the teacher.

TABLE 13.2 Main Elements of a Typical Physical Education Lesson

Student Task	Instructional Function
Enter gym and engage in initial practice task.	Development and teaching of entry routine for practicing familiar tasks
Gather for instruction and receive instruction for a new skill.	Gathering routine and well-planned demonstration that culminates in clear communication of informing task
Practice the informing task.	Guided practice
Disperse for independent practice, and practice task.	Dispersal routine and supervision of independent practice
Refine task being practiced.	Attention routine, clear refinement communication
Extend task by changing conditions of practice, followed by practice.	Attention routine, clear communication of extending task, followed by active supervision
Refine task and continue practice.	Attention routine, clear refinement communication, followed by active supervision
Gather students to explain applying task.	Attention and gathering routines, well-planned explanation and demonstration
Explain organizational format for applying task, and disperse students for practice.	Dispersal routine followed by guided practice
Apply task practice for 10 minutes. Gather for closure.	Active supervision gathering routine followed by closure

TABLE 13.3 Main Elements of a Sport Education Lesson

Student Task	Instructional Function
Enter gym, go to team space, and engage in warm-up skill or skill practice.	Development and teaching of entry routine, teaching student coaches how to guide and supervise practice
Transition to first game is made. Players go to appropriate game spaces. Referees/scorers get equipment and move to assigned spaces.	Gathering routine, teaching coaches how to lead discussion and involve teammates
First game is played.	Transition routines, teaching team managers how to organize equipment and assignment, students fulfilling multiple roles
Game ends and transition to next game is made. New teams, referees, and scorers are named. Results are turned in.	Transition routines, managers guiding team members to appropriate places
Second game is played.	Students fulfilling multiple roles
Game ends and transition to next game is made.	Transition routines, managers guiding team members to appropriate places
Last game ends. Teams return to home place. Statisticians gather all game results. Managers put away all equipment. Coaches debrief teams.	Routines for gathering at home place, game results, and equipment, all roles previously taught
Class gathers for closure: recognition of performance, fair play, and student roles.	Routine for class closure

Learning Experience 13.7

Observe a physical education class, and take note of all tasks in which the students are involved, including managerial and instructional as well as the social tasks that the students pursue. Portray this data much the same as it is in Tables 13.2 and 13.3. Assess whether the teacher is using managerial and instructional routines to their best effect throughout this lesson to support student learning and enjoyment.

Communicating Tasks to Students Effectively and Efficiently

Both managerial and instructional tasks must be communicated to students. If the tasks are informing tasks, the communications will sometimes be fairly extensive. Task communications should be evaluated by their effectiveness and efficiency. **Effective task communication** means that students will attend to and comprehend the information you present and that information will be sufficient for them to initially do the task as it has been described. Efficient task communication means that only as much time as is necessary will be used to ensure effective communication.

Most physical education teachers probably spend more time than is necessary in task communication. They often provide more information than students can use when they begin to practice the task. Most experts agree that students learn most effectively when they have a good general idea of what is to be accomplished and are aware of major technical features of the skill or strategy but not the details. The details of task development are mastered through a series of refining tasks, not by including them all in the informing task.

Learning Experience 13.8

Make an audio recording of yourself teaching a lesson. Sit down in a quiet place following the lesson and listen to how you communicate with students. Is your voice strong and loud enough for students to hear? Is your pitch variable or monotone? Do you provide just enough information for students to follow your directions (what we think of as "need to know" information)? Would you be able to follow your own directions? Do you separate managerial directions from instructional guidelines to avoid confusion? Determine how to improve your communication skills. Practice and record another lesson in a few weeks.

Motor skill and strategy tasks should be introduced by establishing the importance of the task or linking it to previous work. Students should then see what the whole task looks like. They should be told what to look for in terms of the few elements being emphasized for that task practice. Teachers often have students passively watch these task presentations, but there is much to be said for having the students actively involved. Particularly in skill tasks, students can be "shadowing" you as you describe the elements being emphasized.

Before beginning practice, you should check to see if the communication was received accurately. Students can respond as a group, or individuals can be chosen to show or describe an element. This **check for understanding** will serve not only as a signal to you that the task has been communicated effectively but also as an accountability mechanism to keep students attending to your presentation. This check for understanding should include both the elements of the skill or strategy to be practiced and the organizational conditions for practice.

Tasks must be communicated both to students gathered to receive the information and, on other occasions, to students dispersed in some practice format. You should usually gather students for tasks that require new information or more lengthy explanations and demonstrations. This means that these tasks will be preceded by attention and gathering routines. Most refining tasks and some extending or applying tasks can be communicated to students at their dispersed positions, without first gathering them. Communicating tasks to a dispersed class requires you to place yourself where all students can see and hear the explanation. Dispersed task communication also requires that you use a good, strong voice. If the conditions of task practice have been changed, as they often are with extending tasks, then you should check that the students understand them before they return to practice. **Box 13.4** gives suggestions for developing effective task communication skills.

Communicate Learning Tasks Effectively Through Both the Teacher and the Environment

Learning time is a precious commodity that should be used judiciously. Much of the information communicated from teacher to student during class time could be communicated just as effectively but more efficiently as regards using class time. A well-developed handout provides the learner with a permanent record of instructional intent and reduces the possibility of students misunderstanding a verbal presentation. Instructional objectives, rules, diagrams of dance moves and playing fields, defensive/offensive maneuvers and gymnastics routines, and other lesson detail can be communicated to students through handouts. Informational handouts might be posted on the school physical education website or posted on the walls of the gymnasium and sports hall as opposed to printing them out for each student. Of course, it is useless to design and distribute handouts for students if there is no mechanism in your instructional system to ensure that they are used. An informal method of ensuring this is to intermittently ask students questions that pertain directly to the information handouts. For example, if you provide a diagram of a badminton court, you can ask a student to show the back boundary line for the doubles serve, singles sidelines, or the position of the server in singles play. Students' understanding of the material should be formally assessed only if the handout is of sufficient importance to warrant taking time for this. Thus, you might administer a short rules test before beginning actual game competition in a new activity. If students have a handout on the rules and if they must pass a short quiz in order to gain access to the game, then chances are they will learn the material. Thus, the game can proceed at a much higher level because the situations in which rules will need to be clarified will be minimal.

Posters and task cards using cue words to describe the critical elements of the skills that are being practiced can be placed around a gym or distributed to a team so that students can look at them when they need them. Pictures of players with the critical elements emphasized can provide another source of information. Diagrams of strategic movements can also be used. Thus, when students need to have

BOX 13.4 Developing Effective Task Communication Skills

- Be sure about your information. Know your content. Understand what is most important to tell and show students—and what is less important.
- Use language students understand. Take into account their age level and experience with the activity. Teach technical terms carefully so that, when they are used, students understand them.
- Show enthusiasm, but speak clearly and slowly. Students don't know the content as well as you do. They need time to process new information.
- Use metaphors and analogies to bring the new information closer to the student experience. This is what pedagogical content knowledge (PCK) is all about: being able to transform your technical knowledge of content and deliver it to students in ways they can easily assimilate and use.
- Demonstrate (or have demonstrated) the skill under conditions as close as possible to how it will be used in the applied setting. Demonstrate the set pass near the net, goal-keeping skills at the goal. When it is important for students to see the skill from more than one view, provide the appropriate views. For example, to emphasize the appropriate shooting arm elbow position for basketball, show it both from the side view and the front view.
- Make sure the demonstration and explanation are accurate. The demonstration doesn't have to show perfect technique, and the explanation doesn't have to be overly technical. But the critical elements shown and explained should actually be the critical elements and should be shown accurately.
- Remember, you are not demonstrating just a skill or a tactic but also the manner in which you want students to practice it. You should end by demonstrating the practice task itself. Students should know what to do and how they will know if the task is completed successfully.
- As much as possible, involve students during the demonstration/explanation. Passive observing is not as good as shadowing the movements.
- If safety is a particular issue with the task, make sure the dangerous elements are emphasized and appropriate safety rules and routines are clearly understood (e.g., no high-sticking in floor hockey).
- Check to see if students understand what they have seen and heard *before* you disperse them for practice.

this information, they can get it without taking the time of the whole class. For example, if one group is having problems practicing a dance move, it could be sent briefly to a poster and picture to refresh members about which elements to emphasize and see what those elements look like in action.

Learning Experience 13.9

For a unit plan you are currently developing, design a handout for students to take home or access on the school website, a poster to assist students as they practice during class, and a set of task cards to guide student participation. Choose a different activity for each resource.

Choosing Content to Match the Curriculum Model

Once the main-theme curriculum models have been selected and meaningful learning outcomes specified, you must choose the activities that will form program content; design learning experiences for learners to practice application of relevant skills, strategies, and knowledge; and design aligned assessment measures to determine if the outcomes have been achieved. The selection of activities, however, is the point at which program planning often breaks down. Activities are sometimes chosen because they are "attractive" or because it is "that time of year," rather than for the degree the activities lead to expected outcomes. Keep the following points in mind before beginning to plan for and select program activities:

- *An activity is appropriate because it contributes to program outcomes.* "Appropriate" in this case is a relevant term. If your main theme is Tactical Approach to Teaching Games, then team handball and tennis are appropriate activities, as they would be for Sport Education. If you have an Outdoor Education theme, then rappelling and climbing are appropriate activities, especially when built upon an Adventure Education program that emphasizes teamwork and trust. Golf would be an appropriate activity for Sport Education but not for a fitness curriculum. Team orienteering might be appropriate for an Adventure Education program and can also be done in a cross-country season. Any number of activities could be linked across the curriculum in a physical education program focused on the Teaching Personal and Social Responsibility model, just as throwing would be appropriately taught within a Skill Themes model.
- *Successful programs accomplish goals.* If you are to make a mistake in planning, it is wise to make that

error in the direction of trying to achieve too little rather than too much. Limited goals with fewer activities are easier to achieve than a large set of goals and many activities. Doing activity units well takes time. There is reason to question whether a program that attempts to teach some of every activity and content area accomplishes anything of lasting value. If you want your program to be successful, choose a limited number of outcomes, and develop a limited number of activities to achieve them. This assumes, of course, that the outcomes you are trying to accomplish are learning oriented, relevant, and meaningful, rather than merely keeping students busy.

- *Know what you are doing.* The activities you choose become the content of your program. Teachers should know their content well because without that knowledge they cannot develop the appropriate progressions for learning content thoroughly. "Knowing" refers to both the content and how to apply it to specific learners. Choosing activities with which you have limited experience results in inadequately developed content. How much space does the activity take? How can it be modified? How are the skills and strategy best refined? How should equipment be modified? To answer these questions typically requires that you know the activity well. This suggests that, if you include an activity you don't know well, you take the time to research the content and thus enable yourself to design appropriate sequences and learning experiences.

If you choose activities that do indeed contribute directly to the goals implied in your curriculum model, if you know your activities well enough to develop content appropriately for the learners you serve, and if you provide sufficient time for those learners to make meaningful gains in performing the activities, then you will have taken huge strides toward establishing a successful physical education program.

Learning Experience 13.10

Reflect on your strengths and weaknesses when it comes to physical education content. Consider a number of different activity strands (e.g., aquatics, adventure, outdoor, track and field, net games, invasion games, target and fielding games, gymnastics, dance, fitness). Identify the content areas within these strands where you feel confident designing an aligned scheme of work (learning goals, learning experiences and instruction, and assessment). Indicate if you have the knowledge and skill to teach this content at an advanced as well as an entry stage. Now, identify the content areas in which you need to up-skill and investigate where and how you might achieve that up-skilling.

Developing Progressions of Instructional Tasks

Keep in mind what you learned about effective teachers taking time to find out what their students understand about what they are going to learn. In other words, what meanings do they attach to a particular content, and what are the implications for you in your planning? Once you know where you are headed and what you want learners to achieve, you must determine how to meet your goals. To understand how to get there, you should first know your starting point. That is, what will be the students' levels of skill, understanding, and experience when they enter the program? As a trained professional educator, you will know part of this in a general way from your study of motor development and primary and postprimary physical education. This general knowledge will allow you to develop content by planning task progressions that lead to important outcomes. **Progressions** are learning tasks that move students from less complex and less sophisticated tasks to more difficult and complicated tasks. The eventual result is the kinds of meaningful performances that represent the intended outcomes of the program. The application of these progressions, however, will always be specific to the students taught in any particular setting, the experiences students bring with them, and the time available. Experienced teachers know that you can teach two first-year postprimary classes in consecutive time blocks and require very different progressions to adequately meet the developmental differences in each. Nonetheless, designing progressions becomes an important technical skill in developing content. Developing progressions is where knowledge of content and knowledge of teaching come together, what Shulman (1987) has called pedagogical content knowledge, that unique blend of content and pedagogy that is the special expertise of the teacher.

Teachers communicate progressions to students through a series of instructional tasks within a lesson or unit and, from year to year, across units in the same activity or category of activities. Rink's (2009) model for developing progressive instructional tasks continues to be widely used in physical education. Initial tasks *inform* the student of a new skill or strategy. Subsequent tasks *refine* the quality of the performance, *extend* the performance by altering it slightly, and *apply* the skill or strategy.

1. *Informing tasks:* These are the initial tasks to begin a lesson and a sequence of learning tasks. From this initial task the teacher develops the lesson and the subsequent content to be mastered.
2. *Refining performance quality:* Perhaps the most neglected, yet most important, kind of progression is the sequence of learning tasks through which students improve the technical quality of skill or strategy performance, what Rink calls *refinement tasks*. Each skill or strategy task that the teacher introduces will need to be refined. In refining tasks, the conditions of practice do not change. Only the focus of student attention changes as different technical

elements or strategy are emphasized. Teaching primary students to juggle using the cascade technique provides an example. Tossing a juggling ball, or "popping," can be introduced with a demonstration and an explanation of four or five critical performance elements (juggler's box, cupped hands at waist height, count for each pop, figure-eight pattern, keep eyes focused on top of pop) that define the skill (*informing task*). Students can then practice this skill daily as they progress through the juggling unit. However, the skill must be refined if the student is to move on to juggling with three or more implements. Students may tend to break the wrist when they pop the ball, as they should do in other kinds of throws but not in the juggling pop. The pop must be quick, sudden, and short, with no follow-through. Students may try to mimic a juggler who has a smooth, flowing rhythm, yet when learning, they must have sharp and definite movements, sometimes known as *marcato* or *marked rhythm*. It is through a series of refining tasks that students become more aware of the technical components of a good pop so that this critical aspect of juggling improves. Success in skill and strategy requires quality performance, and that should be the teacher's goal. Refining tasks can't always be anticipated. Teachers must use information about the performance of their students to develop progressive refining tasks.

3. *Within-task progressions:* Both skills and strategies need to be simplified to begin with and then gradually made more complex. Think of building content in one of the track and field events, such as the shot put. The basic task, putting the shot, will not change, which means that, right from the outset, a legal put rather than a throw is taught. However, few would begin to teach the shot put by having students start from the back of the circle and then teaching the glide or spin in their mature forms. Instead, a series of *within-task progressions* is taught. Rink (2009) refers to this as *intra-task development*. You might begin with an implement that is lighter than a standard shot and with students in the final putting position, focusing on arm and hand action to "punch" the shot up in the air. Regardless of where you begin, you would have to refine the skill demanded in that task (flick of the wrist as shot leaves the hand) before you extend the skill with a slightly more complex task such as a focus on hip and shoulder rotation to provide force to the put as students punch toward the wall, which would again require refinement (drive the hip toward the target prior to release of the shot) before moving to still another more complex task. Rink (2009) refers to within-task progressions as *extending tasks*, those that change the complexity of performance. At the end of this chapter, we identify a series of methods to modify task complexity, which is essentially a means of extending the movement task. The **extending–refining cycle** repeated over and over again forms the central core of content development in physical education. **Box 13.5** provides an example of appropriate and inappropriate progressions for the overhead set in volleyball. Knowing what to refine and how much to extend for the specific learners you are working with is perhaps the most important ingredient of expert planning. **Box 13.6** provides examples of refining and extending tasks for a one-hand shot in basketball.
4. *Between-task progressions:* When planning a program that begins with either novice learners or young learners, consider progressions between related tasks. For example, moving from a scissors jump to the Fosbury style in developing high jump content, from a horizontal traverse to a vertical climb in developing climbing content, or from three-versus-three strategy in soccer to a full-sided game with more players in a larger space all represent different tasks rather than variations of one major task. The progressions among them become important building blocks in developing content for a program. Between-task extensions need to be thought through carefully. Teachers sometimes assume that tasks are progressions when they are not. To be a progression, one task would have to be related to another in terms of common critical performance elements. For example, we would argue that the underhand serve in volleyball is not a progression for the overhand serve, even though the underhand serve might be used for young or novice volleyball players. The technical demands of the two skills are too different for them to be a skill progression. But the scissors style of high jump contains virtually all the beginning technical elements (curved approach run, plant foot that is away from the bar, drive the knee of the inside leg, and drive the arms up at a 90-degree angle) that students will need when they eventually learn the Fosbury style, so those two form a legitimate progression.
5. *Application tasks:* Providing students with the chance to apply their skills and use strategies in more authentic ways is the intent of application tasks. Application tasks therefore allow students opportunities to participate in the movement through an applied experience or to assess their skill/strategy performance. Small-sided games put students in a setting where they must select and perform skills and game strategies. One partner might be asked to assess the performance of the other partner during a gymnastics competition or to double-check the reading on a heart rate monitor, thus assessing one aspect of his or her own mastery of content. Students might be asked to monitor the number of legal forehand strokes they can perform during a pickle-ball or tennis partner rally. Each of these is an applied task students can perform once they gain adequate skill and confidence. Application tasks need not wait until the final task in a progression. They can be incorporated along the way as a means of providing feedback and allowing students to experience skills and strategies in applied ways.

BOX 13.5 Appropriate and Inappropriate Progressions for the Overhead Set

In each lesson, the teacher has explained and demonstrated the forearm pass and begun practice by having students pass the ball back to a partner from a short underhand toss. Students have already practiced the set pass from a toss in the previous lesson.

Inappropriate task progression by Teacher A:

- *Task 1:* Toss the ball to your partner with an underhand toss from about 10 feet. Your partner passes it back to you with a forearm pass and you catch it.
- *Task 2:* Now let's use the forearm pass in a game. You must use a forearm pass to a teammate before you can send the ball back over the net.

Figure A shows how this progression looks when graphed.

Appropriate task progression by Teacher B:

- *Task 1:* Toss the ball to your partner with an underhand toss from about 10 feet. Your partner passes it back to you with a forearm pass and you catch it with your hands above your head.
- *Task 2:* This time, as you practice, try to get yourself in position to receive the ball before you pass the ball. Get there and get ready.
- *Task 3:* If your trajectory isn't high on the ball after you pass it, what does that mean for where you are hitting it? How can you get a high trajectory? OK, this time get under it more and follow through toward your target (partner's hands above the head).
- *Task 4:* When you and your partner can both pass the ball five times in a row with a high and accurate trajectory, take two or three steps back and try it again.
- *Task 5:* Now let's try a forearm pass followed by a set. Toss the ball to your partner. Your partner will forearm pass the ball to you, you will set it back and your partner will catch it. The sequence becomes toss, forearm pass, overhead set, and catch (toss-pass-set-and-catch).
- *Tasks 6 and 7:* When you can do this five times in a row, move farther away from each other, and see if you can still make it work.
- *Task 8:* In groups of three, one person serves the ball, one does a forearm pass, and one sets the ball. Start with an easy serve, and make the serve more difficult as you are ready.

Figure B shows how this progression looks when graphed.

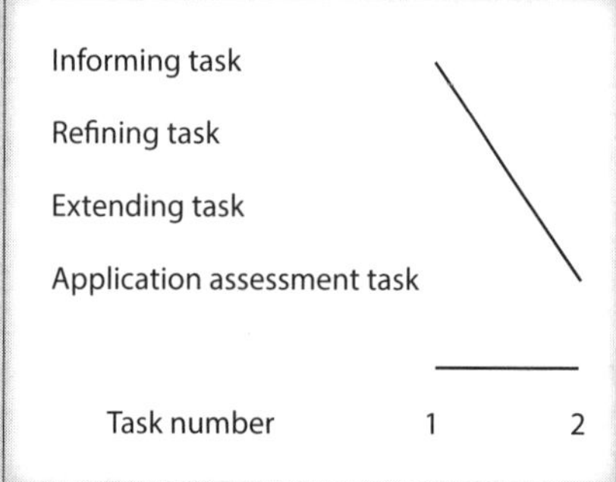

FIGURE A Inappropriate progression steps by the teacher.
Adapted from Rink, J. R. (1998, 2002, 2006, 2009). *Teaching for learning in physical education*. Boston, MA: McGraw-Hill.

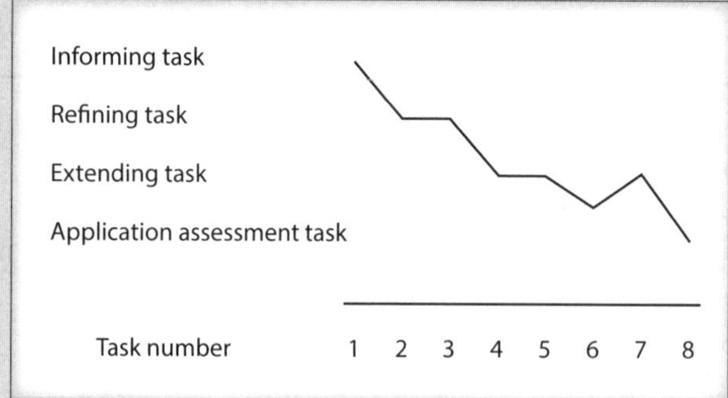

FIGURE B Appropriate progression steps by the teacher.
Adapted from Rink, J. R. (1998, 2002, 2006, 2009). *Teaching for learning in physical education*. Boston, MA: McGraw-Hill.

Adapted from Rink, J. R. (1998, 2002, 2006, 2009). *Teaching for learning in physical education*. Boston, MA: McGraw-Hill.

BOX 13.6 Examples of Refining and Extending Tasks for One-Handed Set Shot in Basketball

Situation: Basketball, one-hand shooting, novice or young learners.

- *Initial informing task:* Square to basket, ball in possession, stationary position, close to basket
- *Refining tasks*
  - Spread shooting hand behind ball.
  - Support with off hand (not pushing or letting go too early).
  - Turn elbow toward basket (not toward side).
  - Keep ball at head level (not brought down).
  - Bend knee to generate force (rather than just with arms).
  - Press toes to generate force (keep ball high).
  - Emphasize wrist snap with ball "rolling" off fingertips.
  - Coordinate knee bend and toe press.
  - Extend wrist and flex elbow as knees are bent.
  - Keep eye on rim.
- *Extending tasks*
  - Pivot away, pivot back to square up position, and shoot.
  - Receive pass from teammate, square up, and shoot.
  - Shoot from different angles but always squared up.
  - Gradually extend distance from basket.
  - With back to basket, pivot, square up, and shoot.
  - Move to spot, receive pass, square up, and shoot.
  - Dribble to spot, square up, and shoot.
  - Shoot from spot, move to next spot, receive pass, square up, and shoot.

Keeping a class shot chart on which students keep track of their shooting practice each day can produce the accountability needed to keep students on task.

Learning Experience 13.11

For a physical education unit that you are currently designing, select one of your learning outcomes and design a lesson progression that demonstrates informing, refining, extending, and applying tasks to move students through an appropriate learning progression. You might also find it useful to develop a table of various refining, extending, and applying tasks that might be used for the different levels of students who might be participating in your class. Use Box 13.6 to guide you.

Developing Tasks for Tactical Awareness in Games Teaching

Although Rink's (2009) extending-refining model may be effectively applied to the teaching of games and game tactics, other approaches have also been used with success in physical education settings. These include Teaching Games for Understanding, a six-stage model developed by Bunker and Thorpe (1982), and the Tactical Games Approach, a three-stage model developed by Griffin, Mitchell, and Oslin (1997) and Mitchell, Oslin, and Griffin (2012). The major focus of Rink's model is designing progressions of skill performance. It begins with an informing task and then utilizes refining, extending, and applying tasks to build skill progressions during content development. The primary focus of the Tactical Approach is on the strategic aspects of performance, rather than on skill components of the game. Motor skill performance is a critical aspect of playing a game, yet knowing what to do and when to do it are equally important. For instance, as students begin to develop their ability to maintain possession of the ball in soccer, they must understand the concept of providing support to their teammates and passing to an open player. As golfers begin to make decisions about hitting the ball the proper distance, they must understand the conditions surrounding the shot: distance from the hole, lie of the ball, and any obstacles between the ball and the hole. The decisions players make prior to the shot (club selection and swing length) are just as important as execution of the shot itself if the ball is to successfully reach the target. These each require tactical knowledge and motor skill to execute. Often, we see physical education classes in which students are taught and practice motor skills yet lack the knowledge of when to use them in a game situation.

Planning for this approach requires identifying tactical problems for different games and getting students to where they know they need the skill to solve the problem. Two critical questions that will help identify these tactical problems have been suggested by Griffin et al. (1997):

1. What problems does the game present for scoring, preventing scoring, and restarting play?
2. What off-the-ball movements and on-the-ball skills are necessary to solve these problems?

This approach emphasizes components of game performance beyond execution of motor skills: decision making, providing support, marking or guarding, covering teammates, adjusting position as the game evolves, and using a base position to ensure court/field coverage (Griffin et al., 1997). The model has four stages that produce a learning cycle (game–practice–game) for game performance: (1) game form (representative and exaggerated), (2) tactical awareness (what to do), (3) skill execution (how to do it), and (4) game form.

1. *Game form:* This approach begins with a modified version of the game and is exaggerated to present tactical problems to students. Let's use net games as

an example and the tactical problem of creating space. In tennis, students may be set up to play a one-point, half-court singles game on a short/narrow court with the goal of becoming aware of space on either side of the net. Conditions require students to alternate serves and use only groundstrokes during the game. In this case, the game resembles the full-court game of tennis, yet the narrower court requires students to play to the back and front of the court to create space and complete the advantage (Griffin et al., 1997).

2. *Tactical awareness:* As previously suggested, the game is modified or exaggerated in such a way that students must determine what to do to succeed in this situation. These conditions must be carefully thought through and developed if they are to encourage students to think in a tactical way. Part of your role as a teacher is to pose to the students questions that will prompt them to problem solve and think both critically and tactically. Planning for questions that will guide students to solve tactical problems takes knowledge of the game and planning. Ask questions about the goal of the game: *What* must they do to achieve that goal (necessary skills)? *Why* are specific skills/movements necessary? *How* can they perform the skills they have identified (Griffin et al., 1997)? The following question/answer example demonstrates the process:
   - *Question:* What was the goal of the game as we designed it for this practice? *Answer:* To become aware of where there is space on both sides of the net
   - *Question:* What did you have to do to win a point? *Answer:* Hit to an open space
   - *Question:* What spaces are there on your opponent's side of the net to hit the tennis ball? *Answer:* Front and back, side to side
   - *Question:* How do you return the ball if it does not come to your forehand side? *Answer:* Backhand

   This line of questioning should lead students to understand the importance of the backhand groundstroke and set the stage for skill instruction and practice on this stroke (Griffin et al., 1997).
3. *Skill execution:* Through game play, teacher questioning, and problem solving, students come to recognize the need for specific skills, and these then become the focus of the lesson. During the skill execution phase of the lesson, the specific skills can be taught, teaching cues can be emphasized, and skill practice can be designed. We again use the tennis example but focus now on backhand groundstrokes. Students might be set up with a feeder and a hitter. The feeder tosses or hits the ball to the hitter, who uses a groundstroke to return it. The ball is stopped and each partner repeats the skill five times. The student, teacher, or partners can use the cues previously emphasized to prompt performance.
4. *Game:* To end skill practice, reintroduce students to a game in which they have the same goal as in the original game. The intent is for them to solve the tactical problem using the skills they have just practiced. In our tennis example, students are put back into a half-court singles game on a long and narrow court with the goal of becoming aware of space on either side of the net. They now know how to return a ball that has been hit to a space on their court that is away from their forehand.

Learning Experience 13.12

Select a game form (e.g., invasion, net and wall, fielding, striking, target), and then identify a tactical problem that students will be presented with and must determine how to solve. Design a lesson using the game form strategy explained previously (e.g., game, tactical awareness, skill execution, game).

How Alignment Fits into Planning Teaching Progressions

Progressions should be thought of as instructional tasks that lead to learning outcomes. We believe it is important to develop learning outcomes that are meaningful and relevant to students outside the instructional setting (that is, playing games well, negotiating wilderness settings, participating in fitness activities, and the like). As tactical problems are posed to students or refining and extending tasks are designed to help their progress toward these meaningful outcomes, instruction must be aligned so that students have the best chance for success.

Instructional alignment exists when there is a match between the intended outcomes, instructional processes, and assessment. In other words, instructional alignment requires a match between goals, practice, and assessment. Substantial evidence suggests that well-aligned "instruction produces achievement results that are two to three times stronger than results of nonaligned instruction" (Cohen, 1987). The concept of instructional alignment requires teachers to think seriously about the nature of the goals they have for their students and how they can arrange task progressions that meet those goals. Using assessment procedures that are closely aligned with the goals helps ensure a better match. "Teach what you assess and assess what you teach" is an old adage in education. It is often violated in physical education.

To effectively refine student performance of skills and to carefully align conditions of outcomes, instruction, and assessment, you must know a great deal about the activity for which you are planning. As Cohen (1987) suggests,

> *Teaching what we assess, or assessing what we teach seems embarrassingly obvious. The fundamental issue is:* What's worth teaching? *This is the same question as:* What's worth assessing? *We can either know what we are doing, or not know what we're doing, but, in either case, we'll be doing something to other people's children. Do we not have an ethical obligation to know what we're up to?*[1]

If instruction is well aligned with goals and assessment procedures, it will allow students many opportunities to practice relevant skills and strategies and solve tactical problems in situations similar to those in which they will be used. Rink (2009) refers to these kinds of tasks as "applying tasks." A particular instructional task can refine a skill or strategy and still be an applying task. That is, the stimulus conditions of practice can be such that they are aligned with outcomes, even though the major purpose of the practice might be to refine or extend the performance of a skill or strategy. Thus, both refining and extending tasks can be defined so that they serve as applying tasks, too. When they do, instructional alignment is more likely.

Modifying Task Complexity

Whether you are planning progressions for use with the skill or the tactical approach, designing tasks so they progress from simple to more complex allows students to initially achieve success and become progressively more challenged with increasingly difficult tasks. The teacher needs to identify factors that impact task complexity, be able to apply them in appropriate learning experiences, and then be able to plan for a progression of experiences that move from simple to complex. We discuss five factors to consider for reducing or increasing task complexity: space, equipment, number of participants, rules, and conditions/tactics/problems. **Box 13.7** describes one way to modify a tennis game using four of these factors.

BOX 13.7 A Modified Game of Tennis

Basic problem of game:

To strike the ball with a racket so it crosses over the net and lands in bounds in such a way that the opponent cannot return it

Modifications:

Space:	Court divided in half (long and narrow)
Equipment:	Use shorter racket for ease in handling
	Use lighter ball to slow pace
	Use "old" tennis balls
	Raise the net to slow pace
Rules:	Eliminate serve; bounce-hit from midcourt
Scoring:	Four-point game
	Alternate serves every point

Space

Moving the volleyball service line towards the net, practicing high jump "backovers" from a raised takeoff platform rather than the floor, shortening or lengthening a playing field, or designing a flat orienteering course with few obstacles all reduce the complexity of an activity. These examples demonstrate how performance complexity can be manipulated by modifying the space or playing area of an activity. A full-sized playing area is inappropriate for most beginners. Modify it to achieve the skill and strategy objectives of instruction. A smaller surface makes a game less strenuous for the novice or less-fit student. If the instructional goal is for students in a three-versus-three soccer game to provide support to the ball carrier, a shortened field will allow them to achieve this without undue fatigue. In fact, they will be able to practice longer. Changing the dimensions of the playing area can increase the complexity as well. Lengthening a pickle-ball or tennis court forces front and back player movement and placement opportunities. Added width forces lateral movement and skill in one aspect of a game. In a game of badminton, players can be challenged by shuttle placement tasks that are the only condition whereby they can score. Modifying space requires that players learn to get into position for a successful response.

Equipment

Using racquetball rackets for tennis, softballs instead of a shot for putting, or larger targets in archery; starting with scarves before moving to balls or clubs in juggling and smaller and lighter balls for basketball; designing an incline climbing wall; providing slower, more rhythmic music for an entry dance routine and a lower balance beam in gymnastics; and lowering the volleyball net for spiking all reduce task complexity. Changing the size or weight of an implement allows progressively more complex tasks to be developed. Novice volleyball players may begin with a balloon and progress to

[1] Cohen, S., *Educational Researcher*, November, 16–20. p. 19, copyright © 1987 by SAGE Publications. Reprinted by Permission of SAGE Publications.

skill practice and game play with a beach ball. The volleyball net can be lowered, and then raised as students become more skilled. These modifications slow down the game, give students time to move to get under the ball, and allow them to get into position to be ready to perform the skill. As they become more skilled, they might move to a large, soft trainer volleyball and eventually use regulation volleyballs. As skills and game tactics develop, task complexity does also.

Number of Participants

One sure way to increase complexity is to add participants. A soccer player may be successfully dribbling and shooting on goal until defenders are added to the game and the tactical demands increase. It is suddenly more difficult to achieve consistent shots when faced with opposition and adapting to others, as opposed to playing on an open field unchecked. Likewise, having to plan for and get eight team members over an outdoor education obstacle adds more challenges than if the team had only five members. Practicing a skill alone is generally easier. Complexity may be added progressively by increasing the number of participants and thus the difficulty. Skill practice or application of a strategy in a three-versus-three field hockey setting allows more opportunities and fewer players with whom to contend than a six-versus-six or full game.

Some skills are difficult or impossible to practice alone. In these instances, the complexity can be altered to achieve the goal. Returning a toss from across the net with a forearm pass is easier than returning a serve. A well-taught toss that is placed accurately and at a constant speed is more easily controllable for the receiver than either an underhand or overhand serve.

Small-sided games allow more student involvement and opportunities. They also set the stage for students to determine what to do and how to do it. Game formations and spatial arrangement can be modified to allow the design of games with a specific focus or adapted for the ability levels of students. A set of small-sided games could have a different focus in each game, from basic skills and tactical problems for the novice players to more complex skills and tactics as skill and experience increase.

Rules

Rules are conditions placed on a game to set boundaries for performance. Primary rules define the main problems to be solved and thus the nature of the game. In field hockey, the main problem to be solved is how to pass and receive the ball with the stick while attempting to put the ball in the opponent's goal. Primary rules should remain intact. Secondary rules, however, can be altered to reduce inhibiting factors and to exaggerate features, strategies, and skills to be learned. These are the rules that can be modified without changing the main problems to be solved in the game, such as increasing or decreasing the number of players who must make contact with the ball or using a shorter or wider playing space. Secondary rules can be modified to change the complexity of the game and opportunities to practice. Offside in soccer and the 3-second rule in basketball are examples of secondary rules. Adjusting how points are scored is a means of modifying rules that has implications for motivation and skill practice, yet does not change the game itself. For example, in tennis, deuce games and four point or no-advantage games can be used. Restarts can be modified so as to speed up play and allow a focus on other skills and strategies.

Conditions/Tactics/Problems

All games have tactical problems that must be solved and associated skills that need to be mastered. The tactical complexity of a game must match the developmental level of your learners. Adding tactical complexity to a game as students' awareness, understanding, and skills increase can do this. Levels of tactical complexity can be identified so that lessons can be designed using appropriately complex tasks for the learners. At the novice level, learners may be required only to understand the importance of maintaining possession of the ball, attacking the goal, and restarting the game and to possess the on-the-ball skills (e.g., passing, receiving, shooting) necessary to solve these problems. As students become more skilled, they can be introduced to the idea of providing support and defending space/goal and the aligned on-the-ball skills (goalkeeping) and off-the-ball movements (marking/guarding) necessary to solve these problems. As the tactical level increases, so do the skills and movements that students must learn and practice.

Learning Experience 13.13

Select an outcome and aligned learning experience for a physical education unit you are currently designing. For each of the five factors that impact task complexity, design a set of tasks that might be used to modify the learning experience you have chosen.

Closed and Open Skills

Most sport performance activities, as well as fitness and outdoor education activities, require efficient execution of both skills and strategies. If the execution of skill and strategy is important content in your sense of appropriate physical education programming, the distinction between closed skills and open skills should affect how you develop that content.

- Closed skills are performed in a fixed environment in which the conditions are unchanged during the performance. These skills tend to be self-paced, repetitive, and routinized. The shot put is a good example. The size of the ring, the weight of the shot, the dimensions of the sector into which the shot is put, and the rules for putting are all fixed.

- Open skills are performed in an ever-changing environment with conditions that are variable. These skills tend to be externally paced. Responding effectively to the changing environment becomes the most important factor when performing open skills. A basketball guard dribbling down court to initiate an offense is a good example. The guard contends with differing defensive configurations, each of which might cue a different set of offensive options. Defensive pressure changes, as do the conditions of the game itself (e.g., time remaining, the score).
- Some skills have stable conditions, yet the performer is often required to perform the skill in different environments. Perhaps the best example of this type of skill is golf, where the basic stroke is the same, yet the player must adjust to different lies on the course, club selection (woods, irons), surfaces (fairway, green, bunker), and distance to the hole.

The closed/open distinction is best understood as a continuum, with the skills performed under most constant conditions at one end and skills performed under most variable conditions at the other. Skills are placed on the continuum according to the conditions under which they are performed, as shown in **Figure 13.1**.

Developing content of closed and open skills differs markedly. The more closed the skill, the more emphasis will be on refining technique that is performed invariably. These skills require consistency in practice so they become routinized and predictable. The more open the skill, the less time will be spent on technique, and the more time will be spent extending tasks that cover the variety of situations in which the skills will be used. The goal is to develop performance that is appropriately responsive to the varying demands of an ever-changing setting. A major error in instructional alignment physical educators make when developing content for open skills is treating them as if they were closed skills, with the conditions of practice constant instead of variable.

Assessing Teaching

As indicated previously, effective teaching is best evaluated by observations of students—their work involvement (process) and what they achieve (outcome or product). When teachers substantially increase the amount of active learning time their students are accruing in physical education on a daily basis, they have, other things being equal, improved their effectiveness. This represents a process approach to evaluating teaching and learning. If students can perform a nearly flawless floor exercise routine at the end of a gymnastics unit, this represents an outcome or product measure of effective instruction. The same is true for students who not only can successfully present folk dances at the end of a unit but also demonstrate new knowledge about the countries in which the dances originated. If the students ask that the folk dance unit be extended because it's so much fun, this too is evidence of effective instruction. Finally, if students take their teams from a Sport Education volleyball season and enter the after-school volleyball league, this is important evidence that effective instruction has occurred.

Evaluating instruction only through observations of the teacher can be misleading. Well-explained tasks and a pleasant rapport with students that do not translate into high rates of work involvement are of little value from an achievement perspective. Do not misunderstand this caution. How teachers instruct is important because it has been shown that some kinds of instruction are more likely to produce effective student work involvement, and effective work involvement has been related to achievement and attitude gains. The point is that evaluating instruction must include evidence about what students do as well as evidence about what teachers do.

Learning Experience 13.14

Select one of the observation tools introduced in the ancillary materials, collect data on a physical education class, and interpret your findings to inform how the observed teacher might improve his or her practice in relation to one of the topics featured in this chapter.

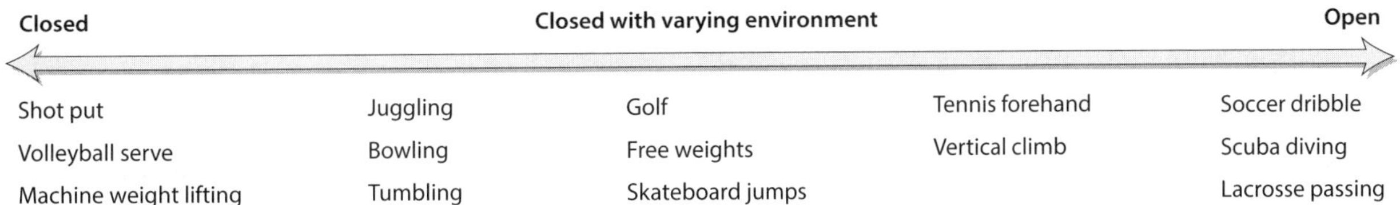

FIGURE 13.1 Closed/open skill continuum.

CHAPTER SUMMARY

The overall purpose of this chapter was to assist the novice teacher in becoming aware of what teachers do to make a difference in student learning and in gaining the skills and knowledge to begin that process in their own practice. We began by describing the characteristics of a professional physical educator and distinguished between learning students and active teachers. Ideas on how to design physically and emotionally safe learning environments where challenging and meaningful learning takes place were discussed. The concept of learning tasks was introduced with examples provided to clarify about why lessons are considered an arrangement of tasks and how to communicate learning tasks effectively to students. A discussion on how to choose content to match the selected curriculum model was provided along with an explanation of how to align teaching with a series of learning progressions. Finally, various principles related to learning tasks were explored from the concept of task complexity to developing tasks for tactical awareness in addition to how to design tasks for open and closed skills.

1. Professional physical educators intend for students to learn, plan for and monitor student enjoyment and progress, manage students to decrease disruptions and increase learning time, organize learning experiences to match student abilities, and are motivated to be competent and caring.
2. The learning student is cooperative, eager to learn and enthusiastic about the opportunity to learn more, and responsible for his or her own behavior; enjoys learning and practices purposefully to improve; and is helpful to peers who are similarly engaged in learning.
3. An active teacher believes he or she can make a difference with students, develops a management system that helps students stay on task, plans and implements an instructional program that keeps students engaged, motivates students to become better learners, and holds them accountable for performance, and does so within a class climate that is supportive and respectful.
4. Within both the managerial and instructional task systems, safety is critical. Students must be taught in a safely engineered environment, taught about safety procedures and practices, and helped to feel safe (emotionally and physically) in this setting.
5. Physical education should be realistic, authentic, and intellectually challenging with students encouraged to question, explore, and solve problems and to express themselves and their reactions to participation in physical activity and receive teacher responses.
6. A lesson can be considered as arrangements of tasks when it is viewed by what students do in the lesson. Remember that every lesson contains managerial and instructional tasks as well as the social tasks students intend to achieve. How these various tasks are developed and combined to orchestrate the classroom will impact student learning and enjoyment.
7. Effective task communication means that students will attend to and comprehend the information you present and that information will be sufficient for them to initially do the task as it has been described.
8. With learning time a precious commodity, the teacher must consider alternative ways to deliver information to students (e.g., well-designed handouts, posters, task cards) that they can access when needed (e.g., to take home, access on school website, posted on gym wall).
9. When choosing activities that contribute to the goals of a model, it is critical that you know the activities well enough to develop content appropriately for the learners and provide sufficient time for those learners to make meaningful gains in performing the activities.
10. Progressions are learning tasks that move students from less complex and sophisticated tasks to more difficult and complicated tasks by adding complexity and difficulty, resulting in meaningful performances that reflect intended program outcomes. These progressions must be specific to the students in a specific context, recognizing the experiences students bring with them and the time available.
11. Rink's (2009) model for developing progressive instructional tasks continues to be widely used in physical education. Initial tasks *inform* the student of a new skill or strategy. Subsequent tasks *refine* the quality of the performance, *extend* the performance by altering it slightly, and *apply* the skill or strategy.
12. The tactical approach focuses on the strategic aspects of game performance, rather than on skill components. Although motor skill performance is a critical aspect of playing a game, knowing what to do and when to do it are equally important. Planning for this approach requires identifying tactical problems for different games and getting students to where they know they need the skill to solve the problem.
13. Instructional alignment is reflected in a program where there is a match between the intended outcomes, instructional processes, and assessment. This alignment requires teachers to consider the learning goals they have for students and how they can best arrange task progressions that meet those goals and use assessment procedures that are closely aligned with the goals.
14. Designing tasks so they progress from simple to more complex allows students to initially achieve success and become progressively more challenged with increasingly difficult tasks. Five factors have been identified for reducing or increasing task complexity: space, equipment, number of participants, rules, and conditions/tactics/problems.

15. When execution of both skill and strategy are important to physical education content, the distinction between closed skills and open skills will affect how content is developed. Skills are placed on a closed–open continuum according to the conditions under which they are performed, with the skills performed under the most constant conditions at one end and skills performed under the most variable conditions at the other.
16. More closed skills require emphasis on refining technique to become routinized and predictable whereas more open skills emphasize extending tasks covering a variety of situations in which the skills are performed.
17. Effective teaching is best evaluated through a process approach involving observation of students, their work involvement (process), and what they achieve (outcome or product).

REFERENCES

Bloom, B. (1984). The 2 sigma problem: The search for methods of group instructions as effective as one-to-one tutoring. *Educational Researcher, 13*(5), 4–16.

Bunker, D., & Thorpe, R. (1982). A model for the teaching of games in secondary schools. *Bulletin of Physical Education, 18*, 11.

Cohen, S. (1987, Nov.). Instructional alignment: Searching for a magic bullet. *Educational Researcher*, 16–20.

Griffin, L., Mitchell, S., & Oslin, J. (1997). *Teaching sport concepts and skills: A tactical games approach.* Champaign, IL: Human Kinetics.

Kelly, L. (1997). Safety in PE. In S. Capel (Ed.), *Learning to teach physical education in the secondary school: A companion to school experience* (pp. 115–129). London: Routledge.

Locke, L. (1975). *The ecology of the gymnasium: What the tourists never see.* Proceedings of Southern Organization for Physical Education of College Women (ERIC Document Reproduction Service No. ED 104823).

Mitchell, S. A., Oslin, J. L., & Griffin, L. L. (2003). *Sport foundations for elementary physical education.* Champaign, IL: Human Kinetics.

Mitchell, S. A., Oslin, J. L., & Griffin, L. L. (2012). *Teaching sport concepts and skills: A tactical games approach.* Champaign, IL: Human Kinetics.

Resnick, L., & Williams-Hall, M. (1998). Learning organizations for sustainable education reform. *Daedalus, 127*(4), 89–118.

Rink, J. R. (2006). *Teaching for learning in physical education* (5th ed.). Boston, MA: McGraw-Hill.

Rink, J. R. (2009). *Teaching for learning in physical education* (6th ed.). Boston, MA: McGraw-Hill.

Shulman, L. (1987). Knowledge and teaching: Foundations of the new reform. *Harvard Educational Review, 57*(1), 1–21.

Wiggins, G. (1989). The futility of trying to teach everything of importance. *Educational Leadership, 47*(3), 44–48.

Yellon, S. L. (1996). *Powerful principles of instruction.* New York: Addison Wesley/Longman.

CHAPTER 14 Selecting Appropriate Instructional Models

Overall Chapter Outcome

To gain skill and knowledge in how to effectively choose and employ appropriate instructional models to facilitate student learning

Learning Outcomes

The learner will:

- Explain the relationship between curriculum and instructional models
- Differentiate between teacher-mediated and student-mediated instruction
- Explain the purpose of, and how to use, guided practice and independent practice
- Describe and provide an example of each teacher-mediated instruction model: direct instruction, task/station/inclusion teaching, and teaching through questions (guided discovery, problem solving, and games-based instruction)
- Describe and provide an example of each student-mediated instruction model: peer tutoring/classwide peer tutoring (CWPT)/reciprocal teaching, small group instruction (cooperative learning and teams), self-instruction (contracting and personalized system of instruction), and service learning

This chapter is about teaching—teaching for student learning. Before we explore what this entails, we believe it is critical to bring curriculum models, instructional models, and teaching and managerial skills and strategies into focus. What do these terms really mean? **Curriculum models** are focused, themes-based, and reflect a specific philosophy. They intend to define a clear focus around the content and aim toward specific, relevant, and challenging outcomes. Once you have selected a curriculum model to develop and promote the type of learning you want young people to experience, you will determine which instructional model will guide instruction and facilitate learning. The **instructional model** organizes instruction and how students will interact with, and practice, content. An instructional model includes a number of non-negotiable strategies and methods used to plan, design, and implement instruction. So, the major difference between curriculum models and instructional models is content versus instruction. A few of the curriculum models are also instructional models (e.g., Tactical Approach to Teaching Games; Sport Education), and in some instances a curriculum model might be linked directly to an instructional model (e.g., Adventure Education) to most effectively reach the intended outcomes. Regardless of which curriculum model or instructional model you select to guide student learning, there are a number of general teaching skills and strategies that facilitate learning within both the managerial and instructional task systems. **Table 14.1** displays the curriculum models, instructional models, and teaching strategies.

BOX 14.1 Key Terms in This Chapter

- *Cooperative learning (CL):* A special variation of small group work that requires the involvement of all members of the group. CL uses questioning to stimulate students to solve problems, think creatively, negotiate, compromise, adapt, and evaluate as they create solutions. CL strategies include (1) pairs–check; (2) jigsaw; (3) think–pair–share; and (4) problem-based learning.
- *Curriculum models:* Provide the framework within which instruction takes place. They are focused, themes-based, reflect a specific philosophy, define a clear focus around the content, and aim toward specific, relevant, and challenging outcomes.
- *Direct instruction:* Provided by the teacher to a whole class or small groups, followed by guided and independent practice in a positive and supportive learning environment set with high, realistic expectations for students for which they are held accountable. Lesson pacing is brisk and teacher controlled, with students getting many learning opportunities and experiencing high success rates.
- *Games teaching:* Incorporates teaching through questions to encourage students to think critically about tactical problems, appropriate skills, and when to use them.
- *Guided discovery:* Characterized by convergent thinking where students respond to a series of task questions/challenges that help them progress toward a specific goal with one correct response.
- *Guided practice:* A period of group practice during which the teacher (1) corrects major errors in performance, (2) reteaches if necessary, and (3) provides sufficient practice so students can move on to participate in independent practice successfully.
- *Inclusion teaching:* Involves students engaging in learning tasks that have multiple levels of performance and allow students choices in selecting their entry levels.
- *Independent practice:* For students to integrate new tasks into previously learned material and to practice the tasks so they become automatic.
- *Instructional models:* How the teacher organizes and delivers instruction and provides practice to students. Each model has a different role for the teacher and students, and how teachers and students interact with one another.
- *Peer teaching and reciprocal teaching:* Characterized by students being arranged in pairs or triads, focused on achieving together the goals of guided practice prior to engaging in independent practice.
- *Peer tutoring:* Used with all young people, and often when teaching students with disabilities. There are two types: (1) when a higher-skilled student tutors a lower-skilled student, and (2) classwide peer tutoring (CWPT) in which all students serve as both tutors and tutees.
- *Problem-solving approach:* Characterized by divergent inquiry that places the learner at the center of the content to be learned, draws out their individual creativity, involves discussion among peers, and stimulates abstract thinking in order to respond.
- *Self-instructional models:* Allow students to progress through a sequence of learning activities without the physical presence, direction, or supervision of a teacher. Models include (1) individualized instruction, (2) contracting, and (3) personalized systems of instruction (PSI).
- *Service learning (SL):* Designed for students to learn about social issues, improve social and interpersonal skills, and develop leadership and positive civic qualities while planning and delivering a service to the community in response to an identified need. Types of SL include (1) direct SL, (2) indirect SL, (3) research-based SL, and (4) advocacy SL.
- *Small-group teaching:* A descriptor for a variety of models where the intent is for students to work in small enough groups that will allow all students to work on and achieve a clearly defined task carried out without the direct and immediate supervision of the teacher.
- *Station teaching:* A subcategory of task teaching where students rotate among stations to experience different learning tasks that are not progressive in nature.
- *Student-mediated instruction:* Includes such models such as (1) peer or reciprocal models, (2) small-group instruction, (3) teams, (4) cooperative learning models, (5) problems-based learning, and (6) service learning.
- *Task teaching:* Organizing the learning environment so that all students can engage in a set of progressive learning tasks simultaneously without changing stations.
- *Teacher-mediated instruction:* Can be delivered (1) directly through group-oriented active teaching models, (2) indirectly through task or station teaching, or (3) indirectly through self-instructional models.
- *Teaching strategies:* General skills and strategies that a teacher uses to facilitate learning within both the managerial and instructional task systems.
- *Teaching through questions:* Challenges students to engage in cognitive processing, explore alternatives, and formulate a response to a question/problem rather than merely replicate a performance.
- *Team:* A special type of small group, teams allow students to take responsibility for their own experiences; thus, in some ways it is a form of self-instruction.

TABLE 14.1 Models to Guide Teaching

		Teaching Strategies				
Curriculum Models	**Instructional Models**	**General**	**Physical, Cognitive, and Affective Tasks**	**Metzler's Teaching During Games**	**Hellison Teaching Personal and Social Responsibility Strategies**	**Management Strategies**

• Developmental physical education models
• Adventure Education
• Outdoor Education
• Sport Education
• Tactical Games Approach for Teaching Games
• Teaching Personal and Social Responsibility
• Social issues models
• Health and wellness models
	• Direct instruction
	• Task/station/inclusion teaching
	• Teaching through questions
	  • Guided discovery
	  • Problem solving
	  • Games-based instruction
	• Peer tutoring/classwide peer tutoring (CWPT)/ reciprocal teaching
	• Small group instruction
	  • Cooperative learning
	  • Teams
	• Self-instruction
	  • Contracting
	  • Personalized system of instruction
	• Service learning
		• Demonstration
		• Explanation
		• Set induction
		• Check for understanding
		• Student task engagement
		• Teachable moments
			• Play–practice–play
			• Experiential learning
			• Drills
			• Game-like tasks
			• Problem solving
			• Critical thinking
			• Brainstorming
			• World Café
			• Predict–observe–explain
			• Know–want to know–learned (K-W-L)
			• Interviews
			• Dialogue
			• Learning log
			• Reflective tasks
			• Varying processing
			• Challenge by choice
			• Risk taking
			• Guided practice
			• Independent practice
				• Chalk talk
				• Walk through
				• Situations
				• Instant replay
				• Player/coach
				• You make the call
				• Controlled scrimmage
				• Television analyst
					• Awareness talks
					• Participation by invitation
					• Behavior modification
					• Self-paced challenges
					• Reflection time
					• Individual goal setting
					• Group meetings
					• Counseling time
						• Lesson focus
						• Instant activity
						• Equipment setup/ dispersal and return
						• Emergency plans
						• Grouping for activity
						• Transitioning students

Instructional Models

Various approaches for teaching physical education continue to be discussed, promoted, debated, and analyzed. These approaches to teaching were first referred to as "teaching styles" by Muska Mosston (1966) when he introduced the spectrum of teaching styles. Mosston's work suggests that teaching is based on a series of decisions teachers make about their teaching behavior and learners are invited to make about their learning behavior. As teachers and learners interact in the teaching/learning process, behavior patterns emerge; these define the different teaching styles that form the teaching spectrum. According to Mosston (1966) and Mosston and Ashworth (1994, 2008), a teacher's choice of teaching style is determined by the series of decisions made, who makes them, how they are made, and for what purpose. These decisions are organized into three sets: decisions about intent that are made prior to face-to-face interaction (pre-impact), decisions about action that are made during a lesson (impact), and decisions about evaluation that will inform subsequent lessons (post-impact). Depending upon who makes these decisions, the spectrum is divided into two clusters of teaching styles: those that seek replication of knowledge and those that seek discovery or creativity of new knowledge.

The spectrum has been applied, studied, and extended for almost 50 years, during which time additional approaches have been developed and promoted. Other physical education scholars have referred to these teaching approaches as instructional formats (Siedentop & Tannehill, 2000) or teaching strategies (Capel, Leask, & Turner, 2001; Rink, 2009). Rink (2009) portrays **teaching strategies** as a delivery system that arranges the learning environment to allow all individuals to learn in a group setting, reminding us that although teaching generally happens in groups, learning occurs within each individual. She suggests that every teaching strategy assigns roles to both the teacher and the learner for different teaching functions within a lesson—content selection, task communication, content progression, and provision of feedback and evaluation (Rink, 2009).

In this text, we refer to the various teaching approaches as "instructional models." It is our contention that an instructional model refers to the ways a teacher organizes and delivers instruction and provides practice to students, how the teacher and student roles change as a result of the different instructional models, and how teachers and students interact with one another. We argue that a teacher does not always make a choice of a particular instructional model for an entire unit, or even a class session. Rather, the model will vary depending on the content being taught, the expected learning outcomes, the abilities and behavior of the students, the curriculum model within which the lesson is a part, how feedback might best be provided, and the decisions the teacher makes in terms of giving students responsibility and choice, and in some cases control of their learning experience. Having said this, there are instances when a chosen curriculum model is closely linked to an instructional model (e.g., teaching through questions and a Tactical Approach to Teaching Games, or cooperative learning and Adventure Education), resulting in the teacher choosing to stay with a particular instructional model throughout a lesson, or even an entire unit when that instructional model produces the strongest learning gains for students.

When selecting an instructional model, we advise teachers to (1) select the content to be taught, (2) determine the outcomes to be achieved in a lesson, and finally (3) select an instructional model that will enable learners to be successful in achieving the learning intent. It is critical to consider the types of learners, their abilities and interests, and the context within which they participate in order to ensure that the selected instructional model is congruent with the developmental level of the learners.

Fortunately, all types of learning, including what Mosston (1966) referred to as reproductive (mirror and replicate) and productive (discover or create), are necessary for learners to achieve across the four learning domains; physical, social, cognitive, and affective. Regardless of the curriculum model chosen to frame a unit of instruction, all activities and content can be taught using various types of instructional models. As noted by Doherty (2010), physical education teachers need to be skilled and knowledgeable at adjusting and revising learning tasks according to the needs and responses of their students.

Understanding the various instructional models and how to select an appropriate model for the learning outcomes identified allows the teacher to use the model most suited for a particular situation and group of learners. There has been some suggestion that the teacher-centered instructional models might be ineffective in maximizing student learning (Cothran, Hodges Kulinna, & Garrahy, 2003). However, we argue that instructional models should not, and cannot, be compared in an attempt to determine which is best or better. If one instructional model is better than another, it is only better within a particular context and with a particular group of learners, and then only because it matches the needs and the context in a particularly effective way. For example, if the outcome of a lesson requires a student to learn a technical skill such as putting the shot, aiming and releasing the arrow in archery, or performing a back handspring in tumbling, modeling and subsequent replication could be necessary. This type of learning, and ultimate performance, might best be developed through a direct teacher-controlled instructional model in the early stages of learning. As learning progresses, the student might improve skill most effectively through more learner-centered types of instructional models such as teaching the skills to a classmate using peer teaching. Whitehead and Zwozdiak-Myers (2007) suggest that how physical education is taught is as important as what is taught for achieving the aims of physical education and the intended learning outcomes for lessons.

Learning Experience 14.1

Observe a physical education class to reveal what the teacher and the learners do during the lesson. Arrive at the physical education class prior to its beginning and find an unobtrusive place to sit where you will not distract either the teacher or the students. Take anecdotal notes on what you observe.

Following the lesson, ask yourself these questions:

- Did the lesson require students to replicate knowledge or create new knowledge?
- Based on your response to question 1, was the teacher's choice for students to replicate or create appropriate to the content being taught?
- Did the teacher appear to have adequate knowledge of the learners and their interests and needs?
- Did the teacher adapt the lesson, and use various instructional models as a result of student responses?
- Did all learners have the opportunity to learn and progress?
- Who made the majority of decisions in the class?
- If students made some lesson decisions, which did they make?
- Would you describe the lesson you observed as teacher-mediated, student-mediated, or a combination of both?
- Do you believe the choice of model was appropriate for the content and the needs of the learners?

Active Teaching Framework

Active teaching is not a recipe that has to be followed exactly; rather, it is a framework for understanding the major skills that effective teachers show in their work. There is substantial room within this framework for the individual styles of teachers to develop. Nor does active teaching mean that there is only one way to design lessons or present content. As you will see, the active teaching framework is applicable across various content areas within all curriculum and instruction models and among varying contexts and learners. This framework is equally applicable to whole-group and small-group teaching and to curricular approaches as diverse as Cultural Studies and Health and Wellness.

Active teaching is related to what has been called direct instruction, explicit instruction, systematic teaching, or effective teaching. The active teaching framework contains the skills and strategies that are suggested for instructional models that employ small-group instruction, cooperative learning, and reciprocal teaching, among others. What all of these approaches share is the development and maintenance of learning students. The active teaching framework provides an understanding of the skills and strategies that are most likely to develop learning students.

Matching Instructional Model to Context

In this chapter, we will describe what a variety of instructional models might look like in practice, providing examples to show how each instructional model could be employed across multiple outcomes and content. We will frame these instructional models within the active teaching framework.

As mentioned previously, education is most effective when teachers adapt instructional models to the contexts within which they teach. Instructional models should reflect sensitivity to (1) the personal skills and preferences of teachers, (2) the characteristics of the learners being taught, (3) the nature of the content being taught, and (4) the context within which teaching takes place. Some teachers feel more comfortable with some models than others. *Teacher personal preference* is a legitimate factor in the teacher's choice of which model to adapt, especially when that preference derives from a professional belief in the validity of a model. Teachers no doubt tend to perform better when they work from a model that they believe to be effective, one with which they are comfortable. Nothing is worse for teachers than to feel they are being forced to adopt an instructional model they do not believe in and cannot employ adequately. We frequently see novice teachers using instructional models that allow them to keep control of most teacher functions as they strive to develop their confidence and skill working with young people in the classroom. Teachers' beliefs about instructional models can change, and teachers can learn to utilize new models, often easily when they become convinced that a different model will better help their students achieve learning goals.

The choice of instructional model should be sensitive to the *characteristics of the learners*. Clearly, when learners have had substantial experience in an activity, you will approach the teaching of that activity differently than if the class were all beginners. Well-behaved students who are able to take responsibility for their own learning and behavior give teachers more options for choice of model than do students who require more attention to behavioral and managerial issues. Children with disabilities, dependent on associated abilities, may require a direct model or warrant consideration when employing a peer teaching or cooperative learning model. Students for whom English is a second language may benefit from a model that is enhanced by teaching tools such as task cards, posters, or materials posted on the school website for reference. It is important to keep in mind that not all students learn in the same way and at the same time. Using different instructional models at different times and for different content will allow students to learn in the way that best meets their needs and also will allow all students to experience various models and come to find them challenging and engaging.

Content is also a factor. Gymnastics, climbing, disc activities, and dance might lend themselves to different instructional models. Teaching basic skills in any activity is a different issue than teaching higher level strategies to learners who already have mastered the basic skills. For example, fitness problem solving in a Health and Wellness unit is best preceded by acquisition of basic knowledge about fitness and basic techniques for measuring it. Thus, a teacher might change from a whole-class active teaching model for basic knowledge and skills to a group-oriented problem-solving model for higher order knowledge and skills, all within the same fitness lesson or unit.

The *context* for teaching is also important to the choice of model, particularly the facilities. If the facility for teaching tennis consists of six courts, all in one row, then the problems of gathering and dispersing students along the row of courts might compel a teacher to use a task or individualized model rather than a games-based model involving teaching through questions where students would need to come together more often. Safety issues in a beginning archery class taught outdoors might suggest active teaching with visible teacher control at the outset and, depending on the students, perhaps throughout the unit.

The effectiveness of any instructional model must be judged in terms of student process and outcomes. Do students achieve the goals of the unit? Are there large amounts of active learning time in the lessons? Do students grow in their appreciation of the activity and their desire to participate? Answers to these questions should determine whether the instructional model meets the needs of the context in which it is used.

Learning Experience 14.2

With a small group of your teaching peers, discuss the four considerations identified previously for choosing an instructional model (personal choice, characteristics of learners, content being taught, and context). Base your discussion on your own beliefs, values, and experiences.

Following this discussion, what do you know about the students you will teach that might influence your choice of models? Do you feel comfortable turning decisions over to students? Are you more comfortable maintaining control? Are you confident in your content knowledge across the many physical education strands taught in primary and postprimary physical education? Are the facilities adequate to allow designing varying learning experiences for students? Does the community in which you will teach hold specific values that will impact your teaching decisions?

Teacher-Mediated and Student-Mediated Instruction

How tasks are mediated in the teaching/learning process defines the categories of instructional models. Teacher-mediated instruction can be delivered (1) directly through group-oriented active teaching models, (2) indirectly through task or station teaching, or (3) indirectly through self-instructional models. There is a growing interest among teachers in student-mediated instructional models such as (1) peer or reciprocal models, (2) small-group instruction, (3) teams, (4) cooperative learning models, (5) problems-based learning, or (6) service learning.

There is no hierarchy of models; each is appropriate for a given context, the outcome and objectives of a lesson, what you want learners to achieve, the content to be introduced, the expectations you hold for learner behavior and growth, and your expertise. These issues will guide your selection of instructional model within either teacher- or student-mediated teaching. Regardless of the instructional model employed, guided and independent practice can play a role in your teaching practices to strengthen the learning of your students.

Guided and Independent Practice

When a new task has been introduced or when the conditions for task practice have been changed substantially, a period of guided practice should occur after the new task has been communicated. **Guided practice** is a period of group practice that functions to (1) correct major errors in performance, (2) reteach if necessary, and (3) provide sufficient practice so students can participate in independent practice successfully.

In **teacher-mediated instruction**, guided practice is most effectively accomplished through teacher-led, whole-group practice. In **student-mediated instruction**, guided practice occurs similarly, except that students lead the practice. Guided practice usually occurs in a whole-group formation with the teacher in a position to see, and be seen by, the entire class. As students practice the task, the teacher provides prompts and cues to emphasize the major technical features of the task and the way the task is to be practiced. The organizational format allows the teacher to check to see if major errors are being made. If so, time is taken to reteach the skill or strategy, emphasizing the elements related to the errors. Checks for student understanding are frequent, both by visually monitoring performance and by asking questions.

Teacher feedback during guided practice typically focuses on the technical aspects of performance, particularly the critical performance elements emphasized during the task communication. Feedback relative to these critical elements should be specific and be balanced between correcting errors and reinforcing appropriate performance. You should also ensure that the conditions for student practice are being followed; that is, student practice is congruent with the task description. For example, if the practice task requires a "feeder" (i.e., a player delivering the throw or pass sets to a partner to practice spiking), the type of feed also should be monitored, with supportive or corrective feedback provided for students feeding correctly and incorrectly.

Response rates during guided practice should be as high as possible, and there should be enough practice trials for you to feel confident that students can be successful when shifted to independent practice. If initial student responses during guided practice result in too many errors, then you should either reteach, emphasizing the elements being performed incorrectly, or shift practice to an *easier* task that will act as a building block for the current task. Once you are sure that tasks can be performed successfully as intended, then students can be shifted to independent practice.

The purpose of **independent practice** is for students to integrate the new task into previously learned material and to practice the task so that it becomes automatic. Students need sufficient practice so they can use the skills confidently and quickly in conditions under which the skill or strategy will eventually be used. Time is a precious commodity in physical education, and many teachers feel that they have to cover a large number of activities. Subsequently, teachers often do not allow enough time for students to practice tasks to the point where they can do them successfully and automatically. The result is that students have covered many skills, strategies, and activities but can't do any of them well enough to enjoy the context in which they are used. Students need to have sufficient command of skills and strategies to utilize them effectively in game and other movement settings. Students need to know dance steps and transitions well enough to do the dances to music without prompts. They also need to be strong and fit enough to perform sustained strength or aerobic activities.

In summary, then, guided practice is used to correct major errors and ensure that students can profit from extended practice; independent practice is used to achieve high rates of successful repetitions of the task. The teaching role (teacher or student) during independent practice is very different than during guided practice. Typically, students are dispersed for independent practice, using all the space and equipment available. The major instructional function during independent practice is *active supervision*. The major purposes of active supervision are to (1) keep students on the assigned task and (2) provide supportive and corrective feedback where necessary (see **Box 14.2**).

Learning Experience 14.3

Design a learning task for both a teacher-mediated and a student-mediated lesson. Develop a description of what guided practice would look like for each learning task and what independent practice would look like. This requires you to consider the teacher's and students' roles in both types of practice. Refer back to the purpose of each type of practice to inform your decisions.

BOX 14.2 Key Features and Elements of Active Supervision

Whether mediated by teachers or students, key elements of active supervision include the following:

- Keep all students within sight. Moving around the perimeter of a space is usually better than moving through a space, especially at the outset when you are trying to establish a strong on-task focus.
- Scan frequently. Don't get caught up for too long with any student or group. Briefly scan the entire class frequently.
- Don't get predictable. Moving down a line of tennis courts or clockwise around a gymnasium gets predictable. Some students, when they can predict you are far away, will be more likely to go off task.
- Use your voice across space. It is important that students know that you are aware of their behavior even though you are not near them. Quick prompts and feedback across space help to accomplish this goal. Try to balance the supportive and corrective comments; that is, don't respond only to the off-task students all the time.
- Be aware of unsafe or disruptive behavior and stop it immediately.
- Try to distribute your attention equitably. Make sure that time and interactions are not predictable on the basis of gender, race, or skill level.
- Use opportunities to build expectations for a successful learning-oriented climate.

Teacher-Mediated Instructional Models

Teachers in an instructional setting generally work with groups of learners. Learning should occur for each member of the group. When designing group instruction, the teacher must decide how to meet the needs of all individuals to facilitate learning: (1) design similar experiences for all learners, (2) provide all learners with appropriate explanations and demonstrations when needed, (3) effectively intervene with each learner as appropriate, and (4) optimize opportunities to respond to all learners.

Direct Instruction

The dominant model used in most physical education programs internationally, especially for children and beginners at any level, is **direct instruction**. Terms that have been used to describe this instructional model include *direct instruction* (Rosenshine, 1979), *interactive teaching* (Rink, 1985), and *explicit instruction* (Rosenshine & Stevens, 1986). Direct instruction also provides the main components for instructional theory into practice, popularly known as the Hunter model (Housner, 1990).

In this model, teachers provide direct instruction, to either a whole class or small groups, followed by guided practice in which major errors are corrected, followed by independent practice in which student work is actively supervised. This all takes place within a supportive climate in which high, realistic expectations are set for student work and students are held accountable for performance. In direct instruction, content is communicated by the teacher, rather than through curricular materials. The pacing of the lesson is brisk and teacher controlled. Students get many learning opportunities and experience high success rates. Direct instruction teachers are skilled managers, relying on managerial routines to optimize time for learning and reduce opportunities for off-task and disruptive behavior.

Direct instruction has been shown to be differentially more effective than other instructional models for well-structured subjects, such as reading, mathematics, and physical education. Part of the success of direct instruction can be attributed to the organizational and supervision aspects of the model that allow teachers to manage student engagement.

In direct instruction, the teacher chooses the content, breaks it down into parts, and arranges the progressions, which are typically sequenced in small steps. Lessons are delivered through clear demonstrations and explanations of both the content and the task to be achieved. Students are held accountable for participation in and achievement of tasks. Feedback and evaluation are done by the teacher, with active supervision as the necessary intermediate function.

Box 14.3 provides a glimpse of an orienteering lesson during which the teacher uses direct instruction to assist students in learning to use a compass.

BOX 14.3 Reading a Compass Using Direct Instruction

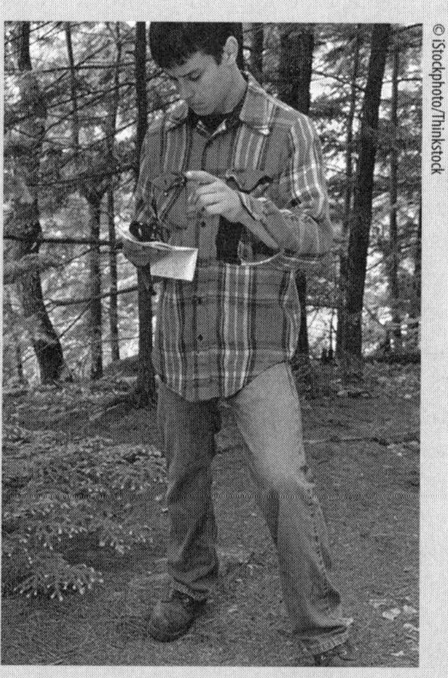

Lesson Outcome: For students to navigate a compass walk

Guided practice:

- Each student has a compass; all are standing a foot apart from one another facing the teacher.
- The teacher has a compass and a large poster of the face of the compass.
- The teacher asks students to set their compass for 155 degrees and face the direction of travel.
- After observing the students, the teacher reteaches/reviews how to set the bearing and how to determine the direction of travel.
- The teacher again asks students to set their compass, this time for 60 degrees, and face the direction of travel.
- After observing the students, the teacher confirms and provides feedback on the task.
- Students are ready to move into independent practice.

Independent practice: Compass walk

Each student is given a task card with the following directions on it:

- Place a coin/marker on the ground between your feet, and set your compass for an arbitrary direction between 0 and 120 degrees (for example, 40 degrees). Face the chosen bearing as directed by the compass and walk this bearing for 20 steps. Stop.
- Look at the compass again, add 120 degrees to the original bearing (for example, 40 + 120 = 160). Set this new bearing on the compass. Face this new bearing as directed by the compass, walk this new bearing for 20 steps, and then stop.
- Again, add 120 degrees to the last setting (for example, 160 + 120 = 280). Reset the compass, determine the new direction to walk, and take 20 steps in the direction indicated by the travel arrow. Stop.
- The coin/marker should be right between your feet if you have used the compass properly and walked exactly. If you did not succeed, try it again with another bearing between 0 and 120 degrees at the start and add 120 degrees at each of the two turns, walking the same distance in each direction. You will succeed in finding your starting point.

Learning Experience 14.4

Select a learning outcome for a content area that you believe would be most appropriately taught using direct instruction. Similar to Box 14.3, design a set of learning progressions that you would use to provide practice for students.

Task Teaching

Teachers often find it useful to have students practicing more than one task at the same time. This is typically accomplished through one of three task-teaching instructional models (task, station, and inclusion). **Task teaching** refers to organizing the learning environment so that different students can engage in different learning tasks at the same time. Task teaching has also been referred to as *station teaching* (Mohnsen, 1995; Rink, 1998), although we would argue that **station teaching** is a subcategory of task teaching because there are ways of doing task teaching without stations. The availability of a climbing wall to accommodate an entire class is an example of task teaching that might prompt a teacher to design a set of related tasks for students to rotate among (see the example in **Box 14.4**).

Although task teaching does allow for station teaching that reduces the need for all students to access the same equipment at the same time, task teaching is not confined to situations in which limited equipment is the dominant contextual factor. Consider the possibilities for teaching strength development or a golf unit. In strength development, several major muscle groups must be worked on regularly. In golf, several different strokes fundamental to the game must be practiced regularly. Both of these could be accomplished with the teacher pacing students through the series of strength and skill tasks, all students doing the same task at the same time. Both could also be accomplished through a model in which various strength and stroke task stations are spread throughout the learning space and students rotate among the task stations during the lesson.

In task teaching, it is usually inefficient for a teacher to communicate the content of each task to students. Teachers sometimes try to describe and demonstrate each task at the outset of a lesson. This strategy, to be effective, requires that tasks be simple and easily remembered. Introducing new tasks is difficult in a task format. Sometimes teachers use active teaching to introduce tasks in the early lessons of a unit and use task teaching to practice these tasks as the unit progresses. Students then know the tasks and can practice them without lengthy teacher explanations and demonstrations.

Most teachers who use task formats design task cards for students or task posters for each station. These communicate the task through brief, simple descriptions. Task posters can also use pictures or drawings. The student reads the task description, perhaps looks at the picture of correct technique, and begins to practice the task. This approach lends itself to either simple tasks or ones with which students are familiar. **Figure 14.1** shows a simple task card, and **Figure 14.2** a more complex task card with diagrams and pictures to aid the students.

One advantage of task teaching is the possibility of accommodating different skill levels at one station. A major problem in teaching large groups of students is that they often have marked differences in ability and experience with the activity. In direct instruction, the teacher typically communicates one task and students respond. Occasionally, very effective teachers find ways to communicate variations in

BOX 14.4 Station Teaching in a Climbing Unit

Students are initially introduced to and have the opportunity to practice a set of climbing-related activities. Following this introduction and practice, these activities become stand-alone stations set up around the teaching area. Each day throughout the 4-week climbing unit, students rotate among the following six stations:

- Cargo net
- Zip line
- Climbing wall
- Horizontal wall
- Soft or Mohawk walk
- Electric fence

Task cards pictorially demonstrate each task and prompt spotting and safety. At the close of each lesson, a debriefing is conducted focused on various aspects of student participation: group support, spotting, fear, conflict resolution, leadership, or enjoyment.

SPRINT STARTS
• Split your foursome into two groups of two.
• One group has a timer and a starter/recorder.
• The second group has two runners.
• Time only the two full effort tasks.
• Groups switch roles after the running group has finished each task, giving time to rest before the next running task.
Task 1: Three starts plus 15 meters at a shuffle
Task 2: Three starts plus 30 meters at a stride
Task 3: Three starts plus 60 yards at full effort
Task 4: Three starts plus 15 yards at full effort

FIGURE 14.1 Simple task card.

Step 1: One ball changing hands

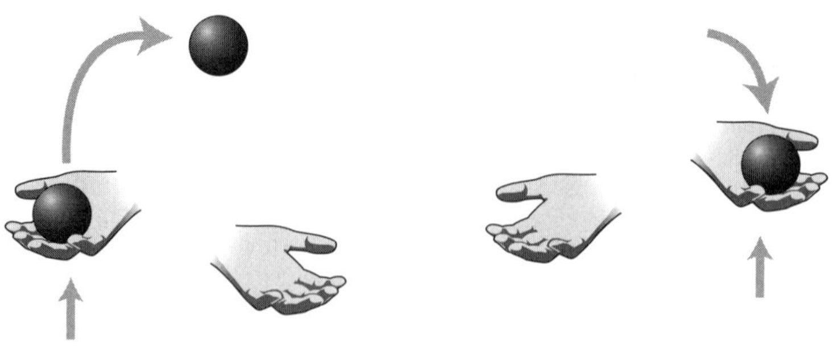

- Toss one ball from one hand to the other.
- Don't toss too high or too far—keep it right in front of you.
- Toss it back to the other hand. Do this until it becomes comfortable.
- Return the ball to the other hand in the same way, tossing it into the air. Do not simply pass it across to your dominant hand.

Step 2: Two ball exchange

The toss *The exchange* *The catch*

- Hold one ball in each hand.
- Toss as before starting with your dominant hand.
- When first ball hits its peak, toss the second ball.
- The up-going second toss travels inside the down-coming ball. Immediately after the second toss catch the first ball. Do not toss too hard; keep them about eye-high.

Next steps: This is the basic skill of juggling. If you can do this with two balls, you can do it with three. Keep practicing exchanging the one in the air for the one in your hand. One, two, catch, catch, stop. One, two, catch, catch, stop. Once you can do this four times in a row, pick up a third ball and follow the same steps.

FIGURE 14.2 A more complex task card for learning to juggle.

the task that accommodate different skill levels. For example, students could be given the option of serving from the end line or center line in volleyball, depending upon their skill level. Stations, however, are perhaps a more effective way of providing for varying skill levels.

Designing tasks that have multiple levels of performance and allow students choices in selecting their entry levels characterizes a special case of task teaching called **inclusion teaching**. Within a given task, there might be options (e.g., skill progressions, physical performance criteria, choice of various implements, size of targets, number of required repetitions), and students would select how and where to begin the task, depending upon their skill level. In hurdling, for example, stations might be set up sequentially, moving students from hurdling a minimal number of hurdles at a low height to increasing the height over an increased number of hurdles. Tasks could be communicated through task cards or self-instructional materials.

Another advantage of task teaching is that teachers can set up their physical space ahead of time in ways that help learners master content. In badminton, for example, a teacher might want specialized learning aids, to help students acquire specific skills. In a direct instruction lesson, these aids would have to be set up and taken down as the tasks changed throughout the lesson. With a task model, they can be set up for the entire lesson, with students rotating through the task stations. One station might be for the short and long serve, with a string stretched above the net to provide feedback for the short serve to increase task difficulty and target areas marked towards the back of the court floor for the long serve. Another station might have similar aids for the clear and drop shots. These stations could be used for individual student practice or set up to allow team practice in three versus three game conditions. A final station might be a computer with an interactive badminton CD to provide students practice at shot selection based on the tactical problem posed. The same activity could be completed on prepared task sheets that denote badminton-specific game play scenarios.

Task progressions between stations are more difficult and represent a general weakness in this instructional model. The problem is that, with six stations and five students per station, all stations have to be used at the outset, with students rotating throughout the lesson. If stations 1 through 6 represent a progression, then some students will be starting at the last stage of the progression and moving to the earlier stations as they rotate. Thus, station teaching is typically used for tasks that do not represent progressions. However, there are instances where three stations can be set up (one on each court) and students can choose where they start with a particular activity (e.g., court A, layup without any approach; B with an approach and carry; and C with a defender). The problem in this case would be if a large number of students all choose a particular station.

Most teachers who use one of the task models signal changes in stations/tasks and have students rotate on a signal or after a set time period. It is possible, however, to have students rotate after having met some particular performance criterion, whether it be volume of practice (25 trials) or quality of practice (five consecutive hits above the line). The problem with criterion-based rotation is that several stations tend to get crowded, with resulting problems of equipment sharing and active involvement.

To use the task models well, students need to have good self-control skills. Teachers can actively supervise task environments just as they would independent practice of any kind. They can provide more feedback and teaching, especially if students are generally well behaved and on task. The task models work best when tasks are clearly described (a situation for performance, the performance itself, and qualitative or quantitative indicators of success or completion) and when there is a strong accountability system other than teacher supervision, such as accumulating points toward individual awards or competition among the rotating groups based on collective scoring.

Learning Experience 14.5

Select a content area (e.g., tennis, gymnastics, flag rugby). Design three different learning outcomes for that same content area and one aspect of a lesson that would employ task, station, and inclusion teaching for each learning outcome. Demonstrate your understanding of the difference among these three task teaching models in your description of how the lesson would unfold.

Teaching Through Questions

Wiggins (1989) suggested that "the aim of curriculum is to awaken, not 'stock' or 'train' the mind" (p. 45), arguing that students need to view questions as a means to go beyond current knowledge to discovery, as a way to deepen meaning, and as a source for stimulating more thoughtful inquiry for which answers must be sought. **Teaching through questions** challenges students to be thoughtful, engages them in cognitive processing, and/or encourages them to explore alternatives. In other words, teaching through questions stimulates the learner to formulate a response to a query or problem rather than merely replicate an example. As Boorstin (1985) said, "Take nobody's word for it; see for yourself."

Teaching through questions refers to an instructional model in which tasks are communicated to students through questions that (1) pose problems that guide student activity toward particular goals or (2) pose problems to be solved or interpreted. In physical education, this approach has been widely used in teaching young children, especially when the focus has been on movement and movement concepts. Teaching through questions when teaching movement to children is really a variation of direct instruction because a whole-group format is typically used, and the teacher tends to control the pacing of the lesson by presenting a sequence of tasks through questions. The questions most often represent refining and extending tasks that allow students to explore options rather than reproduce a skill as shown by the teacher.

The distinguishing characteristic of this model is the way in which the task is presented to students and how that changes the student's role in the learning process. In direct instruction, tasks are described carefully, including the conditions for practice, the task itself, and some measure of success. In teaching through questions, a common strategy is to describe conditions for practice and some measure for success but to leave the performance itself open for student exploration and interpretation. For example, a teacher says, "Maintaining self-space, can you find a different way to balance on three body parts?" Balancing on three body parts indicates the successful completion of the task, but there are several ways students can be successful (e.g., two feet and one hand, two hands and one foot). The nature of the task presentation encourages students to explore different combinations. One

Goal: Students recognize what is needed to "stick" a landing in gymnastics.
Teacher-designed questions might include:
• As you and your partner practice the vault, what might prevent you from stepping forward on the landing?
• What happens when you lower your center of gravity by bending your knees?
• Does it make a difference when you keep your upper body upright and eyes focused on the wall in front of you?
• Which part of the foot is most stable on the landing?

FIGURE 14.3 Questions to guide sticking a landing.

solution might be followed by the question, "Can you find another way to do it?" In this case, the decision of what to do to fulfill the task is left to the student, who does not try to reproduce what the teacher has explained and shown as the right way to do a task.

Guided Discovery: Convergent Inquiry

When teachers prepare a series of task questions that help students progress toward a specific goal with one correct response, the model represents what Mosston described as **guided discovery** (Mosston & Ashworth, 1994). Guided discovery involves convergent thinking where the student is led or directed to the correct answer through well-designed questions. **Figure 14.3** provides an example of convergent inquiry for landing following a vault over a horse.

Learning Experience 14.6

Select a content area. Determine a learning outcome toward which students will strive to achieve with the teacher employing guided discovery. Design a set of convergent questions, or tasks that might be used to move students toward the outcome desired.

Problem Solving: Divergent Inquiry

Both guided discovery (convergent) and problem solving (divergent) may be employed in connection with most instructional models to add a problem-solving component to the learning environment. When teaching through questions is used in connection with other instructional models, the result is most often referred to as a **problem-solving approach**. Teachers can use questioning to help students to solve problems and think critically and tactically through the Tactical Approach to Teaching Games. When content to be learned is intended to place the learner at the center, draw out their individual creativity, involve discussion among peers, and stimulate abstract thinking, then problem solving (divergent inquiry) is appropriate.

Most activity units could be taught using the teaching through questions models. **Box 14.5** shows questions and examples from a basketball unit. Keep in mind that teaching

BOX 14.5 Types and Examples of Questions for Basketball

Questions can be organized into four types according to the cognitive activity involved. Questions from each category are used for different purposes. To use questions as part of an instructional model, make sure they are consistent with the purposes for which they are used.

1. *Recall questions:* These require a memory-level answer. Most questions that can be answered yes or no are in this category.
   - Where should your eyes be when you are dribbling?
   - Which hand should be up on defense against a right-handed dribbler?
   - Which foot should you push off from when cutting?
   - Should you keep your elbow out while shooting?
2. *Convergent questions:* These aid analysis and integration of previously learned material, require reasoning and problem solving, and typically have a range of correct and incorrect answers.
   - Why should you stay between your opponent and the basket?
   - What are your responsibilities if your opponent shoots and moves to the right to rebound?
   - What should you do if the defender steps out to guard you on a pick and roll?
3. *Divergent questions:* These require solutions to new situations through problem solving. Many answers may be correct.
   - What ways could you start a fast break off a steal?
   - What could you do if caught defending a taller player in the post?
   - What passing options do you have when double teamed?
   - What strategies would you suggest when three points ahead with 2 minutes left in a game?
4. *Value questions:* These require expressions of choice, attitude, and opinion. Answers are not judged as correct or incorrect.
   - How do you react when you are fouled but the referee doesn't call it?
   - How do you feel about intentionally fouling opponents at the end of a game?
   - What gives you more enjoyment, scoring a lot or playing on a winning team?

BOX 14.6 Discovering Cardiovascular Fitness

Students come into class and lie on the floor while the teacher explains the expectations of the day's lesson.

Today's lesson will involve a series of individual and partner tasks that can be performed on the field, track, or blacktop surface. As you perform each task you will make a decision on which activities are most suitable for developing your cardiovascular endurance.

- We will first take your resting heart rate and record it on the score sheet.
- After you complete each task, take your pulse and record your heart rate on the score sheet by each activity.
- Between activities, rest until your heart rate is back to resting.

Task 1: Walk for 1 minute.

Task 2: Jog for 1 minute.

Task 3: Skip rope for 1 minute.

Task 4: Walk for 1 minute, jog for 1 minute.

Task 5: Jog the corners of the running track and sprint the straight for two laps.

Task 6: With a partner, play catch with a disc for 1 minute.

Task 7: Count how many times can you pass the disc in one minute

Task 8: Play a game of 1 versus 1 basketball for 2 minutes.

At the end of class, the teacher says, "Let's analyze our data and talk about what we learned from this experience."

- What happens to your heart rate as you change activities?
- Which increases your heart rate more, the activity or the increasing time spent on an activity?
- Are you able to talk while completing some activities more than others?
- How did your heart rates differ from peers'?
- What do you think you need to do to increase your cardiovascular endurance?

through questions is often intended to achieve cognitive goals that are often at least as important as motor skill or strategy goals. **Box 14.6** shows this approach for part of a unit introducing cardiovascular endurance.

Learning Experience 14.7

Select a content area. Determine a learning outcome toward which students will strive to achieve with the teacher employing problem solving. Design a set of divergent questions, or tasks that might be used to move students toward the outcome desired. In designing questions, use recall, convergent, divergent, and value questions.

Games-Based Instruction

Games constitute a huge portion of most physical education and physical activity programs for young people, yet often games are not taught in realistic and challenging ways where young people learn what to do and when to do it at the same time they are learning how to do it. Whether using a Tactical Games Approach or Teaching Games for Understanding, **games teaching** incorporates teaching through questions to encourage students to think critically about tactical problems, appropriate skills, and when to use them. In games teaching, questions are developed based on what you want students to achieve: what, how, when, and where questions are explored (Mitchell, Oslin, & Griffin, 2003).

Learning Experience 14.8

Review the Tactical Games curriculum and instruction model and instructional aspects related to this model. Select content for a particular game and identify the following:

- Tactical problem
- Lesson focus
- Objectives

Then, design the following components of a lesson to achieve these objectives:

- Game: conditions/goal/questions
- Practice task: goals/cues/extension
- Game: conditions/goal
- Closure

Prerequisites for Effective Student-Mediated Instruction

Instructional models that rely on student-mediated instruction are becoming increasingly popular with teachers, and for good reason. Advocates of student-mediated instruction claim that it is effective because it results in the following (Cohen, 1994b):

- More active, engaged, task-oriented behavior than individual work
- More feedback to struggling students
- More opportunities for purposeful practice for students of all skill levels
- Better pro-social behavior development among students
- Strong within-group forces that help students avoid drifting off task
- Better motivation and allegiance to the class because of increased peer interactions
- Equal-status interaction among students

If all these were present, both content and social outcomes would be positively affected through school physical education.

Effective use of the student-mediated instructional models requires that teachers prepare students to be able to take part in them effectively. This is especially true if the students' previous school experiences have been primarily in teacher-mediated, whole-group instructional models. The younger the students, or the less experience they have had working in pairs or groups, the more important is an effective preparation program as a prerequisite for participation in student-mediated instruction.

The goals of a preparation program are twofold: (1) to develop the specific skills students will need to participate effectively in student-mediated instruction and (2) to establish special behavioral norms for working in pairs and groups. The teacher should make it clear to students why student-mediated instruction is important and what they might expect to gain from participating in it. The specific skills needed to participate typically include the following (Cohen, 1994a; Houston-Wilson, Lieberman, Horton, & Kasser, 1997):

- Student capacity to be aware of the different ability and interest levels of their peers
- Communication techniques such as listening skills and providing clear explanations
- Teaching skills such as prompting, showing, observing performance, and giving feedback
- Reinforcement techniques
- Ability to see critical performance elements and common errors in the skills practiced

The behaviors necessary for effective participation in student-mediated instruction group around three important norms: (1) everyone should contribute, (2) no one should dominate, and (3) all should be sensitive to student status within the group. Dominance-avoidance norms are typically achieved by helping students be willing to express their ideas, listen to others so all have a chance, ask others for their ideas, and discuss and give reasons for their ideas. It also is helpful if some means for conflict resolution is taught to students as the appropriate strategy for resolving the differences and disputes that inevitably arise in these instructional models. Students must recognize all the status issues that can marginalize them in physical education (e.g., gender, skillfulness, race, body type, height and weight). The norm of "all getting a fair chance" cannot be achieved without students being fully aware that these status issues often work to the detriment of some of them.

These behavioral norms are identical to those teachers establish as they move from compliance to cooperation to community, regardless of which instructional model is utilized. Cohen (1994a) states that the skills and behavioral norms needed to participate effectively in student-mediated instruction cannot be learned simply through reading about them or listening to someone explain them. She suggests that students best learn these skills and norms through participating in skill builders—games and practice activities designed to allow students to learn to work together. Many of these types of practice activities could be developed through several teacher-mediated (e.g., task teaching, teaching through questions) and student-mediated (e.g., cooperative learning, problem-based learning) models when employed within numerous curriculum models (e.g., Adventure Education, Sport Education, Teaching Personal and Social Responsibility).

Learning Experience 14.9

How would you prepare your students for self-mediated instruction? Refer back to Figure 14.2, which showed three-ball juggling. We are going to extend this task to a student-mediated lesson where students must gain peer approval for skill performance on a task before moving on to the next task. Describe what you must teach the students in order for them to successfully serve as a peer tutor in this case, and how you might achieve that.

Student-Mediated Instructional Models

We have now explained the prerequisite skills and behavioral norms that teachers have to establish among students in order for student-mediated instruction to be fully effective. The question is how effective student-mediated instruction is when it is done appropriately. The answer is clear: Students can teach and learn from each other effectively, and they enjoy it (Cohen, 1994b; Dyson & Ashworth, 2012; Mosston & Ashworth, 2007; Smith, Markley, & Goc-Karp, 1997). There is also evidence that students achieve important social skill benefits through use of these formats (Dyson & Harper, 1997; Strachan & MacCauley, 1997; Sutherland, 2012).

Peer Tutoring/Reciprocal Teaching

As learning groups get smaller, achievement increases (Bloom, 1984), with the most dramatic achievement gains resulting from tutoring. Instructional models that utilize pairs or triads of students as the basic instructional unit are typically referred to as **peer tutoring**, **peer teaching**, or **reciprocal teaching**. These models are particularly useful for achieving the goals of guided practice, which is fundamentally important to putting students in a situation in which they can benefit from independent practice. They also are useful for creating conditions in which students can utilize higher-order thinking skills to solve problems.

In relation to teaching students with disabilities, peer tutoring is typically of two types. One is when higher-skilled students tutor lower-skilled students for the primary purpose of boosting the performance of the latter. This model might prove useful in certain limited situations for short periods of time, but it does not represent a sufficiently general model for use in day-to-day teaching. The more useful, general model is referred to as classwide peer tutoring (CWPT), in which all students serve as both tutors and tutees (Houston-Wilson et al., 1997). CWPT has a long history in physical education, where it is more commonly referred to as reciprocal teaching (RT) (Mosston, 1966; Mosston & Ashworth, 1986, 1994, 2007).

CWPT or RT is typically highly structured, using teacher-developed materials to guide the progress of the tutorials. Tutors benefit from having to teach skills, knowledge, and tactics to classmates. Tutees benefit from individualized attention and feedback. The tutorial pair can progress at a pace conducive to the mastery of content. The key to successful CWPT/RT is the quality of the instructional materials, evaluation, feedback, and encouragement provided by the tutor. An additional benefit to CWPT/RT is that students acquire important interactive skills and also gain knowledge about the learning process through their responsible roles in it.

There is no strong evidence suggesting how student pairs should be formed. Contrary to conventional wisdom, there is evidence that higher-skilled students benefit from peer tutoring as much as lesser-skilled students; thus, mixed-ability pairs might be most useful. What is clear is that tasks assigned to students should be well-structured, unambiguous, and challenging. When students are in pairs, or triads for certain activities, their roles should be clearly defined and understood. When students are tutors, they are teachers. When students are tutees, they are learners. For this model to work, the tutors must be able to evaluate and control their partner's work. Tutors have to have the skills to teach, and students must work cooperatively. When student pairs stay together over extended periods, they can develop a cooperative working relationship of mutual respect. When pair combinations are rearranged within a class, students get new opportunities to learn and teach with other classmates. Thus, there are benefits to both sustaining pairs and switching pairs, and some combination of each is likely to provide the best long-term benefit.

CWPT/RT requires that teachers spend time preparing appropriate well-structured materials that include:

- Breakdown of task and specific steps
- Clear description of task and specific steps
- Critical points to guide tutor observation
- Graphics (drawings, sketches, pictures) of task
- Feedback cues and prompts of appropriate performance

Box 14.7 shows a reciprocal task sheet for use with pairs teaching one another the Macarena; note it starts with the teacher and then the student takes over responsibility. **Figure 14.4** shows a shot putt task sheet for use with triads. Once students have been taught to perform the instructional functions and the necessary managerial routines have been established, the teacher's role during the lesson is to supervise the tutoring process, providing feedback and encouragement to both tutors and tutees. In RT, students work in pairs with one as tutor (teach, observe, provide feedback) and one as tutee (performer), continuing until the task is completed or a signal to switch roles is given by the teacher. Pangrazi and Beighle (2010) suggest the following "pairing principles":

- For effective outcomes (e.g., communication skills, cooperation), allow students to choose partners they regard as supportive.
- When feedback and coaching are important, pair students of higher and lower ability.
- For maximum interaction (problem solving or game strategy), pair students who are compatible in terms of ability.
- For cognitive and affective tasks, gender and ability are not relevant, so pair students based on other factors.
- For tasks that involve pairs against one another, partners should be of similar size, strength, and ability.

Always pair students in ways that do not leave marginalized students to the final pairing; indeed, pairing should be done in ways that advance the community nature of the learning environment and contribute to the goals of anti-bias teaching.

BOX 14.7 Teaching the Macarena (from Teacher to Student)

1. Teacher plays the "Macarena" song to set the stage.
2. Teacher demonstrates the Macarena dance to the music.
3. Teacher teaches Step 1 and has students practice it several times.
4. Teacher teaches Step 2, has students practice it several times, and then adds it to Step 1.
5. Students practice Steps 1 and 2 together several times.
6. Teacher teaches Step 3, has students practice it several times, and then adds it to Steps 1 and 2.
7. Students practice Steps 1, 2, and 3 together several times.
8. Teacher teaches Step 4, has students practice it several times, and then adds it to Steps 1, 2, and 3.
9. Students practice Steps 1, 2, 3, and 4 several times.
10. Students try these steps to the music.

At this point, the teacher turns the responsibility of teaching the final steps (5–8) over to peer tutors. Using the following task card, and working in pairs, students take turns tutoring one another on Steps 5–8 of the Macarena, ensuring that everyone masters the steps. The task card will assist the students in tutoring and being tutored. When all students have tutored and have been tutored, the entire class will dance the Macarena to music.

Macarena steps	Trial 1	Trial 2	Trial 3	Trial 4	Trial 5
1. Dancer stretches right arm forward, palm down, then left arm, palm down.					
2. Dancer turns arms over so palms are up; first right, then left.					
3. Dancer puts hands on own shoulders, first right hand on left shoulder, then left hand on right shoulder.					
4. Dancer puts hands on the back of head, again right, then left.					
5. Dancer places arms on hips, right hand on left hip, then left on right.					
6. Dancer's hands go on their respective hips or rear end, right then left.					
7. Routine finishes with a pelvic rotation in time with the line "Ehhhh Macarena!"					
8. Dancer simultaneously jumps and turns 90 degrees counterclockwise and repeats the same motions throughout the entire song.					

Learning Experience 14.10

Select a content area and a learning outcome for a lesson that requires students to teach one another using reciprocal teaching while in a duo or triad. Design a task card to guide peer interaction in this reciprocal lesson.

Small Group Instruction

Educators are always on the lookout for instructional models that improve achievement while having important social benefits for students. **Small-group teaching** models, including cooperative learning, seem to provide those benefits. We use the descriptor *small groups* as the overall label for a variety of models, of which cooperative learning is one. The intent of small group instruction is for students to work in small enough groups that will allow all students to work on and achieve a clearly defined task carried out without the direct and immediate supervision of the teacher. Group work, as an instructional model, is not the same as ability grouping, nor is it a strategy for teachers to gather special groups of students for short-term intensive instruction. Group work is a fundamental way to organize students for everyday instructional purposes.

There are two key features of small-group work (Cohen, 1994a). The first is that the teacher delegates authority to the group to fashion the nature of its work to accomplish the task the teacher has assigned. The learning process is still controlled by the teacher because he or she evaluates the group's final product, but the manner in which students

1. Doer executes the putt 10 times from the circle toward the retriever using a soft ball.
2. Retriever returns the ball by rolling it back to the door.
3. Observer offers feedback to the doer by comparing the performance to the criteria and graphic provided below.

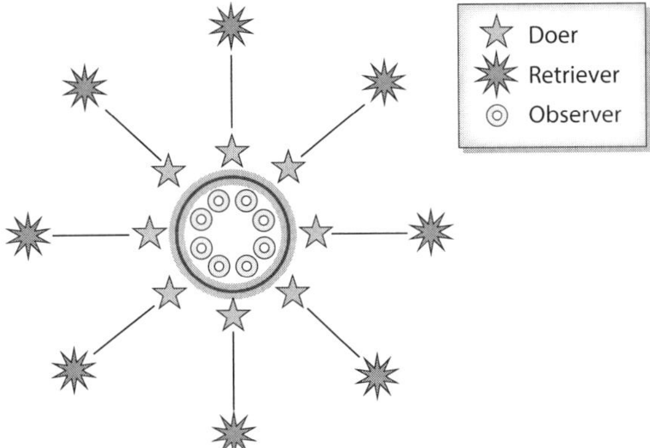

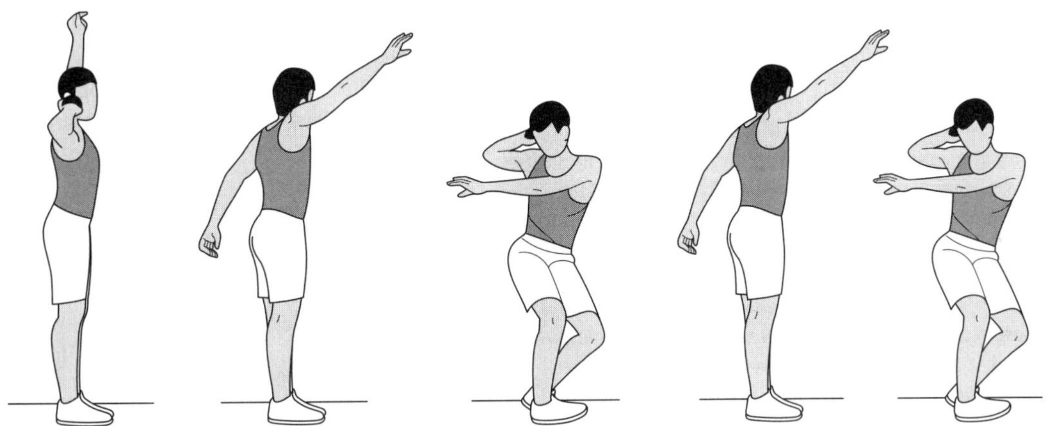

- Standing facing the direction of the putt.
- Grip the shot (ball) with pads of fingers (not resting it in the palm).
- Position the shot (ball) in the soft spot on the neck under the ear of putting arm.
- Putting elbow is held high.
- As putting the shot (ball), lead with hand, not elbow.
- Punch with the putting arm and finish with a flick of the wrist toward the target area.
- Bend and drive through the legs.

FIGURE 14.4 Shot putt task sheet.

fulfill the task is a function of the dynamics within each group. Because of this feature, the teaching functions within the group are largely guided by group decisions and mediated by the students themselves. The fact that the teacher evaluates the final product is the key to the accountability mechanism of group work.

The second feature is that members need each other to complete the task; that is, they can't complete the task by themselves. Group members have to interact to decide how the task assigned by the teacher will be accomplished and who will do what. This requires substantial communication within the group and is the reason communication skills should be pretrained before extensive use of this model. Students will have to listen, ask questions, criticize, disagree, and make collaborative decisions. This process enhances both their thinking and their collaborative skills. Cohen (1994a) suggests that groups of five are optimal for interactive and participatory purposes.

Group work requires interdependence of various sorts. *Goal interdependence* exists when individuals can achieve their goals only when other group members achieve theirs. *Resource interdependence* exists when individuals can achieve their goals only when other group members provide needed resources. *Reward interdependence* exists when rewards to the group are based on contributions of each individual group member. Individual accountability is also important, so that group recognition and rewards are clearly attributable to the cumulative contributions of each group member. The notion of a group reward for which contributions of each member are absolutely clear is especially important for instructional tasks that involve collective and collaborative individual work. When the instructional task is a challenging and interesting group task that requires all group members to contribute to the outcome, the need for individual accountability tracking by the teacher is reduced because the accountability to keep students involved and working hard is embedded within the task itself.

Group work can be powerful in learning for several reasons. The student-to-student interaction within groups requires that all members pay attention and respond. Students also tend to care about the evaluations of their classmates, so they tend to be more task oriented. Members seem not to want to let the group down by not carrying their fair share of the load. Working toward the group goal encourages members to help one another, providing assistance when something is not understood, resources are needed, or technical help with skill or tactics is appropriate.

Groups do not just coalesce and function smoothly on their own. Pre-preparation for associated skills and behavior norms is necessary. It is also helpful if group members have specific roles designed to help the group function more effectively. Once roles are determined, they require preparation and training with modeling, feedback, and clear criteria for how the job is done well.

Learning Experience 14.11

As noted, group work does not always progress smoothly. Often we see young people whose voices are not heard and who are made to feel less valuable than their peers. Status has been identified as a huge issue that impacts young people and their interactions with peers. As a teacher, how might you address this issue with your students prior to involving them in small group work? Design a set of learning experiences that might serve to prepare young people for involvement in group work in such a way that all are included and valued.

Cooperative Learning

Cooperative learning is a special variation of small group work. It has developed as a much-utilized model in both general education classrooms and physical education. The use of cooperative games (in which outcomes are determined by team members to achieve a goal) is common in primary school physical education. However, cooperative learning really refers to an instructional model rather than the activity being pursued (Kagan, 1990).

Cooperative learning is treated here as a special variation because of the specific cooperative learning structures that have been developed and widely tested in schools. Cooperative learning uses questioning to get students to solve problems and think outside the box; negotiating, renegotiating, building on ideas, compromising, adapting, and evaluating are among the higher order thinking skills required. Students are expected to turn obstacles into opportunities while creating solutions.

The types of cooperative learning we have chosen to describe include pairs–check, jigsaw, think–pair–share, and problem-based learning.

- In *pairs–check*, students work together in groups of four with two partner pairs in each group. Student pairs each work on an instructional task with one student coaching the other, as in peer tutoring/RT. The two pairs then get together to check to see if they are achieving the same goal, solution, or outcome, with further feedback as a result. *Pairs–check applied to a lesson:* The class is working on developing a street dance to perform at a parent meeting. Each group of four students is assigned a street dance step. Each pair within the foursome works on learning the dance step. When they feel ready, they get together with their foursome to learn from, provide feedback to, and develop the dance step further.

- In *jigsaw*, a learning task is designed that can be divided into four to six required components. Every member of the class is assigned/chooses a component in which they would like to work. Groups are formed for each component, and members work as a cooperative group to investigate all aspects of that component, becoming an expert in it. After all members become an expert in their component, groups are rearranged so that an expert from each component is now grouped with other component experts, and each shares his or her learning so that eventually all group members know the content. *Jigsaw applied to a lesson:* Each foursome from the pairs–check portion of the lesson now works cooperatively to master their assigned dance step. Each member will become an expert in their dance step and be able to teach it to others successfully. One member of each foursome is now matched with three other students, each representing a different foursome. Each member teaches what they have designed and learned so that each foursome has now learned an entire dance sequence.
- In *think–pair–share*, a learning task or question is posed to the entire class. Students work in cooperative groups to develop their own ideas and build on them with insight, reaction, and brainstorming from peers within their group before sharing them with a larger group or class. *Think–pair–share applied to a lesson:* The class is asked to creatively chronicle their collective learning at the close of a unit of instruction and practice. Students decide to individually reflect on their own learning each day using art as a creative way to conceptualize what happened that day. Pairs get together to discuss and display their learning before sharing it with the entire class and further developing a shared picture of what took place. A class mural on the wall may be the chosen medium through which they will demonstrate their learning.
- *Problem-based learning* is similar to what was originally called coop–coop by Kagan (1990)—students work together in cooperative groups to produce a particular product or outcome to which each group member makes a contribution that can be evaluated. The groups then present their work product to the rest of the class. In some situations, the group outcomes might be combined for a final class product. *Problem-based learning applied to a lesson:* Class members are assigned the task of examining whether sport is delivered equitably in their school. Small groups each select a focus for their research (e.g., gender, race, socioeconomic, ability), which will culminate in a report that presents a picture of sport in their school. Each group will share their report with the entire class and determine how they might move forward in sharing it with the entire school community in an effort to further develop an equitable situation for all.

These cooperative learning models allow learners to be active in their own learning by seeking and clarifying content from, and for, their peers. Frequently, students who need further explanation of a task or concept will be able to grasp it more easily if it is explained by another student, rather than by the teacher. Regardless of the model used, students are generally assigned a task, a problem, or a goal to be solved or achieved as a group. Success at achieving the given task will be determined in part by the students' cooperative skills and willingness to work as a team. These, like any other skills, need to be taught and practiced.

Cooperative learning is intended to produce social and affective outcomes as well as psychomotor content mastery outcomes. When used appropriately, cooperative learning results in social gains among diverse groups and across skill levels as well as more acceptance of students with disabilities and increased friendships among students in general (Slavin, 1990). Teachers often use cooperative learning models for student practice of instructional tasks after having used direct teaching for initial instruction. Cooperative learning, which contains some elements of peer tutoring, could also be used in conjunction with the task model. In this sense, we see the Sport Education curriculum model incorporating a form of cooperative learning in the context of sport.

Size of group is important for cooperative learning. Smaller groups, even pairs, maximize participation and involvement. Keeping the groups small allows more time to practice speaking, listening, and making choices. A variety of techniques can be used to form small groups: self-selection, structured categories procedures, and mixed ability grouping. Depending upon the intent of the cooperative tasks, the number of students in your class, and their interactive skills, each of these strategies can be useful. In cooperative learning, student work is structured so that it requires interdependence in the achievement of group goals but also provides individual accountability for group members.

Learning Experience 14.12

Select a content area, identify a learning outcome for a lesson, and design a cooperative experience that reflects pairs–check, jigsaw, think–pair–share, or problem-based learning.

Teams are a special type of group that we need to mention here because they are frequently used in physical education. Although generally composed of larger groups than those described previously, when used well, teams can result in many of the social benefits described for small groups while allowing students to take responsibility for their own experiences, thus moving teams into the self-instructional models category. One of the strengths of the Sport Education curriculum model is the meaning that students derive from the sport experience as a result of being a member of a team and the personal growth that comes from being affiliated with the same group of individuals over time. As students begin to develop an affiliation with their team and its members, they begin to feel an allegiance to, and responsibility toward, their peers and the team effort. To allow students to take responsibility for their sport experience, the Sport Education model has roles that team members take on and fulfill throughout the season. These roles tend to be more clearly defined because the team is formed for the purpose of competition. Roles include that of participant (everyone), captain or coach, referee, scorekeeper, statistician, and even publicist, manager, trainer, and a sports board. Although each of these roles should be defined so that students know their responsibilities to the team, the decision on who will define them may vary by teacher, experience of students, and context. **Box 14.8** provides an example of roles and responsibilities for a postprimary dance season.

BOX 14.8 Roles and Responsibilities for Postprimary Dance

Master of Ceremonies:

- Introduces team members, dance theme, and music selection
- Attends to management of practice and application tasks

Choreographer:

- Leads team practice
- Assists teacher
- Helps teammates learn dance moves

Fitness trainer:

- Designs appropriate warm-up tasks
- Leads warm-up activities
- Reports injuries to teacher
- Assists teacher with first aid

Dance board member:

- Assists with team selection
- Monitors dance times during competition
- Serves as judge during dance competition

Disc jockey (DJ):

- Maintains audio equipment
- Chooses correct music for dance teams
- Oversees music during dance competition

Reviewer/critic:

- Publicizes reviews via electronic newsletter, posts on bulletin board
- Reports on daily progress to dance team
- Assumes responsibilities for absent teammates

Self-Instruction

Self-instructional models allow students to progress through a sequence of learning activities without the physical presence, direction, or supervision of a teacher. Among the models in this category are individualized instruction, contracting, and personalized systems of instruction (PSI). Self-instructional models embed all the teaching functions in materials and typically use a formal accountability system. Teachers who plan self-instructional lessons spend a great deal of time developing and improving those materials and maintaining records of student performance in an accountability system. As **Box 14.9** indicates, self instruction is one of the instructional models that puts students at the center of the learning environment.

Self-instructional models can be used within a traditional class setting, or they can be used for students to pursue learning independently from a class setting. Self-instructional models are widely used in postprimary physical education for courses that take place away from the school, such as in a local bowling alley, indoor tennis arena, or golf course. The nature of physical education content results in self-instructional models that often require students to work in pairs, triads, or small groups to complete the learning tasks. Thus, self-instructional models are often used in conjunction with peer teaching formats. Also, because of the need to develop clear and explicit materials for learners, self-instructional models take on many of the characteristics of task teaching.

The strengths of self-instructional models are the flexibility allowed to learners and the possibility of matching learning tasks to student abilities more than is possible in a whole-class, direct instruction model. The flexibility of good self-instructional materials is that they can be used within a class or outside a class. There is also much to be said for students having the responsibility of completing a learning sequence on their own by following the materials prepared by the teacher.

Self-instructional models succeed or fail based on how specific and appropriate the materials prepared for students are and the degree to which the accountability system motivates the students to complete the tasks. The self-instructional materials need to be complete and explicit, providing students with the help they need at the point when it is needed. **Box 14.10** shows self-instructional materials for the

BOX 14.9 When Teaching *Least Is* Teaching *Best*

When we think about teaching, our first thoughts typically are about the things teachers do in class. Too often when we think about evaluating teaching, we think about watching what the teacher does. Teachers do not have to be at the center of the stage for good instruction to take place. Indeed, arguments can be made that, for students to become responsible, independent learners, the teacher must move off stage, so that the students themselves can occupy the central roles. There are several instructional models in this chapter that can accomplish that goal.

Responsible, independent learners can no doubt develop from many of the variations of peer tutoring and self-instructional formats. Although responsibility and independence are important qualities, one might argue that learning to work together toward collective goals is also an important, humanizing experience. Some peer models and most cooperative models would be appropriate for this goal.

It is OK for teachers to get off and stay off center stage in the instructional model. Enough is now known about classroom management for teachers to work gradually toward implementing instructional models that not only promote student independence and responsibility but also require collaboration and responsibility for others and allow students to experience the multiplier effect that can be achieved through communal effort toward collective goals.

The models through which these goals can be achieved are not easy to implement. Teachers need highly developed class management skills to develop an orderly environment in which students can learn to function effectively in these student-centered models. Even then, direct instruction might sometimes still be the preferred model because the models need to be adapted to goals and context.

BOX 14.10 Self-Instructional Materials for the Volley in Soccer

Purpose: To redirect an aerial ball strategically
Type of Volley: Foot, knee, shoulder, or head

Skill analysis:

- Align chosen body part with approaching ball.
- Focus eyes on approaching ball.
- Move body and body part toward approaching ball.
- Firmly contact body part to center of ball.
- Follow through in direction of intended flight.

Task learning experiences:

1. Partner A throws the ball towards partner B's shoulder. Partner B volleys the ball, executing a shoulder volley. Repeat five times from a distance of 10 feet. Switch roles and repeat from 15 feet.
2. Repeat task 1, preceding the volley with two or three steps. Switch roles.
3. Repeat tasks 1 and 2, directing the ball to the left, right, and toward center.
4. Repeat task 2 twice, and then task 3, executing a knee volley.
5. Repeat task 2 twice, and then task 3, executing a foot volley.
6. Partner A throws the ball underhand so that it arches and drops toward partner B's head. Partner B executes a head volley. Repeat three times from a distance of 10 feet. Switch roles.
7. Repeat task 6, directing the ball to the left, right, and toward center.
8. Stand 10 to 15 feet from a wall and kick the ball into the wall. Volley the rebound with different body parts according to the level of rebound. For a more forceful rebound, precede the kick with two or three steps. Different levels of rebound can be achieved by contacting the ball at various points below the center. Repeat 10 times.

Adapted from Zakrajsek, D., & Carnes, L. (1986). *Individualizing physical education: Criterion materials* (2nd ed.). Champaign, IL: Human Kinetics.

skill of volleying in soccer. These materials are typical of self-instructional materials to be used within a class.

Contracting

Contracting is a form of individualized instruction in which students sign a learning contract to complete a sequence of learning tasks according to a predetermined set of criteria. Contracting is a popular self-instructional model for physical education courses completed at sites other than the school and under the jurisdiction of persons other than the physical educator. Thus, students might complete a golf unit or a bowling unit at local sites on their own without the supervision of the teacher. The contract specifies the learning tasks to be completed, the amount of practice required, and the criteria for performance necessary for a particular grade or fulfillment of a requirement. An example of a learning contract is shown in **Box 14.11**.

BOX 14.11 Golf Learning Contract

Requirements:

- Practice at a local course for a total of 20 hours.
- Complete a test on golf rules at a score of 90% or better before playing on the course.
- Play 36 holes of golf, submitting completed scorecards.
- Maintain a diary describing problems you encountered in skill practice and play. Submit diary at the completion of the golf unit.
- Play a final 18 holes at the end of the golf unit.

Practice tasks (20 hours minimum):

- On practice range, hit 9 iron, 5 iron, and 1 or 3 wood 20 times each. Utilize a critical element checklist for each practice. If possible, have a partner observe, provide feedback, and complete a checklist.
- On practice green, hit 25 9-iron pitch and chip shots. Utilize a critical element checklist for each practice.
- On practice green, putt 50 putts of varying lengths and slopes.
- As you improve, spend more time practicing the tasks you are having difficulty with.
- Have practice times attested to by a partner or course employee.

Playing tasks (minimum of 36 holes):

- Play at least nine holes at a time.
- Play following official and local rules.
- Complete scorecard and have score attested.
- Record thoughts and reactions in your diary.

Personalized System of Instruction

Personalized system of instruction (PSI) is a self-instructional model in which content is divided into small units students must master before moving on to other units. PSI models require developing specific instructional tasks and clear mastery criteria. Students then practice the tasks until they meet the criteria before moving on to the next task. PSI allows for individual progress through a series of learning tasks. At the end of a PSI unit, students will differ in how much they have learned rather than how well they can perform. Assessment is typically done in terms of how many tasks are completed within the time constraints of the unit. PSI could also be used away from the time demands imposed by class periods and during school days. If so, students who need extra time to master a series of tasks could do so. **Box 14.12** shows two tasks from a PSI disc unit of ultimate, field events, guts, and golf. The unit is composed of a series of such tasks.

Learning Experience 14.13

Identify content for which you might develop a personalized system of instruction for your students. Outline what you envision taking place and develop the expectations, requirements, and steps that will guide student participation.

BOX 14.12 PSI Task Example from a Disc Unit

Self-Caught Flight Events

The disc is thrown and then must be caught with one hand (two hands for beginners). Participants are to challenge themselves to the tasks, record their efforts, and keep a journal of all events as they progress.

Maximum Time Aloft

The disc is thrown and then caught with one hand. The goal is to maximize the amount of time elapsing between the disc being released and being caught. The event demands a powerful and controlled throw and ability to "read" the flight in order to execute the catch. This event tends to be most successful if there is a stiff breeze.

Throw, Run, and Catch (TRC)

The disc is thrown, and then the thrower must run to catch it one-handed. The distance from the point where the disc is released to where it is caught is the score. This event demands good technical ability to throw a long, hovering disc, combined with fast sprinting capability and reliable catching.

Service Learning

Nick Cutforth (2000) describes **service learning** as a "teaching method that provides opportunities for students to acquire academic, career, social, and personal skills through community service projects" (p. 39). He highlights the main reason for including service learning in education programs as being that students "learn best by doing, by serving, and by reflecting on their experience" (p. 41). Service learning intends for students to learn about social issues, improve social and interpersonal skills, and develop leadership and positive civic qualities while planning and delivering a service to the community in response to an identified need. Service learning is a means to set the stage for students to become engaged and involved with various issues in their community, and then bringing them back to the classroom to serve as the basis for academic learning and aligned learning experiences.

The National Youth Leadership Council (see www.nylc.org) identified four types of service learning initiatives in which students can become involved. We have provided examples of these applied to a physical education/physical activity setting.

1. *Direct service learning* involves face-to-face types of projects that directly influence those being served, such as designing and delivering workshops for other students or adults who may be in need.
2. *Indirect service learning* is focused on projects aimed at community or environmental issues rather than the individuals with whom they interact, such as maintaining community activity or playground space or restoring a trail system in the local parklands.
3. *Research-based service learning* involves projects where students are required to locate, access, and analyze information on a given topic and share that information with individuals to impact practices. This might include developing a video to be used in the school fitness center highlighting safety precautions and how equipment is to be used appropriately or using the information gained in the preceding jigsaw assignment on equity in the sport provision at the school.
4. *Advocacy service learning* is intended to influence the community by educating them or bringing issues to their awareness. In the case of physical education, this might include young people investigating and promoting physical activity and healthy eating as a means of educating the public on living an active and healthy lifestyle.

Determining how to employ service learning in physical education is like selecting any other instructional model; it depends on the content being taught, the expected learning outcomes, the abilities and behavior of the students, the curriculum model within which the lesson is a part, how feedback might best be provided, and the decisions the teacher makes in terms of giving students responsibility and choice. **Box 14.13** provides ideas for health and physical education service-learning projects as suggested by the 2007 KIDS Consortium (see www.kidsconsortium.org).

BOX 14.13 Health and Physical Education Service-Learning Projects

Elementary:

- Students decided that their community needed a fun and safe environment to encourage physical exercise, so the students took over the entire planning of the annual fun run at their school and designed markers for the new running path in the area.
- Students learned the basics about nutrition and exercise, including the various winter sport activities that New England has to offer. The students wanted to learn how to snowshoe safely, so they partnered with experts from the Kittery Trading Post. Students then shared what they had learned about snowshoeing with the community through written and oral presentations, in hopes that they would encourage others to engage in healthy activities.
- Students learned about the importance of starting healthy eating and exercising habits at a young age and decided to work with the Jump Rope for Heart Campaign to teach their peers about healthy habits. The students recruited sponsorships and participants for a Jump Rope for Heart fundraiser, which raised over $2,100 for the American Heart Association.
- Students worked with their Public Schools Wellness Policy Committee to help develop, implement, and monitor new nutrition policies. The students also put together a healthy kid-friendly cookbook and held a healthy food fair to share what they learned about nutrition with the whole community.
- Students learned about the number of accidents and injuries that occur because people are not wearing helmets or seatbelts. Students partnered with Life Flight and the local fire and rescue, among others, to address this dangerous problem. The students held a public safety field day and a local health fair, made videos and PowerPoint presentations, and even met with the governor to discuss new safety legislation.
- Students learned that their school needed better sun safety education. The students researched ultraviolet (UV) rays, skin cancer, and sun safety, and then proposed a new school policy about sun safety. They also made and distributed posters and informational brochures to educate others in their community about sun safety.

(continues)

BOX 14.13 Health and Physical Education Service-Learning Projects (*Continued*)

Middle school:

- Working with community health services, physical education students developed age-appropriate exercises for senior citizens. The students then provided a place for seniors to exercise during the winter months and a program for them to follow.
- After learning about public policy, students decided there was a need for better public policy preventing alcohol advertisers from deliberately targeting young people. The students researched alcohol advertisements and proposed new policies, which they presented at two city-wide public forums and in letters to their local elected officials.
- After a student wrote a personal essay about his experience with bullying, he decided to do an independent study project addressing the issue of bullying in schools. Working with the school administration, the school newspaper, and his teacher, the student published his essay in the school newspaper to encourage discussion about the issue and created a computer game to simulate the effect of bullying on all individuals involved.
- Students learning about public policy decided that they wanted to do something about the problem of child abuse and neglect in their community and state. After much research and brainstorming, the students proposed a policy that would require all prospective teachers to be trained in recognizing the signs of child abuse and neglect. The students shared their policy with their local representative, who drafted their policy as state legislation.

High school:

- Students worked with the student council on the annual *Every 15 Minutes* program, an alcohol education and awareness program. The students put together posters with graphs and tabular charts depicting information about blood alcohol content and displayed them in the school during the 2-day program.
- Students learned about Lyme disease, which is a major problem in their area. The students then decided to educate their community about the dangers of Lyme disease through a variety of projects including a radio interview, public service announcement, puppet play, benefit dinner, and webpage.
- Students in a Medical Occupations class were asked by the March of Dimes to educate the community on the importance of folic acid in their diets. The students agreed to work on the project. After doing extensive research on folic acid, they created slideshows, posters, and pamphlets of information on folic acid, which they shared with their peers. They also gave copies of their materials to school nurses and the March of Dimes.
- Students learned that emergency responders in their town needed a more effective and efficient way to identify possible concerns and hazards (overhead electrical wires, staircases, children's bedrooms, etc.) at an emergency scene. The students conducted surveys of potential concerns and hazards in their local community and created a computer prototype that can quickly identify hazards; this prototype was presented to the town council.

The Youth Service of California (2003) highlights the following seven elements it recommends as essential for service learning to be effective:

1. Integrated learning
   - Service-learning goals evolve from knowledge, skills, or values that make up broader classroom and school goals.
   - Service learning and academic learning content is reciprocal.
   - Life skills learned through service learning outside the classroom are integrated into overall learning.
2. Service to community
   - Service responds to an actual community need recognized by the community.
   - Service is age-appropriate and well organized.
   - Service is designed to achieve significant benefits for the students and community.
3. Collaboration
   - Service learning should be a collaboration among students, community-based organization staff, support staff, administrators, faculty, and recipients of service.
   - All partners benefit from the project and contribute to its planning.

4. Student voice
   - Students have a voice in choosing and planning the service project.
   - Students have a voice in planning and implementing reflection, evaluation, and celebration.
   - Students have roles and complete tasks that are appropriate for their age.
5. Civic responsibility
   - Service learning should promote student responsibility to care for others and contribute to the community.
   - Students understand how they impact their community as a result of service learning.
6. Reflection
   - Reflection establishes connections between service experiences and academic experiences.
   - It occurs throughout service learning (before, during, and after).
7. Evaluation
   - All partners are involved in evaluating the service learning.
   - Evaluation measures progress toward learning and service goals.

Learning Experience 14.14

What might a service learning project look like in your physical education program? Identify a need that is apparent in your community and determine how you might build a response to it into your physical education class as a project for the students to complete. Follow the steps outlined to develop the service learning project highlighting where student voice will be invited.

CHAPTER SUMMARY

As we have demonstrated in this chapter, effective instruction comes in teacher-mediated and student-mediated forms. Regardless of age group, curriculum or instructional model, or content selected within the instructional task system, however, we know that maintaining a safe learning environment through an effective managerial task system is essential.

1. Instructional models can be categorized as teacher mediated or student mediated.
2. If one instructional model is more effective than another, it is only within a particular context and with a particular group of learners, and then only because it matches the needs and the context in a particularly effective way.
3. Active teaching is a framework for understanding the major skills that effective teachers show in their work.
4. There is no hierarchy of instructional models; choice of instructional model should be based on (1) personal skills and preferences of teachers, (2) characteristics of the learners being taught, (3) the nature of the content being taught, and (4) the context within which teaching takes place.
5. The purpose of guided practice is to ensure that students understand and can perform a task sufficiently well to benefit from independent practice.
6. The purpose of independent practice is to engage in a sufficient number of successful repetitions to be able to use the skill appropriately in an applied context.
7. Direct instruction is the most frequently used model in physical education; it is successful partly due to the organizational and supervision aspects of the model that allow teachers to manage student engagement.
8. Task teaching refers to organizing the learning environment so that different students can engage in different learning tasks at the same time and includes station teaching (rotating from one station to the next) as well as inclusion teaching (performance options available within each task to accommodate varying ability levels).
9. Teaching through questions is a variation of direct instruction in which student responses are not prescribed, typically taking a guided discovery or problem-solving approach.
10. Students need to be prepared to take part effectively in student-mediated instruction, which includes the particular skills (observing, feedback, etc.) and the appropriate behavioral norms for cooperation.
11. In peer tutoring and reciprocal models, students take on instructional roles, typically in pairs, triads, or small groups, and are prepared to assess peer performance and provide feedback.
12. Small group and cooperative learning involve student work that is structured so that it not only requires interdependence in the achievement of group goals but also provides individual accountability for members of the learning groups.
13. Teachers do not have to be center stage; good instruction and learning often take place with students occupying more central roles.
14. Self-instructional models allow students to progress through a sequence of learning activities without the immediate presence of the teacher, with teacher-prepared materials essential for successful implementation.
15. Contracting and PSI are self-instructional models used in both regular classes and independent study.
16. Service learning intends for students to learn about social issues, improve social and interpersonal skills, and develop leadership and positive civic qualities while planning and delivering a service to the community in response to an identified need.

REFERENCES

Bloom, B. (1984). The 2 sigma problem: The search for methods of group instructions as effective as one-to-one tutoring. *Educational Researcher, 13*(5), 4–16.

Boorstin, D. (1985). *The discoverers: A history of man's search to know his world and himself.* New York: Vantage Books.

Capel, S., Leask, M., & Turner, T. (Eds.). (2001). *Learning to teach in the secondary school: A companion to school experience* (3rd ed.). London: Routledge-Falmer.

Cohen, E. (1994a). *Designing groupwork: Strategies for the heterogeneous classroom* (2nd ed.). New York: Teacher College Press.

Cohen, E. (1994b). Restructuring the classroom: Conditions for productive small groups. *Review of Educational Research, 64*(1), 1–35.

Cothran, D. J., Hodges Kulinna, P., & Garrahy, D. A. (2003). "This is kind of giving a secret away . . .": Students' perspectives of effective class management. *Teaching and Teacher Education, 19*(4), 435–444.

Cutforth, N. J. (2000). Connecting school physical education to the community through service learning. *Journal of Health, Physical Education, Recreation and Dance, 1*(20), 39–45.

Dyson, B., & Ashworth, A. (Eds.). (2012). *Cooperative learning in physical education: A research-based approach.* London: Routledge.

Dyson, B., & Harper, M. (1997). Cooperative learning in an elementary physical education program. *Research Quarterly for Exercise and Sport, 68*(Suppl. 1), A-68.

Housner, L. (1990). Selecting master teachers: Evidence from process-product research. *Journal of Teaching Physical Education, 9*(3), 201–226.

Houston-Wilson, C., Lieberman, L. J., Horton, M., & Kasser, S. (1997). Peer tutoring: A plan for instructing students of all abilities. *Journal of Physical Education, Recreation, and Dance, 6*, 39–44.

Kagan, S. (1990). The structural approach to cooperative learning. *Educational Leadership, 47*(4), 12–16.

KIDS Consortium. Health and physical education service-learning projects. Available from www.kidsconsortium.com.

Mitchell, S. A., Oslin, J. A., & Griffin, L. L. (2003). *Sport foundations for elementary physical education.* Champaign, IL: Human Kinetics.

Mohnsen, B. (1995). *Using technology in physical education.* Champaign, IL: Human Kinetics.

Mosston, M. (1966). *Teaching physical education.* Columbus, OH: Merrill.

Mosston, M., & Ashworth, S. (1994). *Teaching physical education* (4th ed.). New York: Macmillan.

Mosston, M., & Ashworth, S. (2002). *Teaching physical education* (5th ed.). Boston, MA: Benjamin Cummings.

Mosston, M., & Ashworth, S. (1994). *Teaching physical education* (1st ed. [online]). Spectrum Institute for Teaching and Learning. Available from www.spectrumofteachingstyles.org/ebook

National Youth Leadership Council. (n.d.). Home page. Available from www.nylc.org

Pangrazi, R. P., & Beighle, A. (2010). *Dynamic physical education for elementary school children* (16th ed.). San Francisco, CA: Benjamin Cummings.

Rink, J. (1985). *Teaching physical education for learning.* St. Louis, MO: CV Mosby.

Rink, J. (1998). *Teaching physical education for learning.* Boston: W.C. Brown-McGraw Hill.

Rink, J. (2009). *Teaching physical education for learning.* Boston: W.C. Brown-McGraw Hill.

Rosenshine, B. (1979). Content, time and direct instruction. In P. Peterson & H. Walberg (Eds.), *Research on teaching: Concepts, findings and implications* (pp. 28–56). Berkeley, CA: McCutchan.

Rosenshine, B., & Stevens, R. (1986). Teaching functions. In M. Wittrock (Ed.), *Handbook of research on teaching* (3rd ed., pp. 376–391). New York: MacMillan.

Siedentop, D., & Tannehill, D. (2000). *Developing teaching skills in physical education.* Mountain View, CA: Mayfield.

Slaven, R. (1990). Research on cooperative learning: Consensus and controversy. *Educational Leadership, 47*(4), 52–55.

Smith, B. T., Markley, R., & Goc Karp, G. (1997, March). Cooperative learning and social skill enhancement. Annual Meeting of the American Association of Health, Physical Education, Recreation, and Dance, St. Louis, Missouri.

Strachan, K., & MacCauley, M. (1997).Cooperative learning in a high school physical education program. *Research Quarterly for Exercise and Sport, 68*(Suppl. 1), A-68.

Sutherland, S. (2012). Borrowing strategies from adventure-based learning to enhance group processing in cooperative learning. In B. Dyson & A. Casey (Eds.), *Cooperative learning in physical education: A research-based approach* (pp. 103–118). London: Routledge.

Whitehead, M., & Zwozdiak-Myers, P. (2007). Designing teaching approaches to achieve intended learning outcomes. In S. Capel, M. Leask, & T. Turner (Eds.), *Learning to teach in the secondary school: A companion to school experience* (3rd ed., pp. 141–152). London: Routledge-Falmer.

Wiggins, G. (1989). The futility of trying to teach everything of importance. *Educational Leadership, 47*(3), 44–59.

Youth Service of California. (2003). After school service learning: Four profiles of engagement. Available from http://roserbatlle.files.wordpress.com/2009/07/4-exemples-service-learning-in-afterschool.pdf

Zakrajsek, D., & Carnes, L. (1986). *Individualizing physical education: Criterion materials* (2nd ed.). Champaign, IL: Human Kinetics.

CHAPTER 15 Developing Teaching Strategies to Facilitate Learning

Overall Chapter Outcome

To become familiar with the general teaching skills and strategies needed across most teaching contexts, regardless of content choice or which curriculum and/or instructional model is selected

Learning Outcomes

The learner will:

- Explain why it is important for teachers to know how to use managerial strategies in the physical education class
- Describe how and when to use managerial skills and strategies (e.g., transitioning students, equipment setup, behavior and management feedback, teachable moment, lesson closure)
- Explain the purpose of teaching strategy and why it is important to student learning
- Describe how and when to use teaching skills and strategies (e.g., set induction, grouping for activity, checking for understanding)
- Discuss the importance of questioning as a teaching strategy and how it enhances learning
- Describe the various types of questions that can be used in teaching, explaining how and when they are most appropriate
- Explain why the tips for giving feedback are crucial to student learning
- Describe how and why feedback is different during guided practice and independent practice
- Describe the key elements of active supervision
- Discuss the criteria for effective demonstrations and why they are so important
- Explain the strategy of modified games as learning tasks and how Metzler's strategies for teaching during games can be used effectively
- Describe the relationship between a learning experience and teaching strategy
- Describe a learning experience for social, psychomotor, and cognitive development
- Discuss Block's guidelines for modifying task complexity

The managerial, instructional, and student-social task systems interact with and influence one another to develop a learning-oriented and positive classroom ecology where students work to achieve significant learning goals. This kind of ecology requires teachers who have the managerial and instructional skills to support student success. We should not forget that an effective managerial system provides the foundation for effective teaching. An effective preventive management system produces the time and order necessary for students to engage purposefully in the content. Never underestimate the importance of an effective class management system—it provides the opportunity for an instructional system to work. Without it, students are unlikely to engage seriously with the learning tasks, regardless of how well those tasks are planned and delivered.

Effective instructional task systems come in many varieties, ranging from general teaching skills and strategies to the more structured and focused instructional models. Regardless of which skills, strategies, or models a teacher selects within the instructional task system, maintaining a safe learning

BOX 15.1 Key Terms in This Chapter

- *Active supervision:* Designed to keep students on the assigned task and provide supportive and corrective feedback where necessary. It entails the 90–90 principle, scanning frequently, moving unpredictably, using feedback across space, with-it-ness, equally distributing attention, and building on expectations for learning.
- *Behavior and management feedback:* Information provided to the student in response to behavior with the intent of reinforcing, correcting, reducing, or improving a particular behavior that is impacting student learning. It includes prompts, hustles, desists, and praise.
- *Checking for student understanding:* In the management and instructional task system this involves ensuring students understand what they are to do, how they are to behave, and critical elements of a skill or steps in a practice task prior to being disbursed.
- *Equipment dispersal:* Having strategies and class routines to guide distribution of equipment (dispersal and return) and how it is used throughout the lesson.
- *Feedback:* Information provided to the performer in response to a performance with the intent of reinforcing learning, keeping the student focused on the learning task, informing and motivating the student, facilitating learning, and monitoring the student's responses to a task. Both behavior and content feedback can be auditory, visual, written, an outcome, or feelings.
- *Grouping for activity:* The strategies a teacher uses to group students for activity that consider group size, group structure, and procedures for selecting groups to facilitate student learning.
- *Guided practice:* Takes place when a new task has been introduced (informing task) or when the conditions for task practice have changed substantially (extending task), allowing the teacher to correct major errors in performance, reteach if and when necessary, and prepare students to successfully take part in independent practice.
- *Independent practice:* Provides the learner the opportunity to integrate new content and skills into what they have previously learned, practicing until they become confident while the teacher actively supervises.
- *Informal accountability:* Off-the-record practices teachers use to establish and maintain student responsibility for task involvement and outcomes.
- *Instant activity:* A worthwhile and meaningful activity set up for students as they enter the gymnasium.
- *Instructional adaptations:* These modify a task to make it more or less difficult to accommodate both students who are not challenged enough and students who are struggling with achieving tasks.
- *Teaching skills and strategies:* Aimed at achieving a short-term learning goal; they guide student involvement with content throughout a lesson and are characterized by teacher and student tasks.
- *Learning experiences:* The tasks students do to learn and practice content for cognitive development, social development, and physical development.
- *Lesson closure:* The end-of-class time when teachers bring together the parts of a lesson to make it whole for students, to make sure students understood the important elements learned in the lesson, to re-establish the importance of the lesson elements, and to assess and validate students' feelings relative to the lesson.
- *Managerial skills and strategies:* Those skills and strategies that help the teacher maintain flow in the lesson, provide organizational structure, and ensure students have the opportunity to participate in learning tasks, interacting with the content to promote their learning.
- *Pinpointing:* When the teacher stops the class to emphasize or focus on a point by having the class observe one or two students who are working successfully, asking them to demonstrate for the class.
- *Prompts:* Teacher interventions that guide behavior (in the management system) and performance (in the instructional system) in one direction rather than another.
- *Questioning techniques:* Strategies teachers use to clarify student understanding, assess student learning, prompt discussion, seek student insight and perspectives, and encourage students' considering new ideas and content and its application to their lives.
- *Set induction/establishing set:* When the teacher informs the class of what is planned for the day's lesson.
- *Task presentation:* Explicit verbal communication and effective use of accurate visual demonstrations and modeling to allow students to gain information on what, why, and how to complete a skill or task and gain content about concepts, principles, skills, and tactics that they do not currently possess.
- *Teachable moment:* A moment during teaching when the teacher recognizes that a departure from the lesson focus may have benefits for students.
- *Transitioning:* Moving students from one learning task to another through who, what, where, and when statements.

environment through an effective task management system is critical. In this chapter, we consider the general teaching skills and strategies that are necessary for effective teaching in both the managerial and instructional task systems. Whether you choose to utilize a direct, active-teaching model; a small-group problem-based learning model; cooperative learning; or reciprocal/peer teaching, you still need to effectively communicate instructional tasks and help students learn to organize for effective practice in a safe and challenging instructional climate. These and other instructional functions have to be planned and delivered effectively for any instructional model to achieve its goals.

How and When to Use Managerial Skills and Strategies

When considering **managerial skills and strategies**, we are referring to those skills and strategies that help the teacher maintain flow in the lesson, provide organizational structure, and ensure students have the opportunity to participate in learning tasks, interacting with the content to promote their learning. It is imperative that the teacher plans for these managerial strategies and knows when and how to use them while teaching a lesson. Each of the managerial strategies can be adapted or revised to meet the goals of the lesson and remain consistent with the characteristics of the instructional model chosen.

Behavior and Management Feedback

Feedback in the managerial task system refers to information provided to the student in response to behavior with the intent of reinforcing, correcting, reducing, or improving a particular behavior that is impacting student learning. **Behavior and management feedback** can be auditory, visual, written, an outcome, or feelings and includes prompts, hustles, desists, and praise.

A **prompt** is a teacher intervention that guides behavior in one direction rather than another. Prompts are often brief, typically single cue words, actions, or phrases. When initially teaching a classroom routine, the teacher might prompt the students by saying, "When I say 'go' . . ." or checking with the class on an appropriate response, such as "What are you to do when you hear one loud whistle?" In the latter case, the prompts are gradually faded as students learn and respond to the management routines. In some instances behavior feedback might come in the form of a "hustle," where the teacher encourages the students to respond to a task quickly through the use of phrases such as, "Get into formation quickly," counting down from 5 while reducing the number of fingers held above the head, or "Let's go, let's go."

When students are behaving appropriately, responding efficiently to a task or providing support to peers, the teacher might use *praise* as a means of encouraging the behavior to continue. For instance, "Thanks for listening, red team. That makes it easier to keep things moving" or "I really appreciate you putting the equipment down on the stop signal." Alternatively, when a student is behaving inappropriately, the teacher might *desist* that behavior by saying, "Don't sit on the ball as you watch the demonstration, please, because it changes its shape" in an attempt to stop a specific inappropriate behavior.

Learning Experience 15.1

Observe a physical education class. Tally the number of teacher behavior and management prompts that are used.

Prompts *Hustles* *Desists* *Praise*

Analyze the data and determine whether the environment is positive, characterized by students behaving appropriately, or negative, requiring many teacher behaviors to maintain order. What might you do to change the environment so it is a more pleasant place for teachers and learners?

Instant/Entry Activity

Children and youth come to physical education with the expectation that they will be moving and active. We often hear complaints from teachers that students are so slow coming out of the changing rooms that it is difficult to begin class, yet on the other side of the issue we see young people coming to class only to stand around waiting for class to get started. It is our belief that if you have something worthwhile and meaningful up and running as students enter—an **instant activity**—they will be more likely to get to the gymnasium quickly to start activity. During a Sport Education season, students might know to go directly to their team court for warm-up, strategy development, or another team function. In Outdoor Education, students might be charged with setting up a campsite upon entry to class or working with their camping group to practice leaving a marked trail of the route they have taken on their day hike. Primary teachers might have music playing for the children as they enter the gym, asking them to move like an animal to the rhythm of the song, or perhaps have video of a dance performance running while the music plays in the background. Entry activities need not last an extended period of time, should be easy to learn and set up, and should not involve a lot of teacher direction. They should, however, be enjoyable and serve as a draw to get students into class and ready for the day.

One teacher might have an entry routine that involves the same activity each day that is chosen in conjunction with the students and what they enjoy, or is perhaps built into the curriculum model being employed, as in the Sport Education example. Some teachers might have an entry message posted on the changing room door so students know what to expect and what to do when they come to class; another teacher might make arrangements in the previous class session. Regardless of what type of entry/instant activity you choose and how you communicate it, this procedure is intended to bring students into the classroom ready and excited to begin activity, and often prevents them from being off task while they wait for something to happen. It gives young people the opportunity to let off some steam before they settle into the lesson of the day and provides the teacher time for one-on-one interaction with students as they enter class.

Learning Experience 15.2

Select an age group and a content area, and design an instant activity that might be employed to get the class into the facility and involved in appropriate activity.

Equipment Setup/Dispersal and Return

Having strategies and class routines in place to guide **equipment dispersal**, how to respond if equipment goes into someone's space, and what to do with it when the teacher is speaking or demonstrating are crucial for the smooth running of a physical education class. Imagine a group of 25 students being sent to collect a badminton racket and shuttle cock, all of which are kept in one large storage unit at the edge of the courts. This procedure poses safety issues as students push to get their racket and social problems as some students fight over who has which racket. An alternative strategy might involve having rackets in large buckets at several locations around the gym and assigning equipment managers for each court who are responsible for collecting and returning equipment at the start and end of class. If you don't have buckets, hula hoops can serve as a great storage area for almost any type of equipment during class and can be colored for different teams.

As another example, picture the chaos that might ensue if students, who each have a basketball, are standing listening to you give directions, when one student loses her basketball only to have the girl beside her kick the ball as far across the gym as she can. If students had been taught to put the balls on the ground between their feet on the stop signal and to let loose basketballs go until the person to whom it belongs can get it, problems would be greatly reduced.

Transitioning Students

A physical education class may be a single class (30–45 minutes) or double class (60–85 minutes). The amount of time the teacher has for teaching and the students have for learning by being engaged in the content depends on the teacher's planning and the implementation of those plans. A 60-minute lesson may be designed around a series of up to 10 different learning tasks to allow students to successfully achieve the learning goal. As students are **transitioning** from one learning task to another, the speed with which they move and begin a new task is critical if they are to have the necessary time to be successful. Unfortunately, we often see teachers design exciting and relevant lessons yet fail to plan for the transitions between numerous challenging tasks. This wasted time might reach as high as 2–3 minutes between tasks, resulting in up 20 or 30 minutes of management time in that 60-minute lesson.

We like to think of transitions in terms of who, what, when, and where.

- *Who* are you speaking to (e.g., individual or groups)?
- *What* do you want them to do (e.g., form groups, circles, lines)?
- *When* and how quickly do you want them to move (e.g., on go signal and in a specific time frame)?
- *Where* do you want them to move (e.g., specific places in the gym)?

For example, "When I say 'go,' color teams have 20 seconds to move to their team courts and set up for a core volleyball drill." These types of directions are specific and should result in students knowing what to do, when to do it, and how quickly. Letting them know ahead of time what the purpose of the next activity is might also provide a motivational element to comply quickly; the key is to have the next activity ready to go to prevent them from moving quickly, only to stand and wait for further directions.

Learning Experience 15.3

Design task statements that include who, what, where, and when. Determine how you will transition students in a class of 30 into the following formations:

1. Five groups in circle formations
2. Partners with one ball between the two
3. Teams set up in core drills
4. Six shuttle formations

Checking for Understanding

In the previous example where color teams are transitioned to their team courts, the teacher might first check to see if all the students understand what they are to do. For instance, "Jeff, point out your team court." "Regina, can you describe the core volleyball drill?" "Manuela, how much time do you have to get to your court?" Teacher use of time is critical to student learning and enjoyment in the physical education setting, and **checking for student understanding** prior to moving them is one strategy to assist with this aspect of the lesson.

How and When to Use Teaching Skills and Strategies

In this section we provide an explanation and examples of **teaching skills and strategies** that can be employed within the instructional task system and in conjunction with the various instructional models to encourage, facilitate, promote, and aid student learning. As noted by Metzler (2011), a teaching strategy is planned, is aimed at achieving a short-term learning goal and guiding student involvement with content throughout a lesson, and is characterized by teacher and student tasks.

Instructional Prompts

As noted previously, a *prompt* is a teacher intervention that guides behavior (in the management system) and performance (in the instructional system) in one direction rather than another. In both systems, prompts are brief, typically single cue words, modeling actions or phrases. Think, for example, of the prompts used in teaching a folk dance. Handclapping or a drumbeat can be used to accentuate the underlying beat that cues the various steps in a dance. Teachers also often use verbal prompts to cue the steps, especially during initial practice. Transitions from step to step are often highlighted verbally, yet may include the teacher modeling a step for students to see as a reminder of what comes next in the dance. These verbal prompts or modeling can be viewed by students, even from a distance. Although these prompts are gradually faded as students get more proficient and come under the control of the musical prompts, they do not have to be eliminated completely.

Set Induction

We often see students come to the gymnasium for physical education eagerly asking, "What are we doing today?" **Set induction** or **establishing set** is when the teacher informs the class of what is planned for the day's lesson. Set induction lets young people know not only what to expect during class on a given day but also why the lesson has been designed and its importance or relevance to them. This lesson preview can serve to motivate students to take part and help them make connections to previous learning. Examples might include a YouTube segment of students taking part in street dancing, asking students about the athletics competitions they watched on television during the 2012 Olympics, or having students share their experiences of hill walking or camping. The intent of these types of set inductions is to stimulate student interest in taking part and learning more about a particular component of physical education.

Learning Experience 15.4

Select an age group, a content area, and a lesson focus and design a set induction to draw the students' interest into the lesson. What would it look like?

Grouping for Activity

The physical education classroom is a setting where students often work with a partner, a small group, or even a larger group in a team sport activity. Decisions regarding **grouping for activity**—group size, group structure, and procedures for selecting groups—are critical to teachers' decision making. In responding to these questions, teachers must recognize that students in physical education classrooms represent varying characteristics, from gender, size, attractiveness, and ability to experience, race, social skills, and culture. Brock, Rovegno, and Oliver (2009) prompt teachers to become aware of how these characteristics impact student status and how status influences and impacts students in the physical education setting. Tannehill et al. (2012) point out that status matters in group work; students with lower status have limited social interactions, participate less in learning activities, have reduced playing time, and ultimately, have a less positive experience in physical education.

Group size is an important consideration. For example, for invasion games, teams made up of no more than five members allow for small-sided games that are more appropriate for novice and younger players. In many cases, groups of four or five are appropriate because when groups become larger there is more likelihood that someone will be excluded; in contrast, a group of three may sometimes result in two against one. Students working with a partner provides for "pair share" activities, ensuring that the less vocal are in a safer environment in which to interact.

Numerous strategies can be employed in arranging students for group work. We have selected several that you might find useful.

- *Friendship groups:* There are mixed feelings on whether students should be allowed to select their own partners/groups. Cohen (1994) discourages this practice, suggesting that group work should emphasize work and learning rather than play; young people often think of being with their friends as a time to relax and play. Some teachers believe that allowing young people to select their partners/groups will place those who are less social in the position of never being invited to join a group. Another option is to tell the students initially that they may pick groups, but you reserve the right to change them if problems or off-task behavior arises.

- *Attendance/home base groups:* A grid formation is one means of transitioning students among various activities and learning tasks. It allows the teacher to divide the class into partners, and groups of four (grid set), five (colors or rows), or six (lines). We have had a couple of teachers come to recognize the worth of this strategy, and they have commented that it is received well by students because the teacher is not making the group assignments; rather, the grid determines them.
- *Common personal characteristics:* Students can be assigned to partners and groups using the following personal characteristics:
  - Birth month
  - Astrological sign
  - Alphabetical (first or last name)
  - Name (first vowel in name: a, e, i, o, or u)
  - Height (ranges or similarities)
  - Hair color/length/style
  - Eye color
  - Shoe size
  - Glasses/No glasses
  - Color (shoes, socks, shirt, hoodie)
  - Similar shoe types
  - Number (of siblings, of family members, home address, last digit of phone number)
- *Playing cards:* Distribute a playing card to each student. In this way you can group them by suit (clubs, spades, hearts, diamonds), color (red or black), even (2, 4, 6 . . .) and odd numbers (1, 3, 5 . . .), royalty (jack, queen, king), same numbers (9s or . . .), full house (2 of a kind and 3 of a kind), or divisible by a number. Again, this method is not teacher-determined but "the luck of the deal" and causes fewer complaints.
- *Numbered sticks:* Obtain tongue depressors or popsicle sticks and write numbers on them to correlate to the number of groups and number of students in each group you would like to have. So, if there are to be five groups of four students, there would be five sets of 1s, 2s, 3s, and 4s. Keep these stored by the number of groups and students you want so you do not have to redesign them each time you want to use them.
- *Survey choices:* Have your students fill out a survey at the beginning of the school year where they identify their favorite sports, dances, movements, books, songs, music, or subjects. Once this is submitted and collated you will get to know them better and also have numerous choices on how to make groups.
- *Clock buddies:* Clock buddies allows varying of partners. Start with a clock face with a place for names at each hour on the dial. Put the name of one student on each hour of the clock. Each of the other students has this student's name in the matching hour slot on each of their clock sheets. When the teacher wants to quickly pair up students with a different partner, she or he says, "Get with your 10 o'clock buddy." Students go to the clock, pull out their clock buddy sheet, look at 10 o'clock, and then get with the partner designated. When the strategy is set up, partners always have each other's names on their matching hour on the clock buddy chart.

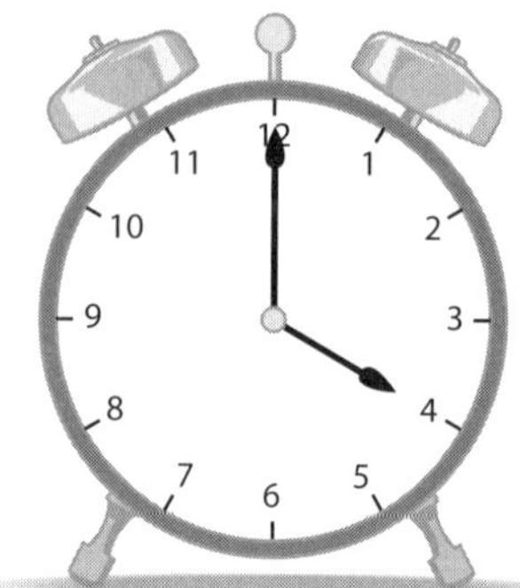

- *Puzzle pieces:* For each group, create a puzzle with the same number of pieces as students to be in that group. Take a picture of the puzzles and laminate them. Cut the puzzle pieces apart, mark the number of students in the group on the back of each piece, and store in a zippered bag. When you want to group your class, select the bag for the size of groups you want, give each student a puzzle piece, and let them find the rest of the people in their puzzle.

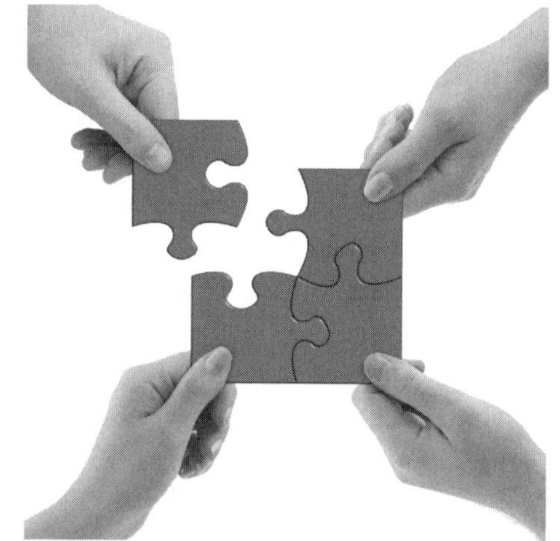

Learning Experience 15.5

Observe a physical education class when a group activity is being employed, noting whose are the dominant voices and what appears to be the experience of the less dominant students. Discuss what you might do differently to allow all voices to be heard.

Checking for Understanding

Checking for understanding within the instructional task system is just as important as in the managerial system. Ensuring that students understand how to progress—either following a demonstration of a skill or practice task, prior to attempting a learning experience that has just been explained, or preceding commencement of a group project—will save time that might be spent repeating yourself to a number of different groups. Frequently, we observe teachers asking, "Do you have any questions?" or "Does everyone understand?" Unfortunately, students may not realize that they don't understand or may be embarrassed to ask a question for fear that others will think them stupid. Checking for student understanding will reduce instructional time and therefore increase activity time, eliminate the need for the teacher to stop activity or practice to re-explain, reduce the likelihood that students will practice incorrectly, increase student knowledge and understanding through repetition (instruction followed by check), and re-emphasize critical points. It is important for teachers to remember that students tend to remember the last thing they see or hear. Numerous strategies have been proposed to check for student understanding (Rauschenbach, 1994).

- *Verbal checks:* Can students verbally describe the task to be performed?
- *Recognition checks:* Can students identify correct technique when observing a performance of the task or skill?
- *Performance checks:* Can students physically reproduce the skill to be practiced?
- *Comprehension checks:* Can students specify a rule or tactic underlying the skill to be performed?
- *Choral responding:* The class verbally shadows or holds up a card in unison (on signal) in response to a question posed about the skill or task.
- *Shadowing:* In unison or in self space, students take the demonstrated stance or slowly go through the motion of the skill.
- *Reiteration:* Students describe (or performs) important parts of a task or skill presentation to a classmate or the entire class to ensure everyone has the same interpretation.

Learning Experience 15.6

Develop a set of questions that might be employed to ensure students understand critical elements of a skill, how to set up for a practice task, or how to undertake a group discussion.

Pinpointing

Pinpointing takes place following demonstration and explanation, checking for understanding, and when students are taking part in the practice task, scrimmage, or activity. The teacher may observe some students struggling to perform a skill or appear to be having trouble interpreting the task once practice has begun. To assist students and to re-emphasize a point, the teacher will stop the class and focus them on one or two students who are working successfully, asking them to demonstrate for the class. "Everyone, look this way and observe how Jeanette releases the disk when it is flat and then follows through to her target; the result is that it flies flat and hits her target." It is important, however, that you know your students and who is not comfortable being on display, and also avoid always using the same student or a highly skilled student to demonstrate. This is a good time to promote those who often struggle but are able to perform the task being performed.

Employing Questioning Techniques

Teachers ask questions. Teachers ask questions frequently. Teachers ask questions to clarify student understanding, to assess student learning, to prompt discussion, to seek student insight and perspectives, and to encourage students to consider new ideas and content and its application to their lives. Questions can be closed (recall of facts or a mere yes or no) or open (to stimulate thoughtful reflexive responses), convergent (lead students to one or two answers) or divergent (lead students to multiple responses). Questions can stimulate understanding or move students toward more in-depth and critical thinking on a topic. It is important to keep in mind that the brain is a muscle, and, if it is to grow and develop, it must be challenged. This suggests posing different kinds of questions to cause students to use all the levels of complexity (from lower-order to higher-order) described by Bloom (1956) in his taxonomy of educational objectives (see **Figure 15.1**).

Zwozdiak-Myers and Capel (2005) suggest that like any effective teaching strategy, a **questioning technique** must be planned. When planning, they encourage teachers to consider the following:

- Why questions are being asked
- What types of questions will be asked
- When questions will be asked
- How questions will be asked
- Who will be asked the question
- How you expect students to respond to the question
- How you will rephrase the question if students do not understand
- How much wait time you will provide for students to respond

How you respond to these questions in your planning and in your delivery of lessons will impact the effectiveness of your questioning to influence student learning and thinking.

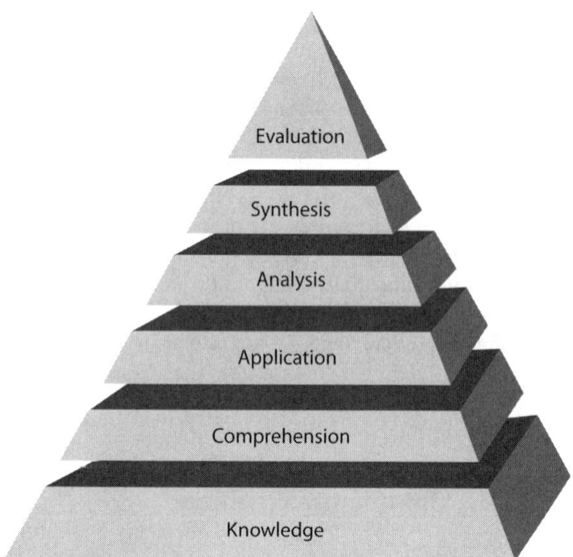

FIGURE 15.1 Bloom's taxonomy of educational objectives.
Adapted with permission of Pearson Education, Inc., from Bloom, B. S. (Ed.). (1956, 1984). *Taxonomy of educational objectives: The classification of educational goals*. New York/Toronto: Longmans, Green, p.18.

Read through the following examples, which are intended to cause you to think about your own questioning style.

1. Reflect on how and to whom you pose questions. Do you call a student's name before asking a question, or do you ask the question and then select a student to respond. Think about how students will react to the two choices. In the first instance, what will many students tend to do if you call one student's name prior to posing the question? Will they continue to listen, beginning to frame their own response, or will they stop listening, relieved that someone else has been asked? If we want to keep all students involved in the critical thinking process, we must leave the question open to all for a response.
2. If the questions we pose are designed to make students think critically and formulate an appropriate response, how long do you wait before seeking a reply, redirecting the question to someone else, sharing your own insights, or rephrasing the question? If you want a thoughtful response, provide adequate *wait time* for students to develop their answers, and remember that follow-up questions can encourage deeper thinking, probe for further insights, and prompt a different perspective.
3. Assuming you provide adequate wait time and a student still does not know the correct answer, how do you react and what do you do? Would the best strategy be to move to another student in the hope of gaining the correct response, ask another student to help the first student in solving the problem, or for you, as the teacher, to assist the first student in coming up with the correct answer? Part of your response will be based on how well you know the students and their reactions to being incorrect, the purpose of your questioning, and what you intend students to gain from the questions. A safe learning environment includes physical, emotional, and cognitive safety; students' thoughts and responses must be valued and treated with care.

Learning Experience 15.7

Either observe a physical education class or ask your cooperating teacher/tutor to observe you teaching a lesson. Write down all the questions that you or the teacher asks during the lesson, indicating who responds to them. Analyze the questions in terms of types of questions asked, how questions were asked, and how students are selected to respond. This will provide you with a glimpse of the questioning approach used and how questions might be used more effectively.

Providing Feedback

Feedback is information provided to performers in response to a performance with the intent of reinforcing learning, keeping students focused on the learning task, informing and motivating the student, facilitating learning, and monitoring students' responses to a task. As with behavior feedback, content feedback can be auditory, visual, written, an outcome, or feelings. Feedback can be intrinsic to the task, where the student is able to gain feedback as a result of the performance (e.g., when the basketball drops through the hoop), or extrinsic to the task, usually in the form of feedback provided by another person with information about the performance, outcome, technique, or effort (e.g., "You followed through to your target well, Marcos"). See **Box 15.2** for explanations and examples of various types of performance feedback that can be used to inform students about their performance.

Despite the plethora of research that has been conducted on feedback in physical education (Rickard, 1991; Silverman & Tyson, 1994; Silverman, Tyson, & Krampitz, 1993), there is no evidence to confirm the relationship between teacher feedback and student learning (Rink, 2009). Regardless, most teacher educators continue to recommend the use of feedback following student skill performance, essentially because it is a form of teacher attention, lets the students know the teacher is observing them, and allows students to gain insight from more than one source (intrinsic and extrinsic and/or verbal and nonverbal). **Box 15.3** provides an overview of tips that will aid the teacher in focusing student performance responses.

BOX 15.2 Subject-Matter Feedback: Types and Examples

- *General positive feedback:* Purpose is to support student effort, motivate, and build a positive learning climate. This general feedback does not give specific information, will not enhance learning, and can become meaningless if overused.
  - Nice shot.
  - Tough defense, Jim.
  - That's better, Jill.
  - Good effort.
  - Yes, terrific, Roberto.
  - Very nice.
  - That's the right idea, Mary.
  - Tremendous pass, Jamal.
  - Squad 1 did really well.
- *Nonverbal positive feedback:* Purpose is to support student effort and build a positive learning climate. It can accompany verbal statements or stand alone. It also can suggest correct or incorrect performance and indicate displeasure or applause.
  - Clapping hands
  - Thumbs-up signal
  - Pat on the back
  - Ruffling hair
  - Raised, clenched fist
  - Smile with nod of the head
- *Positive specific feedback:* Purpose is to provide specific information about what was done appropriately. It is directly related to performance; confirms correct performance, which can be motivational; and provides specific information on what was done correctly.
  - Good pass, Bill, it was exactly the right speed and height.
  - That was creative, Danisha. Your balance was different from everyone else.
  - Beautiful! You really had your knees tucked that time.
  - Everyone did well solving the group challenge and cooperating. Super!
  - Much better. You followed through toward the target that time.
  - Well done, red team. Your timing on the cuts was good.
- *Corrective feedback:* Purpose is to correct errors with specific information. It is directly related to performance and provides guidance on what to change to correct the performance.
  - Denise, you need to keep your position longer before you move.
  - Start from the legs, José; bend the knees deep.
  - You're just shooting with your arms, Brendan.
  - OK, but you did that same stunt last time. Try to find a different one from the same theme.
  - Team Eagles needs to move into the open space; keep control of the ball.
  - Anticipate! Janel, you had an open alley and should have tried a passing shot.
- *Specific feedback with value content:* Purpose is not only to provide information but also to connect performance with outcome. It is directly related to performance and provides *why* a student should do something.
  - Way to help on defense, Pat. When you cover like that, we can take some chances.
  - That's better. When your head is up and eyes focused you can keep your balance more easily.
  - Strong effort, Jamie. When you work hard like that, you will improve very quickly.
  - Thanks, Jessica. When you provide that kind of help, Sonal is going to learn a lot.
- *Feedback sandwich:* Purpose is to provide specific information about what was done appropriately, correct errors with specific information, and end on a positive note. It is directly related to performance, confirms correct performance, provides specific information on how to improve, and is positive, which can be motivational.
  - Your arm platform was flat to receive the ball, now follow through toward the target while continuing to keep your head up.
  - Terrific dance move, but try to keep to the rhythm as you transition to the next step because it is an exciting one.

BOX 15.3 Tips for Giving Feedback

- Give feedback immediately following a performance.
- Correct one error at a time.
- Use a feedback sandwich (corrective feedback couched between two positive).
- Give both individual and group feedback.
- Be specific and congruent in feedback statements.
- Provide feedback across space (with-it-ness).
- Plan feedback by knowing what to look for, critical elements, common errors, and how to correct them (see Box 15.2).
- Use teaching cues as feedback statements.
- Know how to correct errors.

Learning Experience 15.8

Select a content area, choose a skill, and develop a learning experience for students to practice. Design a set of feedback statements to improve student performance. Discuss the type of feedback you have planned.

In many subject areas, student performance provides a permanent record, which allows the teacher to give feedback at a later time. This is not the case in most physical education settings; feedback generally takes place during and immediately after the performance to inform students on how they did. With this in mind, it can be quite useful to the student if the feedback is congruent to the task being practiced. (See **Box 15.4** on correcting student errors.) For instance, if the student is attempting to put the shot while focusing on the "punch" of the arm, and the teacher comments, "Yes, Heath, that punch was sharp and crisp," the feedback was congruent. In contrast, if the teacher suggested, "Heath, you are pulling your head as you release the shot," it would be incongruent.

BOX 15.4 How to Correct Student Errors

Although it seems logical to suggest that teacher feedback should be directed at the main elements of tasks being practiced, it doesn't always happen that way. Occasionally, teachers prompt a student to focus on one element of performance, the student responds successfully, and the teacher corrects another error rather than reacting positively to the successfully performed element. Some have referred to this as the "correction complex" in teaching physical education.

Here are some types of student responses and hints for relating your feedback more appropriately:

- *Student responses that are correct, quick, and firm:* Support positively with brief reactions that do not disturb the momentum of practice.
- *Student responses that are correct but hesitant:* Support positively with brief reactions but add some specific information related to technical elements.
- *Student responses that are "careless" errors:* Briefly correct the error and prompt better concentration or effort.
- *Student responses that show lack of knowledge or skill:* Give *corrective feedback* targeted to specific elements and support for continued effort. Take time to reteach or reassign to component tasks if necessary.

Adapted from Rosenshine, B., & Stevens, R. (1986). Teaching functions. In M. Wittrock (Ed.), *Handbook of research on teaching* (3rd ed., pp. 371–391). New York: Macmillan.

Guided Practice

Guided practice occurs when a new task has been introduced (informing task) or when the conditions for task practice have been changed substantially (extending task). It allows the teacher to correct major errors in performance, reteach if and when necessary, and prepare students to successfully take part in independent practice.

Independent Practice

When students move to **independent practice** they are attempting to integrate new content and skills into what they have previously learned, practicing until they become confident. Students need focused practice if they are to gain the skill and confidence to participate in authentic movement contexts. Teachers must keep in mind that we teach students rather than content, suggesting that our progressions between tasks are dependent on student success and achievement. The teacher role (teacher or student) during independent practice is very different than during guided practice. Typically, students are dispersed for independent practice, using all the space and equipment available. The major instructional function during independent practice is active supervision.

Active Supervision

The major purposes of **active supervision** are to (1) keep students on the assigned task and (2) provide supportive and corrective feedback where necessary. The following are the key features and elements of active supervision, whether mediated by teachers or students: (1) keep all students in sight, (2) scan frequently, (3) move unpredictably, (4) use your voice across space, (5) be aware of and stop disruptive/unsafe behavior immediately, and (6) distribute attention.

Learning Experience 15.9

Observe a class and collect data on teacher movement. At each point the teacher stops, indicate which stop it is (e.g., 1, 2, 3, and so forth) and the reason for the stop. At the conclusion of the lesson, analyze the nature of the active supervision observed.

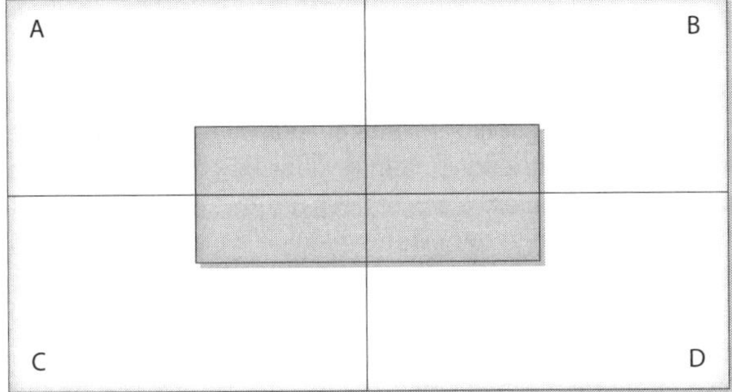

Coding symbols:

I	Position when all are stopped and teacher is giving instruction related to activity.
F	Teacher position when all students are directed to "freeze."
M	Teacher position when giving management/organizational directions.
FB	Teacher position when giving feedback.
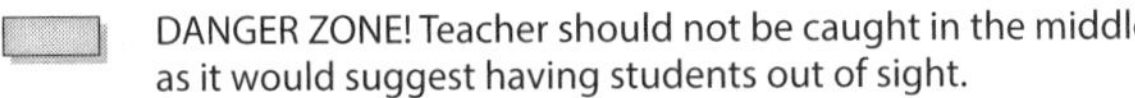	DANGER ZONE! Teacher should not be caught in the middle, as it would suggest having students out of sight.

Task Presentation

Teachers share information and present learning tasks to students frequently throughout any lesson. How this is done varies by lesson intent, curricular model being employed, instructional models selected to support learning, and the role of the learner in the learning process. **Task presentation** involves explicit verbal communication and effective use of accurate visual demonstrations and modeling. Through task presentations, students gain information on what, why, and how to complete a skill or task and gain content about concepts, principles, skills, and tactics that they do not currently possess. With this in mind, communicating tasks to students is perhaps one of the teacher's most important pedagogical skills, requiring selection of relevant content and determining how to share it with students. Whether a verbal explanation or a visual demonstration, several prerequisites should be considered in planning for implementation.

- A cue for gaining learners' attention
- A routine for gathering learners
- A dispersal routine following demonstration
- Equipment set up and ready
- All students paying attention

Verbal Task Presentation

When providing content-focused information to learners, it is most effective to structure the presentation to (1) focus on the content and how to perform a task; (2) limit presentation to one idea at a time, keeping it simple for clarity; (3) recognize that less is more when presenting content—keep it brief and limited to what the learner needs to know to progress; (4) use reminder words or phrases, perhaps a metaphor to aid in visualizing; (5) select appropriate cues to aid observation and feedback; and (6) label activities and learning tasks for students—the name will serve as a prompt for subsequent lessons.

Visual Task Presentation

Visual demonstrations or modeling can be invaluable for students when they are attempting to learn motor skills; they serve several purposes for learning.

- Introduce a skill, strategy, tactic, game, or learning task
- Refine or extend skills/strategies
- Model individual/group feedback
- Emphasize errors or correct procedures
- Introduce creative and cognitive problem-solving tasks
- Emphasize important information about a task
- Provide information on why a skill is performed a certain way
- Improve quality of performance
- Stimulate or motivate students to achieve

Despite the importance of the visual demonstration for learning, we need to acknowledge the limitations of demonstrations for learning. Demonstrations are necessary but not sufficient in and of themselves. More demonstrations are not necessarily better. Spending too much time on demonstration can be counterproductive, and students can only use a limited amount of information at one time.

When planning a visual demonstration the teacher needs to consider who will provide the demonstration, recognizing the importance of the demonstration providing an accurate representation of the skill or tactic. This visual can be provided by the teacher, a student or group of students, a graphic (chart/photo/drawing), moving graphic (video/computer), or floor aids designating movement (poly spots). Demonstrations might be combined with a verbal task presentation, might be shown in slow motion as well as regular speed, or could involve students actively engaged in the demonstration while the teacher explains and demonstrates. Elements of an effective demonstration are presented in **Box 15.5**.

One question we often ask our preservice teachers is: What happens if the teacher demonstrates the skill without demonstrating the task in which the skill will be practiced? The response, of course, is that participants look at each other wondering what to do or they will begin practicing incorrectly. To avoid this situation, we suggest that teachers

BOX 15.5 Elements of Effective Demonstration

- Have all materials ready.
- Perform demonstration where all can see.
- Emphasize safety points.
- Demonstrator is an adequate model.
- Demonstration is directed at students (visually and conceptually).
- Content is accurate and appropriate.
- Language matches learner level.
- Show entire skill first.
- Identify major features performed in sequence.
- Provide what students need to know—keep it simple.
- Show under conditions similar to "real life."
- Show negative and positive instances.
- Link cue words to performance.
- Involve students as demonstration is made.

allow students to walk through the task, thus providing both a verbal and visual view of the task.

Learning Experience 15.10

Design an observation tool focused on visual demonstrations/modeling using the characteristics of effective demonstrations discussed in this section. Ask a peer, your cooperating teacher, or tutor to watch you teach and collect data on your demonstrations. Following the lesson, analyze your data and see what you found. Did you provide demonstrations in line with effective practice? How did students respond to the demonstrations?

Teachable Moment

A **teachable moment** is not planned; rather, it is an opportunity for the teacher to offer an important point, personal insight, or reminder to students. It is a moment during teaching when the teacher recognizes that a departure from the lesson focus may benefit students. Taking advantage of these moments is important because they often have a strong impact on learners; however, caution must be taken to ensure these moments do not evolve into extended discussions; the topic can be revisited at the close of the lesson. For example, during a dance lesson, students might be asked to work in their dance troupe to design an eight-beat hip-hop sequence. The teacher might seize a few moments before moving into this task to seek ideas from the students on the key cooperation behaviors they might use during this activity.

Informal Accountability and Monitoring Student Performance

Instructional task systems are driven by formal and **informal accountability**; in the absence of accountability, the instructional task system can be suspended. What happens to the instructional task system in the total absence of accountability for performance depends on two things: (1) the focus of the managerial system, in which students might have to look like they are making an effort, and (2) the interests and motivations that the students have for the subject being taught.

Accountability refers to all the practices teachers use to establish and maintain student responsibility for task involvement and outcomes. The clearest form of accountability is the grade-exchange opportunity—what we typically refer to as *testing* or *assessment*. Grade exchanges occur infrequently in most physical education classes, often only at the end of a unit. Effective teachers utilize many different kinds of accountability mechanisms to keep students strongly on task and motivate them to improve their performance. Among these accountability mechanisms are the following:

- Public challenges with result reporting, such as "Shoot from the six spots with your partner rebounding," and then "How many made 3? 4? 5? 6?"
- Recording scores, such as keeping records of time on a fitness circuit and recording daily results on a class poster.
- Carefully supervising practice and noting successes publicly, such as monitoring the practice of a volleyball bump-and-set drill and, at the end, noting the several practice groups that did particularly well.
- Actively supervising practice and providing specific feedback and general support, such as monitoring the practice of a gymnastics practice task and providing support for students working hard and technical feedback to students making errors in critical elements of different skills.
- Building accountability into the practice task, such as designing a dribble, pass, trap, and tackle soccer task into a mini-game by providing students a way to keep score.

Learning Experience 15.11

Select an age group, a content area, a lesson focus, and a learning outcome. Design a learning experience that will keep your students on task and motivated to improve their performance.

Lesson Closure

Lesson closure refers to the end-of-class time when teachers bring together the parts of a lesson to make it whole for students, to make sure students understood the important elements learned in the lesson, to re-establish the importance of the lesson elements, and to assess and validate students' feelings relative to the lesson. Many teachers do not plan for or implement closure because they feel it is not important, don't want to waste time with it, or simply run out of time before they get to it. We believe closure is an important ingredient of a lesson and that it should be planned for and implemented carefully.

An effective closure can accomplish many things, although not all of them should be attempted for every class closure.

- *Closure means completion.* Students should be made aware of what was accomplished in the lesson. This can often be done by asking a few pertinent questions, using the answers both to check students' understanding and to underscore their important accomplishments.
- *Closure is an opportunity for recognition.* How did the class as a whole do? Which students did well? Which students provided help to others?
- *Closure is an opportunity to check students' feelings.* Which activity was liked the best? How do students feel about their progress? Use this opportunity to make sure that students feel good about their real accomplishments.
- *Closure can be a review.* What critical elements were learned today? Have a student demonstrate how a cartwheel is done correctly. Students can respond verbally, but they also can *do* the task to show their understanding.
- *Closure can provide a transition from intense activity to locker room or classroom behavior.* Lessons often culminate with an applying task that is often very active and intense. Students then have to go to a locker room to change or return to their class. In either case, closure provides a transition time for students to "cool down" physically and psychologically.

Designing Learning Experiences

A curriculum model is chosen to promote the type of learning you want young people to experience and instructional models are employed to facilitate student learning. In this chapter we have portrayed teaching strategies as general teaching skills used in conjunction with instructional models to assist students in reaching short-term learning goals. So, curriculum models are *the content*, instructional models and teaching strategies are *what teachers do*, and learning experiences are *what students do*. **Learning experiences** can be designed for cognitive development, social development, and physical development. We have selected an assortment of learning experiences across all these categories that might be adapted to different instructional models to meet varying learning outcomes.

Learning Experiences for Social Development

A number of strategies promoted by Adventure Education qualify for facilitating students' social development.

Full-Value Contract

A full-value contract is a learning experience drawn from Adventure Education that asks students to work collectively toward the attainment of group goals and to support each other in meeting individual goals. Key to this experience is students agreeing to work together toward individual and group goals that are revisited at various times during a unit so students can reflect on how they are demonstrating these goals.

Challenge with Choice

Not everyone needs to do everything. Challenge with choice gives individuals a chance to try a difficult or frightening challenge in an atmosphere of support and caring. It is important for students to realize it is OK to back off if self-doubt or pressure is too much, recognizing that the *attempt* is more important than the outcome. In primary physical education, children are often reluctant to hold hands, and you might hear children suggesting that "boys have cooties" and "girls have fleas." To help them, if a task calls for children to be linked, why not give them the choice of holding hands, linking elbows, grasping a sleeve, or gripping a buddy rope (a short rope with a loop at each end for children to put their hands through). In other words, provide them with options that will assist them in moving into more comfortable territory.

Risk Taking

Physical activity experiences often involve an element of risk, not danger. Providing students with experiences where they approach an activity with a challenging level of risk and attempt to conquer it can help students build their confidence. It might help to think of risk as an activity that rests just outside an individual's comfort zone, as shown in **Figure 15.2**. This graphic portrays the risk-taking cycle, in which students move outside their safe and secure *comfort zone* into an area that is unfamiliar and makes them feel a bit unsure. When they are successful in this new *groan zone*, they begin to feel successful and are able to apply new skills to everyday life. Soon, the *growth zone* becomes the *comfort zone*, and they are ready to try a new challenge.

Certainly, many of the learning experiences proposed by Don Hellison (2010) when teaching personal and social responsibility fit the social development category.

Participation by Invitation

Stations with different difficulty levels are set up around the sports hall. Students are invited to begin at a level where they feel most comfortable and will achieve success.

Comfort zone	Groan zone	Growth zone
1. Safe	1. Little familiarity	1. Confidence using new knowledge
2. Known	2. Risky and uncomfortable	2. Integration of skills
3. Familiar	3. Learning and decision making	3. Feelings of mastery
	4. Temptation to withdraw	4. Accomplishment and familiarity
	5. Commit to challenge	
	6. Identify needed learning	

FIGURE 15.2 Risk-taking cycle reflecting the comfort zone, groan zone, and growth zone.

Behavior Modification

These learning experiences are designed around expectations, choices, and the consequences of those choices. Basically, the teacher puts the choice of doing the correct or incorrect thing in the hands of the student using five different strategies.

1. *Accordion principle:* Increasing or reducing the amount of time spent in game play depending on how well the students treat one another.
2. *Self-officiating:* Students are given the responsibility to make the calls in a game.
3. *Five clean days:* A student is given a personal plan at a given behavior level; if behavior stays at that level for 5 days, she or he moves up a level.
4. *Level zero group:* If a student cannot achieve above level 0, he or she has no choices and must stay with the teacher.
5. *Progressive separation from class:* A student is slowly taken away from the group if he or she is not able to reach set expectations that are set individually ahead of time.

Self-Paced Challenges

These learning experiences reflect challenges that permit students to work at their own pace. By encouraging participation through physical activity tasks that have specific goals, it allows the students to work at their own rate to reach the goals. Students can modify their task and challenge themselves appropriately.

Reflection Time

Reflection activities ask students to reflect on their level of respect toward themselves and their classmates and if they were helpful to others and involved in the lesson content. These reflections might be read and discussed with partners, small groups, or the entire class. A reflection might just result in students giving a thumbs-up, thumbs-neutral, or thumbs-down to represent how they viewed their responsibility for the day.

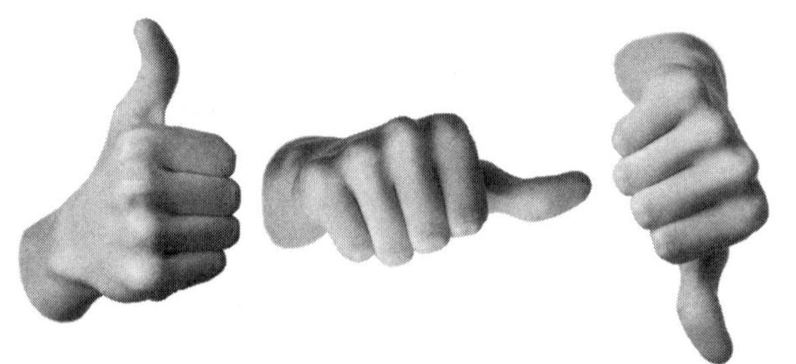

Individual Decision Making

Learning experiences that require individuals to independently negotiate problems, select how they are willing to participate, set their own goals and strategies for achieving them, and determine how much they are willing to give to the class fall into this category.

Goal Setting

Rink (2009) suggests that when students are able to attribute their success to conditions over which they have control, they are generally more active participants in their own learning. Providing students the opportunity to take responsibility for setting goals and striving to achieve them can be done through what has become known as SMART goals (Locke & Latham, 2002). SMART goals are specific, measurable, achievable, relevant, and time-bound.

- *Specific* goals identify exactly what is to be accomplished, why it is important, who it involves, and where it will take place.
- *Measurable* goals have criteria that allow measuring an individual's success toward achievement of the goal.
- *Achievable* goals are realistic and attainable for the individual; the goals are not overly challenging or so low that they are meaningless.

- *Relevant* goals are worthwhile, important, and match what the individual is willing to commit to their achievement.
- *Time-bound* goals are set within a time frame so that the individual knows the target date for their achievement.

Group Meetings

Students work in small groups or with the entire class to share their ideas, opinions, and feelings about class or how to improve the class.

Counseling Time

Students receive one-on-one interaction or counseling time with the teacher, with the intention of assisting an individual student who is struggling, providing support or encouragement, or resolving problems being encountered during class.

Learning Experiences for Psychomotor Development

Specific learning experiences can be designed to assist the student in developing psychomotor skills and movements.

Skill Practice/Drills

Skill practice is designed for students to focus on the technical aspects of a skill and practice it in a controlled setting. Skill practice need not be boring or repetitious; it can be designed in challenging and innovative ways to allow students to focus on a skill and its application to the game, and last a limited amount of time. Often physical education teachers design lessons to reflect a sequence of drill, drill, drill, drill—only at the close of the lesson do students get to participate in a realistic setting. This is not enjoyable for most students. Skill practice should be varied, focused on specific aspects of skill performance and authentic situations, limited in number, and guided by a goal for achievement.

Learning Experience 15.12

Select an age group, a content area, and a learning outcome for an activity of your choice. Design a series of skill practices that might be used within a lesson to challenge students in exciting and meaningful ways.

Stations are designed for small group skill practice. Several stations are set up around the gym and students rotate among the stations, working on the tasks set out at each station. Stations might be guided by task cards, task posters, or demonstrations of what is to be practiced at each station. Students can be directed to make choices of ability level at the various stations and rotate at a given signal or when the task is completed. These types of decisions are made by the teacher depending on the responsibility of the students, the content being practiced, and the design of the lesson.

Modified Games as Learning Tasks

It is possible to utilize small-sided, modified games as learning experiences, that is, to use games rather than skill or tactics drills to provide independent practice for students to improve. Students enjoy games, and their motivation to participate is usually higher in games than in drills. We need to emphasize that, to be useful as learning tasks, games must be sufficiently small-sided to allow for many response opportunities and sufficiently modified that those repetitions can largely be successful. These games are more realistic and allow young people to practice skills, strategies, and tactics in realistic situations.

In a soccer season in a Sport Education unit, for example, teams (usually three for a class of 24 to 27) are introduced to the skills of dribbling, shielding, shooting, and tackling by their team's coach with the help of the teacher. They are also introduced to the tactical concepts of defensive space (stay between your person and the goal) and shooting angles (the goal becomes smaller or larger, depending on the shooting angle). The first competition of the season is a one-versus-one competition played much like half-court basketball. A scrimmage session is held to ensure that students understand the rules and procedures for the game. Play is initiated with a dribble from the back line. As many as eight games can be played simultaneously in an elementary school gymnasium. The games all start and stop at the same signals and are typically of short duration (e.g., 3 minutes). Transitions happen quickly so that the next group of eight games can begin quickly. In a 40-minute period, as many as six or seven groups of eight games can be completed. A round-robin tournament is utilized with points for games won accumulating for each of the three class teams.

The one-versus-one competition is followed by a two-versus-two competition in which the skills of passing and trapping are added and the tactical concepts of tandem defending and offensive spacing are introduced. Again, a scrimmage session is used to ensure that students understand the game and can use the skills and tactics (much like a guided practice session). The round-robin proceeds as in the first competition, with game length extended to 6 minutes (two 3-minute periods to allow for changing defensive position in tandem).

The next competition is three versus three, and throw-ins, corner kicks, and goal kicks are added. Goalie play is also introduced. Most elementary school gyms can accommodate three pitches of sufficient size for the three-versus-three competition. Students experiment with various defensive and offensive combinations, such as two forwards and a defender; one goalie, one defender, and one forward; or two forwards and a defender-goalie.

The season ends with a five-versus-five mini-tournament in which each team competes as a whole. The entire gym space is used, and substitution rules ensure that all players get equal playing time and equal opportunity to play different positions. The amount of time in team practice is kept to a minimum, typically in the first 10 minutes of class, when students enter the gym. Because all players also have to referee and keep score, they tend to learn the rules early and well.

What is important is that you see this approach in the same way you would view a progression of skill tasks that lead up to a five-versus-five soccer game. The series of progressively more complex games provides the independent practice necessary for students to learn the new skills and tactics. Rather than practice each new skill separately in a drill, this approach makes the game a task and gradually adds to the skill and tactical base as the game grows slightly more complex.

Teaching During Games

Many teachers plan to have a culminating event/applying task for each lesson. Units are often planned so that they build to a series of applying tasks toward the end of the unit. Applying tasks can be games, dances, gymnastic performances, and the like. With the approach to planning advocated in this text, the entire unit should be devoted to getting students ready to participate successfully in the applied contexts for which the skills are relevant. However, many teachers design applying tasks, such as games, and then refrain from any teaching while the students are practicing the task.

To consider what teaching functions might be accomplished during applying tasks, first distinguish between the concepts of scrimmage and game. A *scrimmage* is a set of conditions that is very like that of an applied context, such as a game, but in which the teacher stops and starts action to engage in brief teaching episodes and also engages in interactive teaching. A *game* is an applied context in which the stops and starts are determined by the nature of the activity rather than the teacher's judgment. In this general sense, the concepts of scrimmage and game are applicable to activities such as gymnastics and dance. That is, a scrimmage for a dance lesson would be to perform the dance to the musical accompaniment but with brief stops and starts for the teacher to provide instruction; the game would be the dance performed in its entirety without breaks.

Unfortunately, what we described as a scrimmage occurs infrequently in physical education. Most physical education classes move from practice tasks into game conditions without the intervening benefit of scrimmage situations. In contrast, we typically see sport teams using scrimmages frequently. Whether physical education or coaching settings, frequent prompting may be the best teaching function during scrimmages and games. Game play culminating activities, gymnastics routines, and dances are meant to be fun and exciting. Students typically look forward to them, often asking when they enter the gymnasium, "Are we going to play a game today?" There is no reason, however, for teachers to abandon their instructional role during these applying activities. Quite the contrary, these are the activities in which performance needs to be polished and elements put together so that the entire performance is successful, be it a game or a dance. Teachers can prompt behavior and support successful performance without interfering in the activity itself. Likewise, scrimmage tasks can be arranged when game conditions are present, but frequent yet brief teaching episodes can be interspersed to emphasize key points and correct key errors.

Metzler (1990) suggests that teachers need not separate game lessons into isolated skill practice and game play segments; rather, they can combine them using a number of different interaction strategies to help students improve skills and tactical play in more realistic settings. In order to use these strategies Metzler (1990) introduced the idea of the *controlled scrimmage*, where students expect interruptions to occur during game play. These interruptions are intended to assist players in becoming more familiar with game strategies, rules and tactics, and use of skills and to recognize mistakes and violations. In other words, the teacher might focus on any aspect of game play or skill performance and use these teachable moments to help students improve. **Box 15.6** describes seven strategies that can be used by teachers before and during game play.

Performance Video Clips

Video clips can be incorporated into a variety of learning experiences for young people in physical education. In a dance unit, students might be asked to make a daily video clip of their day's progress, which they will review at the start of the next lesson to guide their development of a dance sequence. In gymnastics, students might not feel comfortable performing "live" in front of their peers yet feel quite safe in sharing a video clip of their skill at a concluding event. Using technology is also a way to bring in the media skills of students who might otherwise not be as valued in the physical activity arena.

Learning Experiences for Cognitive Development

As with other types of learning, numerous teaching strategies can be effective in developing students' cognitive knowledge and thinking skills.

Free Write

A free write asks students to reflect on a topic and then respond in writing to a prompt, a quote, or a question. It is a useful tool to encourage students to reflect on their

BOX 15.6 Strategies for Teaching During Game Play

- *Chalk talk* is an interactive approach we typically see coaches using before and during games to remind players of strategies and tactics they should be employing during play. A teacher may use a white board (on a gymnasium wall or handheld) to draw positions or situations or review a play that just transpired. Questioning students on what to do and how to do it increases their involvement and demonstrates understanding.
- *Walkthrough* might be described as a "lived" chalk talk where students are taken through game-related patterns using a slower, quieter, interactive approach prior to game play. This strategy allows students to review and question game patterns before putting them into action in the actual game.
- *Situations* are designed to aid students in understanding, anticipating, and responding appropriately to actual events as they occur during games. During scrimmage play, the teacher uses interactive questions to probe the students (individuals, small groups, teams) on, "What would you do if . . . ?", "How would you respond when . . . ?", "What do you think would occur if . . . ?," and so forth. Follow-up questions will probe more deeply and can seek clarification from students on their initial response.
- *Instant replay* has become popular when watching sports on television because it allows spectators and television viewers to see play repeated several times so they can analyze it or merely watch it again. When using instant replay in teaching, the teacher challenges players to review options they might have for particular plays by stopping the scrimmage, resetting the players, and allowing the play to happen again, encouraging them to consider different options. The instant replay might be considered a form of a teachable moment because it is intended to assist students to learn a new perspective.
- *Player–coach* strategy is used when the teacher wants to clarify, demonstrate, or emphasize a particular skill, game pattern, or movement. The teacher enters the game as a player and proceeds to manipulate play, forcing students to focus on a specific aspect of the game/skill.
- *TV analysts* are knowledgeable about the game and provide insight into many aspects of the game with which the spectator/viewer might be unfamiliar. Rather than share observations with an audience, the teacher can pose interactive questions to the players themselves. This strategy requires the teacher to observe the scrimmage, stop action when she or he sees something occur, share a point of view, and challenge students to determine what happened and how it might be improved. Helping students understand the play and the action is critical to the TV analyst strategy.
- *You make the call* places students in the role of determining game violations, correct signals, and consequences. The teacher takes the role of an official, observes game play, blows the whistle, and then seeks information from the players on why play was stopped and what the consequence of the violation should be.

performance, consider their beliefs and values, and determine how to articulate their findings.

Critical Thinking Challenges

Critical thinking strategies to encourage students to think outside the box can promote creative and innovative thought. Asking students to negotiate, build on their own or others' ideas, compromise, adapt, and evaluate makes them use the higher order thinking skills required to turn obstacles into opportunities and create solutions.

- In *tactical challenges*, students are challenged to determine *what* to do to succeed in a specific situation through questions posed to prompt problem-solving strategies, *why* specific skills are important, and *how* to perform the skills identified correctly.
- In *divergent challenges*, students are challenged to identify a specific solution to a new situation as a result of utilizing problem-solving strategies.
- In *convergent challenges*, students are challenged to approach new material by analyzing and integrating previously learned knowledge through problem-solving and reasoning strategies, resulting in a variety of both correct and incorrect answers.
- In *value challenges*, students are challenged to draw a conclusion based on personal choice, attitude, and beliefs, understanding that their answers will not be judged as correct or incorrect.

Learning Experience 15.13

Select an age group, a content area, and a learning outcome. Design a learning experience for students that would challenge them to think critically using tactical, divergent, or convergent challenges.

Assessing Performance Video Clips

Remember those video clips that students recorded when developing their performance skills? They can be used as a way for students to demonstrate their understanding of a skill, a performance, or the critical aspects of an activity. For example, when they view their daily video clip in dance, they might be encouraged to analyze where they had difficulties and what might be improved and to set goals for the day's practice. When viewing their gymnastics performance, students might use the performance scoring rubric to assess and score their own and a peer's performance, articulating the strengths and weaknesses of what they observed.

Links to the Community

Physical activity and active lifestyles are not linked only to physical education. Written assignments, homework tasks, and group projects are learning experiences that provide students the opportunity to make important connections to the communities in which they live. A group task might see an upper-level class designing and teaching a fitness lesson to a group of elderly citizens at a recreation center or putting on a fun run in the community. Primary students might be asked to select an activity or sport that is a focus within the community and keep a portfolio of the newspaper articles that are written in the local paper on a daily basis. These portfolios might become the data that lead students in a cultural studies lesson and a series of discussions critiquing sport in the community. A variety of learning experiences can be designed as out-of-class tasks to promote the learning taking place and its transfer to life situations.

A number of learning experiences that promote cognitive development are directly linked to the Adventure Education curriculum model and the Cooperative Learning instructional model, including those that require students to process the lesson by recognizing the learning that took place. These learning experiences are referred to as debriefing and include processing around themes, go-arounds, snapshots, and murals.

Processing Around Themes

Questions are focused around a cognitive or behavior theme, asking students to point out when they saw the theme occur during the lesson.

Go-Arounds

This method is used to get a glimpse of how students are feeling after a lesson or for them to respond to any questions that have come up. Student responses might vary from a thumbs-up/down to one-word answers; anyone has the right to not respond.

Snapshots

Every student has an imaginary camera with which they have taken photos of the day. They are each asked to select a photo that portrays something they are proud of, value, or want to remember. Students then describe the picture they have chosen, explaining why it is important to them.

Murals

This is a full class experience that begins with large pieces of art paper covering a wall. Students are invited to either chronicle their learning on a regular basis or on the final day of the unit. Collectively they try to portray the story of their learning through drawing, writing, graphics, or cutting out pictures and words.

Classroom Strategies Adapted to Physical Education

Some teaching strategies that were introduced initially in a classroom setting can be applied and adapted to a physical education setting quite effectively. We have chosen several for which we provide an explanation and example in physical education. Some provide for physical activity; others stimulate different kinds of learning within our content area.

Think–Pair–Share

Students work in cooperative groups to develop their own ideas and build on the ideas of co-learners. Casey and Hastie (2011) propose students design games that are enjoyable and in which everyone can actively participate, following teacher-set parameters. This provides an opportunity for students to engage collectively in a learning task that has social, psychomotor, and cognitive goals.

Debate

Students research a topic and, working in teams, develop their viewpoints, which are then articulated to the class through a debate. A teacher might challenge his or her students to debate the pros and cons of computer games and technology applications, such as the Wii, as appropriate activities for learning in physical education. Students could in this way incorporate physical activity as part of the debate if they choose.

Learning Experience 15.14

Select a number of debate topics that might be used in physical education to assist students in gaining a deeper understanding of the content. Describe how this experience might be incorporated into an entire unit of instruction.

Brainstorming

Students contribute ideas on a topic. The list is then categorized, prioritized, and defended. Brainstorming is one of the strategies used in Adventure Education for students to employ when developing their full-value contract to guide class expectations, and in Sport Education when developing a fair play contract.

Field Experience

Students participate in a planned learning experience to observe, study, and use the community as a laboratory. To assist young people in becoming aware of the types of activities that are available to them in their community, a postprimary teacher might assign students the task of observing physical activity in a community setting of their choice and keeping a journal noting the age group and sex of those who attend, the kinds of activities that seem to draw the most interest and participation, the cost for participation, and how the setting advertises itself to the public.

Predict, Observe, and Explain

The teacher presents the students a situation, and they are then asked to predict what will happen when a change is made. A teacher might employ this strategy to motivate young people to take part in a fitness program designed to increase their physical activity behaviors. They would be asked to predict whether their physical activity behaviors would change as a result of such a program, rationalizing their conclusions. Following this, students would take part in the program, evaluating their prediction.

Jigsaw

Students work in cooperative groups in which everyone becomes an "expert" and shares his or her learning so that eventually all group members know the content. In a hill walking lesson, for example, small groups of students would become experts in one of four areas: (1) using the compass, (2) aligning the compass with a map, (3) leaving no trace, and (4) marking your trail. Once they become experts, the students regroup so that each group has one expert from each category. They then teach each other their skill and go out on a hill walk under the teacher's supervision.

Know, Want to Know, Learned (K-W-L)

Students can use this as an introductory strategy that provides a structure for recalling what students already know about a topic, specifying what they want to know or learn, and finally summarizing what has been learned and what they have yet to learn. Students may be involved in an invasion games unit and are attempting to understand the similarities and differences between all invasion games from skill to game tactics and from on-the-ball skills to off-the-ball movements. This strategy might be employed in conjunction with a Tactical Games approach employed by the teacher. They would discuss, explore, and experience a variety of invasion games while developing their response to the K-W-L.

Learning Log

Students can use this as a follow-up to K-W-L. At different stages of the learning process students respond in written form under the following three columns:

What I think
What I learned
How my thinking has changed

When combined with the K-W-L task, students would come to recognize what they know about invasion games and how to transfer that knowledge to a new game they have yet to play.

Instructional Adaptations

Once learning experiences have been designed to meet the learning outcomes of a lesson, **instructional adaptations** can be used to make tasks more or less difficult to accommodate students who are not challenged enough as well as those students who are struggling with achieving tasks. Block (1994) provides an overview of guidelines for designing appropriate adaptations to meet the needs of all learners (see **Table 15.1**).

CHAPTER SUMMARY

This chapter has focused on the general teaching strategies a teacher employs in the managerial and instructional task systems. Our intention was to assist you in understanding the relationship between learning tasks and teaching strategies, and how teaching strategies can be employed with various instructional models and within several curriculum model frameworks.

1. Teachers matter. Who teachers are and what they do in class affect how much students learn, how they feel about the subject, and how they feel about themselves as learners.
2. Teachers whose students are motivated to participate and use class time well demonstrate effective use of general teaching skills and strategies in the managerial task system.
3. Effective teachers plan for and employ strategies that help maintain flow in the lesson, provide organizational structure, and ensure students have the opportunity to participate in learning tasks, interacting with the content to promote their learning.
4. Teachers who demonstrate effective use of general teaching skills and strategies in the instructional task system are more likely to have students who learn and enjoy that learning.
5. Effective teachers are skilled at using teaching skills and strategies to encourage, facilitate, promote, and aid student learning.
6. Skilled teachers plan for and deliver feedback to students on both their behavior and their skill performance in an attempt to help them take responsibility for their own learning and development.

TABLE 15.1 Adaptions to Meet the Needs of Learners

Variables That Impact the Complexity of a Task or Skill	
• Weight and size of ball • Level of dribble • Direction of ball • Dominant or nondominant hand • Stationary or moving player • Relationship to another player • Directional or nondirectional goal • Direction of locomotion • Speed of movement • Distance of implement from body • Number of people active in one space • Combinations of other skills • Traveling rules	
Exploratory Activities with Kicking as an Example	
1. Effort Awareness	*Force: can you kick . . .* • As soft as you can? • As hard as you can? • So that the ball makes a loud noise when it hits the wall? • Alternating hard and soft kicks? • Stepping forward with a loud noise? *Time: can you kick . . .* • As slowly as you can? • As fast as you can? • By moving your kicking leg as fast as you can? • And twist your body (hips) as fast as possible? *Flow: can you kick . . .* • Using as little movement as possible? • Using as much of your body as possible? • Like a robot? • Like a plastic person? • Without using your trunk? • Using only one other part of your body besides your kicking leg? • As smoothly as you can?
2. Space Awareness	*Level: can you kick . . .* • Up high? • Down low? • As low as you can? • At the wall as high as you can? • At high-, low-, and medium-height targets? • Alternating high and low kicks?

TABLE 15.1 Adaptions to Meet the Needs of Learners (*Continued*)

Exploratory Activities with Kicking as an Example	
	Direction: can you kick . . . • Forward? • Backward? • To the side? • At an angle? *Range: can you kick . . .* • As far as you can? • As near as you can? • With your right leg? • With your left leg? • With both feet? • To the side? • With your leg going through short and long ranges of motion? *Objects: can you kick . . .* • A hard ball? • A fluffy ball? • A small ball? • A large ball? • A football? • A newspaper ball? • A playground ball? • At a target? • Into a bucket? • Over a rope? • From inside a hoop or inner tube?
3. Relationship Awareness	*People: can you kick . . .* • To a partner? • As far as your partner? • As hard or soft as your partner? • The same way as your partner? *Combinations* • Initial experiences should focus on exploring the various aspects of effort, space, and relationships in isolation before you structure experiences involving combinations. For example, "Can you and your partner find three different ways to kick at the target from a far distance?"

Modified from Block, M. E. (2006). *A teacher's guide to including students with disabilities in general physical education.* Baltimore, MD: Paul H. Brookes.

7. Effective teachers develop questioning skills that allow them to probe and query students in an effort to assist them in becoming thoughtful, critical, and innovative thinkers.
8. Teachers who facilitate and encourage student learning demonstrate active supervision skills.
9. Communicating learning tasks to students is one of the teacher's most important pedagogical skills, requiring selection of relevant content and determining how to share it with students; sometimes this skill requires involving students in the decisions on what to teach and how to teach it.
10. If students are to learn, the teacher must hold them accountable for learning, for behavior, and for taking responsibility for their own learning.
11. In-depth and coherent learning in all domains requires well-designed and coherent learning experiences that allow students to interact with content in appropriate and meaningful ways.
12. Effective teachers plan for and implement instruction that provides learning experiences that are adapted for the needs and interests of all students regardless of ability, interest, or special needs.

REFERENCES

Block, M. E. (1994). *A teacher's guide to including students with disabilities in regular physical education.* Baltimore, MD: Paul H. Brookes.

Bloom, B. S. (1956). *Taxonomy of educational objectives, handbook I: The cognitive domain.* New York: David McKay Co., Inc.

Brock, S. J., Rovegno, I., & Oliver, K. L. (2009). The influence of student status on student interactions and experiences during a sport education unit. *Physical Education and Sport Pedagogy, 14*(4), 355–375.

Casey, A., & Hastie, P. A. (2011). Students and teacher responses to a unit of student-designed games. *Physical Education and Sport Pedagogy, 16*(3), 295–312.

Cohen, E. (1994). Restructuring the classroom: Conditions for productive small groups. *Review of Educational Research, 64*(1), 1–35.

Hargraves, A., & Fullan, M. (2012). *Professional capital: Transforming teaching in every school.* New York: Teachers College Press.

Hellison, D. (2010). *Teaching personal and social responsibility through physical activity* (3rd ed.). Champaign, IL: Human Kinetics.

Locke, E. A., & Latham, G. P. (2002). Building a practically useful theory of goal setting and task motivation. *American Psychologist, 57*(9), 705–717.

Metzler, M. (1990). Teaching during competitive games: Not just playin' around. *Journal of Physical Education, Recreation and Dance, 61*(8), 57–61.

Metzler, M. W. (2011). *Instructional models for physical education* (3rd ed.). Scottsdale, AZ: Holcomb Hathaway.

Organisation for Economic Co-operation and Development (OECD). (2006). OECD work on education 2005–2006. Paris: OECD. Available from www.oecd.org.

O'Sullivan, M. (2007). Teachers matter: A framework for professional development in physical education. In P. Heikinaro-Johansson, R. Telema, & E. McEvoy (Eds.), *The role of physical education in promoting physical activity and health* (pp. 45–59). Jyvaskyla, Finland: University of Jyvaskyla.

Rauschenbach, J. (1994). Checking for student understanding: Four techniques. *Journal of Physical Education, Recreation and Dance, 65*(4), 60–63.

Rickard, L. (1991). The short-term relationship of teacher feedback and student practice. *Journal of Teaching in Physical Education, 10*(4), 275–285.

Rink, J. (2009). *Teaching physical education for learning* (6th ed.). New York: McGraw-Hill.

Rosenshine, B., & Stevens, R. (1986). Teaching functions. In M. Wittrock (Ed.), *Handbook of research on teaching* (3rd ed., pp. 371–391). New York: Macmillan.

Silverman, S., & Tyson, L. (1994). Modeling the teaching and learning process in physical education. Paper presented at the annual meeting of the American Educational Research Association (AERA), New Orleans, LA.

Silverman, S., Tyson, L., & Krampitz, J. (1993). Teacher feedback and achievement in physical education: Interaction with student practice. *Teaching and Teacher Education, 8*(3), 333–344.

Tannehill, D., MacPhail. A., Halbert, G., & Murphy, F. (2012). *Applying research to practice.* Oxfordshire, UK: Routledge.

Zwozdiak-Myers, P., & Capel, S. (2005). Communicating with pupils. In S. Capel, M. Leask, & T. Turner (Eds.), *Learning to teach in the secondary school* (5th ed., pp. 105–119). Oxfordshire, UK: Routledge.

CHAPTER 16 Planning to Promote Student Learning

Overall Chapter Outcome

To design a unit plan and accompanying lesson plans to guide delivery of school physical education

Learning Outcomes

The learner will:

- Discuss reasons why teachers plan
- Distinguish between plan-dependent and plan-independent teachers
- Discuss factors to consider when planning
- Outline a well-constructed unit plan
- Encourage the practice of instructional alignment and backward design in planning unit and lesson plans
- Consider a meaningful and realistic goal for students to work towards successfully completing at the end of the unit (big picture goal)
- Provide a matching and worthwhile big picture assessment to determine the extent to which students have successfully achieved the big picture goal
- Explain the purpose of a content analysis (including conducting appropriate procedural, hierarchical, and tactical analyses) and illustrate the construction of a concept map informed by the completed content analysis
- Design learning outcomes that match the big picture goal and big picture assessment
- Consider formative assessments that provide continuous ongoing information and feedback about progress toward learning outcomes
- Consider learning experiences, instructional models, and teaching strategies for learning outcomes and the extent to which learning experiences can also act as formative assessments
- Complete a considered unit plan
- Outline a well-constructed lesson plan that addresses contextual description, timeline, content, organization and management, teaching cues and prompts, and content adaptations
- Complete a considered lesson plan

This chapter focuses on designing unit and lesson plans. The focus of this chapter was chosen for three reasons. First, many teachers consider planning for student learning to be their most important planning task. Many teachers work on a daily basis from their unit plan, rather than having individual daily lesson plans. Second, teachers who prefer to plan at the daily lesson level typically do so by planning all the daily lessons based on the unit plan. Thus, the unit again appears to be the most functional way to think about planning. Third, focusing on unit plans requires that you think about progressions that build across daily lessons and move toward the achievement of unit objectives. Even though a unit is taught

BOX 16.1 Key Terms in This Chapter

- *Backward design:* A method where curriculum design begins with the exit outcomes and proceeds backward to the entry point to ensure that all components are directly related to achieving the outcome.
- *Curriculum plan:* An overall view of all a teacher intends students to experience over a number of years (as part of their physical education experience).
- *Instructional alignment:* When there is a match/consistency among learning outcomes, assessments that determine if students reach those outcomes, and the instructional practices that provide students the opportunity to achieve success.
- *Lesson plan:* Related to the unit plan, this determines what will be taught and how a teacher plans to deliver instruction and practice in a lesson.
- *Plan-dependent teacher:* One who invests a significant amount of time in planning effective units and associated lesson plans.
- *Plan-independent teacher:* One who works from mental recall of previous planning and experience with the activity being taught.
- *Unit (unit of instruction) plan:* Related to the curriculum plan, this specifies what a teacher plans for a content area to achieve the learning goals, assessments, and instruction in an aligned way over a number of weeks.

to students through the daily lesson, it is the series of daily lessons (the unit) that should make sense as a whole.

Why Teachers Plan

Teachers devote time and attention to planning for instruction for a number of reasons (Stroot & Morton, 1989):

- To ensure that a progression is followed both within and between lessons
- To help the teacher stay on task and use time as planned
- To reduce teacher anxiety and help him or her maintain confidence while teaching

In addition to these teacher-focused reasons, it is important to acknowledge that student-focused reasons for teacher planning include ensuring all students have an opportunity to learn and achieve success.

Not all teachers plan for all these reasons, nor do all these reasons influence teachers in the same way. In addition, some school principals encourage teachers to leave their unit plans and block plans in a central space in the school in the event that, owing to illness or some unforeseen emergency, a substitute teacher may be required to teach the class in the short term.

Dependence on Planning

In their study of effective primary physical educators, Stroot and Morton (1989) found what many continually note from observing teachers work. That is, some teachers are very dependent on plans whereas others seem to be nearly independent of plans. They referred to these two extremes as **plan-dependent** and **plan-independent teachers**, respectively. For example, one teacher in their study said, "I would feel incredibly uncomfortable if I did not have them [plans], and I carry them around on my clipboard everywhere I go" (Stroot & Morton, 1989, p. 219). Another teacher taped the daily plan on a wall of the gymnasium where it could be referred to easily if needed, even though observation indicated that the teacher seldom referred to it. Still other teachers go through an entire day's teaching without referring to plans, needing only to glance at them in the morning to remind them about what they intend to do in their classes that day. The difference between plan-dependent and plan-independent teachers seems to be one of personal comfort, reduction of anxiety about lessons, and maintaining confidence as the teaching is actually done. Remember, in this study, these were all effective teachers, so there is no suggestion here that plan-dependent teachers are more or less effective than plan-independent teachers. It seems a matter of personal style, although less-experienced teachers typically tend to be more plan-dependent. We often have heard our preservice teachers comment that they feel more equipped to adapt a lesson if they have planned the lesson thoroughly. The plan-independent teachers do their work from mental recall of their previous planning and experience with the activity being taught.

The same study found, as have most others, that somewhere back in time all the effective teachers had worked hard to plan good units of instruction. The work they did when they initially planned units of instruction is similar to what will be presented in this chapter. Thus, no matter whether the teachers were, at the moment of the study, plan-dependent or plan-independent, they had all gone through extensive planning when initially developing units and they frequently upgraded and modified those initial plans based on their experiences teaching them. If the teachers perceived themselves to be in an activity unit in which their own background was weak, they tended to become more plan-dependent than in those units where their own skills and experiences were stronger.

Considerations When Planning

The problem of planning physical education units, especially when students are grouped by school year level, is that some students will be limited in what they are able to do whereas others will have the physical capacity, skills, and experience for higher-level instruction. Most teachers tend to plan their units at, or just below, what they consider to be the average for their classes. They then attempt to adjust the instructional task system so that it accommodates students who vary markedly in their readiness for those tasks.

Effective programs accomplish real goals, so it makes sense to plan units so that ample time is provided for limited outcome accomplishment. Teachers need to narrow their focus on what goods of physical education they wish to promote and pursue throughout a unit. Many students will need a large number of successful repetitions to develop skills to the point where they can be used in applied settings. Repetitions of skill and strategy practice take class time, often more than planners are willing to allocate. It is through repeated cycles of refining and extending tasks that skill develops and the execution of strategy becomes reliable. This refining–extending cycle takes time, especially if all students are to get enough repetitions to be able to perform the skills and strategies in applied settings.

Levels of Planning

Most physical education teachers will be involved in a number of different levels of planning, sometimes referred to as long-term (curriculum planning), medium-term (unit plan), and short-term (lesson plan). Curriculum planning is when a teacher plans for what they intend students to experience over a number of school years (e.g., primary, postprimary) as part of their physical education experience and acts as a framework to determine the units to be taught. A **unit plan**, which is related to the **curriculum plan**, is what a teacher plans for a content area to achieve the learning outcomes, assessments, and instruction in an aligned way over a number of weeks. A **lesson plan**, which is related to the unit plan, is what and how a teacher plans to deliver instruction and practice in a lesson. Well-planned and organized units and associated lessons have a greater chance of leading to student achievement of the intended learning. This chapter focuses on the unit and lesson level of planning, both of which should be viewed as documents to guide your content and teaching, allowing flexibility to adapt each as you progress in your daily and weekly teaching of the associated content, in line with student needs and progress. As Metzler (2011) comments,

> *Planning serves to facilitate the transfer of content knowledge and general pedagogical knowledge into pedagogical content knowledge (Shulman, 1987)—the ability to teach effectively a specified content to a certain group of learners.*[1]

Metzler also comments that having planned does not always mean a teacher is actually prepared and properly organized for effective instruction, pointing out that you can plan but not be prepared, but if you are prepared, you have planned well enough.

Learning Experience 16.1

Contact a practicing physical education teacher and collect evidence of the sources they identify as informing and guiding their planning of physical education in their school, such as a national syllabus, the school management, facilities and equipment, the areas of expertise of the physical education teacher(s), and/or the student population. At what level of planning do such sources arise (i.e., curriculum, unit, and/or lesson plan)?

Considering a Unit Plan

This chapter provides the reader with a proposed outline for a unit plan (see **Box 16.2**) before unpacking each element. There is no best way to actually write a unit plan. Eventually, teachers adopt formats that prove to be most useful for them in their daily teaching. Remember, it is the class lesson that gets taught to students. The unit plan, therefore, should be constructed using a format that provides the necessary guidance at the lesson level. The unit plan shared in this chapter focuses on providing an example appropriate for any curriculum model. Once the complete unit plan has been shared, we will engage with planning and designing lesson plans. Before this, it is imperative that the reader understands two concepts, backward design and instructional alignment, that guide the design and planning of the unit. **Backward design** encourages us to consider (1) What do we want students to know and be able to do as a result of participating in our programs? (i.e., curricular goals); (2) How will we know when they have been successful? (i.e., assessment); and (3) How

[1] Reproduced from Metzler, M. W. (2011). *Instructional models for physical education* (3rd ed., p. 131). Arizona: Holcomb Hathaway.

BOX 16.2 Outline for a Unit Plan

- Contextual description
- Big picture goal
- Big picture assessment
- Concept map
- Learning outcomes
- Formative assessments
- Instruction: instructional model, learning experiences, teaching strategies, instructional adaptations
- Resources
- Structure of self-appraisal
- Preventive management
- Block plan

can we get them there in the most challenging and engaging ways possible? (i.e., instruction) (Lund & Tannehill, 2010; Wiggins & McTighe, 1998). **Instructional alignment** is evident in a meaningful and coherent physical education program when there is an alignment among (1) learning goals, (2) assessments that determine if students reach those goals, and (3) the instructional practices that provide students the opportunity to achieve success (Cohen, 1987; Lund & Tannehill, 2010).

Designing a Unit Plan

This section will work through the elements of a unit plan proposed in Box 16.2. To enhance the reader's understanding of how one element informs the next, and to demonstrate the effectiveness of instructional alignment, we have chosen to work through a specific unit plan based on the Outdoor Education curriculum model. The unit plan can be physically pieced together by the reader extracting, in turn, all the boxes titled as *Unit Plan* (i.e., contextual description, big picture goal, big picture assessment). In instances where some of the concepts related to an element require further unpacking, we provide additional examples outside of the Outdoor Education unit plan. This chapter strongly encourages the reader to complete each Unit Plan step in sequence, resulting in the reader developing and completing, in the first instance, a unit plan, and then a lesson plan by the end of the chapter.

Needs Assessment and Contextual Description

When beginning to plan a unit, the teacher (and students) should identify factors to be considered, from available equipment and the range of student ability, to prior learning, to understanding students' interest in the content and its relevance to them (i.e., a needs assessment). Once this is considered, it is imperative to provide demographics of the context in which the proposed unit plan is to be delivered.

UNIT PLAN 16.1 Contextual Description to Be Established Before Planning a Unit

Specific topic/area of study: Outdoor Education
Name of the class: 3A (third year postprimary)
Number of students: 23
Number of lessons: 6
Length of lessons: 80 minutes
Rationale for the topic: This is the first time the class has undertaken Outdoor Education and provides an opportunity to build on skills students previously experienced in their first year of postprimary when they undertook a 6-week unit in Adventure Education. The focus of the Adventure Education unit was on team building, communication, cooperation, and trust, focusing mainly on low-level initiatives.

Unit Plan: Step 1

Select a specific topic/area of study, identify a group of students you are likely to teach in the near future, and complete a contextual description similar to that provided here, identifying the specific topic and the rationale for the topic you intend to introduce to the group along with number of students, number of lessons, and length of lessons.

Such information includes the specific topic/area of study (e.g., athletics, dance) to be covered throughout the unit, the name and year of the class, the number of students in the class, the number of lessons, the length of lessons, and the rationale for the topic. An example of such demographic information is provided in **Unit Plan 16.1**.

Big Picture Goal

Designing a big picture goal entails considering a goal for a unit of instruction students will work towards successfully completing by the end of the unit. That is, what do you want the students to learn/achieve? The choice of a big picture goal is important because it forms the basis of unit planning. Therefore, the big picture goal should be defined with the entry-level status of learners clearly in mind and with a realistic appraisal of what can be accomplished in the time available. Depending upon your program, your view of student learning, and students' role in determining what is meaningful for them to learn, you may in some cases involve students in designing the big picture goal.

A big picture goal is

- Developmentally appropriate
- Something worth achieving

BOX 16.3 Innovative Ideas That Reflect a True Big Picture Goal

- *Big picture goal for gymnastics:* Students will safely demonstrate an ability to select, create, and perform a short gymnastic sequence.
- *Big picture goal for gymnastics:* Students will demonstrate key gymnastic skills through a group performance that is directed by assigned student roles and responsibilities.
- *Big picture goal for health-related activity:* Students will demonstrate an understanding of health-related activity through a variety of unique and challenging sports and activities.
- *Big picture goal for health-related activity:* Students will demonstrate their understanding of why it is important to develop and maintain adequate levels of physical activity and fitness by participating in health-related activity lessons and creating a subsequent health-related activity lesson focused on the effects of exercise on the body.

- Realistic
- Achievable
- Relevant to daily life
- Meaningful to young people
- Exciting and challenging

A big picture goal should also allow for exploration and opportunities to make sense of experiences. Samples of big picture goals that we have seen designed for student learning are shared in **Box 16.3**. The big picture goal chosen for the exemplar unit of instruction in this chapter and related to the demographics provided in Unit Plan 16.1 is noted in **Unit Plan 16.2**.

UNIT PLAN 16.2 Big Picture Goal

For students to work cooperatively to successfully complete an overnight trip at an outdoor center and participate in a day hike and orienteering.

Unit Plan: Step 2

Revisiting the specific topic and rationale for the topic noted in Unit Plan Step 1, consider an appropriate big picture goal that the students will work towards successfully completing by the end of the unit.

UNIT PLAN 16.3 Big Picture Assessment

Students will cooperatively and successfully complete an overnight trip at an outdoor center and participate successfully in a day hike and orienteering event.

Unit Plan: Step 3

Revisiting the big picture goal identified in Unit Plan Step 2, identify a matching and worthwhile big picture assessment that will provide evidence on the extent to which students have successfully achieved the big picture goal. Design a scoring tool to accompany this big picture assessment.

Big Picture Assessment

Frequently, we see teachers who are not sure where they are going with student learning and so teach the wrong thing or misalign what they teach, what students practice, and what they assess as having been taught (Cohen, 1987). In order to provide evidence on the extent to which students have successfully achieved the big picture goal, a matching and worthwhile big picture assessment needs to be determined. In other words, the assessment should not be a surprise or intended to take the students off guard but an opportunity for them to demonstrate success at achieving the big picture goal. The big picture assessment chosen for the exemplar unit of instruction, and related to the demographics and big picture goal provided in Unit Plans 16.1 and 16.2, respectively, is noted in **Unit Plan 16.3**.

Content Analysis and the Concept Map

Returning to our exemplar unit plan for Outdoor Education, once a big picture goal and associated big picture assessment have been determined, the next step is to consider what students need to learn to achieve the big picture goal. That is, what are the possible areas of content that students should be taught to prepare them adequately to achieve the big picture goal? Building on the big picture goal and assessment noted in Unit Plans 16.2 and 16.3, respectively, there are a number of content areas that could be considered as appropriately contributing to students being able to work towards successful completion of the big picture goal. These content areas are illustrated in **Unit Plan 16.4**.

Content analysis is a technique to determine all aspects of content that must be taught and learned (i.e., physical, tactical, social, and cognitive) if students are to reach the big picture goal (outcome). In other words, what is the specific content students are expected to perform to demonstrate successful achievement of the intended learning. Each of these components will also be further analyzed and broken

UNIT PLAN 16.4 Possible Content Areas Related to the Big Picture Goal

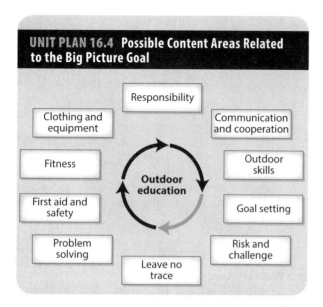

BOX 16.4 Content Analysis in Sport Education: High Jump

Goal: Using the flop technique, students will achieve a height commensurate with their height and weight during a class track meet.

Assessment: During a class track meet students will compete in a high jump competition, competing in ability flights.

At this point, the teacher needs to ask the task analysis (TA) question: "What does the learner have to do to perform this task?" The answer will come from the content analysis the teacher carries out, the start of which is identified in the following list of components to be learned:

- Physical
- Tactical
- Social
- Cognitive
- Technical skill performance
- Height to start
- Team player
- Rules of flop technique
- Height to pass
- Fair play
- Etiquette
- Ritual

Once this outline of components to be learned is determined, each can be further analyzed and broken down as the pre-requisite skills/knowledge the student should possess prior to entry into unit/season. This process is achieved by continuing to ask the TA question for each component.

down to allow the development of instructional sequences and the design of learning experiences. **Box 16.4** provides an example using a track and field event (high jump) in a Sport Education season.

Procedural and Hierarchical Analyses

Two kinds of content analysis are used in planning, the *procedural analysis* and the *hierarchical analysis.* A procedural analysis describes a chain of events that together define a meaningful unit of performance. Activities such as bowling, cascade juggling, vaulting in gymnastics, running a three-lane fast break in basketball, and the long jump in track and field are typical of those skills for which a procedural task analysis is useful. Procedural analyses of the long jump and fast break are shown in **Figure 16.1** and **Figure 16.2**, respectively.

For skills in which a procedural task analysis is useful, the individual elements of the chain (the foot plant, the take-off, and so on) can be learned somewhat independently and then put together to form the chain. Usually, the individual elements of the chain are fairly easy to learn. The putting together represents the crucial aspect of the instruction. The final outcome requires that each element of the chain be performed smoothly and in an integrated fashion. A breakdown at any element tends to ruin the entire performance.

A procedural task analysis is useful for identifying the points at which instruction should be focused, both in identifying the elements of the chain and in pinpointing the crucial spots at which the elements have to be linked smoothly for a skilled performance. The long jump represents a short, fairly simple chain, whereas rebounding and initiating a fast break in basketball represent a considerably more complex set of elements. A procedural task analysis of a fast break is shown in Figure 16.2. Notice how the analysis allows the designer or planner to identify the important learning tasks (the elements of the chain) and *also* the points at which they need to be put together smoothly for a skilled performance.

Hierarchical analysis is a description of all the subskills that must be learned to perform the terminal skill. In a hierarchical analysis, there is a necessary relationship among the skills. One skill must be learned before the other can be learned (unlike in the procedural analysis, in which elements can be learned independently). In a hierarchical analysis, the planner starts with the instructional goal and asks the task analysis question: What will the students have to be able to do in order to accomplish this task? This question is asked again and again until the basic entry skills for the task are learned. A hierarchical analysis is shown in **Figure 16.3**.

The hierarchical analysis identifies only those skills necessary for accomplishing the higher-level skill. With practice, designers and planners become able to identify subskills and adjust the size of the subskill steps to best suit learners' needs. The size of steps from one subskill to another is

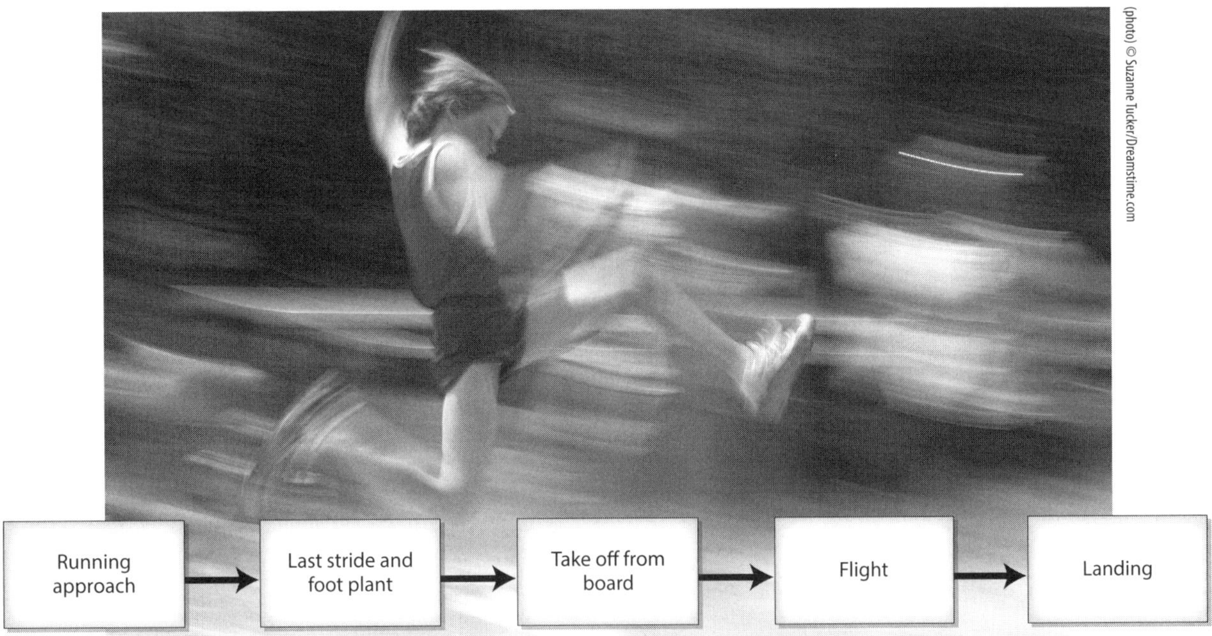
Goal: Long jump with proper approach, takeoff, and landing.
(photo) © Suzanne Tucker/Dreamstime.com
Running approach
Last stride and foot plant
Take off from board
Flight
Landing

FIGURE 16.1 Long jump procedural analysis.

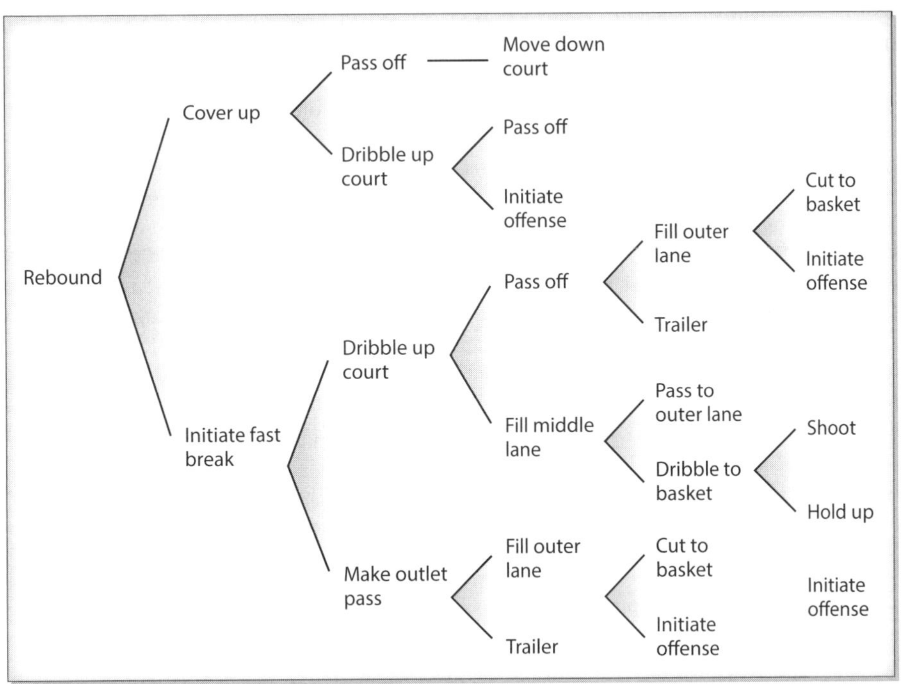

FIGURE 16.2 Some possible fast-break chains of events for a basketball player rebounding.

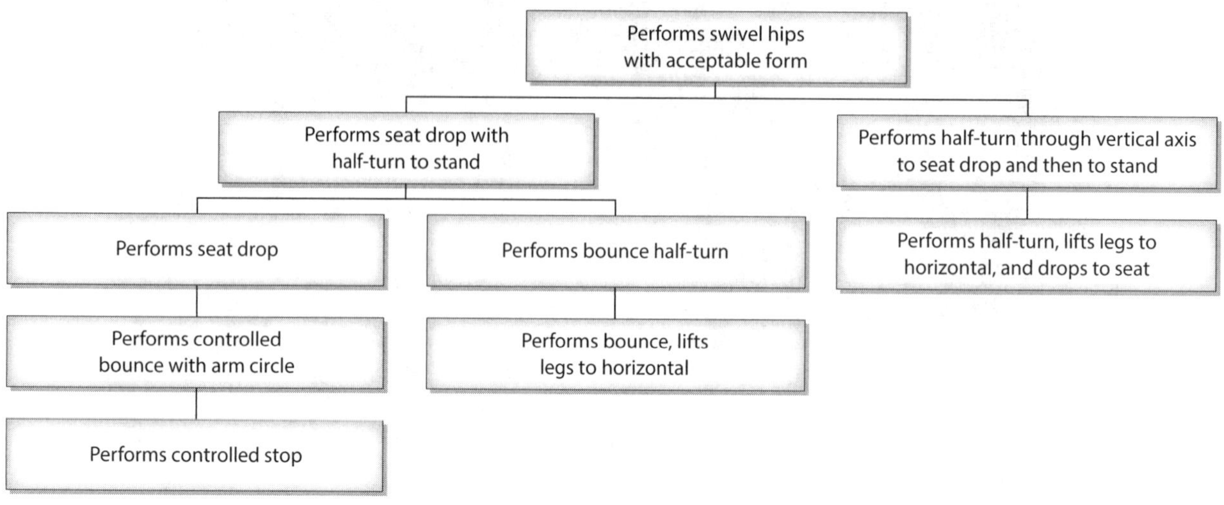

FIGURE 16.3 Hierarchical analysis.

crucial to the success of the design. If the steps are too large, students will experience failure too often and lose interest and enthusiasm. If the steps are too small, they might become bored. The planner works to establish steps that are large enough to be continually challenging and small enough so that students achieve frequent success.

Social and cognitive goals are likely to require a hierarchical rather than a procedural analysis. If the goal is that students will correctly call their own fouls and violations in modified games without arguing, the teacher has to ask her- or himself what tasks need to be designed to achieve that goal by the end of the unit. The goal involves a cognitive component because the students must know the fouls and violations and the appropriate consequences when they are committed. The goal also involves a social component in that the students are willing to make calls on each other without arguing. The teacher might decide that students will routinely call their own violations and fouls in all skill drills. This introduces the need for students to know the rules and to become accustomed to acting in less-intense situations than an actual game.

Tactical Analysis

A *tactical analysis* can take either of the forms just described. If you are using the Tactical Approach to Teaching Games, developing game frameworks to identify and break down tactical problems would be more appropriate. A game framework identifies the tactical problems that must be solved in three categories, (1) scoring, (2) preventing scoring, and (3) restarting play. In addition, each tactical problem will involve off-the-ball movements and on-the-ball skills that are critical to success in game play. **Table 16.1** provides an example of a game framework for soccer.

The choice of tactical problems depends on the readiness of your students and the level of their tactical understanding and skill in a game. Griffin, Mitchell, and Oslin (1997, 2006) suggest that the task analysis question in this case becomes: How tactically complex do I want the game to be? Asking this question allows the planner to develop levels of tactical complexity to meet the needs of the students and outlines a progression of tactical complexity to follow in designing instruction (see **Table 16.2**).

Once you have identified instructional goals and completed relevant analyses, most of the actual content for the unit is developed. If you are using a skill progressions approach, the subskills and elements identified become the informing and extending tasks for the unit. Most tasks will require refining along the way. Applied tasks should be inserted regularly to sustain the students' enthusiasm and show them how they are developing skills and strategies.

Returning to our Outdoor Education example, once the teacher has considered which content areas are most pertinent to meet the big picture goal (taking into consideration the demographics of the context in which the unit is to be

TABLE 16.1 Tactical Problems, Movements, and Skills in Soccer

Tactical Problems	Off-the-Ball Movements	On-the-Ball Skills
Scoring		
Maintaining possession of the ball	• Supporting the ball carrier • Dribbling for control	• Passing: short and long • Control: feet, thigh, chest
Attacking the goal	• Using a target player	• Shooting, shielding, turning
Creating space in attack	• Crossover play • Overlapping run	• First-time passing: 1 versus 2 • Crossover play • Overlapping run
Using space in attack	• Timing runs to goal, shielding	• Width: dribbling 1 versus 1, crossing, heading • Depth: shielding
Preventing Scoring		
Defending space	• Marking, pressure, preventing the turn, delay, covering, recovery runs	• Clearing the ball
Defending the goal	• Goalkeeper: positioning	• Goalkeeping: receiving the ball, shot stopping, distribution
Winning the ball		• Tackling: block, poke, slide
Restarting Play		
Throw-in: attacking and defending	Corner kick: attacking and defending	Free kick: attacking and defending

Reproduced with permission from Griffin, Mitchell, & Oslin. (1997). *Teaching sport concepts and skills: A tactical approach* and Mitchell, Oslin, & Griffin. (2006). *Teaching sport concepts and skills: A tactical games approach, second edition* (table 2.1, p. 10). Champaign, IL: Human Kinetics.

TABLE 16.2 Levels of Tactical Complexity for Soccer

	Levels of Tactical Complexity				
Tactical Problems	**I**	**II**	**III**	**IV**	**V**
Scoring					
Maintaining possession of the ball	Dribble Pass and control: feet	Support player who has ball		Pass: long Control: thigh, chest	
Attacking the goal	Shooting	Shooting Turning	Target player		
Creating space in attack			First-time passing	Overlap	Crossover
Using space in attack				Width: dribbling, crossing, heading	Depth: timing of runs
Preventing Scoring					
Defending space		Marking, pressuring the ball	Preventing the turn	Clearing the ball	Delay, cover, recover
Defending the goal		Goalkeeper position, receiving, throwing			Making saves, kicking/punting
Winning the ball			Tackling: block, poke	Tackling: slide	
Restarting					
Throw-in	Throw in				
Corner kick	Short kick		Near post		Far post
Free kick			Attacking		Defending

Reproduced with permission from Mitchell, Oslin, & Griffin. (2006). *Teaching sport concepts and skills: A tactical games approach, second edition* (table 2.2, p. 11). Champaign, IL: Human Kinetics.

UNIT PLAN 16.5 Concept Map Related to the Content Areas Noted in Unit Plan 16.4

Communication and cooperation (Task Analysis)	• Support • Encouragement • Positive interactions		Skill Analysis
Clothing (Task Analysis)	• Layering • Shoe selection • Changing weather		Skill Analysis
Leave no trace (Task Analysis)	• Plan ahead and prepare • Respect wildlife—carry in and carry out • Leave what you find		Skill Analysis
Outdoor skills (Task Analysis)	• Hiking (Skill Analysis)	• Pacing yourself • Leaning in to hill on up incline/Dig in heels on downhill • Walk with a partner	Further Skill Analysis
	• Orienteering (Skill Analysis)	• Using a compass (direction of travel arrow, shooting bearings) • Reading compass with map (thumbing, identifying landmarks)	Further Skill Analysis

Unit Plan: Step 4

Consider what students need to learn to achieve the big picture goal noted in Unit Plan Step 2 by compiling a list of all the possible areas of content that students could be exposed to in order to prepare them adequately to achieve the big picture goal. Once you have considered which content areas are most pertinent to pursue to meet the big picture goal (taking into consideration the demographics of the context in which the unit is to be delivered), construct a concept map.

delivered), the teacher then begins to construct a concept map. The chosen content areas are termed as "task analysis," and the unpacking of the content areas into associated content for teaching purposes are termed "skill analysis." **Unit Plan 16.5** denotes a concept map that is developed from the content areas noted in Unit Plan 16.4. In this instance, the teacher has chosen four content areas/task analyses (i.e., communication and cooperation, clothing, leave no trace, and outdoor skills) that they deem appropriate to prepare students to be able to effectively complete the big picture goal. The teacher has then systematically broken down each task analysis into more specific content foci (i.e., skill analysis). Teachers are encouraged to further unpack at the skill analysis level into more detailed teachable episodes/learning experiences, as illustrated for hiking and orienteering in Unit Plan 16.5.

Learning Outcomes

Once you have established the concept map that denotes the task and skill analysis for each chunk of content you plan to include in the unit plan, you need to consider at least one matching learning outcome for each chunk. A learning outcome is what students are expected to do and know as a result of participating in the activities in a program. In other words, what are the significant lessons that are the intent of instruction and match your big picture goal and big picture assessment? What will learners need to know and be able to do for each aspect of the content analysis? They should be valid, meaningful, and relevant leading to achievement of the larger big picture goal. In other words, the learning outcomes in the unit plan directly inform the learning outcomes in the associated lesson plans. In some instances the same learning outcome may be apparent in both the unit plan and lesson plan. In other instances, where the unit plan learning outcome is particularly broad, an associated learning outcome in the lesson plan is likely to be more specific in terms of the learning context and identified aspects of quality. In other instances it may take several lesson learning outcomes to help the student achieve the larger unit outcome, or big picture goal. **Unit Plan 16.6** lists a learning outcome for each chunk of content identified in the concept map noted in Unit Plan 16.5.

Breckon and Gower (2006) encourage teachers to consider the inclusion of an action verb in every learning outcome to describe what students will know, do, and understand (e.g., acquire, develop, select, recognize, plan, describe).

UNIT PLAN 16.6 Learning Outcomes to Match the Concept Map

- Students will work together to achieve the goals of the overnight trip (Communication and Cooperation).
- Students will select appropriate clothing to suit the weather on the overnight trip (Clothing).
- Students will participate in an overnight trip following leave no trace concepts (Leave No Trace).
- Students will successfully participate in hiking and orienteering (Outdoor Skills).

Unit Plan: Step 5

Referring back to your concept map, note at least one matching learning outcome for each task analysis heading/chunk of content. Remember that learning outcomes are what students are expected to do and know as the result of participating in the activities in the unit.

Learning Experience 16.2

Consider the following big picture goal and assessment and derive four potential learning outcomes related to achieving the big picture goal:

- *Big picture goal:* Students will safely demonstrate an ability to select, create, and perform a short gymnastic sequence.
- *Big picture assessment:* Students will select gymnastics skills to create and perform a short sequence.

Revisit your four learning outcomes and identify the verbs that you have used in each. Consider the extent to which you would be able to assess if students had been successful in achieving each learning outcome. Are there particular verbs that make it easier to assess students having completed the learning outcome successfully? What does this imply about the choice of verbs when compiling learning outcomes?

Formative Assessments

The best way to ensure a high degree of instructional alignment is to have the learning outcomes match the assessment measures. As you have learned, designing authentic outcomes allows students to strive for assessments that are worthwhile and relevant. If teachers set skill, tactical, social, and cognitive goals, these should be included at this point with a means of assessing when they are achieved. As we sometimes tell our students, "If it is worth teaching, it is worth assessing." Teaching towards an assessment is desirable if the assessment matches the intended outcomes. Formative assessments provide continuous ongoing information and feedback (for student and teacher) about progress toward learning outcomes, act as a learning experience for students, and motivate students to improve their performance. Consequently, the outcomes from such assessments can inform any changes to the planned unit plan. In deriving formative assessments you need to ask yourself the following:

- How will I know when a student has been successful?
- How will a student know when he or she has been successful?
- How can I best design an assessment that matches the learning outcome and provides appropriate choices to all learners?

It is important to note that formative assessments are different from summative assessments, which provide a final judgment on learning, determining how well students have achieved the big picture goal. Formative assessments to match each of the learning outcomes noted in Unit Plan 16.6 are shared in **Unit Plans 16.7 to 16.10**. A rubric that can be used by individuals and peers to assess the extent to which the group is working together (the learning outcome to match with the communication and cooperation content identified in the concept map) is noted in Unit Plan 16.7. The members of the group, listed in the first column, can keep score of the extent to which they believe they and their peers have contributed to working as part of a group during each activity (i.e., packing appropriate equipment, preparing

UNIT PLAN 16.7 Formative Assessment for the Learning Outcome "Students Will Work Together to Achieve the Goals of the Overnight Trip" (Communication and Cooperation)

Reflect on and score yourself and each member of your hiking team in the four categories identified below.
3 = consistently works as part of the team
2 = sometimes works as part of the team
1 = infrequently works as part of the team

	Equipment	Meals	Transport	Clean-up Duties
Eileen				
Martha				
Michelle				
Elena				

UNIT PLAN 16.8 Formative Assessment for the Learning Outcome "Students Will Select Appropriate Clothing to Suit the Weather on the Overnight Trip" (Clothing)

Students will take part in an orienteering event. Teams will designate one person as the "hiker" and will do the following:

- Select clothing for the 3-day trip.
- Navigate the five control point course.
- When arriving at each control point, dress their hiker for the weather.
- Note their clothing decisions on the task card.

Once the teams have completed the event, a whole class final debrief of their clothing decisions will guide where learning is still needed.

UNIT PLAN 16.9 Formative Assessment for the Learning Outcome "Students Will Participate in an Overnight Trip Following Leave No Trace Concepts" (Leave No Trace)

In small groups, students will compile a hiking, fishing, or camping scenario. Students will then swap their scenario with another group of students and determine if the participants in the other group's scenario are following the leave no trace principles. If not, they should be able to share with the class what they were doing incorrectly. The other groups in the class will assess each group's analysis of the scenario.

UNIT PLAN 16.10 Formative Assessment for the Learning Outcome "Students Will Successfully Participate in Hiking and Orienteering" (Outdoor Skills)

Orienteering Tasks	Always	Sometimes	Occasionally
Using a compass: direction of travel arrow			
Using a compass: shooting bearings			
Reading a compass with a map: thumbing			
Reading a compass with a map: identifying landmarks			

Unit Plan: Step 6

Design a formative assessment for each of the learning outcomes identified as an outcome to Unit Plan Step 5. Try to introduce a mix of self-, peer, and teacher assessments.

meals, organizing transport, and responsibilities for cleaning up). Each student would score a 3 when consistently working as part of the group, a 2 when sometimes working as part of a group, and a 1 when infrequently (if ever) working as part of a group.

Unit Plan 16.8 provides a formative assessment of an orienteering event that will allow students and the teacher to assess the extent to which students are able to select appropriate clothing to suit the weather (the learning outcome to match with the clothing content identified in the concept map). The idea of the teacher preparing an outdoor scenario that students would engage with in order to assess students' understanding of leave no trace (the learning outcome to match with the leave no trace camping content identified in the concept map) is shared in Unit Plan 16.9.

Unit Plan 16.10 contains a scoring rubric to ascertain each group of students' appropriate participation in orienteering. A similar task can be constructed for hiking (the learning outcome to match with the outdoor skills identified in the concept map). At this point, keep in mind that you will need to prepare students to work cooperatively in a peer tutoring task where they are providing assessment and feedback.

Instruction

The next phase of the unit plan is to consider how you will teach, and students will practice, the learning outcomes. For each learning outcome, you should identify the following:

- Instructional model (e.g., direct teaching, task/station teaching)
- Learning experiences (e.g., informing, extending, refining, and applying tasks; tactical tasks for games teaching)
- Teaching strategies (e.g., demonstrations, feedback, closure)
- Instructional adaptations (i.e., to make a task more or less complex)

Learning experiences need to be sequenced in such a way as to allow all students to progress towards successfully fulfilling the associated learning outcome. Two learning experiences related to the learning outcome "Students will select appropriate clothing to suit the weather on the camping trip," as well as a related instructional model and teaching strategies, are noted in **Unit Plan 16.11**. Learning experiences can also act as a form of assessment, and it is possible to consider assessment tools that assess whether the learning experiences have been met. Learning experiences can therefore enable you to observe progress formatively throughout the lesson but also assess the extent to which such learning experiences have contributed to the achievement of the intended learning outcome. An assessment tool for each of the learning experiences is also noted in Unit Plan 16.11.

Instructional Adaptations

Modification of Equipment

The achievement of learning outcomes and associated instructional tasks can be made easier or more difficult by modifying the equipment students use. Successful repetitions are often difficult to achieve with full-sized equipment. It is much easier to learn good stroking skills in net games with rackets that are shorter and lighter. Slightly deflated soccer balls or foam balls make it easier to learn kicking and trapping. Any game or activity that requires students to anticipate the flight of an object can be made easier by slowing down the object or causing it to stay in the air longer. Students can often execute skills in controlled settings (partner pass) but not when the action goes more quickly. The problem is that they do not have sufficient experience to anticipate the flight of the object and move to be in position to execute the skill. Thus, using beach balls for beginning volleyball-type skills or raising the net in badminton-type games to keep the object in the air longer gives students more time to anticipate and move to the proper position. The overall point is that student performance outcomes for units often depend on the equipment used.

UNIT PLAN 16.11 Learning Experiences, Instructional Format, Teaching Strategies, and Instructional Adaptations

- *Learning outcome:* Students will select appropriate clothing to suit the weather on the camping trip.
- *Learning experience 1*: Students will work in groups of three. Students will read a scenario of a day hike event (e.g., weather conditions, temperature, time of day and time of year), and from a stack of clothes dress one hiker appropriately.
  - *Instructional model:* Teaching through questions; cooperative learning.
  - *Teaching strategies:* Employing questioning techniques; experiential learning; active supervision.
  - *Instructional adaptation:* If the task is too challenging, a task card might have prompts on suitable clothing for various types of weather to guide the student. If not challenging enough, the skilled student might serve as the "sherpa" to give feedback on each group's response.
  - *Matching assessment:* At the end of class, the teacher asks the students to share their responses. As a group they discuss the appropriateness of the various responses.
- *Learning experience 2*: Individually students are to determine what is missing from prepacked day-hike packs identified as suitably accommodating specific weather conditions.
  - *Instructional model:* Teaching through questions.
  - *Teaching strategies:* Equipment setup; feedback and questioning; experiential learning.
  - *Instructional adaptation:* If the task is too challenging, a checklist might be provided to guide the student. If not challenging enough, the students might be asked to pack the backpacks for the initial task.
  - *Matching assessment:* Students complete a self-assessment or peer assessment comparing responses to the scorecard for the prepacked day-hike pack.

Optimizing Equipment with Student Numbers

Optimizing equipment/student ratios is another resource consideration. Few instructional factors influence student response rates as much as the ratio of available equipment to students. More good responses lead to more achievement. Other things being equal, students in class with a 2:1 student–equipment ratio will get twice the number of response opportunities as those in a class with a 4:1 ratio. The equipment–student ratio should be a major factor in planning unit performance outcomes. The higher the ratio, the less you can expect students to achieve. This is an especially important factor for all individual skill practices. When skill practice purposely takes place in groups, then the appropriate consideration is the equipment–group ratio. This factor needs to be kept in mind when designing applied tasks such as games.

Resources

The unit plan should not only note any further resources required (e.g., posters, charts, ribbons, homemade certificates) but also include a copy of each. The resources required for the unit plan presented in this chapter are denoted in **Unit Plan 16.12**.

Unit Plan: Step 7

Compile two learning experiences and associated instructional models, teaching strategies, instructional adaptations, and a matching assessment for each learning outcome identified in Unit Plan Step 5.

UNIT PLAN 16.12 Resources for the Outdoor Education Unit Plan

- Maps
- Compasses
- Bags of sticks and stones
- Prepacked day packs
- Maps of school grounds
- Assessment scoring rubrics and pencils
- First aid kit
- Water bottles

Unit Plan: Step 8

List the resources necessary for the running and completion of the unit plan developed in Unit Plan Steps 1 to 7.

UNIT PLAN 16.13 Structure of Self-Appraisal

Upon completion of each lesson, the teacher will reflect on the following:

- Clarity and effectiveness of explanations and demonstrations
- Quality of teaching cues and prompts
- Use and appropriateness of higher order questioning
- Appropriateness of activities, challenges, and adaptations
- The extent to which the teacher checked for understanding throughout the lesson and the effectiveness of classroom management.

Unit Plan: Step 9

Include a list of prompts/questions that convey how you intend to reflect, and on what, at the end of each lesson and the unit.

Structure of Self-Appraisal

The unit plan should include how the teacher intends to reflect on what happened at the end of each lesson and the unit. An example of such a structure is noted in **Unit Plan 16.13**. Teachers might choose to use prompts such as, Did I achieve my objectives? Did I structure the content in a coherent fashion? What would I do differently if I had to teach this lesson again? How will this lesson affect my future planning? Alternatively, or in addition, teachers may choose to use a standard checklist to grade their teaching under a number of different headings such as teacher enthusiasm, questioning skills, quality of demonstrations, pace of the lesson, and variety of instructional strategies practiced.

A focus on self-appraisal should not diminish the importance of assessing student learning as a means to evaluate the effectiveness of your teaching. As Gower (2004) advises,

> *Evaluation of teaching must be informed by assessment of pupil learning if it is to be at all meaningful and impact upon the quality of response by both the learner and the teacher. Knowledge and understanding of learners' responses should help to adapt and change many aspects of your teaching. Therefore, planning structures should prompt you to assess pupil learning and use this data to reflect critically on how to improve pupil learning and also your approaches to teaching. In any evaluation all the questions are focused around one important factor: "What did the pupils achieve?"*[2]

[2] Reproduced with permission from Gower, C. (2004). Planning in PE (p. 48). In S. Capel (Ed.), *Learning to teach physical education in the secondary school: A companion to school experience* (pp. 27–50). Oxon: RoutledgeFalmer.

TABLE 16.3 Preventive Management Plan

Rules	Routines	Student Expectations	Teacher Expectations
• No talking when others are talking. • Touch equipment on teacher's direction.	• Stop on whistle. • Attendance card entry. • Gather on raised hand. • Disburse on "Go."	• Dressed for activity. • Give best effort. • Respect self and others. • Listen to others.	• On time to class • Prepared for lesson • Approachable • Knowledgeable • Caring

We encourage you to add several questions to the previous self-assessment list that will cause you to consider how students responded to the lesson, interacted with one another and the content, and overall reacted to you and the learning experiences.

Preventive Management

The best preventive class management systems are developed as social contracts between teachers and their students. Involving students in the development of the system of rules, procedures, and routines facilitates their taking ownership of the class and their behavior. Taking the time to establish rules and procedures, and allowing students to practice those behaviors and consistently enforcing consequences for breaking rules, is time well spent. A sample preventive management plan is displayed in **Table 16.3** and a sample contingency management plan might look like that in **Table 16.4**.

Accountability Mechanisms

Your unit plan should also allude to the creation of accountability mechanisms to ensure high rates of on-task behavior and achievement of goals. Two kinds of accountability need to be considered when planning: (1) daily accountability aimed at on-task behavior and (2) unit-level accountability aimed at achievement of end-of-unit outcomes (i.e., the big picture goal). Teachers need to hold students accountable for staying on task on a daily basis. Some activities, such as a checklist for gymnastics stunts, lend themselves to peer monitoring of performance. Some activities lend themselves to group challenges with resulting public recognition. Some teachers rely on active supervision, prompts, and feedback to keep students on task.

When planning the unit plan, other issues to consider that will hopefully result in the teacher addressing issues at the beginning of the unit to ensure high rates of on-task behavior and achievement of goals include (1) anticipating safety issues and establishing special rules, (2) class entry and exit outcomes to guide class time boundaries and allow activity, (3) specification of special managerial routines for the unit, and (4) organizational arrangements to save time. Although these issues are not necessarily listed on the unit plan, it is important for the teacher to consider them when planning the unit. Over time as a teacher, and in building relationships with particular groups of students, you will develop routines, rituals, and relationships that minimize potential problems and maximize on-task behavior. These could already be part of your preventive management plan that you have shared previously with the class of students (see Table 16.4 as an example).

TABLE 16.4 Contingency Management Plan: Consequences for Misbehavior

Offense	Consequence for Misbehavior
1st offense	Warning
2nd offense	2-minute timeout to reflect on behavior
3rd offense	5-minute timeout with explanation to teacher as to why sent to timeout
4th offense	5-minute timeout and talk to class head teacher
5th offense	After-school detention

Block Plan

You cannot construct a good unit by simply starting at the beginning of the content analysis and moving toward the end. Remember, the unit is a series of lessons. Each lesson should make sense on its own. The unit plan should have anticipated instructional tasks blocked by lesson so that day-to-day teaching progressions will be clear, and each lesson can be judged as an independent entity as well as being part of a series of lessons comprising the unit (see **Unit Plan 16.14**). The intention of a block plan is to allow for a degree of flexibility in accommodating and adjusting expectations as you progress through teaching the unit, while noting the intended

Unit Plan: Step 10

Consider a preventive management plan suitable to the unit plan you have been developing in previous Unit Plan steps, conscious that the development or reinforcement of already agreed-upon routines, rituals, and relationships will minimize potential problems and maximize on-task behavior.

UNIT PLAN 16.14 Block Plan

Week 1:	*Week 2:*	*Week 3:*
1. Start lesson with a cooperative activity. 2. Introduce elements of hiking through a series of walking tasks including options on how best to dress for the weather.	1. Start lesson with a communication activity. 2. Introduce leave no trace through a walking trail that shows abuse by people. 3. Discuss appropriate attire, including footwear.	1. Introduce students to tracking signs to allow them to stay found (i.e., not get lost).
Week 4:	*Week 5:*	*Week 6:*
1. Start lesson with a trust activity. 2. Introduce orienteering (map and compass).	1. Start lesson with a team-building activity. 2. Develop previous walking/hiking skills through an orienteering course (star, line, or landmark).	1. Take part in a mock event where students demonstrate they have the skills and knowledge to undertake the overnight trip (working as a team, appropriate clothing, demonstrating leave no trace through hiking and orienteering).

Unit Plan: Step 11

Complete a block plan that outlines what you plan to teach on a weekly basis in order to have students be in a position to successfully participate in the big picture goal of the unit you have been working on in previous Unit Plan steps. Remember, this block plan can be flexible and helps direct the content of weekly lesson plans.

focus and content for each lesson in the unit plan. We therefore strongly suggest that teachers plan and prepare lesson plans on a weekly basis to allow them to take account of what did or did not take place in the previous lesson and accommodate this accordingly in the next lesson. This allows the teacher to revisit after every lesson where students are in terms of their learning, where you want them to be at the end of the unit, and how your next lesson is going to contribute to getting them there.

Designing a Lesson Plan

In a bid to strive for effective teaching and learning, designing an appropriate lesson plan is as important as designing a unit plan with respect to creating the confidence that comes with having a good plan to refer to when needed. Whereas the unit plan is an outline/framework for the delivery of a specific big picture goal, lesson plans provide the specifics of content and instruction for each lesson intended to contribute towards the achievement of the big picture goal by the end of the unit. As alluded to earlier in the chapter, the planning for daily lessons, although strongly aligned to the unit plan, is not overtly tied to the details of the unit plan but rather is relatively flexible to accommodate for what has or has not been achieved in the previous lesson. By preparing lesson plans on a weekly basis rather than as a full complement of lesson plans to accompany the unit plan at the start of the unit, lesson plans can appropriately develop the content and associated learning experiences from the previous lesson. This supports the use of assessment from one lesson to establish the quality of leaning and to inform the planning of the next lesson, potentially resulting in adaptations being made to the unit plan, and in particular the block plan (see Unit Plan 16.14).

There may be instances where a unit plan for a particular content area and year group services more than one physical education class in that particular year group. This is perfectly acceptable if weekly lesson plans are drawn up for each class to accommodate the different rate of learning and individual needs of the group, potentially leading to noting different levels of challenges and extension of progressions to the content noted in the unit plan.

Although there is general consensus on what should be noted in a lesson plan, there is no one definitive lesson plan template (examples include Gower, 2004; Metzler, 2011). The format used should reflect specifics of your teaching and student participation and does not need to be prescribed. It will vary by teacher as well as across content areas. This section will work through the elements of a suggested generic lesson

BOX 16.5 Outline for a Lesson Plan

- Contextual description
- Timeline
- Content
  - Set the stage
  - Lesson content (warm-up and learning experiences/activities)
  - Lesson closure
- Organization and management
- Teaching cues and prompts
- Content adaptations

plan template proposed in **Box 16.5**. There is consensus that a lesson plan should reflect the following:

- The anticipated progression of tasks with a time allotment for each task (It is most helpful to the teacher if the time allotment is listed cumulatively for the length of the lesson.)
- Descriptions for how each task will be communicated to students (Some feel that, at the outset, the exact words should be written on the lesson plan.)
- The organizational arrangements for each task and how they will be implemented.
- Any teaching cues or prompts the teacher wants to remember to help the students master the task (These might be critical elements of skills or just reminders to "speak slowly and enunciate clearly" if you have been experiencing difficulty with students understanding your explanations and directions.)
- Some way of recording reactions to what took place so that the next time the lesson is taught or when the unit is revised, you have information about what went well or what might be changed.

To enhance the reader's understanding of how one element informs the next, and to demonstrate the effectiveness of instructional alignment, we have chosen to work through what could potentially be a lesson plan related to the Outdoor Education unit plan discussed in this chapter. In instances where some of the concepts related to an element require some further unpacking, we provide additional examples. A template of a lesson plan is noted in **Figure 16.4**, and we work through each element in turn before presenting a completed lesson plan (see **Table 16.5**) for the third lesson of the Outdoor Education unit of work. As you read across Figure 16.4, the alignment and logical link across the timeline, content, organization and management, teaching cues and prompts, and content adaptations should be evident.

Timeline	Content	Organization and management	Teaching cues and prompts	Content adaptations
	Setting the stage Lesson content Lesson closure			

FIGURE 16.4 Template for a lesson plan.

TABLE 16.5 Outdoor Education Lesson Plan

Physical Education Lesson Plan
Date: October 16, 2014
Name of class: 3A (third year postprimary)
Number of students: 23
Lesson length: 80 minutes
Lesson number: Third of six
Students' previous knowledge/skills/experience: Students completed a 6-week Adventure Education unit in their first year where they experienced team building, communication, cooperation, and trust, focusing mainly on low-level initiatives. The first two lessons of this Outdoor Education unit introduced students to basic hill-walking skills, the concept of leave no trace, and the need for using a compass and map.
Lesson focus (i.e., content area): Staying found—students will learn how to use tracking signs to design and navigate a trail/course
Lesson outcomes:

- Students will work in groups as they use tracking signs to design and navigate a trail/course.
- Students will cooperate and communicate with their group members as they work together to follow a trail set up by another group.
- Students will recognize and solve problems and issues encountered while designing and navigating a trail/course.

Resources/equipment: Four bags of sticks and stones (three groups of six and one group of five) and a map of the school grounds
Safety considerations: Jewelry removed and students suitably dressed for outdoors. Students to stay in their groups working cooperatively throughout the lesson and stay within the school grounds.

Timeline	Content	Organization and Management	Teaching Cues and Prompts	Content Adaptations
0 to 10 minutes	*Setting the stage:* • Allow class to arrive and change into appropriate clothing. • When in their home base, they should familiarize themselves with the map of the school. • Ask students if they can orient the school map to locate their current location. • Make sure to explore the map and ensure you know the different points on the map.	• Students sit in their home areas in their already established groups on entry to the gymnasium.	• Check the orientation. • Where are you now?	
10 to 20 minutes	*Lesson content:* • In groups, students will work their way through the six tracking signs noted on the associated card: this way, no entry or danger, turn left or turn right, water ahead, obstacle ahead, and gone home. They will be encouraged to use the stones and sticks in their bag to physically copy the signs from the card and understand what each sign conveys.	• Each group is to be given a bag of sticks and stones and a tracking signs card (see www.world-scouts.com/index.php/codes-a-signs/380-tracking-signs for a resource). Each group is to work in their home areas.	• Make sure the signs are distinctive (e.g., an arrow looks like an arrow).	• If necessary, assign roles in a group to facilitate cooperation.

20 to 25 minutes	• Recap on what is important to consider when constructing the signs: What do you need to consider when striving to accurately convey the tracking signs? Do any problems arise? How do you suggest solving such problems?	• Students come together to sit around the whiteboard on the wall of the gymnasium.	• Does anyone else have another idea? • Did you encounter the same problem?	• If students are unable to identify problems, introduce prepared scenarios to prompt response.
25 to 45 minutes	• Each group will be allocated a section of the school grounds on which to design a trail/course using the tracking signs. Students are to mark their trail/course on the school map to serve as a key. Students are not to work outside the allocated section.	• Students are allocated a section of the school grounds where they go to meet with their group and plan their trail/course.	• Where is your trail/course boundary? • Respond to students' ongoing trail/course design.	• Locate any group with behavior or health issues closer to the school building.
45 to 60 minutes	• Each group will be given the opportunity to follow the trail/course set up by one other group.	• Students will move to another part of the school grounds to complete another trail/course.	• Refer students to the school map and card to decipher the trail/course. • Encourage working together.	• In instances where students struggle with relying solely on tracking signs for navigation, prompt them by using the trail/course key developed by the associated team.
60 to 70 minutes	*Lesson closure:* • Debrief on today's lesson by asking: • What are the six tracking signs we used today? • What do you need to consider when using the tracking signs on different terrain? • How does communication and cooperation aid your team in designing a trail/course? • What makes a trail/course that you are unfamiliar with easier or harder to follow?	• Students come together to sit around the whiteboard on the wall of the gymnasium/sports hall.		
70 to 80 minutes	• Allow for students to shower and change their clothes.			

Contextual Description

It is essential that each lesson plan notes information that is pertinent to the class for which the lesson plan is prepared. Although some lesson plan information should be duplicated from the demographics noted on the associated unit plan, additional information is necessary for the individual lesson. Remaining with the Outdoor Education unit plan demographics (see Unit Plan 16.1), information included in the first associated lesson plan for that unit is noted in **Unit Plan 16.15**.

UNIT PLAN 16.15 Contextual Description to Be Included at the Start of the Lesson Plan

Date: October 16, 2014
Name of the class: 3A (third year postprimary)
Number of students: 23
Length of lesson: 80 minutes
Lesson number: Third of six
Students' previous knowledge/skills/experience: Students completed a 6-week Adventure Education unit in their first year where they experienced team building, communication, cooperation, and trust, focusing mainly on low-level initiatives. The first two lessons of this Outdoor Education unit introduced students to basic hill-walking skills, the concept of leave no trace, and the need for using a compass and map.
Lesson focus: Staying found—students will learn how to use tracking signs to design and navigate a trail/course.
Lesson outcomes: (1) Students will work in groups as they use tracking signs to design and navigate a trail/course; (2) Students will cooperate and communicate with their group members as they work together to follow a trail set up by another group; and (3) Students will recognize and solve problems and issues encountered while designing and navigating a trail/course.
Resources/equipment: Four bags of sticks and stones (three groups of six and one group of five), tracking worksheet, and a map of the school grounds
Safety considerations: Jewelry removed and students suitably dressed for outdoors. Students to stay in their groups working cooperatively throughout the lesson and stay within the school grounds.

Unit Plan: Step 12

Revisiting the unit plan developed in completing Unit Plan Steps 1 to 11, choose which lesson week you are going to prepare a lesson plan for (acknowledging students' previous knowledge/skills/experience in the unit) and complete the contextual description to be included at the start of the lesson plan.

The lesson focus will be determined by the block plan included in the unit plan (Unit Plan 16.4), and the lesson outcomes can be taken directly from the unit plan (or informed by the outcomes noted on the unit plan) (Unit Plan 16.6), with between one and three lesson outcomes tending to be sufficient for one lesson.

Timeline

A timeline denoting the length of time you plan to spend on each section of the lesson plan should be included to help keep the teacher within certain time limits. This can include the time allocated to students getting changed for physical education, individual sections of the lesson being taught, lesson closure, and students showering and changing at the end of the lesson. Teachers need first to consider what they want to accomplish on a given day. What are the expected outcomes? This requires analyzing the tasks required to achieve these outcomes (i.e., How many tasks will it take? How many repetitions do students need to perform the task well? How much time is available?). Once teachers have this information, they can begin to determine how much can be accomplished and what a time schedule might look like to include all the tasks necessary for success. The timeline acts as a guide to the pacing of the lesson and can be adjusted throughout the lesson to accommodate instances where more or less time is needed to successfully complete a specific task. This said, keep in mind that as teachers, we do not teach the plan, we teach students. So, when we move from one task to another should not be based on the timeline noted on the plan but rather the response and success of our students.

Content

There are three main elements that fall under content: (1) setting the stage, (2) lesson content (warm-up and learning experiences/activities), and (3) lesson closure.

Setting the Stage

In setting the stage, you are concerned with sharing with students what you have planned for the lesson and what you expect from them.

Content: Warm-up

The warm-up component of the lesson content includes noting the entry message with directions. For example, reinforcing the entry practices you have set for the class such as entering the gymnasium and beginning activity in small groups. Where a warm-up is used, the warm-up section of the lesson plan should include a detailed warm-up routine/associated warm-up activities, directly related to the focus of the lesson where possible, and also instructions on how students are to complete the warm-up.

Unit Plan: Step 13

Informed by your block plan completed in Unit Plan Step 11, compile the content for the lesson plan and denote a timeline for each area within the three elements of setting the stage, lesson content, and lesson closure.

Content: Learning Experiences

The learning experiences/activities element of the lesson content entails including for each learning experience, (1) the critical elements to reinforce in encouraging the related skill technique, (2) who will provide demonstrations and explanations and what will be said related to each, and (3) related skill practices or drills and how they are to be completed.

Lesson Closure

Lesson closure is an opportunity to recap what was completed throughout the lesson, review and check for student understanding by posing specific questions, and acknowledge what has been accomplished and how this is to inform the following week's lesson.

Organization and Management

The organization and management component of the lesson plan notes how students will be organized (usually noted through formation diagrams) and how equipment is arranged and where it is to be arranged. One critical component that should be included in the plan is the teacher's decision on how the organization will be implemented. For example, if you merely write on the plan, "students will be in pairs," it is important that you have determined how they will be put into pairs. If you suggest that groups of five will work at each station, make sure you note how the groups will be developed, which station will be the starting point, and how the rotation will be conducted. Frequently we see teachers who indicate what is going to happen in the management portion of the plan yet they have not considered how it will happen. The result is a lot of wasted time and, in many cases, students waiting for something to happen.

Teaching Cues and Prompts

The teaching cues noted in the lesson plan are typically in bullet format and are the critical elements/features/key points of a skill. Teaching cues can also include behavior prompts and reminders of previous teaching cues. Teachers can also include diagrams or pictures under teaching cues where appropriate.

Content Adaptations

The content adaptation element of the lesson plan prompts the teacher to consider how they will adapt the content of the lesson to suit all children. This can include (1) changing the size of the court/activity area; (2) introducing modified equipment; (3) encouraging student choice; (4) having the students work individually, in partners, or in small groups; and (5) considering your own positioning as a teacher in the class. Modifying task complexity provides insight into how adaptations might best be made to increase or decrease the complexity of a given task.

Unit Plan: Step 14

For each content/task identified in response to Unit Plan Step 13, note corresponding organization and management elements, teaching cues and prompts, and content adaptations. On completion of the lesson plan, read across the five columns and check for alignment and a logical link among the timeline, content, organization and management, teaching cues and prompts, and content adaptations.

CHAPTER SUMMARY

This chapter clarified the steps in planning a unit of instruction through examples and clarification of designing a full unit plan and accompanying lesson plan to guide teaching. Three reasons are discussed as critical to planning at the unit level: (1) teachers' belief that planning for student learning is critical with many choosing to teach directly from their unit plans as opposed to individually designed lesson plans, (2) teachers who plan daily lessons tend to do so based on a thoroughly developed unit plan, and (3) teachers suggest that focusing on unit planning requires considering progressions that build across daily lessons and move toward achievement of broader unit objectives. Considering these points suggests that the unit level appears to be the most functional way to think about planning, and the steps outlined in this chapter will assist the teacher in achieving this important task.

1. Teachers plan to ensure progressions within and between lessons, to use time efficiently, and to reduce anxiety and build confidence.
2. Although teachers may be plan dependent or plan independent as they teach, evidence suggests that all effective teachers originally plan units thoroughly.
3. Three levels of planning are commonly referred to as long-term (curriculum planning), medium-term (unit plan), and short-term (lesson plan).
4. Backward design occurs when curriculum design begins with the exit outcomes and proceeds backward to the entry point to ensure that all components are directly related to achieving the outcome.
5. A meaningful and coherent physical education program reflects an alignment among learning goals, assessments

that determine if students reach those goals, and the instructional practices that provide students the opportunity to achieve success, commonly referred to as instructional alignment.

6. Designing a big picture goal entails considering a goal for a unit of instruction students will work toward successfully completing at the end of the unit. In order to provide evidence on the extent to which students have successfully achieved the big picture goal, a matching and worthwhile big picture assessment needs to be agreed upon.
7. A content analysis is a technique to determine all aspects of content that must be taught and learned (i.e., physical, tactical, social, cognitive) if students are to reach the big picture goal (outcome). A procedural analysis describes a chain of events that, taken together, form a meaningful unit of performance. A hierarchical analysis is a description of all the subskills necessary to perform the instructional goal.
8. Learning outcomes are what students are expected to do and know as a result of participating in the activities in a program. The learning outcomes in the unit plan directly inform the learning outcomes in the associated lesson plans.
9. For each learning outcome, you should identify learning experiences, instructional format, and teaching strategies.
10. A focus on self-appraisal should not diminish the importance of assessing student learning as a means to evaluate the effectiveness of your teaching.
11. An already established preventive management plan that addresses routines, rituals, and relationships that minimize potential problems and maximize on-task behavior enhances the effectiveness of the delivery of the unit and lesson plans.
12. Lesson plans should be prepared on a weekly basis to allow them to take account of what did or did not take place in the previous lesson and accommodate this accordingly in the next lesson.

REFERENCES

Bloom, B. (1980). The new direction in educational research: Alterable variables. *Phi Delta Kappan*, 61(6), 382–385.

Breckon, P., & Gower, C. (2006). Medium- and short-term planning in physical education. In S. Capel, P. Breckon, & J. O'Neil (Eds.), *A practical guide to teaching physical education in the secondary school* (pp. 40–49). Oxon, UK: RoutledgeFalmer.

Cohen, S. A. (1987). Instructional alignment: Searching for a magic bullet. *Educational Researcher, 16*, 16–20.

Gower, C. (2004). Planning in PE. In S. Capel (Ed.), *Learning to teach physical education in the secondary school. A companion to school experience* (pp. 27–50). Oxon, UK: RoutledgeFalmer.

Griffin, L., Mitchell, S., & Oslin, J. (1997). *Teaching sport concepts and skills: A tactical games approach.* Champaign, IL: Human Kinetics.

Lund, J., & Tannehill, D. (2010). *Standards-based physical education curriculum development* (2nd ed.). Sudbury, MA: Jones and Bartlett.

Metzler, M. W. (2011). *Instructional models for physical education* (3rd ed.). Scottsdale, AZ: Holcomb Hathaway.

Mitchell, S., Oslin, J., & Griffin, L. (2006). *Teaching sport concepts and skills: A tactical games approach.* Champaign, IL: Human Kinetics.

Shulman, L. S. (1997). Knowledge and teaching: Foundations of the new reform. *Harvard Educational Review, 37*, 1–22.

Stroot, S., & Morton, P. (1989). Blueprints for learning. *Journal of Teaching in Physical Education*, *8*(3), 213–222.

Wiggins, G., & McTighe, J. (1998). *Understanding by design.* Alexandria, VA: Association of Supervision and Curriculum Development.

CHAPTER 17 Supporting Technology for Teaching Physical Education

Overall Chapter Outcome

To optimize the knowledge and use of technology for the purpose of planning, implementing, and assessing the physical education program, as well as promotion and advocacy efforts

Learning Outcomes

The learner will:

- Explain the general influence of technology on people's lives
- Understand the potential benefits and potential harmful effects of technology on children and youth
- Explain the evidence on the use of active video games
- Discuss the considerations for selecting appropriate technologies to support program management, instructional delivery, and student learning
- Know how technologies can be used to aid physical educators in their teaching
- Explain how technologies can be used to support students' learning experiences

Most will agree that in the last three decades, few trends have influenced life in developed countries as much as the emerging digital technologies. As recently as 1992, few people would have understood the following statement: "After I completed the review of the text file, I converted it to a PDF and attached it to an email I sent via my webmail." Terms such as *DVI/HDMI Adapter*, *USB*, *Firewire*, *Ethernet*, and *social media* simply did not exist in the 1980s. Because of the pace with which new technologies emerge, revolutionary new technologies can end up outdated within a short amount of time. For example, the personal digital assistant (PDA) was a terrific type of handheld technology in the mid-2000s. Within only a few years, other more advanced handheld devices with more capabilities quickly surpassed the PDA.

In this digital age that we find ourselves in, it is increasingly more common for students to be more familiar with and better versed than their teachers in using a multitude of technologies. Palfrey and Gasser (2008) reminded us that today's generation of "**digital natives**" is the first to grow up in this age of rapidly evolving digital technologies. This only serves to highlight the need for those teachers born well before the digital era to develop and maintain currency with existing and emerging technologies that are especially pertinent to teaching physical education.

In this chapter we highlight the degree to which technology in postprimary is influencing everyday life, education, and physical education. We will also share some evidence regarding the positive and negative impacts technology is having, especially as it relates to the various health risk behaviors of children and youth. Considerations for selecting technology are presented next. We then provide several ways in which teachers can employ technology to enhance their own teaching and to support students' learning experiences. We close the chapter with a brief glimpse at the future of technology in physical education programs.

BOX 17.1 Key Terms in This Chapter

- *Active video games:* Also referred to as "exergames." An activity combining exercise with electronic game playing. Examples include Dance-Dance-Revolution, Wii, and X-Box Kinect.
- *Device staying power*: The degree to which use of a technology device or program is sustained over time.
- *Digital natives:* The generation of youth that has grown up during the emerging era of digital technologies.
- *Educational technology:* Use of technology in support of teaching and/or learning.
- *Listserv:* A program that automatically sends messages to multiple email addresses on a mailing list.
- *Operating platform:* Software that directs the operations of a computer, controls and schedules the execution of other software programs, and manages storage, input/output, and communication resources. Examples include Windows for PCs and OS X Mountain Lion for Apple devices.
- *Podcast/Vodcast:* Audio and/or video broadcasts that a user can download from the Internet and play on computers and most other handheld devices.
- *Screen time:* Time spent being sedentary while looking at a computer or television screen.
- *Video gaming:* Electronic and interactive games played using computers or computer consoles.
- *Web browser:* Software program that allows users to explore, retrieve, and present information resources on the World Wide Web. Examples include Apple Safari, Microsoft Internet Explorer, and Mozilla Firefox.
- *Wi-Fi:* Short for "wireless fidelity", this refers to wireless networking technology that enables computers, tablets, and the like to communicate using a wireless signal.
- *Wiki:* A website that allows users to add and update content on the site using their web browser. (The word has its roots in the Hawaiian phrase "wiki wiki," which means superfast.)

Influence of Technology

Technology has affected people in very positive ways across countless facets of their lives. Many more people can access valuable information easily; people who lost their legs can now be fitted with prosthetics that allow them to walk again; and sport performance has improved, in part, because of improved equipment designed using new technologies. Perhaps the most recognizable example of how improved technology combined with effective conditioning practices (and human spirit!) can impact human life in positive ways is reflected in the Paralympics as well as veterans of war. Athletes with sometimes-severe physical disabilities are outfitted with high-tech prostheses and other supporting devices that allows them to participate and compete successfully at world level. Veterans of war who lose one or multiple limbs also benefit from more advanced rehab protocols where they learn to use artificial limbs. Moreover, how we communicate with others, listen to music, search for information, and the like is fundamentally different today because new technologies continue to emerge and improve at a seemingly dizzying pace.

Education also has seemingly benefitted from technology. As recently as 2000, former U.S. President Bill Clinton noted the following in his State of the Union address: "In 1994, only 3 percent of our classrooms were connected. Today, with the help of the Vice President's E-rate program, more than half of them are, and 90 percent of our schools have at least one Internet connection" (American Presidency Project, 2000). One of the key problems in education with regard to keeping up with rapidly emerging new technologies is the cost associated with not only purchasing the technology but also installing the needed hardware, training the entire teaching staff on how to use it, and maintenance. Previously, certain technologies became obsolete after a few years. Today, a seemingly revolutionary new technology may actually be obsolete in a matter of months. This places enormous responsibility on school managers when deciding on which technologies to invest in for their schools or districts.

Technology applications and equipment in schools vary internationally. Today, most primary and postprimary schools in the United States have elaborate computer labs or classrooms. **Wi-Fi** access provides teachers and students constant and reliable access to the Internet with their laptops, tablets, or iPads. Many schools and school districts in the United States employ system-wide software to track student information, performance, and progress. Parents can monitor their child's performance in school whenever and from wherever they want.

The empirical study of the effects of **video gaming** on various health behaviors (e.g., sedentary behavior, physical activity, aggression) and other variables (e.g., school performance, desensitization to violence, decreases in pro-social behavior) is a relative new line of inquiry. The popular belief is that the increased time that youth spend playing computer games causes them to engage in violence and other negative health behaviors. Yet, there is also a growing body of evidence showing that the relationship is more complex, in that it can also offer important benefits. For example, based on their recent review of 38 published research papers, Primack et al. (2012) reported that the use of video games improved outcomes in various clinical settings, including psychological therapy (69% of outcomes), physical therapy (59%), health education (42%), pain distraction (42%), and disease self-management (37%). Thus, the type of technology and the purpose for which it is used can make important contributions. There is also evidence that video games can support health-related behavior change efforts (Baranowski, Buday, Thompson, & Baranowski, 2008).

Learning Experience 17.1

To appreciate the impact of technology on everyday life, select a 48-hour period during which you turn off/avoid using all forms of computer hardware and software technology, television, wireless phones, and the like. Avoid asking others to use the technologies for you. During this period, use a written diary to log all instances where you find yourself limited or hampered in any way in engaging in life's activities. After the 48-hour period, reflect on and explain in writing (again without use of any form of computer technology) how you addressed and overcame these limitations. If you did not or could not overcome them, explain what you did instead.

One area of technology that is especially pertinent to the field of physical education is the meteoric rise of sport-related computer gaming in the last decade (even though these games, with few exceptions such as Wii, are not widely used in physical education). It has become a major form of entertainment for youth (and adults). Video gaming technology is now very sophisticated and reinforcing to children and youth. Specifically with regard to how children and youth spend their discretionary time, games like Call of Duty: Black Ops, Madden NFL 2013, and FIFA Soccer 2013 are immensely popular. **Table 17.1** includes sales numbers for all computer games between 2006 and 2011 across various countries and regions.

Although sales dropped in most countries during the recent economic recession, during 2011 in the United States alone, sales of computer video games, hardware, and accessories still reached almost $25 billion (Entertainment Software Association, 2013).

TABLE 17.1 Video Games Sales

Country/Region	Sales in Billions (most recent year available)
Asia	$14 (2006) and $20 (2009)
Japan	$20 (2009)
Europe	$18.9 (2007)
United States	$18.6 (2010)
China	$6 (2011)
United Kingdom	$5.6 (2008)
France	$4 (2008)
Germany	$3.8 (2008)
Canada	$2.1 (2008)
Netherlands	$1.9 (2008)
South Korea	$1.7 (2008)
Australia	$1.3 (2008)
Mexico	~$1 (2008)
Italy	~$1 (2007)

This table uses material from the "Video Game Industry" article on the Video Game Sales wiki at Wikia and is licensed under the Creative Commons Attribution-Share Alike License.

Undoubtedly, one key reason for their popularity is the realism and authenticity of the games' designs. The game designers have created game experiences that, albeit virtual, are exciting, provide authenticity, are challenging, allow for creativity, and of course, provide ample reinforcement. To paraphrase Bunker and Thorpe (1982), they know how to "get a good game going . . . and keep it going." Along with other forms of computer entertainment such as fantasy football, sport video games are especially serious competition for school physical education programs because they provide youth with the opportunity to pretend to be playing the real game and pretend they are the real athletes (albeit in a virtual reality). Contrast this with asking students in physical education to stand stationary apart from each other and practice the basketball chest pass or bounce pass, first in late primary and then again in each year of postprimary. As teachers, we should not act surprised that students get bored and fail to see the meaning of it all.

The sedentary nature of extended **screen time** is also a threat from a public health perspective, in that it is associated with developing obesity and inactivity (Lanningham-Foster et al., 2006). In addition, the playing of video games is also linked to poor school performance (Gentile, Lynch, Linder, & Walsh, 2004).

Learning Experience 17.2

Choose 3 consecutive days, and estimate how much time you believe you will be engaged in sedentary activities using all forms of technology, including television, computers (desktops, notebooks, or tablets), and your mobile phone. Then, using a simple time log and a stopwatch, mark down the time that you spend sedentary using these same devices at any time over the course of those 3 consecutive days. Also, mark down how many hours you spent asleep during each of the 3 days. After the third day, and not counting the time that you spent asleep, calculate the percentage of time for each day that you spent using/interacting directly with technology.

Reflect on these results, especially given the estimates you made beforehand. Were the actual percentages higher, lower, or right on? If you over- or underestimated the percentages, what might have caused that?

On the positive side, there is evidence that children and youth engaging in "active" video games expend more energy than those interacting with "inactive" video games (e.g., Foley & Maddison, 2010; Graves, Stratton, Ridgers, & Cable, 2007; Lenzer, 2010; Maloney et al., 2008). Some policy makers are starting to make significant financial investments in the use of **active video game** hardware and software for use in school physical education programs. For example, Schiesel (2007) reported that all of West Virginia's primary and postprimary schools would be outfitted with the Dance-Dance-Revolution hardware and software.

In a recent review of the available research literature on the effects of active video games on measures of energy expenditure, Biddiss and Irwin (2010) found that, although active video games will increase light to moderate physical activity levels, not all games are created equal. Games emphasizing mostly upper body use resulted in significantly less energy expenditure than those requiring mostly lower body movements. Barnett, Cerin, and Baranowski (2011) completed a similar review, but included an assessment of the degree to which active video game use is sustained over time by youth. They concluded that although active video games can and do contribute to youth reaching recommended physical activity levels, most of them do not sustain their play even after a short period of time.

Most recently, Active Healthy Kids Canada (see www.activehealthykids.ca) completed a comprehensive analysis of all available evidence on active video games (also known as "exergames"). Their conclusion:

> *Active Healthy Kids Canada does not recommend active video games as a strategy to help kids be more physically active.*
>
> - *Playing active video games doesn't lead to increased overall daily physical activity levels.*
> - *Active video games may get heart rates up, but they're not significantly helping kids get to the 60 minutes of moderate- to vigorous-intensity physical activity required each day.*
> - *Kids find active video games appealing, but the appeal wears off over time and many don't stick with them.*
>
> *Active video games don't offer the fresh air, vitamin D, connection with nature and social interactions that come with outdoor active play. (Active Healthy Kids Canada, n.d.)*

Teachers' Receptivity to Incorporating Technology

People approach learning to do something new in varying ways. It is no different for learning about and learning how to use new technology. Some teachers will embrace technology with open arms. They are willing to invest significant amounts of time and energy to learn about it, are comfortable with technology in general, are eager to implement it, and are able to see how it would work best in their own situation. Others may be more hesitant and prefer to see how well it works when colleagues use it before they take the plunge. Still others have a mindset that (for varied reasons) reflects an outright unwillingness to even consider learning about new technology tools, let alone using them. For example, Fernández-Balboa (2003) and Stidder and Capel (2010) reported that some physical education teachers see any uses of technology or innovation as detracting from the core purpose of our field, increasing physical activity for the purpose of learning.

According to Rogers (1995), the following conditions must be present if teachers are to embrace and successfully build technology into their teaching. First, teachers should have the opportunity to utilize technology on a trial basis before it is implemented full scale. Trying out the technology on a small scale allows teachers to become more comfortable with it and see the possible value. Second, teachers should be able to readily see observable results of using the technology. Third, it must have an advantage over other technologies or other traditional approaches of doing one's work. Fourth, the technology must be relatively easy to figure out. If the device or software is too complex, teachers are much less likely to use it. Finally, the technology must be compatible with other existing practices. Similarly, there is evidence that if preservice teachers see technology modeled by program faculty, get frequent opportunities to use the technology throughout the program, and receive support from instructors and peers, they are more likely to have a more positive attitude toward employing different forms of technology and are more likely to adopt it in their teaching (e.g., Crowe, 2003; Crowe & van 't Hooft, 2006; Hunt & Bohlin, 1995; Keiper, Harwod, & Larson, 2000; Mason & Berson, 2000).

Learning Experience 17.3

Describe what forms of technology you are currently using on a regular basis while teaching groups of students in physical education settings. (If you are not currently teaching physical education classes yourself, approach a physical educator and request the opportunity to observe him or her.) Explain the reason(s) why you (or the observed teacher) are or are not using technology.

Technology: To Use or Not to Use

The information presented thus far offers a picture of how technology is not inherently beneficial or detrimental to teachers and students. As Bill Gates once implied, it is teachers themselves who ultimately are the most important people in deciding how and if the tool of technology may be best utilized and how to infuse technology into lessons in ways that will actually benefit their own teaching and/or their students' development.

One of the difficulties surrounding the infusion of technology is that it is assumed that, because instruction is computer-based, it must inherently be of better quality than "traditional" approaches to instruction, and that we should bank on technology with blind faith. As well, those who strongly believe in technology are often so passionate that they may portray a new piece of technology or software program as a "silver bullet" that will solve all problems that teachers face.

Learning Experience 17.4

You have just received notice that you and your colleagues in your school can apply for one of ten $25,000 grants for infusing technology that will support your physical education program. Draft a proposal on how you would invest these funds. Your proposal should include the following:

- Type of equipment/device/software
- Cost per item (or set)
- Vendor/supplier
- Rationale for each item on your list of purchase requests (i.e., how you will use each item and how each item impacts your ability to deliver your program and/or support your students' learning experiences)

A related contradiction is the fact that despite the enormous expense, in some countries and communities new technology continues to be infused into today's classrooms. At the same time, other areas in school budgets are reduced, resulting in larger class sizes, teachers being laid off, and reduced weekly minutes allocated to music, art, and physical education (Richtel, 2011). Especially in older school buildings, outfitting, repairing, maintaining, and upgrading technology infrastructure take up a significant portion of the overall investments. Depending on the technology equipment itself or the building structure, simple teacher tasks such as sending student attendance records to the main office in postprimary schools may be hampered by inconsistent or slow transmission, potentially even forcing physical educators to copy electronic records onto paper and have a student bring them to the office. Perhaps one area that is often neglected is the need for teachers to get professional development and training on how new equipment or other technology devices and software can/should be implemented.

Heavy financial investment in technology does not automatically translate into improved teaching and/or student learning. One example is a school district of 19 primary and 6 middle schools in Arizona that invested almost $33 million to equip all its classrooms with tablet computers, interactive smartboards, software, and other components, all aimed at improving student performance in reading and math. At the same time, physical education periods were reduced to only once a week for 45 minutes, and periods in art and music were also reduced. Despite these efforts, student scores in math remained flat, whereas similar districts' scores have improved (Richtel, 2011).

Regardless, physical educators should at the very least continue to stay up-to-date on what new technologies are available and how they work, so they can make more informed decisions on which to infuse into their program. This will help them determine that some types of technology may be too expensive for individual teachers to purchase, whereas others are quite reasonable. Some may require additional training in order to become sufficiently familiar with their use, whereas others are so intuitive that teachers can implement them immediately.

There is some initial evidence that technology can be very beneficial for student learning. For example, Casey and Jones (2011) reported that students described as "problem" students improved their understanding of throwing and catching and reported feeling less marginalized through the use of video technology. However, Thomas and Stratton (2006) conducted a national assessment of physical educators' use of information communication technology in the United Kingdom. Their findings are a sobering reminder that physical educators are slow to embrace the many available technologies. The most widely used piece of technology was the CD player (a rapidly disappearing technology in recent years given the available digital music technology). PowerPoint was the presentation software of choice, when that type of software was used. Moreover, although digital cameras were readily available in nearly all schools, physical educators rarely employed them in their teaching.

In this section, we offer a series of questions that teachers can and should ask when considering guidelines and criteria to determine the efficacy and worthiness of technology, as well as guidelines for easing the process of embracing and implementing the various technology tools. Right or not, education in general is often criticized for using antiquated approaches to teaching. Yet schools increasingly invest heavily in implementing computer technologies for the purposes of data management and tracking students' performance. In addition, companies continue to develop new software programs for use in instruction in classroom subjects. Technology tools for use in physical education are also becoming increasingly prevalent. Mohnson (2012) provides an expansive overview of possible technology uses in teaching physical education, including basic word processing, spreadsheet and database management, photography, digital video, audio systems, Internet, software, measurement devices (e.g., body composition, strength, GPS, cardiovascular capacity), and online learning. Additional examples of relatively new technologies include iPads, Wi-Fi, exergaming (e.g., Dance-Dance-Revolution, Wii systems, the X-box Kinect games), iPhone and/or Android applications for smartphones, and the use of global positioning systems (GPS) for geocaching (a modern day treasure hunt game; see www.geocaching.com).

The following are four key questions teachers can ask when considering using different technologies in their teaching:

1. *Is the cost of the technology worth it in terms of its potential impact on student learning?* In order to determine what the actual advantages and disadvantages are, teachers must take time to become familiar with the tool or equipment, and test it out. Many companies will allow a 30-day free trial of a particular type of software. When considering the purchase of new computer or video game hardware, be sure to determine whether the equipment can be returned within a certain time period without penalty. This will afford teachers the chance to try out the equipment and determine whether it meets the needs of their students or themselves. Only then will you be able make a sound cost–benefit determination.

   Importantly, Casey and Jones (2011) noted that teachers would be wise to carefully review the multiple technology choices. Given the needs of the teacher, investing in the lower cost ones may prove to be the better choice.
2. *Will the technology work effectively in the physical education teaching environment?* The physical education environment is fundamentally different from classroom settings. While in classrooms, students spend most of their time in seats, and each student may have access to a computer. In physical education, the emphasis is (or should be) primarily on movement. Various types of technology are now so commonplace that their efficacy is no longer questioned (e.g., data projectors, heart rate monitors, pedometers). However, new technologies (and their newer improved versions) are brought to market at such a high rate that it may not be clear immediately whether a piece of equipment or software can be used and how it could best be used. One example is the recent emergence of Apple's iPad. This small tablet has a broad range of uses. For example, Sinelnikov (2012) described how teachers can use the iPad in creative ways within Sport Education and help shift responsibilities and ownership to students. As of the summer of 2012, well over 100,000 apps had been developed specifically for use with iPads. Importantly, the PEGeek website (see www.thepegeek.com) keeps physical educators current on the latest app developments for mobile devices. An excellent example is Coach's Eye (available through iTunes), which is an app that enables physical educators and sport coaches to provide quick video-based feedback to learners. It is similar to video analysis programs like Dartfish (see www.dartfish.com) but at a much lower cost. Another example of a low-cost app is Highlights Sports Recorder (available on iTunes). This app may be especially useful for showing learners their actions during game play as part of using the freeze replay strategy (Launder & Piltz, 2013). Learners can see a retrace of their movement instantaneously, which teachers can then use as a springboard for briefly discussing other options or reinforcing quality game play. Perhaps one of the most attractive features of such mobile device applications is that teachers can carry the mobile devices around in their pocket and employ them at any time throughout the lesson. Quickly capturing, storing, and retrieving photo or video images will require some practice by teachers, but this type of technology can offer powerful support to students. Although policies and laws will differ across countries, physical educators always must be mindful of them relative to having consent from parents and guardians to photograph and/or video their students.

   Moreover, the PEGeek website continues to produce more apps specific to teaching physical education. The key for teachers is to determine which apps are user-friendly in the context of teaching physical education. A related issue is the ease with which a piece of technology can be set up or removed. From a time management perspective, it is essential that the setup and startup of the equipment do not take away valuable class time and time for other critical teaching functions such as instruction and assessment. Effective teachers will develop routines where they can overlap the equipment setup with learning activities and/or have students assist with the setup.

3. *How much of a learning curve will there be before you are comfortable using it to its fullest extent within your teaching?* The efficacy of any technology tool is influenced by how easy it is to master its use. If it takes weeks or months to reach the point where a teacher can use the tool seamlessly, the risk of a teacher losing interest will likely increase. Related to this, teachers have to be willing to spend time outside of teaching to become familiar with the specifics of a technology tool.
4. *How much of a "novelty effect" is there among students when using the new technology?* As noted earlier, the initial data on whether students will continue to use certain types of active video games are not promising as yet. Thus, teachers will want to be mindful of the potential risk of initial enthusiasm and excitement for a new tool, device, or game wearing off and interest waning after a period of time. No doubt the rapid advances in technology in other aspects of life reinforce students' seeming insatiable appetite for newer and more exciting technology, which renders last year's technology as "old and boring." When choosing technology that students would use, one of the key criteria is **device staying power** (i.e., the degree to which use of a technology device or program is sustained over time).

Examples of how technology can be used in a physical education teaching setting include: (1) keeping attendance, (2) storing and retrieving fitness test scores, (3) filing electronic lesson plans, (4) keeping inventory, (5) grading, (6) tracking student physical activity levels, (7) recording student performance in the various learning domains (e.g., psychomotor, cognitive, affective), (8) performing assessments of various skills and behaviors associated with learning, and (9) expanding available resources via Internet capabilities. In the next section, we provide several examples of how teachers can utilize technology to support their various instructional efforts, student learning experiences, and other related aspects of their work.

Technology for Enhancing Instruction

Physical educators have countless forms of technology available to enhance the quality of their instruction. First and foremost, the Internet provides a wealth of resources that teachers can use to stay abreast of the latest developments in the field (see **Tables 17.2 through 17.9** for examples). Internet use for professional purposes ranges from lesson plan development to content selection and design, obtaining information for use in advocacy when addressing policy makers, remaining current on trends and issues, finding new activity resources, and reading about the latest research on teaching and coaching in physical activity settings. Moreover, with the increasing presence of social media such as Facebook, Twitter, and blogs, teachers can stay connected and receive updated information as it becomes available. A noted physical education technology expert in the United Kingdom, Casey (personal communication) noted that physical educators would describe this as the best form of professional development they have engaged in. The following Twitter hashtags offer physical educators a highly interactive means of conversing with colleagues about virtually any professional questions: #PEgeeks, #pechat, or #Physed; #edchat and #ukedchat are hashtags for those interested in discussions around general education issues.

TABLE 17.2 Teaching and Curriculum Sites: Be Connected

ABC of Rock Climbing	www.abc-of-rockclimbing.com
Be Active New York State	www.beactivenys.org/mfl
The Art of Coaching Volleyball	www.theartofcoachingvolleyball.com
EPEC	www.michiganfitness.org/epec
Essential Tennis	www.essentialtennis.com
Expert Village	www.expertvillage.com
Fuzzy Yellow Balls	www.fuzzyyellowballs.com
Health and PE	www.awesomelibrary.org/health.html
Healthy Kids Challenge	www.healthykidschallenge.com
Healthy People	www.healthypeople.gov/2020
Howcast How-Tos	www.howcast.com
Let's Move	www.letsmove.gov
PE Central	www.pecentral.org
PE4life	www.pe4life.org
Physical Education Software	www.pesoftware.com
The Physical Educator	www.thephysicaleducator.com
Play Sports TV	www.playsportstv.com
SPARK	www.sparkpe.org
Take 10: Classroom-based physical activity	www.take10.net
Teach PE	www.teachpe.com
Tennis Instruction	www.tennis.com/instruction
TV Turn off Network	www.tvturnoff.org
U.S. Tennis Association (for schools)	www.usta.com/Youth-Tennis/Schools/SchoolsHome

TABLE 17.3 Advocacy and Policy-Related Target Sites: Be Connected

Active Living Research	www.activelivingresearch.org/toolsandresources/all
American Alliance for Health, Physical Education, Recreation and Dance Advocacy and Legislative Action Center	www.aahperd.org/whatwedo/advocacy
The Council of State Governments	www.csg.org
FirstGov.gov	www.usa.gov
Healthfinder.gov	www.healthfinder.gov
National Association of State Boards of Education Healthy Policy Database	www.nasbe.org/healthy_schools/hs
National Conference of State Legislatures	www.ncsl.org
National Governors Association	www.nga.org
National School Boards Association	www.nsba.org
Society of State Leaders of Health and Physical Education	www.thesociety.org
U.S. Conference of Mayors	www.usmayors.org
U.S. House of Representatives	www.house.gov
U.S. State Senate	www.senate.gov
The White House	www.whitehouse.gov

TABLE 17.4 Professional Organizations and Development Sites: Be Connected

Action for Healthy Kids	www.actionforhealthykids.org
American Alliance for Health, Physical Education, Recreation and Dance	www.aahperd.org
American College of Sports Medicine	www.acsm.org
American Council on Exercise	www.acefitness.org
Association for Supervision and Curriculum Development	www.ascd.org
Institute of Medicine	www.iom.edu
International Association for Physical Education in Higher Education	www.aiesep.ulg.ac.be
International Council for Health, Physical Education, Recreation, Sport, and Dance	www.ichpersd.org
National Academy of Kinesiology	www.nationalacademyofkinesiology.org
National Association for Sport and Physical Education	www.aahperd.org/Naspe
National Board for Professional Teaching Standards	www.nbpts.org
The President's Council on Fitness, Sports and Nutrition	www.fitness.gov

TABLE 17.5 Adapted Physical Education and Sport: Be Connected

American Association of Adapted Sports Programs	www.adaptedsports.org
Courage Center Sports and Recreation	www.couragecenter.org/sports
Deaflympics	www.deaflympics.com
Disabled Sports USA	www.dsusa.org
Dwarf Athletic Association of America	www.daaa.org
International Federation of Adapted Physical Activity	www.ifapa.biz
National Beep Baseball Association	www.nbba.org
National Center on Health, Physical Activity and Disability	www.ncpad.org
National Center on Physical Motor Opportunities Via Education (Move)	www.move-international.org
National Consortium for Physical Education and Recreation for Individuals with Disabilities	www.ncperid.org
National Sports Center for the Disabled	www.nscd.org
National Wheelchair Basketball Association	www.nwba.org
Palaestra	www.Palaestra.com
Paralympics	www.paralympic.org
Special Olympics	www.specialolympics.org
Sport in Society	www.northeastern.edu/sportinsociety
USA Deaf Sports Federation	www.usdeafsports.org
U.S. Association of Blind Athletes	www.usaba.org
U.S. Paralympics	www.usparalympics.org
U.S. Quad Rugby Association	www.quadrugby.com
Wheelchair Sports USA	www.wsusa.org

TABLE 17.6 Related Health and Fitness/Sport Sites: Be Connected

Alliance for a Healthier Generation	www.healthiergeneration.org
American Obesity Association	www.obesity.org
Centers for Disease Control and Prevention, Division of Nutrition, Physical Activity, and Obesity	www.cdc.gov/nccdphp/dnpao
Centers for Disease Control and Prevention: Fruits and Vegetables	www.cdc.gov/nutrition/everyone/fruitsvegetables/index.html
ExRx.net: Exercise Prescription	www.exrx.net
Human Kinetics	www.humankinetics.com
National Alliance for Youth Sports (NAYS)	www.nays.org
National Coalition for Promoting Physical Activity	www.ncppa.org
National Strength and Conditioning Association	www.nsca-lift.org
The Nemours Foundation	www.kidshealth.org
Sports and Fitness Industry Association	www.sgma.com
USDA Team Nutrition	www.teamnutrition.usda.gov
U.S. Olympic Committee	www.teamusa.org

TABLE 17.7 Children and Youth Sport: Be Connected

National Alliance for Youth Sports	www.nays.org
American Sport Education Program	www.asep.com
Center for Sports Parenting	www.sportsparenting.org
Character Counts	www.charactercounts.org
Mom's Team: Youth Sport Parenting Information	www.momsteam.com
National Council of Youth Sports	www.ncys.org
North American Youth Sports Institute	www.naysi.com
Positive Coaching Alliance	www.positivecoach.org
Sport for All	www.s4af.org
St. Louis Sports Commission Sportsmanship Initiative	www.sportsmanship.org
Youth Sport Network	www.myteam.com
Youth Sport Trust	www.youthsporttrust.org

TABLE 17.8 Women's Sport: Be Connected

Empowering Women in Sports	www.feminist.org/sports/index.asp
National Association for Girls and Women in Sport	www.aahperd.org/nagws
Title IX—Equity Online	www.edc.org/womensEquity
Title IX—National Women's Law Center	www.nwlc.org
Title IX—Office for Civil Rights	http://www2.ed.gov/about/offices/list/ocr/index.html
Women in Sports	www.Makeithappen.com/wis
Women in Sports Careers	www.WiscFoundation.org
Women's Sports Foundation	www.womenssportsfoundation.org

TABLE 17.9 Supplementary Information Sites: Be Connected

American Academy of Pediatrics: Overweight and Obesity	www.aap.org/obesity/index.html
Amateur Athletic Union	www.aausports.org
American Association for the Child's Right to Play	www.ipausa.org
Brain Gym International	www.braingym.org
Centers for Disease Control and Prevention: Physical Activity Facts	www.cdc.gov/HealthyYouth/PhysicalActivity
Coordinated School Health Initiative	www.cdc.gov/healthyyouth/cshp
Dr. John Ratey	www.johnratey.com
Energizing Brain Breaks	www.brainbreaks.blogspot.com
The Eunice Kennedy Shriver National Institute of Child Health and Human Development	www.nichd.nih.gov
International Association of Athletics Federations	www.iaaf.org
National Association of Sports Officials	www.naso.org
National Institute for Fitness and Sport	www.nifs.org
Centers for Disease Control and Prevention: Healthy Youth	www.cdc.gov/HealthyYouth/shpps/index.htm
Physical Education Update	www.physicaleducationupdate.com
Responsible Educators Accountable for Learning	www.supportrealteachers.org
Sports Media	www.sports-media.org
VERB (a national advertising campaign for PA)	www.cdc.gov/youthcampaign

Learning Experience 17.5

Use the Internet resources provided in the Tables 17.2 through 17.9 to develop a short presentation that you can use to advocate for and/or promote physical education as a program to a group of constituents (e.g., parents, school management). The focus could be on a variety of topics, such as the role/importance of physical education in schools, the benefits of physical activity, the national guidelines/recommendations for physical activity in your respective country, how the program is linked with other programs in the community, or the like.

One example of an excellent reference website is the online technology newsletter for K–12 physical education teachers on Dr. Bonnie Mohnson's website, www.pesoftware.com/technews. Teachers can find information about the latest developments in computer and video hardware and computer software and the varied uses of such technology tools.

A similar resource for remaining abreast of the latest trends and issues is the pelinks4u website (see www.pelinks4u.org). This website provides a free monthly newsletter of sorts that includes information sections on adapted physical education, sport coaching, primary physical education, post-primary physical education, and health, fitness, and nutrition.

Importantly, this site also offers additional web links to other related Internet sources.

In the United States, perhaps the most popular resource website for physical educators for over 15 years has been the PE Central website (see www.PECentral.org). Started by George Graham and its current website manager Mark Manross, it includes information resources for students and teachers, as well as parents and school managers. Examples of resources that are available range from class management to lesson plan ideas, assessment, job listings, and use of various media. A recent addition to the site is the "Log it" link, which allows students to track their own physical activity levels. PE Central also includes links to other sites offering important informational resources. Evidence of the site's popularity is the number of site visits. In recent years, PE Central has averaged approximately 150,000 unique visitors per month.

There are also countless software programs that individual teachers or schools can use to handle managerial and organizational tasks such as student grading. Examples include Gradekeeper (see www.gradekeeper.com), Class Mate Gradebook (see www.classmategrading.com), Easy Grade Pro (see www.easygradepro.com), and Gradebook (see www.thinkwave.com). Some are free, whereas others offer a free 30-day trial period. Some can be used on both PC and Apple **operating platforms**, whereas others work on only one. Increasingly, most school systems have moved to employing centralized software systems such as Genesis (see www.genesisedu.com), which is used in New Jersey. In addition to tracking students' grades, such comprehensive software programs enable schools to manage student registration, attendance, class scheduling, student medical records, and so on.

Software programs for word processing, spreadsheets, and presentations have been part of the technology landscape since the early 1980s. Most students are introduced to using these programs in primary and postprimary schools, and the programs are now so commonplace that for most students they are second nature. If prospective teachers are still not familiar with their basic uses, interactive tutorials and workshops are readily available on the Internet. A quick Internet search using the software name (e.g., "Excel tutorial") will direct teachers to an extensive array of tutorial options.

Some curriculum programs now also come with extensive web-based resources to aid teachers in planning and implementing their lesson activities. Examples include the Active and Healthy Schools program (see www.activeandhealthyschools.com), the SPARK program (see www.sparkpe.org), and the Sport Education model. The latter provides web-based resources that enable teachers to plan and implement authentic and developmentally appropriate sport experiences. The resources range from tournament forms to team banners, fair-play prompts, team binder materials such as coach guidelines, score sheets, and other supporting materials for the various nonplayer roles (e.g., coach, referee, scorekeeper, manager, statistician). All resources can be downloaded and modified so teachers can customize them to fit their own teaching contexts. As physical educators build their digital resources to support their teaching (especially when they start employing digital video), they should be mindful of the issue of storage capacity either on their computers or in the cloud (online). Whereas 15 years ago a consumer-level 1-gigabyte hard drive might have been considered excessively big, today's digital video technologies require storage capacities that easily exceed 1 terabyte.

Building Your Content and Pedagogical Content Knowledge Using Technology

Siedentop (2002) argued persuasively that physical educators can never develop credible pedagogical content knowledge (PCK) without having a strong knowledge of the content being taught; that is, without knowing about the techniques, tactics, rules, history, safety, and/or etiquette of archery, dance, tennis, or weight training, you will not be able to teach it. The Internet has become an extensive resource to learn about content. It offers a variety of excellent activity-specific websites that can help improve teachers' content knowledge of specific activities. Combining verbal and visual information, these websites offer users good insight into the critical elements for proper execution of techniques in sport, fitness, and/or outdoor pursuits (as well as common errors among beginners). Examples of such websites include www.fuzzyyellowballs.com (for tennis), www.revolutiongolf.com (for golf), and www.abc-of-rockclimbing.com (for rock climbing). These sites give teachers access to content experts who are steeped in the content. Although these experts may not work with children and youth, they provide teachers with important knowledge about *what* to teach. Some of these websites offer free access during which certain content may be accessible for a limited amount of time (e.g., 3 days). A nominal annual fee enables the user to have unlimited/continued access.

Physical educators have various types of hardware available to enhance their instruction. They include smartboards, very compact video cameras such as GoPro cameras, tablets (e.g., iPads), and smartphones. Smartboards are anchored to classroom walls and offer interactive features enabling teachers to switch among multiple software programs during instructional episodes. With some practice, compact and lightweight equipment such as GoPro cameras, tablets, and smartphones are easy to use. Tablets and smartphones allow teachers to show video examples of how to execute a particular technique, videotape students in action and provide immediate feedback, and/or collect data on student performance during classes for the purpose of formal assessment. No doubt the continuing growth of available apps for tablets and smartphones will include more and more options specific to the physical education teaching/learning environment.

With the limited amount of weekly class time available for physical education, one of the key dilemmas for physical educators is how to balance class time between instruction (where students are largely sedentary/inactive) and activity (where students are actively engaged in learning activities). However, technology can play a powerful role in bringing students in direct contact with pertinent information outside of class time. Out-of-class (homework) assignments can be developed using a variety of technologies. For example, Google Docs, **podcasts**, and **vodcasts** (i.e., video-on-demand casts) enable teachers to share key content knowledge with students beyond the class meetings. Vodcasts are video clips that are accessible online just like podcasts. Use of each of these technologies will require some instruction and practice, but numerous Internet-based tutorials can be readily found by using one of the following websites, by typing in "creating vodcasts," which then offer search options and step-by-step directions on creating vodcasts:

- Google (www.google.com)
- YouTube (www.youtube.com)
- SchoolTube (www.schooltube.com)
- TeacherTube (www.teachertube.com)

As is the case in classroom subjects, physical educators do need to build some type of accountability mechanism into the course to ensure that students do access and study the material made available beyond the class period.

Wikis are another tool that teachers can use to foster learning outside of class time. A wiki is essentially a website that enables users to develop, add, edit, change, and/or delete its content, using a regular **web browser** (e.g., Firefox, Safari). Wikis can be used for taking notes and managing new knowledge. One example of using a wiki in physical education could occur during a Olympics competition within Sport Education, when team members could work together on building a country profile. In a recent project, Hastie, Casey, and Tarter (2010) reported that during a unit on student-designed games, the use of wikis helped students develop better quality games.

Other ways in which technology can extend a physical education program include the use of **listservs**, enabling teachers to communicate with groups of students quickly, again beyond the regular class times. For example, in Ireland, a physical education listserv is available to all teachers who choose to discuss, pose questions, or consult one another on topics related to any aspect of teaching in physical education. Other ways of communicating information to students include electronic message systems such as bulletin boards, where individuals can post and read messages, and chat rooms, where students can converse on issues related to their classwork. Of course, a physical education program webpage is also a powerful means of communicating not only with student and parents but also with the broader surrounding community. This is especially pertinent in the context of comprehensive school physical activity programs where the school is the community's hub for physical activity. In addition, social media such as Facebook and Instagram are another means of conveying information to students, parents, and other constituents.

A relatively new option for teachers to engage in informal continuing professional development, and to learn, converse, and share information is the Physical Education Practitioner Research Network (see www.peprn.com). The site seeks to encourage interactions between school- and university-based physical education professionals. Through blogs, RSS (Really Simple Syndication) feeds, and Twitter, professionals can learn about and stay current on new developments, and share perspectives regarding a variety of topics and issues in school physical education.

Technology can also be used to extend the physical education program in interesting ways. For example, during the Winter and Summer Olympics, a program could be organized around the Olympics theme. In addition, physical education classes in the United States have linked with classes in the host countries to discuss issues involving the games. In the 1990s, a student group in a Nebraska postprimary school used only email to organize a track meet involving 17 schools from around the world. Each school conducted similar meets and compared times, distances, and heights for each event. Overall results and standings were then distributed to each school (Mills, 1997).

Learning Experience 17.6

Using Internet resources provided in Table 17.2, develop a set of five instructional aids (e.g., skill task cards, fitness task signs) that you can use to highlight key concepts, terms, or other directions for how to do the selected activities that you describe.

More recently, primary classes in Auburn, Alabama, participated in a Sport Education season with similar school classes in Spain and Portugal. The competition included three divisions: the Wildcats, Birds, and Reptiles. Each division contained teams such as Snow Leopards, Pink Panthers, Screaming Eagles, Spitting Cobras, and so on. Each team contained players from all three countries. Their respective team scores (e.g., games won, fair play points) were pooled to determine team/league standings across countries. The season's team standings and team performance statistics were kept up-to-date and posted on a dedicated website. During the season, team members from different countries would Skype with each other each Friday and discuss their games. Although a language barrier was present, it was overcome because students in the three countries were sufficiently multilingual (Hastie, personal communication).

Finally, with the emergence of programs like Skype and FaceTime, physical educators can invite outside speakers and other experts to join a class. Consequently, students gain more exposure to outside expertise, which can thus enrich the learning environment.

Technology and Continuing Professional Development

We want to highlight how technology plays a key role in continued professional development (CPD). For example, an increasing number of departments of physical education (or exercise science or human movement) in the United States are offering a master's degree program in an online format (e.g., Jacksonville State University, Central Washington University, University of Utah). Although there is no evidence as yet that fully online (or hybrid version) degree programs are equal to, better than, or worse than a traditional face-to-face program in terms of outcomes, no doubt other universities around the globe will follow suit.

In addition, a number of advanced digital video analysis systems are available today that enable users to do more fine-grained analyses of teaching performance (and student performance) (e.g., www.dartfish.com). Digital video technology has made the development of videos of teaching episodes much easier, and, with some practice, software programs such as iMovie (for Apple computers) and Windows Movie Maker enable users to develop high-quality video-based portfolios of one's teaching. In addition, systematic observation software such as The Observer (see www.noldus.com) allows teachers and researchers to collect data on teaching events, producing immediate data summaries.

Learning Experience 17.7

Using the Internet resources provided in Table 17.4 or other related websites, find out what the professional development opportunities and other benefits are of the national professional organization or society in your country.

Technology for Enhancing Student Learning

Many of the technology examples noted in the previous section are aimed at enhancing instruction, yet they can also (directly or indirectly) enhance students' learning experiences. In this section we highlight several that can support the learning of key concepts and help shape physically active lifestyles. We highlight the following: heart rate monitors, pedometers, exercise equipment, computers, and the Internet.

Heart Rate Monitors

Heart rate (HR) monitors enable students to track and monitor exercise patterns and learn how varying activity intensity affects the heart. Depending on the type and quality of HR monitor, data can be downloaded and saved to computers, where students can graph, analyze, and interpret them, including changes over time. As is outlined in the various health-related physical education curriculum models (e.g., Fitness for Life, SPARK), one of the key outcomes is for students to conduct personal fitness assessments relative to health-related fitness components. Tools such as HR monitors, along with the Trifit 700 System (see www.PolarUSA.com), are an integral part of numerous physical education programs throughout the United States.

One of the better-known examples of how a school physical education program incorporated such technologies occurred at Naperville (Illinois) North High School. In the 1990s, the physical education department mounted a sustained effort to rebuild the physical education program based on a health-club approach with a strong health-related fitness focus. Through grants and other fundraisers, the school's physical education staff acquired the needed equipment and computer support enabling students to engage in health-enhancing physical activity and teaching them to monitor their own fitness and physical activity levels.

One excellent example of a program embracing deliberate infusion of technology throughout physical education is the Dyffryn Taf School in Whitland, Carmarthenshire, in Wales. The teachers at this school have woven technology throughout all classes. Students regularly can be seen using hardware; software such as spreadsheets; Moodle; blogging; podcasts; handheld devices such as iPhones, iPod Touch, and iPads; Skype; and skill performance analysis software. The teachers have developed a program website (see www.dyffryntaf.org.uk/sports) with extensive information and updates for both students and their parents. Students are encouraged to use handheld devices to videotape their performance, which is then used for feedback and self-reflection. They use iMovie to develop performance records that include narratives and written materials in support of the video records. They also use spreadsheet programs to record their heart rate levels (Blain, 2012).

Pedometers

Students' fitness levels are influenced by a number of variables other than their physical activity. Two prime examples are the type and quantity of food and beverages, and genetic endowment (Bouchard, Blair, & Haskell, 2012). Physical activity has been shown to have important health benefits relative to reducing a number of health risks. This evidence has been an important impetus for the promotion of physical activity among children, youth, and adults. Along with this information has come improved pedometer technology, to the point where it is now an accepted device for use in both applied/clinical settings (e.g., personal use, physical education) and formal research. Compared to other physical activity tracking devices (e.g., accelerometers, GPS), pedometers are easy to use and relatively low in cost.

Cheap pedometers are often given away as part of promotions in fast food restaurants, provided at conferences, and available through sporting goods stores or online vendors. Teachers should avoid purchasing cheaper pedometers because they are more prone to breaking down and/or being inaccurate. There is extensive evidence that Yamax (see www.yamax.com) and Walk4Life (see www.Walk4Life.com/home/default.aspx) build quality pedometers.

Depending on the type, pedometers can be used to count steps, time spent in physical activity, and distance traveled (depending on the stride length set). In the latest designs, pedometers can be set so they can provide an estimate of light, moderate, and vigorous levels of physical activity based on the cut-points set for steps per minute. That is, the higher the number of steps per minute, the higher the intensity. Some pedometers even provide the user with verbal encouragement and/or reinforcement based on the accumulated step count.

As with HR monitors, students can use pedometers to track their own physical activity levels per lesson, per day, and/or per week. Students can wear the pedometers over the course of several days. The resulting information can then be compared to national guidelines/recommendations and/or to set personal physical activity goals. There are also useful resources available to assist physical educators with implementing pedometers in physical education lessons (e.g., Pangrazi, Beighle, & Sidman, 2007).

Exercise Equipment

Incorporation of computer technology continues to improve fitness/activity equipment as well. The computer software built into treadmills, stair climbers, and elliptical bikes includes expansive features that allow users to customize the type, intensity, and duration of the activity; connect to televisions; and choose from various video-based challenges and sceneries, allowing the use to bike or jog through the Alps while actually exercising in their gym. Other examples of software-supported exercise equipment are those where body movement controls movements on the screen using a plug-and-play video game controller. Examples include the GameBike (see www.gamebike.com), Wii Fitness, and Dance-Dance-Revolution.

Mobile Technology

The aforementioned iPads enable students to develop their own videos of their performances in a variety of activities. Such video clips can become part of students' portfolios. In Sport Education, sport broadcasters can use the iPad to give a running account of the game's action while also videotaping the game. These are all authentic learning experiences that provide direct artifacts of learning. Other examples of how students can demonstrate their learning from a public health perspective are Runkeeper (see www.RunKeeper.com) and the Nike+ (see http://nikeplus.nike.com/plus). Both are apps for mobile devices that allow students to track their own activity levels. Such tools may be quite powerful in helping develop credible evidence of student learning, which is increasingly important in today's high-stakes accountability climate in many countries.

The Internet

As is the case for teachers, the Internet is an endless resource of information for students to aid in possible learning assignments. Historically, physical education programs have not included the use of formal homework assignments, however, the Internet and other software programs can put students in direct contact with ways to acquire important knowledge about activities and develop greater understanding. For example, the history and development of sports and other activities, sport etiquette, and the like can all be found on the Internet. During an outdoor pursuits unit (e.g., hiking), in preparation for certain lessons, students can be grouped and directed to use the Internet to learn about various steps involved in preparing for a multiday trip, the needed equipment, safety measures, first aid, and emergency procedures. Or as part of a strength-conditioning unit, students could be directed to web-based information to learn about the role of performance-enhancing drugs (PEDs). Other examples include out-of-class assignments where students use interactive tutorials on fitness concepts or sport instruction. Through these websites, students can learn how the heart works, or learn the rules of, and strategies for, a variety of sports.

Learning Experience 17.8

Design a homework assignment for students that requires them to access the Internet to find information pertinent to the current activity unit or season. Explain how it would connect with the unit and how it would enhance students' knowledge. How will you make sure that the students actually complete the assignment?

The advent of websites like YouTube (as well as Teacher Tube) has also given rise to an endless array of video clips on activities that teachers can have students watch (either during or outside of class) showing the technical execution of individual techniques. Because these are open websites where anyone can post videos, teachers need to decide which videos are appropriate in terms of content quality. Teachers who are teaching badminton, rock-climbing, or track-and-field can now easily direct students to specific YouTube links that highlight key information about the technical execution of the techniques at hand. Simply typing in "badminton drop shot technique" or "shot put glide technique" results in a wide array of examples of video models across a range of skill levels.

Learning Experience 17.9

Using YouTube, select a sport or other activity with which you are unfamiliar. Using the available video clips, develop a file (hard copy or electronic) with pertinent information that would strengthen your content knowledge specific to that activity. For example, if you wanted to learn some basic information about orienteering, plug in search terms such as "orienteering basics" or "map and compass use."

Assessment of Student Learning with Technology Tools

Students can be assessed on meaningful content using a variety of technology tools, as you have seen throughout this chapter. These tasks might range from one-time event tasks, such as interacting with the technology using heart rate monitors, recording scores in a computer program, or coding their own performance from a videotape, to more extensive assignments in which they design and present a multimedia project on selected physical education content. The extent to which these kinds of assessments can be implemented depends upon access to computers and other technology hardware within the school setting as well as teacher comfort with and training in the use of technology applications. Some schools have computer labs for students to access; others may have one computer per teacher or department. Still others may have only a computer for teachers to access through the library. There may be access to a variety of technology equipment (e.g., scanner, video camera, digital camera, Internet access, presentation programs, authoring programs) that can be scheduled on alternating or specific days, weeks, or even for a unit during which students rotate among equipment stations to develop their projects. These types of projects might be left wide open for student decisions or be more structured to meet specific intents of instruction.

For example, in a Sport Education soccer season, students performing the various roles for each team may be responsible for developing a presentation for the class to assist them with their responsibilities. The officials may access the Internet and search for examples of official score sheets, samples of how to keep game statistics, and a set of the official soccer rules. These materials could be pulled into standard presentation, spreadsheet, and/or word-processing software and used to teach a how-to session to the class, with hard copies developed and printed. The teams' publicists might design a newspaper template with a desktop publishing program, so they can publish stories on the soccer season as it progresses. If students have been introduced to basic web design in a different class, they might be asked to develop a team website where they can present the many kinds of artifacts of their team's performance (e.g., team motto, player profiles, action photos, game reports). Depending on student access to computers, they could choose to publish their newspaper using PowerPoint or Prezi (a relatively new cloud-based presentation software program; see www.prezi.com). They might also find some helpful tools to design awards using clip art and banners to add festivity to the season. Captains and coaches might work together to design, print, and post daily practice workouts along with a checklist for students to note when they have completed tasks. Trainers may have their teams alternately wear heart rate monitors to assess and record the amount of time they spend within their training HR zone during activity. The possibilities go on and on.

Simons Middle School in Birmingham, Alabama, has integrated technology into its physical education program in numerous ways with assessments that appropriately meet the challenges they set (Chestnutt, 1997). The school developed a course that provides students the opportunity to select and conduct an in-depth technology-based study of a sport or activity of their choice, culminating in a multimedia presentation summarizing their results and learning. Students may select from a variety of resources to assist in their research or presentation: heart rate monitors, video editing, digital cameras, interactive programs, and nutritional software. Students work individually and in small groups throughout the 9-week course, spending 3 days per week in activity and 2 days in research on their sport or activity. As students delve into their own sport or activity, they create an electronic and written portfolio that includes a series of specific tasks designed to assist them in their analysis, including the following:

- Heart rate analysis of five activities utilizing a spreadsheet, word processing, and HR monitors
- Multimedia reports (e.g., print, video, other graphic) around a topic pertinent to a specific sport/activity utilizing Hyper-Studio (see www.mackiev.com/hyperstudio/select.html)
- One self-selected task chosen from such tasks as reading biographies, interviewing, videotaping, developing practice plans, and designing a conditioning or nutritional plan
- A 5- to 7-minute final presentation to the class of a multimedia summary of research about the chosen sport/activity in video or slide format (i.e., PowerPoint, Persuasion)

Teachers' use of technology in teaching and assessing student performance is limited only by availability, access, and their own creativity and comfort with its use. Ask the students for help and ideas. In many cases they may be well ahead of you in terms of level of comfort with employing different forms of technology. As a physical educator you may be amazed at what they already know and can do with technology. Remember that being able to have students present such work to parents, other teachers, and school managers is a powerful tool to demonstrate that students are learning relevant and important skills.

The Future of Technology in Education

In 1980, few could have imagined how much technology would be affecting daily life and education to the extent it does today. Similarly, it is difficult to predict what new technologies will be commonplace in 2020, let alone 2030. In education, no doubt the ongoing development of new technologies will force schools and teachers to continuously replace, update, and/or upgrade their infrastructure to accommodate the new technology tools. Barber (2012) recently reported on what experts see as some current trends in **educational technology**. First, experts anticipate an increased emphasis on personalizing students' learning environments, which aligns with the continued call for student-centered instruction.

Second is the availability of improved mobile devices and digital content. This is contributing to a BYOT (Bring Your Own Technology) trend where schools are now increasingly encouraging student use of mobile devices so they can connect to virtual learning sites that can supplement in-class instruction (Ringle, 2012). Thus, K–12 students will be more likely to have constant access to tablets, smartphones, and netbooks anywhere, anytime. Though speculative, it is not hard to envision that following enormous investments, separate computer labs in schools will become obsolete in the next decade. In the United States and many other countries, mobile devices are starting to replace textbooks. For example, South Korean authorities recently allocated $2 billion to replace textbooks with tablet devices in primary and post-primary schools (Barber, 2012). Online tutoring technology is reaching the point where gaps in students' knowledge can be more easily determined, and subsequent learning tasks can be individualized. Related to this is the emergence of the field of *learning analytics*, which focuses on the development of software that supports personalized student learning not only by adapting to the needs of the students but also by providing teachers and school managers better insight into assessing student needs. This is closely related to the need for better formative assessment of student learning.

The notion of "Bring Your Own Technology" does bring with it the issue of equity and access to technology across all students. Economically disadvantaged families will be less likely to be able to afford the types of devices that other families might. Not unlike how the clothing worn to school by students can create differences, schools and teachers will need to consider this issue with care as they contemplate how far to push this BYOT approach because it can create and perpetuate social standing differences among students. School managers and policy makers must do all they can to manage technology investments in ways that ensure equity in access (Casey & Jones, 2011). BYOT also increases the odds that students will start multitasking by using the technology to text, check email, browse the web, and so on. Teachers will want to ensure that the in-class tasks and activities are designed such that students are less likely to lose focus and stray.

Third, digital learning environments will become more commonplace. This will constitute an advancement beyond e-books, which in many cases are PDF versions of the hard copy text. Digital learning environments add video and websites, simulations, and other visualizations to the learning experience.

A fourth trend is a focus on better bridging the digital divide between high-income and low-income technology users. Low-income families continue to be disadvantaged in terms of having consistent and reliable access to the Internet. For example, the U.S. government recently provided start-up funding for a program called Digital Promise aimed at (1) improving the process of bringing technological breakthroughs into classrooms, (2) supporting research and development around technology innovation in school environments, and (3) increasing the number of low-income households that can connect to the Internet (Barber, 2012).

Future classrooms will likely switch from being solely physical to more of a hybrid of a physical and virtual one. Given the continuing economic malaise in many countries, funding for supporting continued technology infusion in schools will most likely come from a variety of sources, including grants, technology fees, foundational donations, parental contributions, and regular operating budgets. Professional development for teachers to support the increased use of technology will continue to be a key need. Physical educators would be wise to keep abreast of developments in the areas of technology specific to physical education. The resources noted in this chapter should help in that effort. Moreover, keeping a finger on the pulse of various funding opportunities that support technology will position physical educators so that they can respond to such opportunities. This can only help them in terms of how their school managers view their professional development efforts.

One of the future trends specific to physical education may well be the move toward online physical education. Recently, Daum and Buschner (2012) reported that despite the limited empirical research and inconsistent results about its effectiveness to produce student learning, online learning is changing the overall landscape of education. In a survey of U.S. high school physical educators who teach online, they found that the educators generally focus on delivering a concepts-based fitness curriculum. Moreover, most online courses in physical education (75%) do not meet the postprimary school national guidelines of 225 formal physical education minutes per week; the majority of courses required physical activity on only 3 days per week, and some required no physical activity at all. The surveyed teachers' views on using an online mode of delivery ranged from support, to hesitation, and in some cases opposition to online physical education. What remains largely unknown is the efficacy of online delivery of physical education experiences and whether it would do better in promoting physically active lifestyles beyond school than face-to-face physical education programming.

CHAPTER SUMMARY

What do all these trends mean for physical education programs? Physical educators might question why these trends are noteworthy. In no small part because of the constant pressures in most industrialized countries to improve students' performance in classroom subjects, much of the emphasis on infusing technology in schools will continue to target improvements in classroom subjects. Schools will continue to see more money being made available for additional technology infusion. Physical educators must remain vigilant in staying abreast of opportunities for appropriate and well-thought-out technology infusion.

1. In the last three decades, technology has changed numerous aspects of life in general.
2. Education has benefitted from the rapid advances in technology.
3. Computer technology has been shown to have important benefits relative to improving health but also has had negative consequences.
4. Technology contributes to the increasingly sedentary lifestyles of children, youth, and adults, which in turn are associated with developing obesity.
5. Active video games may make a small contribution to increasing physical activity levels but appear to have a "novelty effect."
6. Teachers are more likely to adopt use of a particular technology if (1) teachers can try out the technology before full-scale implementation, (2) they can see immediate observable results of using the technology, (3) they can see the advantage over other technologies or other traditional approaches, (4) they can figure out the use of the technology with relative ease, and (5) the technology is compatible with existing practices.
7. Preservice teachers will be more receptive to infusing technology if they see it modeled by program faculty, get frequent opportunities to use the technology throughout the program, and receive support from instructors and peers.
8. It is frequently assumed (incorrectly) that instruction that is computer-based is inherently of better quality than "traditional" approaches to instruction.
9. Infusion of technology in an education setting is very cost-intensive and does not automatically translate into improved teaching and/or student learning.
10. Questions that should be asked when weighing investments in technology for physical education include: (1) Is the cost of the technology worth it in terms of its potential impact on student learning? (2) Will the technology work effectively in the physical education teaching environment? (3) How much of a learning curve will there be before you are comfortable using it to its fullest extent within your teaching? and (4) How much of a novelty effect is there among students when using the new technology?
11. Sample technologies for enhancing instruction include the Internet, computer software, and hardware (e.g., apps, mobile devices).
12. The Internet is a prime source of information for strengthening physical educators' content knowledge.
13. Technology can support physical educators' continued professional development in multiple ways.
14. Technology can personalize student learning through the Internet, devices, and software that help track physical fitness and physical activity.
15. Technology can extend physical education programs by putting students in direct contact with content knowledge beyond the scheduled class periods.
16. The Internet provides extensive information that can support students' learning across the psychomotor and cognitive learning domains.
17. Hardware, such as tablets (e.g., iPads), mobile devices, and exercise equipment, increasingly includes advanced computer technology enabling teachers to enhance their instruction both within and beyond class time.
18. Future trends for technology in education will likely include personalizing students' learning environments, the availability of improved mobile devices and digital content, digital learning environments becoming more commonplace, improving access to the available technology innovations for economically disadvantaged students, and classroom environments becoming more virtual than just a physical place to meet.
19. Physical educators must remain vigilant in staying abreast of opportunities for appropriate and well-thought-out technology infusion.

REFERENCES

Active Healthy Kids Canada. (n.d.). Active Healthy Kids Canada's position on active video games. Available from www.activehealthykids.ca/active-video-games-position.aspx

American Presidency Project. (2000, Jan. 27). William J. Clinton: Address before a joint session of the Congress on the state of the union. Available from www.presidency.ucsb.edu/ws/index.php?pid = 58708

Baranowski, T., Buday, R., Thompson, D. I., & Baranowski, J. (2008). Playing for real: Video games and stories for health-related behavior change. *American Journal of Preventive Medicine, 34*, 74–82.

Barber, D. A. (2012). 5 K–12 ed tech trends for 2012. *The Journal.* Available from http://thejournal.com/articles/2012/01/10/5-k-12-ed-tech-for-2012.aspx?sc_lang = en

Barnett, A., Cerin, E., & Baranowski, T. (2011). Active video games for youth: A systematic review. *Journal of Physical Activity and Health, 8*, 724–737.

Biddiss, E., & Irwin, J. (2010). Active video games to promote physical activity in children and youth: A systematic review. *Archives of Pediatric and Adolescent Medicine, 164*, 664–672.

Blain, D. (2012). Team of the year. *Physical Education Matters, 12*, 62–64.

Bouchard, C., Blair, S. N., & Haskell, W. (2012). *Physical activity and health* (2nd ed.). Champaign. IL: Human Kinetics.

Bunker, D., & Thorpe, R. (1982). A model for the teaching of games in the secondary school. *Bulletin of Physical Education, 10*, 9–16.

Casey, A. (2013). Personal communication.

Casey, A., & Jones, B. (2011). Using digital technology to enhance student engagement in physical education. *Asia-Pacific Journal of Health, Sport and Physical Education, 2*, 51–67.

Chestnutt, C. B. (1997). *Personal sport and technology ... Now more than a course!* Paper presented at the National Conference on Technology in Physical Education and Sport. Ball State University, Muncie, IN.

Crowe, A. (2003). Integrating technology into a social studies education course: Problems and possibilities. In C. Crawford et al. (Eds.), *Proceedings of Society for Information Technology and Teacher Education international conference 2003* (pp. 3467–3470). Chesapeake, VA: AACE.

Crowe, A., & van 't Hooft, M. (2006). Technology and the prospective teacher: Exploring the use of the TI-83 handheld devices in social studies education. *Contemporary Issues in Technology and Teacher Education, 6*(1), 99–119.

Daum, D. N., & Buschner, C. (2012). The status of high school online physical education in the United States. *Journal of Teaching in Physical Education, 31*, 86–100.

Entertainment Software Association. (2013). Industry facts. Available from www.theesa.com/facts/index.asp

Fernández-Balboa, J. (2003). Physical education in the digital (postmodern) era. In A. Laker (Ed.), *The future of physical education: Building a new pedagogy* (pp. 137–152). London: Routledge.

Foley, L., & Maddison, R. (2010). Use of active video games to increase physical activity in children: A (virtual) reality? *Pediatric Exercise Science, 22*, 7–20.

Gentile, D. A., Lynch, P. J., Linder, J. R., & Walsh, D. A. (2004). The effects of violent video game habits on adolescent hostility, aggressive behaviors, and school performance. *Journal of Adolescence, 27*, 5–22.

Graves, L., Stratton, G., Ridgers, N. D., & Cable, N. T. (2007). Comparison of energy expenditure in adolescents when playing new generation and sedentary computer games: Cross sectional study. *British Medical Journal, 335*, 1282–1284.

Hastie, P. A. (2012). Personal communication.

Hastie, P. A., Casey, A., & Tarter, A. (2010). A case study of wikis and student-designed games in physical education. *Technology, Pedagogy and Education, 19*, 79–91. DOI: 10.1080/14759390903579133

Hunt, N., & Bohlin, R. (1995). Events and practices that promote positive attitudes and emotions in computing courses. *Journal of Computing in Teacher Education, 11*(3), 21–23.

Keiper, T., Harwood, A., & Larson, B. (2000). Pre-service teachers' perceptions of infusing computer technology into social studies education. *Theory and Research in Social Education, 28*, 566–579.

Lanningham-Foster, L., Jensen, T. B., Foster, R. C., Redmond, A. B., Walker, B. A., Heinz, D., et al. (2006). Energy expenditure of sedentary screen time compared with active screen time for children. *Pediatrics, 118*, e1831–e1835. DOI: 10.1542/peds.2006-108

Launder, A. G., & Piltz, W. (2013). *Play practice* (2nd ed.). Champaign, IL: Human Kinetics.

Lenzer, J. (2010). U.S. Heart Association endorses active video games. *British Medical Journal, 340*, c2802.

Maloney, A. E., Bethea, T., Kelsey, K. S., Marks, J. T., Paez, S., Rosenberg, A. M., et al. (2008). A pilot of a video game (DDR) to promote physical activity and decrease sedentary screen time. *Obesity, 16*, 2074–2080.

Mills, B. (1997). Opening the gymnasium to the world wide web. *Journal of Physical Education, Recreation, and Dance, 68*(8), 17–19.

Mason, C., & Berson, M. (2000). Computer mediated communication in elementary social studies methods: An examination of students' perceptions and perspectives. *Theory and Research in Social Education, 28*, 527–545.

Mohnson, B. S. (2012). *Using technology in physical education* (8th ed.). Big Bear Lake, CA: Bonnie's Fitware, Inc.

Palfrey, J. G., & Gasser, U. (2008). *Born digital: Understanding the first generation of digital natives*. Philadelphia: Basic Books.

Pangrazi, R. P., Beighle, A., & Sidman, C. (2007). *Pedometer power: Using pedometers in school and community* (2nd ed.). Champaign, IL: Human Kinetics.

Primack, B. A., Carroll, M. V., McNamara, M., Klem, M. L., King, B., et al. (2012). Role of video games in improving health-related outcomes: A systematic review. *American Journal of Preventive Medicine, 42*, 630–638.

Richtel, M. (2011). Technology in schools faces questions on value (print title: In classroom of future, stagnant scores). *New York Times*, September 3. Available from www.nytimes.com/2011/09/04/technology/technology-in-schools-faces-questions-on-value.html?pagewanted = all

Ringle, H. (2012). Valley schools telling students to B.Y.O.T. (Bring Your Own Technology). *Arizona Republic*, 2012, Aug. 10, B1, B5.

Rogers, E. (1995). *Diffusion of innovations* (4th ed.). New York: The Free Press.

Schiesel, S. (2007). P.E. classes turn to video game that works legs. *New York Times*, Apr. 30. Available from www.nytimes.com/2007/04/30/health/30exer.html?fta = y

Siedentop, D. (2002). Content knowledge for physical education. *Journal of Teaching in Physical Education, 21*, 368–377.

Sinelnikov, O. A. (2012). Using the iPad in a sport education season. *Journal of Physical Education, Recreation & Dance, 83*(1), 39–45. DOI: 10.1080/07303084.2012.10598710

Stidder, G., & Capel, S. (2010). Using information and communications technology to support learning and teaching in PE. In S. Capel & M. Whitehead (Eds.), *Learning to teach physical education in the secondary school* (3rd ed.; pp. 183–196). London: Routledge.

Thomas, A., & Stratton, G. (2006). What we are really doing with ICT in physical education: A national audit of equipment, use, teacher attitudes, support, and training. *British Journal of Educational Technology, 37*, 617–632.

Wikia. (n.d.). Video game sales wiki. Video game industry. Available from http://vgsales.wikia.com/wiki/Video_game_industry

SECTION IV The Reality of Teaching Physical Education

Introduction

William Ayers (1993) reminds us that, "teaching is not something that one learns to do, once and for all, and then practices, problem-free for a lifetime" (p. 126), suggesting that teaching is a process of growth and development through self-renewal, continued learning, and recognizing that educators are both teachers and students. These final two chapters introduce the reality of teaching school physical education to preservice teachers and encourage novice teachers to develop/maintain (1) strong program administration, (2) a plan of action for professional development, and (3) an ongoing program promotion/advocacy agenda for their physical education subject. It is through these endeavors that the quality of physical education continues to improve and provide worthwhile and challenging experiences for young people delivered by qualified and exceptional teachers—teachers who matter.

REFERENCE

Ayers, W. (1993). *To teach: The journey of a teacher.* New York: Teachers College Press.

CHAPTER 18 Professional Development: Staying Alive as a Teacher

Overall Chapter Outcome

To examine the opportunities for teacher professional development across all stages of a teacher's career, from initial teacher education to induction into the teaching profession and ultimately to the continuing professional development available to teachers

Learning Outcomes

The learner will:

- Describe professional development opportunities available across a teaching career (initial teacher education, induction, and inservice/continuing professional development)
- Consider how to access and engage with professional development opportunities at different stages in the career (e.g., mentoring, school ethnography, self-assessment of teaching, teaching portfolio)
- Discuss the guidelines suggested for becoming a professional physical educator and why this is an important aspect of initial teacher education
- Describe your understanding of being a change agent and the implications for the physical education delivered to young people
- Consider the purpose of developing a professional development plan as you enter your first year of teaching
- Discuss the purpose of a community of practice and how you might become involved in such a professional group
- Consider the implications of a school–university partnership on all stakeholders including teachers, preservice teachers, and university faculty

Professional development should happen across a teacher's career (Armour, 2011), involve teacher change (Guskey, 1995), promote teachers as active learners (Breckon & Capel, 2005), support reflective practice (Attard & Armour, 2006), and ultimately develop teacher effectiveness in working with young people in the classroom (Chung Wei et al., 2009). Hargreaves (2001) suggests that teachers' ongoing learning, known as **continuing professional development**, is "about enriching the quality of the lives of teachers themselves and their intellectual and moral excellences" (p. 493).

Teacher professional development in education and physical education, as we know it, has a long history, and one in which we have seen little change. Key characteristics of this traditional professional development include it being (1) delivered as generic in-service days or one-time workshops with little or no follow-up, (2) housed in out-of-school venues with little relationship to school contexts or the students served, (3) disconnected from previous and subsequent professional development opportunities, (4) provided by external experts charged with designing and disseminating materials and strategies selected by the school higher echelon, and (5) intended for teachers to accept and adopt practices transmitted to them. As a consequence, typically we see these professional development opportunities as mandatory, passive events that many teachers in all subject areas dread and find irrelevant to their practice. This type of professional development, or teacher learner, is contrary to what we learned early on from Dewey (1958), when he concluded that education is

BOX 18.1 Key Terms in This Chapter

- *Change agent:* A person who acts as a catalyst for change, challenging and questioning the status quo while taking action to bring about improvements.
- *Community of practice:* "When you see a group of teachers sharing and critically interrogating their practice in an on-going, reflective, collaborative, inclusive, learning-oriented, growth-promoting way" (Stoll & Seashore Louis, 2007, p. 2).
- *Continuing professional development (CPD):* Lifelong teacher learning. It includes a range of educational experiences designed to enhance teachers' professional skills, knowledge, understanding, application, and capabilities throughout their careers.
- *Continuum of teacher education:* The stages through which a teacher passes in their career: initial teacher education, induction into the profession, and early continuing professional development.
- *Critical friends:* Typically two people who trust and value each other's viewpoints and are willing to work together to share, critique, and challenge one another to produce personal and professional growth.
- *Induction program:* Designed to support the induction of newly qualified teachers into the teaching profession.
- *In-service education/training:* A common form of professional development for teachers to help them improve their knowledge and practice. In-service training usually is one size fits all, offered to teachers of all subject areas in one workshop, designed by outside agencies or to meet an administrative agenda, and is mandatory.
- *Mentoring:* Traditionally involves two professionals (usually a mentor and a mentee) working together for the purpose of the mentor providing guidance to the mentee. More recently, mentoring is viewed as a form of professional development shared between two or more colleagues working together for the development of each other.
- *Professional development:* Involves gaining the skills, qualifications, and experience that allow teachers to progress across their career.
- *Professional development plan:* A tool preservice teachers use to reflect on their current practice, set goals for improving that practice, and identify a timeline and the means by which that improvement will take place.
- *Reflection:* For a teacher, this is the process of thinking back on a lesson, the teaching of the lesson, and the students' response to the lesson to allow preservice and practicing teachers to consider their practices and the learning of their pupils in order to make improvements.
- *School–university partnerships:* Typically take the form of a formal partnership arrangement between higher education institutions and schools to provide structured support and guidance to preservice teachers during teaching practice. Recently, school–university partnerships are expanding to include a shared perspective on professional development for professionals in both the school and the university context.
- *Teaching practice/student teaching:* An extended period of time in which a student teacher is placed in a host school to practice teaching prior to graduating from teacher education.

a continual process of becoming, acknowledging that some learning experiences actually hinder rather than promote learning.

Teacher education might be viewed as a continuum that includes initial teacher education, induction into the profession, and early continuing professional development. Ideally, these stages should seamlessly align with one another to ensure ongoing and continuous professional development and support to all teachers. Unfortunately, in many countries, teacher education tends to place the emphasis on initial teacher education as the setting where new knowledge is introduced and opportunities are provided to practice application of that knowledge in artificial (peer or micro teaching) as well as realistic applied settings (teaching practice). Although still not available in all contexts, efforts to design formal and informal teacher induction programs are frequently being implemented internationally following guidelines that are based on research in best practices. However, continuing professional development opportunities beyond induction and into the later stages of a teacher's career are less frequent, less well-developed, and typically characterized by the attributes of traditional professional development as outlined previously. On a positive note, and perhaps one that will push the agenda forward, the European Commission (2010) stated that, "The education and professional development of every teacher needs to be seen as a lifelong task and be structured and resourced accordingly" (p. 12). Requirements for teacher professional development vary from state to state and country to country. For example, in the state of Delaware, full-time physical education teachers need to complete 90 clock hours every 5 years to maintain certification; 18 of these clock hours each year *must* be specific to physical education and not simply in-school faculty meetings. In some states and countries, professional development is now included as a part of formal assessment programs examining teachers' up-skilling and development.

In this chapter we intend to provide insight on what continuing professional development might look like across the **continuum of teacher education**. Although we concur with Hargreaves (2001) that professional development needs to be designed by and with teachers, we recognize that the opportunity for teachers to be involved in this development is an evolving process. We therefore provide ideas, strategies, and examples of what the novice, entry, and veteran teacher might do to ensure they are able to develop personally and professionally across their entire teaching careers, recognizing that there will necessarily be overlap across and between the stages.

Strategies for All Stages Across the Teaching Continuum

Mentoring

Mentoring is traditionally viewed as a one-on-one relationship in which a senior person works with a younger protégé to provide guidance and assist with the protégé's professional development (Dodds, 2005; Higgins & Krams, 2001; Tannehill & Coffin, 1996). A more recent iteration of mentoring defines it as a process to support professional development; it can be viewed as an active and emotionally close relationship that develops between individuals, reflects a focus on pedagogy, supports professional development, and produces teacher change (Parker et al., 2010). This mentoring relationship might be developed between two preservice teachers, or a preservice teacher and his or her cooperating teacher, lecturer, teaching practice supervisor, or even a parent. Parker et al. (2010) prompt us that a mentoring relationship evolves through social interaction with others, suggesting that mentoring relationships may develop and change throughout a teacher's career. In some instances, a teacher might seek multiple mentors to meet various professional needs, resulting in what Higgins (2000) refers to as mentoring networks.

If we are to view multiple mentoring relationships as a meaningful form of professional development, then providing preservice and practicing teachers with opportunities to develop these relationships is critical. **Critical friends** might be viewed as one example of a mentoring relationship that can be developed through a teacher education program. Costa and Kallick (1993) define a critical friend as

> *A trusted person who asks provocative questions, provides data to be examined through another lens, and offers critiques of a person's work as a friend. A critical friend takes the time to fully understand the context of the work presented and the outcomes that the person or group is working toward. The friend is an advocate for the success of that work.*

However, helping prospective teachers identify and select a peer to serve as a critical friend is a challenging task. When we place preservice teachers, or practicing teachers for that matter, in a partner learning experience where they are asked to challenge one another by providing critically reflective feedback on some aspect of teaching, we often find them providing nothing but unquestioning support. In contrast, a critical friend is one who is invited to provide critical, constructive, and developmental commentary through a collaboratively developed personal and professional relationship that is willingly established by mutual selection. Thus, it is the willing mutual selection that cannot be forced if the critical friend process is to be beneficial. If a teacher educator is able to provide a foundation and the experiences where collegial relationships develop, reflective practice is encouraged, and preservice teachers are able to confront difficult issues by taking and receiving critique, then critical friends might develop. This would provide opportunities to both solicit and give feedback in a manner that promotes reflective learning. **Box 18.2** shares ideas promoted by Brookfield (1995) to encourage critical conversations about teaching.

Learning Experience 18.1

With a partner, determine how a meaningful group discussion of the following teaching task might be developed:

Preservice teachers select a peer with whom they feel comfortable co-planning and co-teaching a physical education program to primary children once a week for 5 weeks. As a teaching team they will co-design the five lessons, co-develop teaching aids as necessary, co-teach the lessons, debrief following each lesson, co-inquire through critical conversation how the lesson progressed, identify evidence of student learning, and determine in what ways the lesson might have been designed, taught, and managed to more effectively impact student learning and enjoyment.

School Ethnography

A school's ethnography (see **Box 18.3**), which includes community mapping, examining the school's ethos, and both a teacher and student study, might provide you with key information for your development as a teacher during teaching practice, when moving into your first teaching job, and in later years when gaining employment in a new teaching setting. We may teach in a community yet fail to recognize the experiences of many members of the community, acknowledge what is available to young people in the community, or even notice the links, or lack of links, between the school and the community. Cockburn et al. (2001) remind educators that the relationship between the school and community must be developed and maintained because both have something to

BOX 18.2 Developing Preservice Teachers as Mentors

Designing practices to develop mentoring groups in teacher education is problematic. As noted previously, although social interaction is a key element of mentoring and an important component of learning, teacher educators attempting to force mandatory collegiality will result in contrived relationships as opposed to mutually selected peers committed to the growth and well-being of one another through in-depth and critical reflection. Brookfield (1995) prompts us that holding critical conversations is difficult in what we frequently see today as a culture of competitiveness and individual ownership. He suggests a sequence of activities that must be experienced for partners or groups to take part in reflective, critical conversations that allow participants to engage in important discussion of their personal teaching practices.

1. Allow groups to spend time developing ground rules to guide how democratic discussion among members will occur.
2. To get initial discussion started, introduce nonintrusive-type questions for members to share information about themselves or their teaching.
3. Ask groups to share critical incidents that occurred during their teaching to serve as points of discussion. These incidents might be positive or negative and reflect a classroom event that had a significant impact on their teaching or an experience that caused them to question their ability as a teacher.
4. A critical response discussion intends to encourage active listening and attending to a group discussion while developing a shared perspective. Select a topic, allow each individual 2 uninterrupted minutes to share their viewpoint, and once all have spoken, open the discussion for general reactions.
5. To avoid status issues developing where some voices are heard more frequently or valued more, a discussion might be stopped and a "circle of voices" called where each individual who has yet to respond shares his or her perspective on a topic.
6. Having every member of a group hold a different conversational role on a rotating basis in discussions can encourage everyone's voice to be heard. Brookfield (1995) suggests problem poser, reflective analyst, devil's advocate, theme spotter, and umpire.

Adding a structural framework to a discussion provides guidelines to the group so that discussion does not end without providing any useful insights. For example, there could be a storyteller (who introduces an incident for discussion), the detectives (group members focused on helping improve the practices of the storyteller), and an umpire (a member who keeps the group focused on solving problems, not placing blame) assigned as a discussion group. Groups ultimately determine the usefulness of the conversation to practice.

offer young people. It is up to the teacher to gather information about the community and make use of that information to inform both teaching and student learning. Developing a school's ethnography is one method for gaining an informed perspective and understanding of the community where your school is situated and determining how you can most effectively use this information in your lessons and the learning of your students. We have found it interesting, and perhaps a bit distressing, that when our students return from conducting a school ethnography in their teaching practice setting, they frequently have other teachers in the school comment that the preservice teacher knows more about the community than they themselves do, who have been teaching in the setting for many years.

Self-Analysis

Analysis of your own teaching, which we know is based on how and what students do in the learning situation, is an initial and ongoing step in your development as a teacher and improving teaching practices and ultimately student learning. Breckon and Capel (2005) encourage teachers to become aware of what is happening in their lessons and to use their professional judgment to make appropriate decisions on how to respond to, adapt, and revise the learning context to facilitate student learning. One way to begin practicing this is to video record one of your lessons, after which you sit down with the video to observe, collect data, and interpret what happened and how it might be changed to impact student learning more effectively. Often we focus on what we are doing rather than how students are responding and how we might facilitate their learning and development. As you progress through your teaching career you will tend to focus first on yourself as a teacher and then evolve to focusing on the student and finally on what you as a teacher might do to influence what you observed in the students' response to the lesson.

BOX 18.3 School Ethnography

The school ethnography is to include the following:

- Community mapping assignment
- Case study of a teacher
- Case study of pupils
- Review of the school ethos

Community Mapping

Mapping the neighborhood with a camera, taking photos, observing the neighborhood, and interacting with the people who work and live in the neighborhood should allow you to "see" the community with new lenses. You will map the local area (size should be walkable if in a city or you may need transportation if in a suburban or country school), collecting information and talking to people. You will create an electronic collage and map of your journey and experiences.

School Ethos (Policies, Mission Statement, Climate of School)

Talk with members of the school staff including teachers, secretaries, administrators, and custodial staff. Examine teacher handbooks, materials provided to pupils and parents, and any written documentation that portrays a picture of the school and its environment. Attempt to identify what makes the school tick. In other words, develop your understanding of the school ethos and climate and the role of teachers, administrators, and pupils in developing it. Reflect upon the implications of this school ethos for your own teaching at this site.

Case Study of a Teacher

This task is twofold

1. Identify a teacher with a reputation as a highly effective teacher and obtain permission to observe teaching. Observe at least one class and talk to the teacher before and after your observation. Design a set of questions that you wish to ask the teacher to help you learn from what is done so effectively.
2. Observe your physical education cooperating teacher (CT). Take note of the rules and routines that are set for the class, how these are taught to pupils, and if they are reinforced and maintained from one lesson to the next. Document the teaching behaviors that your CT uses when teaching. How are pupils treated and do they seem to enjoy class? Take the time to find out from your CT how the curriculum is designed. Is it in line with state and national expectations? Is it taught with a variety of methods using various curricular and instructional models?

Based on what you learn from these two case studies, draw the implications that this information has for your own teaching and classroom management. Capel (2007) states that observation of other teachers is not meant to provide you with a model to copy, but to give insight on different pedagogies teachers use and how they impact students in varying contexts and allow you to make decisions that fit your own teaching values and beliefs as well as the needs of your specific learners.

Case Study of Pupils

Identify at least two pupils and obtain permission to observe them for part of the school day (different days for each pupil). Pick pupils you find interesting and with different backgrounds from your own. Take notes that will help you to recall significant events or comments during the day. Do your best to get to know the pupils and understand their feelings about the school and teachers. What is school like for these students, and what did you learn that will influence your work with these young people? Draw insight from their voices, experiences and feelings about life in their school, what it means to their learning, and how you might facilitate their growth and development.

Adapted from O'Sullivan, M., Tannehill, D., & Hinchion, C. (2010). Teaching as professional inquiry. In R. Bailey (Ed.), *Physical education for learning: A guide for secondary schools* (pp. 54–66). London, UK: Continuum Press.

During Initial Teacher Education

Teacher education varies significantly across countries worldwide. The Organisation for Economic Co-operation and Development (OECD, 2010) reports that the length of initial teacher education programs varies substantially among OECD countries, with the trend being for the length of initial teacher education to increase. Generally, initial teacher education programs range from 3 years (e.g., for some primary teachers in Ireland and Spain) up to 6.5 years for some teachers in Germany, 7 years in some programs in the Slovak Republic, and 8 years for some postprimary teachers in Italy. Regardless of the length of time spent in initial teacher education, much can be achieved in this stage of your career-long journey of continuing professional development (CPD).

Tannehill, MacPhail, Halbert, and Murphy (2012) suggest that "it is through sustained engagement in CPD that we can develop the skills and dispositions that are central to being a professional" (p. 156). They suggest that this journey to becoming a lifelong learner who actively seeks and participates in learning opportunities must begin in initial teacher education. Cooperative learning is the foundation of continuing professional development, and preservice teachers who leave teacher education with these skills and dispositions will strengthen the ongoing teacher learning opportunities for themselves and their colleagues.

Teaching Portfolio

A *teaching portfolio* often is part of initial teacher education programs that require preservice teachers to document evidence of their success in achieving performance-based learning outcomes (e.g., National Association of Sport and Physical Education [NASPE] Beginning Teaching Standards in the United States [1995, 2004]; Teaching Council Learning Outcomes in Ireland [2011]). These teaching portfolios may be linked to completion of a course of study or initial teacher licensure. In some instances, these collections of work are referred to as reflective portfolios because they require not only evidence of learning outcomes achievement but also a demonstration of understanding how the chosen evidence relates to effective practice (see **Box 18.4**). This might include (1) for each learning outcome, evidence that demonstrates achievement of one or more aspects of the specific outcome; (2) for each piece of evidence, a detailed description of its relationship to the learning outcome; and (3) for each piece of evidence, a reflective summary demonstrating understanding of the relationship of the evidence to what we know about effective practice. This teaching portfolio will most often become a growing body of evidence that moves through a teacher's career documenting development of teaching at each stage.

BOX 18.4 An Example of a First-Year Preservice Teacher's Reflective Portfolio Entry for One Component of the Irish Teaching Council's Learning Outcome 1: Knowledge

Outcome

1. Knowledge: breadth/knowledge: kind
   - Ethical standards and professional behavior
   - Education and the education system
   - Key principles of planning, teaching, learning, assessment, reflection, and self-evaluation
   - Subject knowledge and curriculum process and content
   - Communication and relationship building

Evidence

Lesson plan for peer teaching lesson using a peer-mediated instructional model. Copy of lesson plan and task cards included in portfolio.

Description of Performance Evidence

A lesson was designed to teach an appropriate sequence of tasks that would allow students to reach a specific learning goal using a peer-mediated instructional model. The learning goal in this volleyball season lesson was for students to demonstrate skill in using a forearm pass to the setter in preparation for an offensive hit. This lesson was delivered in a gym setting with three volleyball courts during a 45-minute time period. Key points for each of a series of six tasks as well as critical elements of skills/tactics, teaching strategies, teaching cues, and adaptations to facilitate individual students are highlighted in the plan. Detailed task cards, with performance diagrams and critical elements, were developed to guide peers in providing appropriate feedback and assistance. How to use these task cards and provide peer support and feedback are planned through the pedagogical practices outlined in the plan. Specific guidance for management and safety are also detailed in the plan.

BOX 18.4 An Example of a First-Year Preservice Teacher's Reflective Portfolio Entry for One Component of the Irish Teaching Council's Learning Outcome 1: Knowledge (*Continued*)

Relationship of Evidence to Standards and Competencies

One of the knowledge outcomes is *subject knowledge and curriculum process and content.* Within this outcome is the expectation that the novice teacher has knowledge and understanding of the *subject matter, the pedagogical content*, and *related methodology of the relevant curricula/syllabi and guidelines*.

This lesson plan on the volleyball forearm pass included critical elements of skill that demonstrate my knowledge of the content and a suitable sequence of activities/learning experiences for students to reach a specific learning goal that reflects appropriate pedagogical content knowledge. It also included teaching cues that were identified to assist the student in visualizing the correct technical performance of the skill and prompt the correct performance through interactive feedback and modeling from the teacher. The skill chosen and the teaching strategies are in line with the Junior Cycle Physical Education (JCPE) syllabus outlined by the National Council of Curriculum and Assessment (NCCA).

Reflection on Relationship of Evidence to Effective Practice

A teacher must know what he or she is teaching. The critical elements can be used as teaching cues to guide instruction, as prompts for students to think of while watching a demonstration or practicing a skill, and as cues for the teacher to use when providing feedback (Oslin, 2002). The combination of appropriate teaching cues based on critical elements of the skill to be learned and a well-designed set of learning experiences in a developmentally appropriate sequence will facilitate student learning (Siedentop & Tannehill, 2000). Knowing the critical elements of the skill allows the teacher to observe student performance as a means of determining when they are ready to move on.

Pedagogical practices matter. An appropriate learning sequence is important and allows learners to develop skills in a step-by-step fashion; when they are successful at one level they can move to the next. Hellison (2002) encourages teachers to design lesson adaptations that provide options for students to meet their needs—more complex adaptations to challenge those who are more skilled and less complex adaptations for those who are struggling.

In some cases, student-mediated instruction is useful in helping students recognize what a performance should look like and internalize how to improve that performance. Metzler (2011) shares key aspects of peer teaching that encourage students to observe, assess, and provide feedback to one another to improve practice. Although the teacher still delivers the content, it is typically done through explicit and detailed task cards that guide peer tutoring.

The lesson plan guides the teacher through the lesson in order to assist learners in reaching the learning goal. If a teacher is going to assist a learner in reaching a learning goal, he or she must plan and then deliver lessons and learning experiences in a safe environment, use materials that are meaningful and will assist students in understanding and progressing through a skill/activity, provide demonstrations and explanations that are accurate models of what the student is trying to learn, provide relevant and accurate feedback in the form of instructional cues and critical elements, and deliver the instruction using a format that matches the content, the learners, and the setting. If learning is the goal of instruction, then the teacher must have all aspects of the lesson planned appropriately and in detail. This can be done through both teacher-mediated and/or learner-mediated instruction.

Reproduced from the curriculum materials from the Professional Diploma in Education–Physical Education, University of Limerick, Deborah Tannehill, PhD.

Learning Experience 18.2

Select one of the beginning teacher outcomes/standards that guide initial teacher education in your own context, and

1. Select a piece of evidence that demonstrates achievement of one or more aspects of the specific outcome.
2. For this piece of evidence, provide a detailed description of its relationship to the learning outcome.
3. For this piece of evidence, write a reflective summary demonstrating your understanding of the relationship of the evidence to what we know about effective practice.

You also may provide an outline of what evidence you might select for other outcomes/standards for which you are to be held responsible.

Becoming a Professional

Becoming a professional is one of the first criteria that initial teacher education often emphasizes to preservice teachers. Tannehill et al. (2012) maintain that being a professional across all stages of a teacher's career is important, suggesting that professional development is inherent within that professionalism. Becoming a professional requires teachers, at all stages of their careers, to be willing to collaborate with one another, yet it must be recognized that they need the space and the tools to collaborate effectively. This might start during initial teacher education when preservice teachers are helped to view themselves not just as teaching peers in their education, but more as colleagues in the teaching profession.

This might begin with preservice teachers being invited to join the professional organization for physical education. In the United States, the professional organization to which most physical education teachers affiliate is the National Association for Sport and Physical Education (NASPE), which is affiliated with the American Alliance for Health, Physical Education, Recreation and Dance (AAHPERD) and provides numerous benefits to preservice and practicing teachers (see **Box 18.5**). Similar professional organizations are available

BOX 18.5 AAHPERD Membership

The associations of AAHPERD are designed for professionals in elementary, secondary, and higher education, administration, research, youth programming, dance, coaching, sport medicine, health education, public health, fitness, choreography, therapeutic programs, parks and recreation services, and other careers in movement-related fields or focused on improving quality of life. The content thread among these professionals is an interest in promoting healthy and active lifestyles for all.

AAHPERD membership entitles professionals to many services:

- Access to five national associations (American Association for Health Education [AAHE], American Association for Physical Activity and Recreation [AAPAR], National Association for Girls and Women in Sport [NAGWS], National Association for Sport and Physical Education [NASPE], and National Dance Association [NDA]); six district associations, all of which hold an annual convention (Central, Northwest, Midwest, Eastern, Southern, and Southwest); and the Research Consortium, whose mission is to advance and disseminate research in physical education, physical activity, and health.
- Access to national convention registration, products, and continuing education (all accessible on the AAHPERD website [see www.aahperd.org]).
  - Journals: Members receive one journal of their choice from AAHPERD's four key journals with membership (Journal of Physical Education, Recreation and Dance; Strategies, A Journal for Physical and Sport Educators; American Journal of Health Education; and Research Quarterly for Exercise and Sport). Additional online and print journals are provided and can be accessed on the website.
  - Newsletters: Members receive UpdatePLUS, in addition to newsletters from each of the associations selected as part of membership.
- Professional recognition and program development such as grants, scholarships, and awards are available through all AAHPERD associations. In physical education, NASPE provides details of what is available in terms of grants, scholarships, awards, and recognition on its website at www.aahperd.org/naspe. For example, grants that are available include:
  - Head Start Body Start: Head Start Body Start intends to increase physical activity, outdoor play, and healthy eating among Head Start and Early Head Start Center children, families, and staff.
  - ING Run for Something Better: This grant seeks to increase physical activity in students and help fight childhood obesity nationwide through the creation of school-based running programs.
  - Research Grant Program: The purpose of the NASPE Research Grant Program is to provide substantial funding for critical applied research related to K–12 physical education, school-based physical activity and sport programs, or youth sport that is relevant to a large number of NASPE members.
  - Carol M. White Physical Education Program (PEP): The purpose of the Carol M. White Physical Education Program (PEP) grant is to provide funds to local educational agencies and community-based organizations to initiate, expand, and improve physical education programs.
- Networking and career resources such as access to an online membership directory, social networking, online forums, blogs, webinars, and face-to-face interaction at the national convention, workshops, and meetings.
- Personal benefits that include financial programs such as health, auto, and liability insurance; identity theft protection; and equipment discounts.

to physical education teachers in most countries and offer similar benefits to their members (Association for Physical Education [afPE] in the United Kingdom [see www.afpe.org.uk], Physical Education Association of Ireland [PEAI, see www.peai.org], Australian Council for Health, Physical Education and Recreation [AHPER, see www.achper.org.au], and Physical Education New Zealand [PENZ, see www.penz.org.nz]). These organizations provide the teaching professional with access to conferences and workshops, publications, and resources; grant and scholarship opportunities; a professional listserv or discussion blog; the latest research-based pedagogical strategies; advocacy events; and information and details regarding current educational issues that impact teaching and learning.

Beliefs About and Philosophy of Teaching

Preservice teachers' reflection on and development of their *beliefs about teaching and learning and design of a teaching philosophy* (e.g., teaching metaphor, critical friend, change agents) are frequent components of initial teacher education. We know that after 12 years as students in schools, preservice teachers enter teacher education with preconceived perspectives about teaching and learning that tend to guide their own practice (Lortie, 2002; Sugrue, 2004). We also know that unless preservice teachers are confronted with their held beliefs and challenged about them through commanding and focused learning experiences, they will not alter these beliefs as a result of teacher education (Britzman, 1991; Feiman-Nemser & Remillard, 1996). With this in mind, many teacher education programs ask their preservice teachers to develop a teaching philosophy to reflect their beliefs about teaching and learning as a means of guiding their work with young people, to demonstrate their growth as professionals, and to frame their challenging of these held beliefs. In line with other scholars in education (Britzman, 1991; Bullough & Gitlin, 2001), Tannehill and MacPhail (2012) propose that examining teaching metaphors might be another way for teacher educators to help young teachers recognize their preexisting beliefs about teaching and learning and help them to reflect on and examine these beliefs and how they impact both their teaching and their students' learning. They describe how learning experiences can be designed to challenge teaching metaphors and encourage preservice teachers to acknowledge, explore, and modify their beliefs through community discussion and examination of whether their teaching behaviors are consistent with and reflect the beliefs they have portrayed in their metaphor (see **Box 18.6**). Ayers (1993) suggests that "of all the knowledge teachers need to have, self-knowledge is most important (and least attended to)" (p. 129). Critical friends, as discussed previously, might be consulted to pose challenging and provocative queries as a means of encouraging reconsideration of their beliefs.

Learning Experience 18.3

Write a metaphor of yourself as a teacher. Begin by visualizing your ideal classroom: what are you doing, what are the pupils doing, what is the climate, how does it feel, what kinds of learning do you see, and what is your role? Jot down your thoughts after you visualize, read through them, and see if some image comes to mind. As these images evolve, attempt to articulate them in the form of a metaphor.

Being a Change Agent

From our perspective, becoming a **change agent** is a critical aspect of initial teacher education that is often overlooked. O'Sullivan (2003) prompts physical education teacher education (PETE) programs to consider the criticism directed at them for holding a narrow focus on developing teachers able to follow change, rather than lead change. Likewise, Fernandez-Balboa (1997) proposes that the inability of PETE programs to educate preservice teachers with the knowledge and skills to lead change in schools and communities has resulted in what he refers to as a crisis in physical education. Recently, MacPhail and Tannehill (2012) studied how PETE can help preservice teachers assess and revise the assumptions they hold about themselves as new teachers and change agents, and how they might explore the taken-for-granted school practices and processes that students and teachers encounter on a daily basis. They suggest that,

> *Encouraging PSTs to interact effectively with teachers to allow them to explore worthwhile teaching and learning strategies, learning to work collaboratively as part of a community and advocating for physical education, is the sort of exposure and experience PSTs need to equip them with the ideas, and hopefully the stamina, to persevere in their teaching of physical education. (p. 311)*

These are the types of issues preservice teachers must be aware of if they are to develop into knowledgeable practitioners.

At the NASPE PETE conference held in October 2012, Steve Mitchell and Connie Collier shared their insights on the Ohio Benchmark Assessments that were to be implemented across the state of Ohio in autumn 2012 (Mitchell & Collier, 2012). They shared the legislation that placed the Benchmark Assessments on the school report card, development and implementation of the assessments, and the potential impact of the assessments on physical education in Ohio. Through this session, the presenters led the audience in a discussion of the challenges we face in promoting physical education as a subject for school-wide assessment. They successfully employed the "Yes, but . . ." "Yes, and . . ." strategy (see **Box 18.7**) to demonstrate what can be achieved through a positive, challenging, and solution-focused discussion while encouraging the "naysayers" to think differently.

BOX 18.6 Example of a Preservice Teacher's Confirmed Teaching Metaphor

As a teacher I am a rock. A rock has a hard surface, yet it still allows water to pass through it. As a teacher I aim to slowly allow more and more water (knowledge) to pass throughout my career and use this water to help my students. A rock is part of a group of rock formations and belongs to a broader picture in geology, the make-up of the planet. Rocks can be chipped down into something new. As a teacher I will be chipped at and broken down on several occasions, but will remain strong and determined to stay strong and dedicated to holding the pillars of the school ethos in place. If one wave crashes against this rock, the rock will be slightly damaged, but will still stay strong for the remainder of the waves. If a rock is carved, as opposed to chipped, the rock can then be used to build the most magnificent things. In my teaching, if the students listen and are willing to learn, we can then build a new structure together. My students will be the fossils contained within this rock. Each fossil offers something new and unique to a rock. No two rocks are the same, just as no two fossils are the same. A rock can be displaced in many different locations. Learning to accept and nurture these new situations allows the rock to bind into its new location. Some fossils need a rock to feed off, some don't. Some fossils exist because of a rock, others don't. As a teacher I aim to reach out to each and every child. Like a rock helps moss to grow, I aim to help each and every student to also do so. Each fossil tells its own personal story. Some are there by accident, some are there by choice. As a teacher I aim to nurture each fossil and allow them to learn to accept their place in the rock formation. If each rock (and its fossils contained within) works together like a farmer works his barren land into a blossoming blooming field, this rock formation can create a gasping, eye catching cliff face.

As a result of my own learning experiences, teaching practice, and peer discussion and challenges, I feel my teaching metaphor has not changed; rather it has been reinforced. My view on teaching has changed and been expanded, but I still feel what I wrote back at my entry into teacher education still applies to how I feel now. I feel the line, "Some fossils need a rock to feed off, some don't" and leading into my desire "to reach out to each and every child" is still one in which I passionately believe and has consistently influenced my teaching this past year. I now aim to frame this metaphor and use it as a reminder of where I have come. These thoughts and feelings about teaching reflect how I did, and do still feel about teaching. I now wish to start a new chapter in my life as a NQT [newly qualified teacher] and feel I will refer to this on many occasions. I know in time my metaphor will change, but right now, I feel this still plays a significant role in highlighting to me my stance and feelings on teaching.

Reproduced with permission from a preservice teacher's assignment highlighting how and why his metaphor confirmed his beliefs about teaching throughout his 1-year initial teacher education.

BOX 18.7 "Yes, but" and "Yes, and" Discussions

When involved in a group discussion, "yes, but . . ." is a way of agreeing but really disagreeing with someone, and often turns into looking at the negative side of an issue. For example, a group of teachers are discussing the possibility of allowing pupils to have a voice in the physical education curriculum in which they will take part.

"*Yes*, I agree that might be useful with young people, *but* I am not sure I feel comfortable giving them that much voice in the lesson."

"That's a great idea, *but* when you really examine it you can see that it will cause other problems with facilities."

"*Yes*, we could do that, *but* I really don't want to."

Basically, these types of responses tend to serve as discussion stoppers, and they are difficult to respond to because they often bring more reasons why something will not work or is inappropriate. Thompson (2004) suggests that "yes, but . . ." statements "allow excuses rather than possibilities" to guide discussion. He suggests that instead of looking at the downside of an issue, we look at the possibilities it might encourage. This can be done through what is known as "Yes, and . . ." discussions—statements that tend to push dialogue forward and invite new ideas and alternatives to surface.

"*Yes, and* it might also serve to get more students involved in class because it meets their needs and interests."

"*Yes*, it might be interesting, *and* would provide me with a reason to gain support from my principal for up-skilling myself in new areas."

"*Yes*, we could give it a try, *and* it might help us get to know our students better as well. However, it does kind of scare me."

An interesting strategy for thinking creatively was proposed by Thompson (2004). He suggested asking a group of school staff to examine some "rules" that tend to be considered important in most education systems (see **Table 18.1**) and determine if they believe these rules stifle the discussion that might take place in the classroom. If the teachers agree that the rules do inhibit both their ideas and those of their students, ask them to come up with new guidelines that might aid them in being creative in solving problems. Examples of what teachers might come up with are displayed in Table 18.1.

In the Irish education system, students are required to complete 3 years of postprimary education through junior cycle (the lower secondary level) between the ages of 12 and 15. They then proceed to senior cycle (upper secondary level) from ages 15 to 18 years, where they choose from a range of programs over a 2- or 3-year cycle, depending on whether students choose to take an optional Transition Year in the first year of senior cycle before they follow the 2-year Leaving Certificate program. The National Council for Curriculum and Assessment (NCCA) developed two options for schools at the senior cycle in physical education:

- Senior Cycle Physical Education (SCPE) Framework: nonexaminable
- Leaving Certificate Physical Education (LCPE) Syllabus: examinable

Nonexaminable SCPE is designed to provide schools with a framework within which they can design a physical education program for those students who do not choose to take physical education as part of their Leaving Certificate. The draft framework for SCPE was approved for consultation by the NCCA in January 2011. The ensuing consultation process was designed to ensure appropriate and meaningful engagement with different groups and individuals. It consisted of a number of different elements:

- An online questionnaire and opportunity for submissions
- Focus groups with practicing physical education teachers facilitated by the Physical Education Association of Ireland (PEAI)
- Focus groups with five groups, including preservice physical education students, Leisure and Recreation students, and post-Leaving Certificate students in sport and leisure courses
- Consultation meetings with interested bodies

The consultation meetings were designed on a regional basis and conducted in conjunction with the PEAI. The experiences of senior cycle are designed with the learner at the center, which prompts us to consider what this means for what we teach and how we teach physical education. The role of the teacher in senior cycle is to facilitate students' learning, encouraging them to be self-directed and focused in their learning. With this in mind, the consultation meetings were designed to probe teachers on how physical education might be linked to the curriculum planning; co-curricular activities; qualification, training, and resources for teachers; links with the community; and promotion of physical activity. These consultation meetings took the form of a World Café, as outlined in **Box 18.8**, and revolved around a set of seven focused questions to which participants responded.

1. What kinds of innovations or curriculum strategies might you use to influence the physical education you offer in your school?
2. What ideas could we share to promote or develop inclusive practices in physical education and physical activity for all learners (disabilities, gender, ethnicity)?
3. In what way can national governing bodies (NGBs) be brought in to enhance physical education and physical activity?
4. What type of professional development opportunities could we get involved with, and how could we share these with colleagues?
5. How might we become aware of what is going on in the community? How do we make links with the community? How do we inform young people of what is available to them in the community and how to access it?
6. What kinds of events can be organized/promoted in our schools to advocate for physical activity, promote young

TABLE 18.1 Guidelines for Creative Problem Solving

Old Rules of School	Guidelines for Creativity and Innovation
1. The teacher is always right.	1. Solicit opinions from those doing the work.
2. There is only one answer.	2. There are several correct answers.
3. Keep your eyes on your own paper.	3. Collaborate and share ideas.
4. Raise your hand.	4. Don't measure everything.
5. Grade by report cards.	5. Allow for divergent thinking.
6. Stay on the subject.	6. Form self-directed teams.
7. Work alone.	7. Envision problem as solved, work backwards.
8. Stop daydreaming.	

BOX 18.8 World Café Discussion Strategy

According to Rainmaker Coaching, World Café is a collaborative dialogue that draws on the collective thoughts and knowledge of a group, shares and builds on that knowledge, and encourages creative solutions to challenging issues. The environment for a World Café is set up like a café with people sitting in small groups (four or five to a table). The group holds a series of conversational rounds lasting from 20 to 30 minutes, centered around one specific question at each table. At the end of each round, one person remains at each table as the host (recorder/informant) while the others move to separate tables. Table hosts welcome newcomers to their tables and questions, sharing an overview of that table's previous conversation. Newcomers bring their own thoughts to the table, and thus conversation continues, deepening as the round progresses. Individuals moving to new tables, with new members and a new focus throughout several rounds, allows ideas and themes to begin to link and connect. Sometimes a new or probing question that helps to explore the topic may be posed during one of the rounds of conversation. At the conclusion of several rounds, individuals return to their original tables to synthesize their discoveries and conclusions. The entire group is then invited to take part in sharing their insights; patterns are identified, collective knowledge is developed, and action items are explored further.

Adapted from Rainmaker Coaching. Knowledge café workshops. October 15, 2010. Available from www.rainmaker-coaching.co.uk/worldcafeknowledgecafe

peoples' healthy lifestyles, and celebrate their opportunities?

7. How might we involve student voice in developing and enhancing our physical activity and physical education programs?

From our perspective, if change is to take place in schools, teachers must position themselves to be open to change; be willing to consider change; be proactive in observing students and other teachers to learn from them; be responsive to issues that come up in physical activity settings, recognizing and gaining ideas and new insights; and be willing to grapple with new practices, even those outside their comfort zone, and bringing the students in to help them grow if necessary. Key to this change, of course, is support from colleagues and administrators if the change is to be achieved and valued. It takes time and is driven by a plan.

Student Teaching

During **teaching practice/student teaching**, preservice teachers are in a setting that has the potential to provide them with the first steps in their professional development. Preservice teachers are typically assigned a cooperating teacher and university supervisor with whom they can collaborate in a safe and consistent learning environment. Through this *supervisory mentoring* relationship, preservice teachers gain information on their teaching and their students' learning, seek and share ideas to impact lesson design and managing of student behavior, reflect on and challenge their perceptions on teaching strengths and weaknesses, and seek advice on how to handle difficult situations. Throughout this mentoring process, we encourage preservice teachers to develop a **professional development plan** to work toward in improving personal teaching practices and student learning. Consult your mentors in designing the goals for this professional development plan and a method to monitor progress toward achieving these goals that includes a time frame for improvement as well as identifying specific pedagogical practices and/or strategies that will assist in achieving these goals (see **Box 18.9**).

Learning Experience 18.4

Using the guidelines noted in Box 18.9, design your own professional development plan. Share it with a teaching peer, seeking insight on your choice of goals, strategies to achieve your goals, and the reality of the timeline you have outlined.

During the First Few Years: Induction

Research (Day et al., 2007; Day & Gu, 2010) shows that one of the main reasons early career teachers leave the teaching profession in the first few years is unsupportive working conditions and contexts and a lack of support. Hargreaves and Fullan (2012) suggest that keeping teachers beyond the first 3 years requires individual support "through well-led, dynamic, strongly supported schools where there is a belief in student success, a knowledge of how to bring it about, and a willingness and eagerness for everyone on the staff to keep learning and improving—inexperienced and experienced alike" (p. 70). There is even speculation that new teachers are influenced more by the experiences in their first teaching setting than by their teacher education program. This highlights that it is critical that the culture of the schools be changed if new teachers are to be impacted and retained in the profession and have an influence on the learning of young people.

BOX 18.9 Professional Development Plan

Develop a professional development plan that details how you intend to continue your development as a teacher. Based on your meetings with your supervisory tutors and your own reflections on areas where you need to improve, design at least one goal for each of the following categories: teaching, professional development, and being a member of the educational community. You may choose from the example areas provided or select a focus that meets your current needs. Once you have designed your goals, identify strategies you intend to use to assist you in reaching each goal and a date to assess your progress.

Category	Goal	Detailed Strategy	Assessment Date
1.			
2.			
3.			

Teaching:

- Effective teaching practices, preventive management strategies, and/or assessment strategies to monitor student learning
- Effective development and maintenance of a positive, student-focused learning environment
- Effective design of a challenging curriculum that is developmentally appropriate
- Effective demonstration of culturally sensitive teaching
- Effective use of student achievement and performance information to advise and involve students, parents, and the education community
- Effective integration of technology in teaching and learning
- Effective collaboration with parents, the school, and the community to impact the learning of young people

Professional development:

- Designing effective ways to evaluate your teaching
- Identifying appropriate resources for developing your teaching practices
- Responding to current issues in education
- Demonstrating effective application of current ideas on best practice
- Developing and monitoring teaching practice and student learning
- Designing an effective means of gaining knowledge on effective teaching practices

Member of educational community:

- Designing a personal participation strategy within the school and community
- Taking responsibility for aspects of curriculum development in the school
- Designing a physical education advocacy initiative
- Planning for involvement in a professional organization
- Planning for attending to the needs of all learners
- Developing communication and skills for working as part of a school community

Induction Programs

As a means of retaining newly qualified teachers and assisting them in their development, **induction programs** are being designed on different levels, from local schools and school districts to state and national initiatives. Induction has been described as "a comprehensive, coherent, and sustained professional development process aimed to train, support and retain new teachers and represents the first part of a lifelong professional development programme" (Wong, 2004). The Northwest Territories in Canada set the following goals for teacher induction (see www.newteachersnwt.ca/index.html):

1. Improve teacher performance.
2. Retain competent teachers in the profession.
3. Promote the personal and professional well-being of the new and beginning teacher.
4. Build a foundation for continued professional growth through structured contact with mentors, administrators, and other veteran teachers.
5. Transmit the culture of the school and teaching profession.

In addition, they have identified the perceived benefits for new and beginning teachers:

1. Accelerated success and effectiveness
2. Greater self-confidence
3. Heightened job satisfaction
4. Improved personal and professional well-being
5. Enhanced commitment to students, school, and profession
6. Increased opportunity for building connections with the community
7. Improved level of comfort and support

In Ireland, the National Induction Programme for Teachers (2010) has been designed to support the induction of newly qualified teachers (NQTs) into the teaching profession in primary and postprimary schools. This program intends to promote the professional development of NQTs through systematic support in their first year of teaching, followed by subsequent professional growth and development. One of the key characteristics of the program is providing NQTs with an experienced mentor teacher in their school or in a neighboring school who has undergone professional mentoring education. In addition, a whole school approach to induction is promoted with induction activities including mentor meetings, scheduled planning time, planned observation of other teachers teaching, making connections with the National Induction Services, and professional development workshops.

Ayers (1993) prompts educators to recognize teaching requires teachers and students to be partners in the learning environment. He suggests that to develop this partnership entails first establishing a positive learning environment where both partners are allowed to grow and develop. He describes becoming a teacher as an endeavor that is never finished, noting that it "demands an openness to something new, something unique, something dynamic" (p. 129), highlighting that what teachers need to know will be discovered as they teach. He proposes a set of guiding principles that maintain a focus on the student and student learning, including (1) being self- and peer critical on behalf of students; (2) finding allies and building alliances to benefit students; (3) developing audacity and humility in your teaching; (4) holding onto your ideals about teaching and learning, while working with others to improve education; (5) caring about, feeling compassion for, and offering guidance and advice to students, but not being their friend; and (6) operating on the principle of less is more, and implementing the strategies that make sense for your teaching context and your students.

Keay (2006) writes that during early induction into teaching, novice teachers' voices need to be heard and valued as they settle into the teaching profession. Although we recognize that newly qualified teachers can learn much from experienced and veteran teachers, a novice teacher has equally as much to share and contribute to a school, the teaching environment, and ultimately the learning of young people. Building collaborative relationships between and among teachers from all stages of their careers will make the teaching and learning environment a richer and more supportive place in which to work.

Mentors

Finding a mentor who is a qualified teacher to support and encourage the NQT in a teaching position in a school that does not provide an induction program is essential. This mentor needs to be someone with whom the new teacher can talk, seek guidance, share frustrations and concerns, and gain support. The mentor must be someone the new teacher trusts and who is directly linked to the context of the school, enabling support in working through situations specific to the setting. A mentor need not be a member of the same teaching department or content area; it may take time to identify an appropriate person as the new teacher transitions into a new role in the school. If you are a beginning teacher and the only physical education teacher at your school, Tannehill et al. (2012) suggest that you ". . . seek out a like-minded teacher in another subject department. Good practice is good practice irrespective of subject area" (p. 164).

Reflection and Self-Assessment

Reflection and self-assessment have been highlighted as important skills for a NQT to possess and practice. Posner (1989) suggests that nonreflective teachers are passive in the learning environment, uncritically accepting the norms they encounter in the school culture, seeking quick fixes and efficient means to achieve ends. They are influenced by their own impulses and known traditions as opposed to reflecting on their own practice. Developing teachers as reflective practitioners is a common goal of many current teacher education programs and requires teachers to consider the circumstances of their teaching, whether students are learning, and if changes are needed to ensure a quality learning experience. As you come to know yourself as a teacher, gain confidence in your ability to teach, and come to know your students and their needs and the learning environment in which you teach, your skill at reflecting on your teaching and student learning will be enhanced. "Taking time to reflect can help you to observe, gain perspective, make decisions, be critical, act in a particular way, challenge beliefs and values, and ultimately to better understand your circumstances" (O'Sullivan et al., 2010, p. 59). This suggests that when learning to teach, reflection can be viewed as one way to facilitate your development as a teacher. We would argue that finding a method of reflection with which you are comfortable and are willing to undertake on a regular basis is essential.

As a result of their research on reflection, Tsangaridou and O'Sullivan (1994) concluded that specific reflective pedagogical strategies can be learned, and when used over time can help preservice teachers in reflecting on and improving their own practice. They found that preservice teachers initially tend to focus on technical skills of teaching, which is not surprising when novice teachers first begin to teach. However, Tsangaridou and O'Sullivan encourage preservice teachers to view their teaching from a variety of perspectives, developing the skill to do so progressively as they move through their teacher education. As a result, they developed the Reflective Framework for Teaching in Physical Education (see **Box 18.10**). This model describes both the focus and level of preservice teachers' reflection on teaching and has been shown to be a useful tool for preservice and practicing teachers to consider their practices and the learning of their pupils. This model is most effectively employed in conjunction with a supervisory process that reflects an indirect approach to encouraging reflection.

BOX 18.10 The Reflective Framework for Teaching in Physical Education (RFTPE)

The focus of reflection:

- *Descriptive:* Describe information about an action/event.
- *Justification:* Focus on the logic or rationale of an action/event.
- *Critique:* Explain and evaluate an action/event.

Levels of reflection:

- *Technical:* Instructional or managerial aspects of teaching; focuses on application of effective teaching skills
- *Situational:* Contextual issues of teaching; results from meaningful situations that occur and on which teachers must make a decision
- *Sensitizing:* Social, moral, ethical, or political aspects of teaching; relates to issues around social construction of class (gender, race), moral actions (bullying), or political aspects (power, authority)

How to write reflections using the RFTPE framework:

- *Describe the event in detail:* What happened? What did you do? What did the students do?
- *Provide the logic or rationale for your actions:* Why was this event important or significant? Why did you react as you did?
- *Critique what you did:* How do you feel about what you did? What did you learn from this event? How do you plan to follow up regarding this event?

Learning Experience 18.5

With a teaching peer, read the following scenario and determine whether it is technical, situational, or sensitizing and if it reflects descriptive, justifying, or critique.

Scenario: When building shelters in adventure today, I prompted the students to make sure the sides of the shelter were taut and they just looked at me without responding. So, I said it again and still no response. At first I panicked, and then I realized that they did not know what "taut" meant. So, I told them to pull the sides of the shelter tight so that water would move down and not puddle. They understood this explanation and moved to pull the sides of the shelter so they were, in fact, taut.

After spending a number of years in a formal teacher education program, a new teacher undoubtedly has received frequent feedback (formal and informal) on their teaching practice from instructors, tutors, and even preservice teaching peers. They have taken part in group discussion focused on best practice, pedagogical strategies, and how they facilitate student learning and developed protocols for improving their practice. When beginning to teach in schools, new teachers no longer have university faculty and peers readily available with whom they can seek information on their teaching. Assessing your own teaching is a skill that you will need to develop while drawing on the assistance of colleagues and administrators, and even using technology to assist you in your efforts.

During the First Few Years: Postinduction

Think about your new and emerging professional development needs and consider how these might be developed. Clarify opportunities available to you in your own school context, with the state and/or national professional organizations accessible to you, and perhaps by informally seeking support from a colleague. The strategies identified in this chapter that take place during teacher education might be continually developed as you move through both the early and later stages of your teaching career.

In response to Keay's (2006) work on collaborative learning in teachers' early career development, Tannehill et al. (2012) conclude that perhaps the focus should be on teachers' professional learning, which they describe as "more sustained and collaborative engagement with learning" (p. 163) rather than professional development, which connotes something "being done to teachers" (p. 163). To promote professional learning, they urge all of us as physical education professionals to focus on building collaborative professional learning environments in all school settings at every educational level, suggesting that this is the responsibility of every educator. This begs the question, is professional learning part of your job as a teacher? We would argue that it is one of the most significant parts of your job as a teacher. If so, then how can we bridge the gap between professional development and professional learning for experienced teachers? Perhaps through interrogation of teacher as learner and encouraging teachers to pursue professional learning across their career.

Ongoing Throughout Your Teaching Career

Induction and early professional development span a relatively short time in the continuum of a teacher's career, whereas continuing professional development is needed to support the remainder of the teacher's career. In recognition of this, the lifelong learning and career development of teachers is emerging as a key priority internationally (OECD, 2005; Scottish Executive, 2004). This learning is considered critical for ensuring that teachers are able to meet the challenges and demands of a changing society and education systems.

Teacher professional development not only impacts teachers' practices, their beliefs about teaching and learning, and what physical education looks like in schools but also ultimately and perhaps more importantly influences the learning of their students. In professional development, the teacher is the learner. It is critical that professional development providers, be they outside agencies or teachers themselves, consider how teachers learn and recognize that, like students, in order for deep learning to occur, teachers must want to learn. In other words, professional learning is all about teachers being professional and committed to the improvement of their own practice throughout their teaching careers. We argue that continuing professional development should be school based, teacher designed, and gently facilitated through guidance and challenge. We encourage all teachers to commit to locating, accessing, and engaging in ongoing professional development. This might be through a community of practice, choosing to become part of a school–university partnership, or in-service education.

Community of Practice

A **community of practice** is a form of continuing professional development where experiences are led by teachers rather than something that is done to them. When working effectively, a community where teachers work together toward a common goal, share insights, challenge one another's perspectives, and grapple with issues that have an impact on their work can add depth to the learning of each teacher. From our reading of the literature (Armour & Yelling, 2004; Deglau & O'Sullivan, 2006; Parker et al., 2010), we argue that a community of practice as professional development has the following characteristics:

- Sustained over time rather than a one-off course.
- Focused on the needs of the community rather than the agenda of others.
- Involves meaningful and purposeful discourse around the reality of teaching in schools.
- Learning with the community is achieved together and from one another.
- Shared commitment and empowered teachers result from the group taking ownership of the community.
- Developed relationships through personal interaction sustain the community throughout the ups and downs of teaching.
- Occurs in the teaching setting.

A community of practice might evolve as the result of an issue about which a group of teachers becomes concerned (e.g., bullying), dissatisfaction with current professional development opportunities (e.g., that do not meet teachers' needs), through identification of a common initiative that a group of teachers chooses to investigate (e.g., developing a curriculum around Sport Education or Cultural Studies), at the suggestion of like-minded teachers in your area (e.g., helping young people take responsibility for their own learning), or through an initiative proposed by your professional organization (e.g., assessment for learning). Regardless of how a community evolves, all physical educators have the opportunity to become involved to the extent they are willing to source and access a community and then commit to the group and its focus.

School–University Partnerships

School–university partnerships are being encouraged at many education levels internationally, with the development of these partnerships becoming a key feature of redesigned initial teacher education (OECD, 2005). School–university partnerships typically take the form of a formal partnership arrangement between higher education institutions and schools to provide structured support and guidance to student teachers during teaching practice. These partnerships span a continuum from a work placement model (school playing a host role) to a partnership model (shared responsibility between the school and the higher education institution) to a training school model (school providing the entire training). Patton (2012) tells us that "school–university partnerships require extensive collaboration, trust, reflection and continued revision on the part of those involved to make a positive impact" (p. 14).

Developing a relationship between physical education teachers and teacher educators, between physical education preservice teachers and practicing teachers, and as a collective of these individuals might provide many benefits to each, as well as to how physical education is delivered in schools. As noted, the relationship that develops among all stakeholders in the teaching practice/student teaching experience is the most common link between schools and universities and in some cases is not well developed, outlined, or pursued, resulting in really no relationship at all. Alternatively, a practicing teacher might work with a researcher to design and conduct an action research project in physical education with the goal of impacting the learning of a group of postprimary students. A teacher educator might approach a practicing teacher seeking help in understanding some of the behavior issues that are most frequently occurring in schools as a means of better preparing prospective teachers. Each of these relationships must be developed by interested teachers, preservice teachers, teacher educators, and even administrators if they are to produce outcomes that impact teaching and learning in schools. Some will be initiated by the university and others by a group of teachers, and in some cases perhaps pursued as a result of a professional organization initiative. Recognizing all that we can learn from one another is the first step in developing these relationships.

The *Journal of Physical Education, Recreation and Dance* (JOPERD) recently published a feature focused on four school–university partnerships that were collaboratively developed in the United States with the intent of promoting physical education program reform and professional development for the teachers in these programs (Patton, 2012). In concluding this feature, Parker, Templin, and Setiawan (2012) share the five dimensions that emerged as critical to the development and maintenance of the school–university partnerships. They discuss each of the following five dimensions, suggesting that "reform is about positive relationships between partners with a commitment to change" (p. 33):

- The advantages of partnerships are reciprocal.
- Overcoming inequalities and differential power is necessary for the relationship to be successful.
- Recognizing and accepting knowledge and practice differences between settings will allow the designing of effective programs.
- Shared leadership among both partners is essential for change and accountability.
- Through change and sustainability renewal, rewards and positive benefits will accrue for both teachers and students.

In-Service Education

In-service education/training is a common form of professional development for teachers to assist them in building on their knowledge with current and up-to-date applications. Feiman-Nemser (2001) suggests that in-service training for teachers can be thought of as either the actual learning opportunities and activities to which teachers are exposed (OECD, 2009) or the learning that occurs during these sessions to change teaching practice (Winkler, 2001).

In-service education for teachers can take the form of lectures, workshops, or activity sessions, yet is typically "one size fits all," offered to teachers of all subject areas in a school, designed by outside agencies or to meet an administrative agenda, and mandatory. The focus of in-service education might range from assessment practices to differentiated learning to handling disruptive students. Although there are certainly nuggets of information that might prove useful to any teacher attending the in-service, the fact that they are not geared toward a particular context is problematic. It is quite different to manage a group of 30 students in a classroom setting as opposed to those same 30 students in a gymnasium or athletic field.

Like other education subjects, Bechtel and O'Sullivan (2006) note that in physical education, rather than teachers experiencing consistent and coherent professional development, they take part in fragmented opportunities to improve their teaching practice offered through various avenues across their careers. The result often is many teachers not perceiving this professional development as beneficial to their improvement as teachers or the learning of their students. They do highlight and acknowledge that some teachers want to learn, want to improve their teaching practice, and want to advance the learning of their students, striving toward this by taking whatever opportunities they can find to assist them in this development. Armour (2011) argued that continuing professional development should focus on supporting teachers in developing progressively, as learners, throughout their careers, noting that teachers need to refocus on themselves as career-long learners. This is consistent with what many scholars have begun telling us in recent years (Hargreaves & Fullan, 2012). Teachers must be given the opportunity and responsibility for development of the profession, and education policy makers and administrators must provide them with the time, the support, and the autonomy to achieve their goals for both teaching and learning.

In response to Armour and Yelling's (2004) paper on bridging the gap between professional development and professional learning, Tannehill et al. (2012) highlight a number of steps to ensure that continuing professional development opportunities in which teachers become involved will ultimately support the learning outcomes designed for students in physical education. Before selecting a professional development event in which to participate:

1. Consider what you believe are the key learning outcomes for physical education.
2. Consult your teaching colleagues to ensure the outcomes embrace all students in your program.
3. Compile a list of the professional development experiences you have recently undertaken, identifying the outcomes they supported and those they overlooked.
4. Discuss with a teaching colleague how you might apply the knowledge you have gained at the relevant continuing professional development events to your own practice and student outcomes.
5. Consider how you might seek continuing professional development to address the outcomes you have noted as overlooked.

6. Let your voice be heard regarding the types of in-service and continuing professional development opportunities that are and are not available so that the experiences designed might better meet the needs of you as a teacher and ultimately your students.

CHAPTER SUMMARY

The focus of this chapter is to highlight the opportunities available for professional development across all stages of a teacher's professional career. We provided insight on what continuing professional development may look like across the continuum of teacher education, including initial teacher education, induction into the teaching profession, and continuing professional development available to practicing teachers. Ideas, strategies, and examples of what the novice, entry, and veteran teacher may do to ensure they are able to develop personally and professionally across their entire teaching careers were discussed, recognizing that there will necessarily be overlap across and between the stages.

1. Teacher learning should be ongoing across a teacher's career, with teachers being active, reflective learners, involved with teacher change and improved teaching effectiveness.
2. Traditional professional development is characterized by generic in-service days housed in out-of-school venues, disconnected from other forms of professional development, provided by external experts, and intended for teachers to accept and adopt without question.
3. Teacher education is a continuum including initial teacher education, teacher induction, and early continuing professional development that are seamlessly aligned with one another.
4. Traditional continuing professional development opportunities beyond induction typically are not frequent or well-developed.
5. Mentoring is a process to support professional development involving an active and emotionally close relationship between individuals, reflects a focus on pedagogy, supports professional development, and produces teacher change.
6. Critical friends are one example of a mentoring relationship where trusted colleagues challenge and support one another.
7. A school's ethnography is intended to provide a teacher with key information about the community, school, and those who spend much of their lives in the school in which you work.
8. Analysis of teaching is based on how and what students do in the learning situation and can inform teacher development and improvement.
9. Cooperative learning is the basis of becoming a professional and of the continuing professional development of teachers.
10. A teaching portfolio requires a teacher to document evidence of their success in achieving standards and/or outcomes.
11. Preservice teachers enter teacher education with preconceived beliefs about teaching and learning that will guide their own practice. Until confronted and challenged about these beliefs, teacher education will not alter them.
12. Teachers who are change agents are able to lead change rather than follow or avoid change; for change in schools to occur, teachers must be open to and proactive in leading change.
13. A professional development plan is intended for teachers to design plans to work toward improving personal teaching practices.
14. Induction programs are comprehensive and sustained professional development programs designed to train, support, and retain new teachers.
15. Reflective teachers consider their own practice, the learning of their students, and how to improve their practice.
16. A community of practice is a form of continuing professional development where teachers work together toward a common goal, share insights, challenge one another's perspectives, and grapple with issues that have an impact on their work.
17. School–university partnerships can range from a work placement model (school playing a host role) to a partnership model (shared responsibility between the school and the higher education institution) to a training school model (school providing the entire training).
18. In-service training is the actual learning opportunities and activities that teachers undertake or the learning that teachers gain during in-service sessions.

REFERENCES

Armour, K. M. (2006). Physical education teachers as career-long learners: A compelling agenda. *Physical Education and Sport Pedagogy, 11*(3), 203–207.

Armour, K. M. (2011). *Sport pedagogy: An introduction for teaching and coaching*. Englewood Cliffs, NJ: Prentice Hall.

Armour, K., & Yelling, M. (2004). Continuing professional development for experienced physical education teachers: Towards effective provision. *Sport Education and Society, 9*(1), 95–114.

Attard, K., & Armour, K. (2006). Reflecting on reflection: A case study of one teacher's early-career professional learning. *Physical Education and Sport Pedagogy, 11*(3), 209–229.

Ayers, W. (1993). *To teach: The journey of a teacher.* New York: Teachers College Press.

Bechtel, P. A., & O'Sullivan, M. (2006). Effective professional development—what we now know. *Journal of Teaching in Physical Education, 25*, 363–378.

Breckon, P., & Capel, S. (2005). Extending your expertise as a teacher. In S. Capel (Ed.), *Learning to teach physical education in the secondary school* (2nd ed., pp 203–218). London: Routledge-Falmer.

Britzman, D. (1991). *Student makes student: A critical study of learning to teach.* New York: SUNY Press.

Brookfield, S. D. (1995). *Becoming a critically reflective teacher.* San Francisco, CA: Jossey-Bass.

Bullough, R. V., & Gitlin, A. (2001). *Becoming a student of teaching: Methodologies for exploring self and school context* (2nd ed.). Madison, WI: Brown and Benchmark.

Chung Wei, R., Darling-Hammond, L., Andree, A., Richardson, N., & Orphanos, S. School Redesign Network at Stanford University. (2009). *Professional learning in the learning profession: A status report on teacher development in the United States and abroad.* Stanford, CA: National Staff Development Council and the School Redesign Network.

Cockburn, T., Treadwell, P., & Cockburn-Wootten, D. (2001). The politics of community: Challenges in digital education. *Campus-Wide Information Systems, 18*, 187–194.

Costa, A., & Kallick, B. (1993). Through the lens of a critical friend. *Educational Leadership, 51*, 49–51.

Day, C., & Gu, Q. (2010). *The new lives of teachers: Teacher quality and school development.* Abingdon, UK: Routledge.

Deglau, D., & O'Sullivan, M. (2006). The effects of a long-term professional development program on the beliefs and practices of experienced teachers. *Journal of Teaching in Physical Education, 25*, 379–396.

Dewey, J. (1958). *Experience and education.* New York: Macmillan.

Dodds, P. (2005). Physical education/teacher education (PE/TE) policy. In D. Kirk, M. D. Macdonald, & M. O'Sullivan (Eds.), *Handbook of research in physical education* (Section IV, Chapter 6). London: Sage.

European Commission. (2008). *European qualifications framework for lifelong learning.* Luxembourg: Office for Official Publications of the European Communities.

European Commission. (2010). *Teachers' professional development: Europe in international comparison. An analysis of teachers' professional development based on the OECD's Teaching and Learning International Survey (TALIS).* Luxembourg: Office for Publication of the European Union.

Feiman-Nemser, S. (2001). Helping novices to learn to teach: Lessons from an experienced support teacher. *Journal of Teacher Education, 52*, 17–30.

Feiman-Nemser, S., & Remillard, J. (1996). Perspectives on learning to teach. In F. B. Murray (Ed.), *The teacher educator's handbook* (pp. 63–91). San Francisco, CA: Jossey-Bass.

Fernandez-Balboa, J. M. (1997). Knowledge base in physical education teacher education: A proposal for a new era. *Quest, 49*, 161–181.

Guskey, T. R. (1995). Professional development in education: In search of the optimal mix. In T. R. Guskey & M. Huberman (Eds.), *Professional development in education: New paradigms and practices* (pp. 253–267). New York: Teachers College Press.

Hargreaves, A. (2001). The emotional geographies of teaching. *Teachers College Record, 103*(6), 1056–1080.

Hargreaves, A., & Fullan, M. (2012). *Professional capital: Transforming teaching in every school.* New York: Teachers College Press.

Hellison, D. (2002). *Teaching responsibility through physical activity* (3rd ed.). Champaign, IL: Human Kinetics.

Higgins, M. C. (2000). The more the merrier? Multiple developmental relationships and working satisfaction. *Journal of Management Development, 19*, 277–296.

Higgins, M. C., & Krams, K. E. (2001). Reconceptualizing mentoring at work: A developmental network perspective. *Academy of Management Review, 26*, 264–286.

Irish National Teachers' Organization. (2010). *National induction programme for teachers.* Dublin, Ireland: Irish National Teachers' Organization.

Keay, J. (2006). Collaborative learning in physical education teachers' early-career professional development. *Physical Education and Sport Pedagogy, 14*, 323–334.

Lortie, D. (2002). *Schoolteacher* (2nd ed.). Chicago: University of Chicago Press.

MacPhail, A., & Tannehill, D. (2012). Helping pre-service and beginning teachers examine and reframe assumptions about themselves as teachers and change agents: "Who is going to listen anyway?" *Quest, 6*(4), 299–312.

Metzler, M. (2011). *Instructional models for physical education* (3rd ed.). Scottsdale, AZ: Hathaway.

Mitchell, S., & Collier, C. (2012, Oct.). Ohio physical education assessments. Paper presented at the NASPE Physical Education Teacher Education Conference, Las Vegas, Nevada.

National Association for Sport and Physical Education. (1995). *Moving into the future: National standards for physical education.* Reston, VA: Author.

National Association for Sport and Physical Education. (2004). *Moving into the future: National standards for physical education* (2nd ed.). Reston, VA: Author.

Northwest Territories Teacher Induction. (n.d.). A program for beginning teachers. Available from www.newteachersnwt.ca/index.html

Organisation for Economic Co-operation and Development. (2005). *Teachers matter: Attracting, retaining and developing teachers.* Paris: OECD.

Organisation for Economic Co-operation and Development. (2010). Higher education and adult learning: Education at a glance 2009—OECD indicators. Available from www.oecd.org/edu/eag2009

Oslin, J. (2002). Sport education: Cautions, considerations and celebrations. *Journal of Teaching in Physical Education, 21*, 419–426.

O'Sullivan, M. (2003). Learning to teach physical education. In S. J. Silverman & C. D. Ennis (Eds.), *Student learning in physical education: Applying research to enhance instruction* (2nd ed., pp. 275–294). Champaign, IL: Human Kinetics.

O'Sullivan, M. (2006). Principles of professional development. *Journal of Teaching in Physical Education, 25*, 441–449.

O'Sullivan, M., Tannehill, D., & Hinchion, C. (2010). Teaching as professional inquiry. In R. Bailey (Ed.), *Physical education for learning: A guide for secondary schools* (pp. 54–66). London, UK: Continuum Press.

Parker, M., Patton, K., Madden, M., & Sinclair, C. (2010). From committee to community: The development and maintenance of a community of practice. *Journal of Teaching in Physical Education, 29*, 337–357.

Parker, M., Templin, T., & Setiawan, C. (2012). What has been learned from school–university partnerships? *Journal of Physical Education, Recreation and Dance, 83*, 32–35.

Patton, K. (2012). The dynamics of promoting sustained school–university partnerships. *Journal of Physical Education, Recreation and Dance, 83*, 13–14.

Posner, G. J. (1989). *Field experience: Methods of reflective teaching.* New York: Longman.

Rainmaker Coaching. (2010, Oct 15). Knowledge café workshops. Available from www.rainmaker-coaching.co.uk/worldcafeknowledgecafe

Scottish Executive. (2004). *Building the foundations of a lifelong learning society: A review of collaboration between schools and further education colleges in Scotland.* Edinburgh: Scottish Executive.

Siedentop, D., & Tannehill, D. (2000). *Developing teaching skills in physical education.* Mountain View, CA: Mayfield.

Stoll, L., & Seashore Louis, K. (2007). *Professional learning communities: Divergence, depth and dilemmas.* Berkshire, UK: Open University Press.

Sugrue, C. (2004). Rhetoric and realities of CPD across Europe: From cacophony towards coherence? In C. Day & J. Sachs (Eds.), *International handbook on the continuing professional development of teachers* (pp. 67–93). Berkshire, UK: Open University Press.

Tannehill, D., & Coffin, D. (1996). Mentoring in physical education teacher education in the USA. C: Research trends and developments. In M. Mawer (Ed.), *Mentoring in physical education: Issues and insights* (pp. 217–238). London: Falmer Press.

Tannehill, D., & MacPhail, A. (2012). What examining teaching metaphors tells us about pre-service teachers' developing beliefs about teaching and learning. *Physical Education and Sport Pedagogy Journal.* [in press]

Tannehill, D., MacPhail. A., Halbert, G., & Murphy, F. (2012). *Research and practice in physical education.* Oxfordshire, UK: Routledge.

Teaching Council of Ireland. (2011). Teaching council learning outcomes in Ireland. In: *Initial teacher education: Criteria and guidelines for programme providers.* Maynooth, Ireland: Author.

Thompson, C. (2004). Yes, but . . . Available from http.//innovationsupplychain.com/files/yesbutebook.pdf

Tsangaridou, N., & O'Sullivan, M. (1994). Using pedagogical reflective strategies to enhance reflection among preservice physical education teachers. *Journal of Teaching in Physical Education, 14*, 13–23.

Winkler, G. (2001). Reflection and theory: Conceptualising the gap between teaching experience and teacher expertise. *Educational Action Research, 9*, 437–449.

Wong, H. (2004). Induction programs that keep new teachers teaching and learning. *NASSP Bulletin, 88*, 43. Available from www.NewTeacher.com

CHAPTER 19 Advocating for and Promoting Your Program

Overall Chapter Outcome

To optimize the knowledge for developing and implementing a deliberate program promotion and advocacy plan

Learning Outcomes

The learner will:

- Demonstrate understanding of the need to employ marketing and promotion strategies to increase awareness of the critical role of school physical education programs among key constituents
- Demonstrate understanding of the current trends and issues facing school physical education
- Demonstrate skills to provide constituents within and beyond school settings with the latest and best available knowledge about quality physical education, physical activity, and its role in promoting health and wellness
- Develop understanding of the need for and strategies to proactively advocate for physical education in school to key constituents, such as parents, policy makers, and other members of the community

Ask 100 physical educators what they believe to be the overarching purpose of school physical education, and most will respond with a statement along the lines of: "To provide students with the skills, knowledge, and dispositions that will lead them toward a physically active lifestyle." Your formal teacher preparation program should give you the opportunity to develop essential skills through focused practice and feedback on your progress. Some of these essential skills and areas of knowledge include program development, curriculum design, instructional delivery, assessment, and the interplay between them. What is equally important is that, as your teaching career unfolds, you become vigilant and skillful in advocating for and promoting your program. With few exceptions (e.g., Finland), physical education is not considered a "core" subject in primary and postprimary schools. Consequently, it is a "marginalized" school subject. Thus, everyone in the field (including teaching professionals, university faculty, and professional organizations) plays a central role in demonstrating that physical education is, in fact, an indispensible part of every student's formative education. This chapter focuses on the various program promotion and advocacy aspects of your job as a professional physical educator.

BOX 19.1 Key Terms in This Chapter

- *Advocacy:* Any effort aimed at informing, persuading, and/or changing existing beliefs or views with the intent to support new or change existing formal rules/mandates/legislation.
- *Best available knowledge:* The most current/up-to-date evidence available that can be used in support of stated claims, beliefs, and positions.
- *Constituents:* People who have a vested interest in and concern about particular issues, programs, and the like.
- *Policy:* A set of rules aimed at governing the behavior of people within a particular setting (e.g., class, program, school, school system, state, country). "Stronger" policies are those that come with consequences, oversight, and funding. If one or more of these are not present, they are considered "weaker" policies, with the consequence that the policy is less likely to be followed.
- *Policy makers:* People in positions who review, consider, and vote on proposed new (or changes to existing) formal rules, mandates, and/or legislation. Examples include school managers, school system board members, and local, provincial/state, or national legislators.
- *Program promotion:* Any effort aimed at informing, educating, or building awareness in others about aspects of the physical education program. Analogous to marketing.

Learning Experience 19.1

Together with four classmates, use community mapping to develop a physical activity profile of a community (or portion thereof) to answer the following questions:

1. In addition to school physical education programs, what free or fee-based, public or private (i.e., commercial) programs and facilities are available to children, youth, adults, and older adults?
2. How prevalent are shared-use agreements between groups or agencies that are in the business of providing physical activity opportunities for children and youth?

Based on the profile you develop, determine the following:

1. Which population groups appear to be at an advantage in terms of access to physical activity?
2. What is the balance between public and private/commercial opportunities?
3. What is the balance of free versus fee-based physical activity opportunities for children and youth?

Physical education has been a part of schools in most countries for over a century. In earlier times, the field received increased attention during times of warfare, when it became evident that the fitness levels of military personnel were well below where they needed to be. Over the last two decades, there have again been frequent calls for increased time and need for physical education in schools; however, this recent attention is rooted in the public health problems surrounding increased levels of overweight and obesity across most layers of the population in most developed countries.

Ironically, today's school physical education has perhaps never faced a greater dilemma. On the one hand, time allocated for physical education has been squeezed because of ongoing educational reform efforts to improve students' academic performance (e.g., Center on Education Policy, 2007). Moreover, the recent global economic recession continues to reverberate throughout many nations; coupled with the increased focus on improving academic performance, this has resulted in significant budget cuts and reduced time allocation for physical education and other non-"core" subjects.

Simultaneously, today's wide variety of physical activity choices has never been greater. The 20th century saw the emergence of a sport culture in most developed countries, and today sport is arguably one of the most powerful and influential cultural institutions. But sport is by no means the only form of physical activity. For example, the fitness movement re-emerged in the 1970s. According to Lauer (2006), U.S. participation levels in fitness exercise among adults peaked in 1990, but have declined significantly through 2005 (see **Table 19.1**). Table 19.1 also reflects trend shifts in the types of activities in which adults engage. Other examples of alternative forms of physical activity include what were first called "extreme sports" in the 1980s. Activities such as skateboarding and BMX reflect a rejection of the values typically espoused in team sport (e.g., teamwork, cooperation, uniformity, and subordination to leadership). Instead they reflect values of individualism, creativity, and the like. Interestingly, aided in no small part by U.S. cable television giant ESPN, these activity forms have quickly become

TABLE 19.1 Sport Participation Trends in the United States from 1998 to 2004

Exercise Type	1998	2000	2004	Change (%)
Pilates		173,900	1,100,541	+506.2
Stationary cycling	1,076,500	2,879,500	3,143,100	+2.8
Weight machines	1,526,100	2,518,200	3,090,300	+102.5
Free weights	2,555,300	4,449,400	5,205,600	+130.8
Treadmill exercise	439,600	4,081,600	4,746,300	+979.7
Fitness walking	2,716,400	3,798,100	4,029,900	+48.4
Running/jogging	3,713,600	3,615,200	3,731,000	+0.5
Aerobics	2,122,500	1,732,600	1,576,500	-23.7
Fitness swimming	1,691,200	1,454,200	1,563,500	-7.5
Home gym exercise	390,500	757,700	934,700	-139.4

Data from Lauer, H. (2006). *The new Americans: Defining ourselves through sports and fitness participation.* Fort Mill, SC: American Sports Data.

highly institutionalized in the form of today's summer and winter X Games competitions that are held annually throughout the globe (Siedentop & van der Mars, 2012). Finally, the Adventure Education arena presents another broad menu of activity choices. Activities such as rock climbing, whitewater rafting, hiking, and mountain biking are now also well-established means of enjoying physical activity.

On the other hand, physical education programs have been identified as a central point of intervention in efforts to promote physical activity. Globally, numerous organizations and government agencies have highlighted the critical role of schools in promoting health through school physical education, increased opportunities for physical activity throughout the school day, and so on. These initiatives are all based in part on the efforts to reverse the trends in overweight and obesity among children and adolescents. A recent Gallup survey study on levels of overweight and obesity in England showed that one in every four Britons 18 years and older is obese (Mendes, 2011). In the United States, Ogden, Carroll, Kit, and Flegal (2012) reported that almost 17% of children and adolescents are obese. They also noted a positive development in that from 2007–2008 to 2009–2010, obesity levels had begun to level off. **Figure 19.1** shows the levels of overweight and obesity among European boys and girls (ages 11–15).

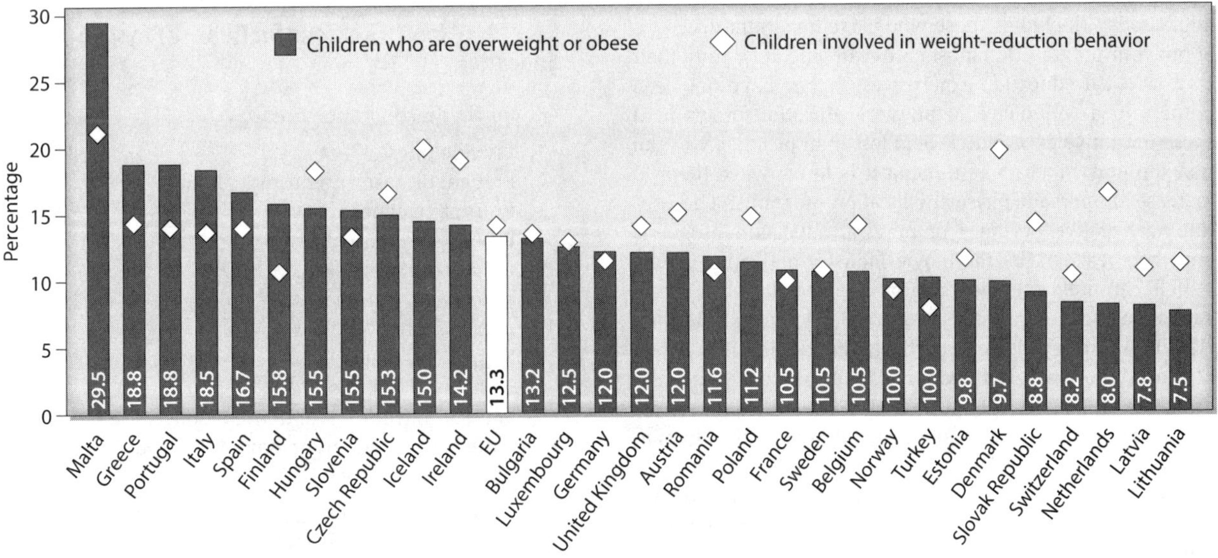

FIGURE 19.1 Percentage of European 11- to 15-year-olds who are overweight or obese, by country, 2005–2006.
Reproduced from OECD. (2010). Health at a glance: Europe 2010. OECD Publishing. http://dx.doi.org/10.1787/health_glance-2010-en. Reprinted with permission.

The emergence of the concept of the "Bewegte Schule" (i.e., school on the move) in the 1990s in Germany and Switzerland (e.g., Schmidt-Millard, 2003) and, more recently, the Comprehensive School Physical Activity Program model (NASPE, 2008) in the United States reflect the push for school environments to support and promote access and opportunity for physical activity throughout the school day for *all* students. This represents a fundamental shift, in that delivering a physical education program in schools encompasses more than just teaching one's lessons of the various instructional units throughout the school year. As we have noted, school physical education programs do not have a monopoly on providing opportunities for physical activity that can contribute to that "physically active life." Thus, physical educators not only have to demonstrate that they have relevance to co-teachers in their school, their school managers, and parents but also have to demonstrate the same to the broader community. As physical educators, we understand how important our programs are and why; however, in the end it matters little what we believe about our own profession's role in education and the community beyond (Sallis & McKenzie, 1991). The key is what the relevance of our field is in the eyes of the public at large. That is where program promotion and advocacy come in.

Physical Educators' Unrealized Role

Physical educators perform many roles beyond teaching their lessons. Promotion of and advocacy for one's program is one of these. One way of conceptualizing your role as program promoter and advocate is to view it as informing and educating your **constituents** about the need for and value of quality school physical education. Remember as well that most adults today (including those who make important decisions about your program!) in most cases can only draw from their own physical education experiences, if they have not been witness to a well-delivered physical education program. If those formative experiences were less than positive, you can imagine how much more difficult it is to convince them to increase support for physical education programs. The continuing negative portrayal of physical education programs and their teachers by the movie industry and other media outlets certainly does not help to change the public's perception of school physical education (McCullick, Belcher, Hardin, & Hardin, 2003). Of particular importance is the view of those who make key decisions about physical education programs in schools: **policy makers**. These include school managers, school board members, and government legislators at the various levels.

There is evidence in the United States that relative to their own primary physical education program, school managers (i.e., principals) (1) are significantly more satisfied with their own physical education program than are their physical education teachers, (2) have little familiarity with their programs, and (3) are rarely involved in any form of evaluation of their programs (Lounsbery, McKenzie, Trost, & Smith, 2011). This suggests that there is little incentive for school managers to invest more resources into improving the quantity and quality of school physical education and, thus, represents a barrier for moving the field forward. In light of the increasing emphasis on improving students' academic performance, Sallis (2010) argued that in the United States:

> *It is likely school principals, school board members, superintendents, and state and federal education officials are unfamiliar with the consistent findings that active, fit, and lean children do better in school. It is counterintuitive that spending less time in the classroom and more time in PE might improve learning. (p. 697)*

It should be obvious that beyond educating children and youth, the public must become better informed about what quality physical education programs can and should accomplish. Le Masurier and Corbin (2006) offered insight into defensible arguments that physical educators can make when advocating for quality physical education in schools (see **Box 19.2**). These can be supported with empirical evidence when speaking with policy makers and other constituents. The remainder of this chapter is devoted to providing an overview of the various strategies that physical educators can use to accomplish this task. In the next sections we will show how program promotion and advocacy go hand in hand in that promotion efforts lay the foundation for advocacy.

BOX 19.2 Top 10 Reasons for Quality Physical Education

Quality physical education can . . .

1. Provide physical activity
2. Prevent disease and promote health
3. Promote wellness
4. Promote lifelong fitness
5. Help prevent obesity
6. Teach skills including self-management (i.e., behavior change) skills
7. Support academic achievement
8. Be economically sound practice
9. Support development of the whole child
10. Count on broad endorsement from outside agencies and professional societies

Reproduced from Le Masurier, G. C., & Corbin, C. B. (2006). Top 10 reasons for quality physical education. *Journal of Physical Education, Recreation and Dance, 77*(6), 44–53. With permission of the publisher (Taylor & Francis Ltd., www.tandf.co.uk/journals).

Learning Experience 19.2

Select five of the reasons listed in Box 19.2 and develop an articulate and persuasive written statement that could be used when speaking before a group of constituents (e.g., parents, school board). Be sure you use appropriate supporting literature. The presentation should be no longer than 4 minutes.

Program Promotion Strategies

Arguably, few school subjects suffer as much as does physical education from the "teaching is easy" claim. Former athletes who choose to coach a team of youngsters quickly find out that quality teaching or coaching requires more than just having been a skillful player. Even fewer people can appreciate the skillfulness needed by teachers to aid diverse groups of learners in becoming more competent and literate movers in enjoyable ways so that they are more likely to continue seeking out physical activity. In addition, ask yourself the question: Do others (i.e., parents, school managers, co-teachers) really know what I do in my program?

Above all, planning, delivering, and evaluating a quality physical education program is the most important contribution teachers can make toward promoting their program. But your students, their parents, and your school's managers are all key people who should know details about your program's mission, the curriculum, and what students are actually learning. Although students' school report cards will give some indication of their progress in physical education, a grade alone does not offer much detail. Typically, parents (and as noted previously, school managers) will have great interest in their children's performance in classroom subjects. Thus, beyond delivering a quality physical education program, the field as a whole must find ways to be "on the radar" of these constituents. The question for individual programs is: How will you and your colleagues show that you are making critical contributions?

Program promotion has three fundamental purposes: (1) increase the program's visibility on and beyond campus; (2) inform parents, school managers, and the public at large about the good things that happen in the program; and (3) improve and maintain the program's credibility. Creating Comprehensive School Physical Activity Programs (CSPAPs) (NASPE, 2008) in the United States or Active Schools in Ireland (see www.activeschoolflag.ie) are important steps toward increasing physical education's visibility and making the program a more integral part of the school. However, two preconditions are necessary for any other program promotion efforts to get traction with constituents. First, teachers must develop credible information about the program. Second, teachers should maintain currency in the constantly emerging knowledge base relative to instructional and curricular practices, and current trends and issues in the field and beyond.

Developing Credible Information to Share About Your Program's Accomplishments

First and foremost, you have to be able to show that your program is accomplishing its goals and objectives. Nothing will make the public (including policy makers) doubt the program's value and relevance more than when physical educators make claims about their program's many goals and objectives, but cannot offer any credible evidence that they are accomplishing any of them. Formal assessment of student learning is a central teaching function/responsibility of all physical educators. Developing an evidence base around the various program objectives (as described in content standards) by employing ongoing formal formative assessment should go a long way toward providing you with the needed information. Like it or not, the increasing emphasis on having teachers' performance evaluations based in part on evidence of student learning will require physical educators to increase their attention to assessing their students' performance on an ongoing basis. Recently, McKenzie (2012) went so far as to argue that

> *. . . [the] profession also needs to move beyond "standards-based" PE to actually deal with "evidence-based" PE. Currently, we have little evidence that PE makes any difference in the lives of children or to society, especially related to social and emotional outcomes. We need to teach potential teachers how to gather evidence and how to use it to evaluate their programs relative to the objectives that are established.*

Maintain Currency with Current Trends, Issues, and Best Available Knowledge

Today's context for school physical education, education in general, and society at large is fundamentally different from three decades ago. Similarly, not unlike the field of medicine, the knowledge base underlying the delivery of school physical education programs evolves continuously. As part of making sure that the school management, policy makers, and the broader public are informed about physical education, it is imperative that physical educators can convey the latest developments in their field. Staying current about new developments, trends, and issues in the field is a central goal of teachers' continuing professional development efforts.

In the last four decades, sport pedagogy has emerged as a legitimate area of inquiry that focuses specifically on the study of the teaching and learning processes in physical activity settings such as school physical education, sport coaching at all levels, and the fitness club industry (e.g., personal training, group exercise classes) and the role of the many variables that may be influencing these processes. Physical educators now can get access to multiple professional journals, and professional organizations offer regular workshops, conferences, webinars, and the like, all aimed at helping professionals stay current.

Maintaining currency is critical because when physical educators are called upon for their opinion/expertise (or when they recognize the need to change misconceptions in others), they want to be in a position where they can provide informed advice that is based on the **best available knowledge**, rather than just based on "how they feel." Consider the following sample questions:

- What is the relationship between students' physical activity and their performance on fitness tests?
- What are the health benefits of physical activity? What are its economic benefits?
- What do we know about the relationship between the time in physical activity (including physical education) and students' academic performance?
- What are the current local, state, provincial, or national policies in effect relative to the delivery of physical education? Recess? Physical activity as a form of punishment?

These are legitimate questions whose answers should be at the fingertips of physical educators because this information forms the basis for educating the public and policy makers. And for each of these questions there is now a substantial evidence base. How would you answer these questions?

Learning Experience 19.3

Working in groups of three or four, and using legitimate resources (e.g., professional and research journals, websites of professional organizations, position and policy documents, etc.), answer the four sample questions listed. Develop a professional two-page brief that provides a synopsis of the available evidence that can answer these questions.

When physical educators can demonstrate that (1) their program does contribute to the development of students and (2) they are informed and up-to-date on current trends and issues in the field, program promotion efforts will improve greatly.

Inform, Communicate, and Educate the Public

Being current and knowledgeable about the field and the evidence that supports school physical education programming is important in that it can inform teachers' own instructional and curricular practices, and thus impact their students' learning experiences. However, the public at large generally has dated (and often negative) perspectives on school physical education based in no small part on their own experiences as students. We recommend that teachers use the following strategies continuously to ensure that the students' and program's accomplishments are continuously on the radar with parents, school managers, and others:

- Formal presentations
- Informal information sharing
- Newsletters and website announcements
- Inviting key people to visit your program
- Using local print and television media
- Connecting with community organizations
- Fundraising
- Special demonstration events

Any combination of these strategies can help increase program visibility both on campus and beyond and help convey the important role that physical education plays in the lives of children and youth.

Formal Presentations

Sharing key highlights, activities, and accomplishments about your program is vital to increasing the visibility and credibility of physical education in schools. The point here is that you want to be prepared to do this at any time, anywhere, and to anyone. Physical educators have numerous forums as potential outlets, including staff meetings, school board meetings, parent–teacher organization (PTO) meetings, parent–teacher conferences, school open houses, curriculum nights, family fitness nights, and/or physical education program demonstration nights. In addition, community organizations such as Chambers of Commerce, Lions Clubs, and the like are also potential targets for promoting the important role of school physical education programs in ensuring that children and youth develop the behaviors that lead to a healthy lifestyle. As we will show in more detail, such presentations can form the foundation for seeking supplemental funding for the program. These venues and events are prime opportunities to highlight your students' performance. One effective strategy would be to develop a "boilerplate" presentation that, with minor adjustments, can be used with different audiences.

The key is to understand that you have only a limited amount of time to showcase (1) what you and your students do in the program, and (2) what your students can do and know. Thus, you will want to have a plan for what you wish to emphasize. For example, based on your data related to students' physical activity levels, you can show the percentage of students in the program and how this trends across class levels and time. Other examples would be to show the degree to which students know about the FITT—Frequency, Intensity, Time, and Type—principles, their performance in officiating games (i.e., refereeing, scorekeeping), applying safety precautions with rock climbing, or proper preparations for a 2-day outdoor hike. Typically, presentations at faculty meetings, school board meetings, or with other policy makers can be no longer than 3–5 minutes. Thus, the message you want the audience to take away must be focused and crystal clear.

Learning Experience 19.4

Daily sessions of recess in schools are a critical part of the school day for multiple reasons. In many cases, time for recess has been scaled down or, worse, eliminated altogether. Your task is twofold: (1) Gather information about the evidence supporting the time for recess and (2) develop a short and persuasive 3- to 5-minute presentation that you and your peers could present before a group of policy makers who are considering shortening the weekly minutes for recess. The presentation should be professional and demonstrate the need for daily recess. Be sure you can support the presentation using appropriate evidence from the research on recess.

In addition, develop a one-page brief that offers a clear overview of the key messages in the presentation that can be left with the target audience.

The keys to making these short presentations persuasive are to know your audience and find a way to make an emotional connection with that audience. Presentations that include photos or very brief video clips of students in action, such as recent Sport Education seasons, strength conditioning sessions, an outdoor hiking trip, or even selected students sharing their reactions, are powerful means of showing what students know and can do.

Such presentations also educate the attendees that your program goes beyond the experiences that they might have had. Sharing your efforts and accomplishments with classroom colleagues during faculty meetings (or in passing) also improves their awareness/knowledge of your program's mission and accomplishments. Your active engagement in such meetings will be noticed (as would your lack of involvement or absence).

"Once is not enough" is the adage to live by when it comes to educating and persuading the broader public about your program's accomplishments, the need for quality physical education, and physical activity programming at schools in general. Program promotion is quite similar to commercial advertising in that a company does not expect the customer to buy into the product advertised after just one wave of advertising. Companies will employ multiple promotion strategies to connect with potential customers. Similarly for physical education programs, the goal of program promotion is to repeatedly connect with the many constituents. That is where the next strategy can be effective.

Informal Program Promotion Opportunities

Brief and often chance encounters with school managers and/or parents around campus before or after school or in the community are great opportunities to let them know what is going on in your program and report on their son's or daughter's successes. Related to this, we know of teachers who every week make it a point to make four to five phone calls home to the parents/guardians of a small group of their students and share the students' accomplishments. Imagine the surprise of parents to receive such news! The key point is that physical education teachers come to view promoting their program as something that has no off-season. It can and should take place anytime, anywhere, and with anyone.

Schoolwide Announcements

Daily public announcements that are common in most postprimary schools are an excellent strategy for when students, classroom teachers, and school managers are the target audience. Announcements are made through either the public address system or the closed circuit school television. This is an excellent means for announcing open gym times (e.g., before school, at lunchtime) or special after-school events such as an upcoming fun run challenge or sending out reminders about the scheduled after-school staff fitness/wellness sessions, community-based physical activity-related events, and the like. Schools will likely have a protocol for submitting the information so the announcement is included at the appropriate times. The advantage of the closed-circuit school television is that announcements can be up for several days and the target audience is more likely to see it.

Another way in which students can be reached quickly is through announcements made by classroom colleagues. Physical educators can email all classroom colleagues with pertinent information included and request that the classroom teachers make an announcement in their classes. Although schools may have policies in place prohibiting or limiting the use of social media, it is a potentially powerful means of spreading information because social media (e.g., Facebook, Twitter) are an increasingly popular means of communication among youth.

Newsletters and Websites

Beyond face-to-face meetings, physical educators have multiple additional venues through which they can reach constituents beyond the school campus. Most schools send out monthly newsletters to parents. In most cases today, newsletters are delivered in web-based formats. Typically, newsletters include updates from the school manager, announcements of special events, important deadlines, and the like. Physical educators can request that they have a section devoted solely to news, events, recent developments, and announcements specific to the physical education program, healthy living, and physical activity promotion beyond the campus. Schools typically have a staff person dedicated to compiling the information needed for each newsletter issue, and today most are produced using desktop publishing software. Thus, physical education teachers can focus mostly on deciding what should go into the newsletter. For example, physical education programs can share the upcoming instructional units and other key announcements.

Including photos of students in action on the website is another powerful way of sharing experiences during units just completed. Teachers can recruit students to assist with shooting photos. Announcements of upcoming events in the community are an excellent way of promoting physical activity among the students (and their family) beyond the campus as well. For example, local organizations frequently will organize special events such as annual 1K/5K/10K walk/jog/runs. Physical educators who are connected with other community organizations such as sport clubs, sporting goods stores, and the like can then encourage students and their families to sign up for such events. Providing frequent prompts on school bulletin boards and school websites on how students can be encouraged to seek out physical activity at home on weekends are another example of promoting physical activity beyond the confines of the school campus. Photos of students in action that are hung around the school's hallways are another means of creating a culture of an active and healthy campus.

In the United States, another approach is to use the school district's website to provide information and resources to students, teachers, administrators, parents, and the public at large, specific to physical education programs and physical activity. One example is Arizona's Chandler Unified School District website, which includes an area dedicated to physical activity promotion throughout the school day (see www.mychandlerschools.org/Page/1246). It offers resources for all the district physical educators and classroom teachers to promote physical activity beyond physical education lessons. Some include plug-and-play videos and other resources for classroom teachers to build physical activity breaks into their classroom instruction, as well as resources for promoting active recess periods and before-school activities.

Invite Significant People to Visit Your Program

Classroom colleagues, parents, school managers, and policy makers all have busy work schedules; however, each of them needs to become more informed about the current trends and issues in our field and how their school's physical education program is contributing. In primary schools, classroom teachers typically use the physical education period for their own planning. However, they also need to know specifically what it is that physical educators try to accomplish. This will happen only if they come and witness how their students do in physical education or during other physical activity–related special events. They will learn about the complexities of managing large groups of children in a movement-oriented environment and the complexity of designing appropriate learning tasks. Moreover, they get to see their students in a different environment, which may help inform their teaching approaches in their own classroom.

Parents in primary schools will frequently visit the school and observe their children in class events. Seeing their child actively engaged in a well-managed and high-energy physical education lesson is a powerful way of showing what such experiences mean to their child. It is here where physical educators can bring the messages about active lifestyles to life that parents read about in the school newsletter or on the physical education program website. Once they witness the energy, passion, and enthusiasm with which students participate in the lessons, they will become more aware of your programmatic efforts. They may be willing to serve as volunteer assistants and can also become powerful allies in terms of advocating for the program before policy makers. Finally, at every opportunity, invite school managers to come see the action in your classes, and invite them to special events that you have planned.

From an educative perspective, it is important that physical educators provide context for what visitors are witnessing. The purpose of the activities and how they are organized may be perfectly clear to physical educators, but it may not be that obvious to the layperson. Once students are engaged in the activity, teachers can provide visitors with a brief explanation. For example, in a team-building lesson with students engaged in problem-solving activities, you can briefly explain the purpose of problem-solving activities, how these align with your program mission, and how the skills that students develop transfer to other aspects of life. In a Sport Education lesson you can highlight the multiple roles that students have beyond player, how these are legitimate learning outcomes, and how learning these roles contributes to a better and deeper understanding of sport. Playing matches that are part of your culminating events during a school assembly is another excellent way of demonstrating what your students have accomplished. Imagine their reaction when school managers and other adults see motivated, self-directed students who demonstrate well-played matches or performances. Good administrators will recognize and remember such efforts.

The typical physical education lesson in a gymnasium is a more public setting than a typical classroom where math instruction is taking place. Contrary to their reaction to, perhaps, the science classroom, outsiders generally feel more comfortable walking in during a physical education lesson. With the increased focus on teacher evaluation, there is a good chance that school managers will make unscheduled stops during lessons. These instances again are a good opportunity to educate and inform.

In the case of a special event, such as a schoolwide fun run (or walk), physical educators could invite school managers, parents, and/or school board members to join the event as participants. Remember that a one-time invitation will likely not suffice. Their schedules will be such that they cannot attend each event you hold. But, if teachers make these public figures part of the standard list of invitees, then at some point they can and will attend. Physical educators in the Kyrene school district in Arizona hold an annual "Turkey Trot" right before the Thanksgiving Day holiday. When possible, some of the schools will map out a route for this run/walk event that takes them right past the home of the school manager and/or one of the school system's board members. Again, these are effective ways to make a program more visible to important people.

Using Local Print and Television Media

Whenever possible, invite the local newspaper or television stations to the program. Notwithstanding its history of negatively stereotyping physical education teachers, the media can be an important ally in promoting the "good" in school physical education. The important role of the media was recognized in that it was one of eight societal sectors that contributed to formulating strategies and tactics for promoting the importance of physical activity as part of the 2010 National Physical Activity Plan in the United States (see www.physicalactivityplan.org/media.php). Especially in the United States, the local print and television media (and even the national media) pay substantial attention to interscholastic sport, because of the strong draw that it has created among the public. In other countries, the club system forms the main structure through which children, youth, and adolescents participate in sport. There, too, the print media will allocate space to report on accomplishments. Thus, there is no reason why school physical education programs cannot make use of these media to help inform and educate the public. **Figure 19.2** shows an example of how a postprimary school in Ahwatukee, Arizona, connected with a local television network affiliate to share its news about a before-school physical activity program.

Local media are always in search of stories of local interest, and this places physical education front and center in terms of promoting its broader mission and the efforts underway to make the mission a reality. Invitations for media visits need not be for just formal or special events. For example, an ongoing feature in the local print and/or television media could focus on how the program is gradually adding the various CSPAP features such as before school programs, active recess periods, or infusion of physical activity breaks in the classrooms. The public would thus learn about how today's school physical education program looks fundamentally different from the one that the public experienced years earlier. Special events like family fitness nights or open houses are also excellent opportunities to bring in the local media. Again, photographs in the local newspapers (and videos on their websites) are an excellent means of advertising the

HOME NEWS MORNING SHOW WEATHER SPORTS TRAFFIC LIFESTYLE VIDEO SEEN ON TV

Mountain Pointe High School Physical Activity Program

Posted: May 07, 2010 11:19 AM EDT

Earlier this week, President Obama unveiled the first physical activity plan for our country. It's the first big attempt to curb the obesity rate, which is at an all-time high.

Part of the plan is to get high school students more active.

Here in the valley, Mountain Pointe High School in Phoenix is already hard at work.

The program is free and open to all the students.

Phil Abba Dessa has the details.

On the Net:

Mountain Pointe High School - www.tuhsd.k12.az.us/mtp

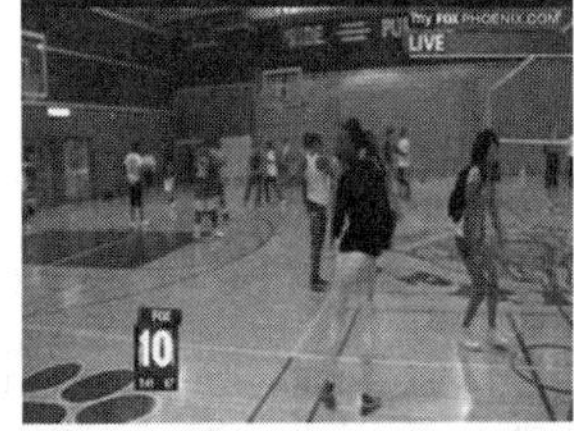

FIGURE 19.2 Local television media visit an Arizona postprimary school.

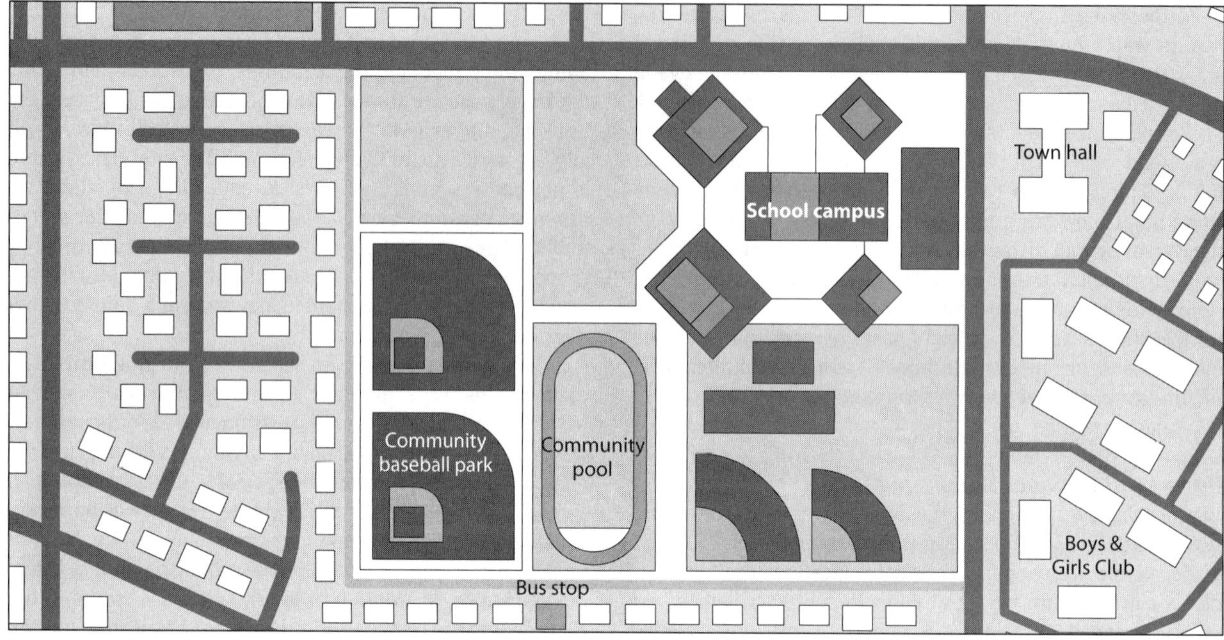

FIGURE 19.3 School proximity to community facilities.

good things that are going on in the program. On the day of the media visit, students could be recruited and interviewed about their experiences.

Connecting with Community Organizations

Countless community organizations are potential partners for school physical education. For example, local sport clubs could be excellent partners in that the physical education program can promote the availability of the clubs, their programs, and events. At the same time, sport clubs can be great sources of expertise for activities for which physical educators may not have sufficient content knowledge, but would like to build into their school programs. For example, in U.K. school physical education programs it is increasingly common that for certain units of instruction the delivery is outsourced to outside content experts from local sport clubs.

Community-based sport and recreation facilities like parks and recreation, public golf courses, bowling centers, swimming centers, and the like also are potential sources for collaboration with physical education programs. In the United States and many other countries, outside organizations dedicated to youth development and school campuses are actually neighbors. This opens up all kinds of opportunities for shared use of the physical activity venues by both organizations. For example, **Figure 19.3** shows how a municipal swimming pool, a Boys and Girls Club recreation facility, and a postprimary school are located right next to each other. The school physical education program makes use of the recreation facilities and vice versa. Both are within approximately 300 feet of the swimming pool. **Figure 19.4** shows a photo of a municipal indoor multiuse gymnasium in The Netherlands that the school physical education program from a nearby school uses during school hours, while the local sport club, which includes indoor soccer, basketball, and

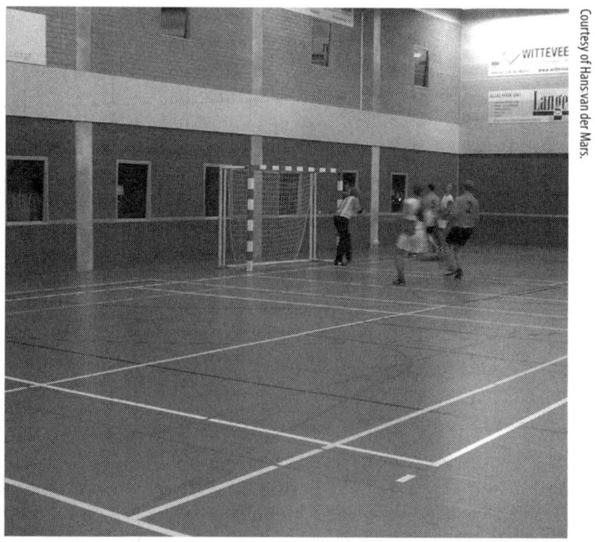

Courtesy of Hans van der Mars.

FIGURE 19.4 Municipal multiuse facility shared by school physical education programs and sport clubs.

volleyball divisions, uses it in the late afternoons, evenings, and on weekends.

Another source of connections could be local vendors of sporting equipment. For example, many local stores that sell outdoor equipment (e.g., skis, rollerblades, mountain bikes) also may offer equipment rental programs. Physical educators could make arrangements with such programs to expand the content offerings and clue their students in on the various opportunities for outdoor physical activity.

Especially for postprimary schools, making connections with local health clubs offers varied opportunities for the physical education program. Again, the expertise of the employees at the health clubs can be a great supplement to the physical education program. Schools could seek to build arrangements where students who have completed an Introduction to Strength Conditioning course become eligible to receive a discount on junior memberships at the health club with limited privileges. For example, they would be able to use certain sections or amenities of the health club during times when the volume of business is lower (e.g., mid-afternoon on weekdays, Sundays). If they enroll in other physical education classes beyond the required courses, access to the health club would be increased. If such collaborations between physical education programs and local health clubs become more established, it not only adds visibility to the former but also demonstrates that the program is actively encouraging physical activity engagement beyond just physical education classes. It can help encourage those who complete their postprimary education to maintain a health club membership over the long term, which in turn benefits local health club businesses.

It should be easy to see how collaboration with such community organizations and programs are win–win situations for both sides. Community mapping provides an excellent resource for physical education programs to seek out potential partners in supporting the development of physically active lifestyles for children and youth throughout a community. Physical education programs (and their students) gain by being able to expand program offerings, obtain more equipment, add content expertise, and so on, while the community organizations and local businesses gain by increasing participation levels, recruiting future clients, and/or providing increased business. Importantly, local organizations and businesses are also potential sources of sponsorship and other fundraising efforts.

Special Program Demonstration Events

Schools organize schoolwide curriculum nights or open houses where parents can get to know the teachers and their program. Such events are typically held at the beginning of the school year and offer an excellent opportunity for teachers to showcase their program. Another example of a special event that is specific to physical education and might target families of early primary and postprimary students is an event that is sometimes called "family fitness night." This event focuses on what the program does to encourage physical activity during physical education lessons, during other school day times, and on weekends; activities that families can engage in on weekends; how the program is weaving physical activity throughout the day; and so on.

Fun runs are another example of how programs can gain visibility. Fun runs are typically held during the afternoon after school hours. Students sign up to participate, and on the day of the event remain at school. They gather in an outside area (e.g., running trail, athletics track). Physical educators can recruit classroom teachers and parents to assist with the planning and implementation of such events, which may be held on a set schedule throughout the year (e.g., twice in the fall and twice in the spring; once a month).

Teachers should not be surprised or discouraged that such events may not draw a lot of attendees during the first few times. It may require a few trials for such events to become more well-known and more popular. Once established, students will likely come to expect these events to be held.

Fundraising

A final strategy that can support program promotion is fundraising. School budgets are strained, especially during times of economic recession. Consequently, budgets for school physical education programs are generally very limited. However, this does not mean that there are no solutions. Increasingly, and in part because of the increased interest in the health of children and youth, professional organizations, and private foundations are making funds available for which individual schools can apply. Motivated teachers have been very successful over the course of several years to add new equipment and initiate before and after school programs. The key is that every small additional grant or sponsorship helps increase the program's capacity to influence students' physical activity experiences.

School parent–teacher organizations (PTOs) often hold fundraisers that create funding support specifically for requests by individual teachers in a school. Depending on the amount of funds available in a given year, teachers can request as much as $2,000. The key is that physical educators periodically attend the organization's meetings and actively participate. Once the leadership in the school's parent organization sees that the physical educator is genuinely interested, a request for funding is more likely to be viewed favorably.

Importantly, when requesting funds for the purchase of certain equipment items, support for funding a field trip, or funding a guest instructor with specific expertise, physical educators need to ensure they provide the following: (1) a clear description of what the request is (i.e., name, how many, cost per item, etc.), (2) how they plan to use the items, (3) which students will get to use them, and (4) how it will benefit the students (and thus the program). This information should be prepared in writing (between one and two pages). When making the case for this request in person to the organization, teachers should be prepared to respond to questions from the organization's board. We have seen countless examples of schools where physical educators have not tapped into this source of support.

In the United States, over the last decade the federally funded Carol M. White Physical Education Program (PEP) grant initiative has provided extensive funds to school districts (and other community-based organizations) across the country. In 2011, the program provided grant funding ranging from $100,000 to over $700,000. This competitive program is aimed at helping physical education programs restructure so that they can better help students meet state standards. Examples of funded proposals have included (1) building evidence-based programs, (2) integrating technology into physical education programs, (3) building ropes courses to aid in focusing on social/life skills outcomes, and (4) changing curricular foci from traditional team sports to lifetime physical activities. A central expectation for those programs that get the funding is that they have to develop evidence that the grant funding has produced the desired outcomes. In many cases, school districts have contracted with physical education teacher education programs in the region to provide assistance with various aspects of the grant program such as grant preparation, implementation of the new program initiatives, and data collection.

The chances of receiving such large grants improve if the grant proposal (1) abides by the proposal submission rules, (2) clearly conveys the need for the funding, (3) has a clear focus with a persuasive rationale showing how the funds will benefit the students, (4) has a well-defined assessment protocol that can show how students are progressing toward meeting the standards, and (5) demonstrates that the district has the human capital to successfully implement the program initiative. Many of the grants that were funded employed an outside (or school district–level) grant writer to assist with developing the grant.

One of the key preconditions is that the physical education teachers themselves, as a group, are actively involved in the entire decision-making process of proposing, implementing, and evaluating the grant program. Having buy-in from all teachers will improve the odds that appreciable program changes will result. **Box 19.3** includes several examples of websites for grant and fundraising opportunities in the United States, as well as grant locators. A number of the websites include resources aimed at assisting in the grant writing process. There are also other possible funding sources that are more regional in focus. Many hospitals or other health organizations have foundations that put out calls for proposals to nonprofit organizations. Finally, many large corporations have foundations that are aimed at connecting with community organizations (including schools) and have as their charter to support efforts to improve the health and lives of children and youth.

BOX 19.3 Examples of Funding Opportunities and Funding Source Search Engines

Carol M. White Physical Education Program	www2.ed.gov/programs/whitephysed/index.html
ING Run for Something Better	www.orangelaces.com
Girls on the Run	www.girlsontherun.org
Head Start Body Start	www.aahperd.org/headstartbodystart
Fuel Up to Play 60	www.fueluptoplay60.com
Peaceful Playgrounds	www.peacefulplaygrounds.com/grants.htm
Jump Rope for Heart	www.heart.org/jump
Hoops for Heart	www.heart.org/hoops
International Walk to School	www.iwalktoschool.org
These websites offer teachers access to new and continuing funding opportunities as well as tips and guidelines for successful fundraising and grant funding initiatives.	www.tlfoundation.org www.gophersport.com/resources/index.cfm?PAGE_ID=24 www.flaghouse.com/grantwriting.asp www.sparkpe.org/grants/grantfunding-resources www.pecentral.org/professional/fundraisers.html

Learning Experience 19.5

Find a potential funding source that offers an opportunity for improving students' physical education experiences. Seek out a connection with a physical education teacher in a local school. Determine his or her interest in obtaining supplemental funding for the program. Determine the funding program's focus and qualifications. Working with that teacher, write a persuasive proposal (i.e., strong rationale, clear purpose, reasonable budget), and submit it to the funding organization.

In summary, the fundamental goal of physical education program promotion on the school campus and beyond is to (1) make it more visible among the broader school population, (2) help inform the public about its value and role in the development of students, and (3) improve its credibility among other teachers, school management, and parents. Physical educators' efforts in doing program promotion are within reach if they choose to work together and develop a plan of action. By informing and educating the key constituents through program promotion, teachers can lay the foundation for program advocacy, which is the focus of the next section.

Advocacy for Physical Education Programs and the Profession

Advocating for the program and the health of students is perhaps the most critical noninstructional function for physical educators in today's education environment. The ultimate goal of **advocacy** in physical education is to develop new or change existing policies that influence its delivery. It is very much linked to the aforementioned program promotion efforts. The latter focuses on informing key constituents, and making them more knowledgeable about the field. When people are more informed about our field, the hope is that they develop more favorable attitudes toward school physical education programs and how they are delivered. Once the community at large is more informed, teachers are in a much stronger position to advocate for strong policies related to physical education and physical activity. Without that, the likelihood of developing new or changing existing policies and/or laws is slim to none.

A **policy** (or law) is a statement/directive that directs people to act in accordance with a set of rules specific to the setting (e.g., rules of conduct). Policies are set across many levels. If there is no policy or law in effect at the national level, then individual states or provinces may decide on them. If there is none in effect at the state/province level, then school districts may set them, and so on. Policies at one level are superseded by and cannot be in contradiction with those in effect at the level above; that is, if a policy or

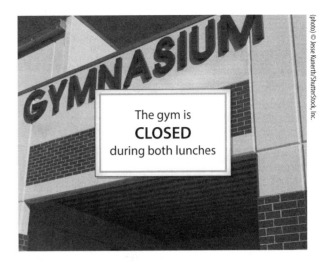

(photo) © Jesse Kunerth/ShutterStock, Inc.

FIGURE 19.5 Physical education program policy affecting physical activity.

law is in effect regarding the number of weekly minutes of physical education instruction or recess at the state/province level, the policy at the district level must specify at least that many minutes.

At the program or school level, physical educators and/or school managers get to set policies for such things as dress, on-time behavior, and use of facilities, some of which will actually suppress students' physical activity opportunities (see **Figure 19.5**). Schools and school districts will have policies for student conduct ranging from smoking, drugs, and violence to passing time between classes. Policies specific to teachers' conduct and performance are generally agreed upon as part of collective bargaining agreements (CBAs) between the teachers' union and the school district. These range from the number of personal days that teachers can take to the number of professional development days, the number of times that teachers are to be evaluated formally, and so on. Beyond those agreed upon in the CBA, there are district policies that affect instruction. For example, the number of minutes allocated to physical education is typically decided on at the district level. States or provinces will have policies related to teacher qualification/certification, teacher evaluation, the number of instructional days per school year or which school subjects in which all students are to be assessed.

One might question whether having district-, state-, and/or national-level policies in place supporting physical education and/or physical activity makes a difference; however, in other health behavior–related areas, inroads are being made relative to policies on food and beverage consumption in schools (e.g., Johnston, O'Malley, Bachman, & Schulenberg,

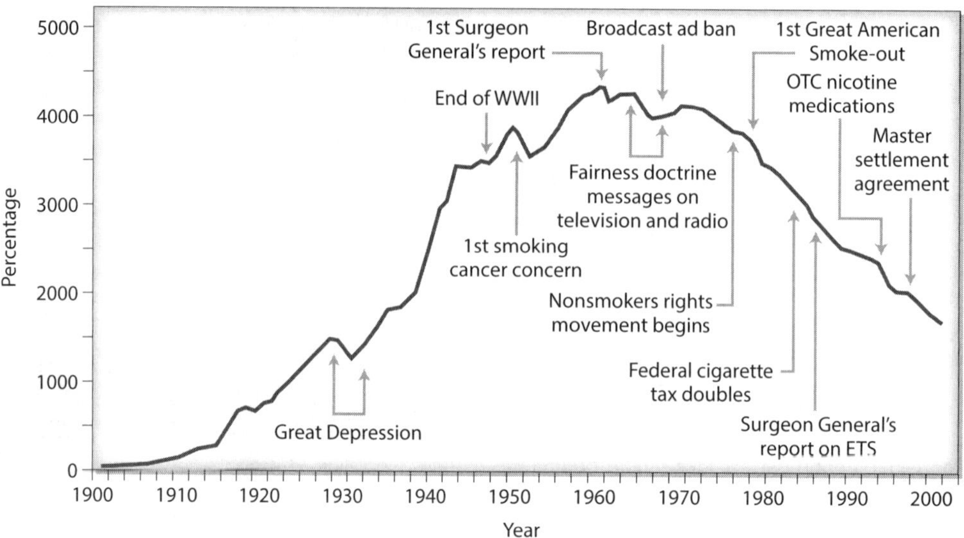

FIGURE 19.6 U.S. adult per capita cigarette consumption trends and major smoking and health events between 1900 and 2005.
Courtesy of Gary A. Giovino.

2010; Trust for America's Health, 2011) and smoking (e.g., Pentz et al., 1989). A good lesson on the time needed to appreciably change an unhealthy behavior at the societal level can be learned from seeing the impact of important health events on the cigarette smoking behavior of U.S. adults between 1900 and 2010 (see **Figure 19.6**) (Giovino, 2012). Initial concerns about the link between smoking and lung cancer were raised in the early 1950s. The resulting brief dip in cigarette consumption was followed by a steep increase until its peak in the early 1960s. The publication of the first Surgeon General's report on the dangers of smoking in January 1964 (followed by subsequent antismoking campaigns and policy efforts) produced a gradual drop in cigarette consumption. All the while, the tobacco industry has continued to find new ways to encourage this potentially deadly behavior. Consequently, it took almost 46 years after the release of the report for smoking levels to reach those seen during the Great Depression.

The Relative Contribution of Policies/ Legislation Support in Education and Physical Education

As part of a comprehensive analysis of over 270 reviews and syntheses of research studies on the contribution of numerous variables to students' learning, Wang, Haertel, and Walberg (1993) demonstrated that all contribute differentially to student learning; that is, no single variable affects student learning appreciably, including the contribution of school, district, state, or government policies. As can be seen in **Figure 19.7**, classroom management is the prime contributor to student learning. The relative contribution of policies was found to be smaller. Ultimately, it is the combined effects of numerous variables that together play a major role in fostering student learning.

Historically, the field of physical education has paid little attention to the role of policies and legislation at different levels of governance and their impact on the field. However, in recent years, interest and attention has increased significantly. For example, physical education–specific policies could target the number of minutes of physical education per week, teacher certification requirements, formal assessment requirements, number of credits required for graduation, and so on. In the United States, there is wide variation across the 50 states in the degree to which physical education–friendly policies and laws are in place (National Association for Sport and Physical Education and American Heart Association, 2012; Thomas, 2004). Specific to physical education and physical activity promotion, there is now a growing body of research that shows how policies can directly impact physical education and physical activity programming (e.g., Barroso et al., 2009; Cawley, Meyerhoefer, & Newhouse, 2007; Evenson, Ballard, Lee, & Ammerman, 2009; McKenzie & Lounsbery, 2009; Slater et al., 2011).

For example, Slater et al. (2011) found that U.S. schools located in states or school districts with laws or policies in place requiring 150 minutes of physical education per week significantly improved their odds of actually meeting this requirement. They reported a similar trend for daily recess. In the same study, the authors reported a possibly unintended

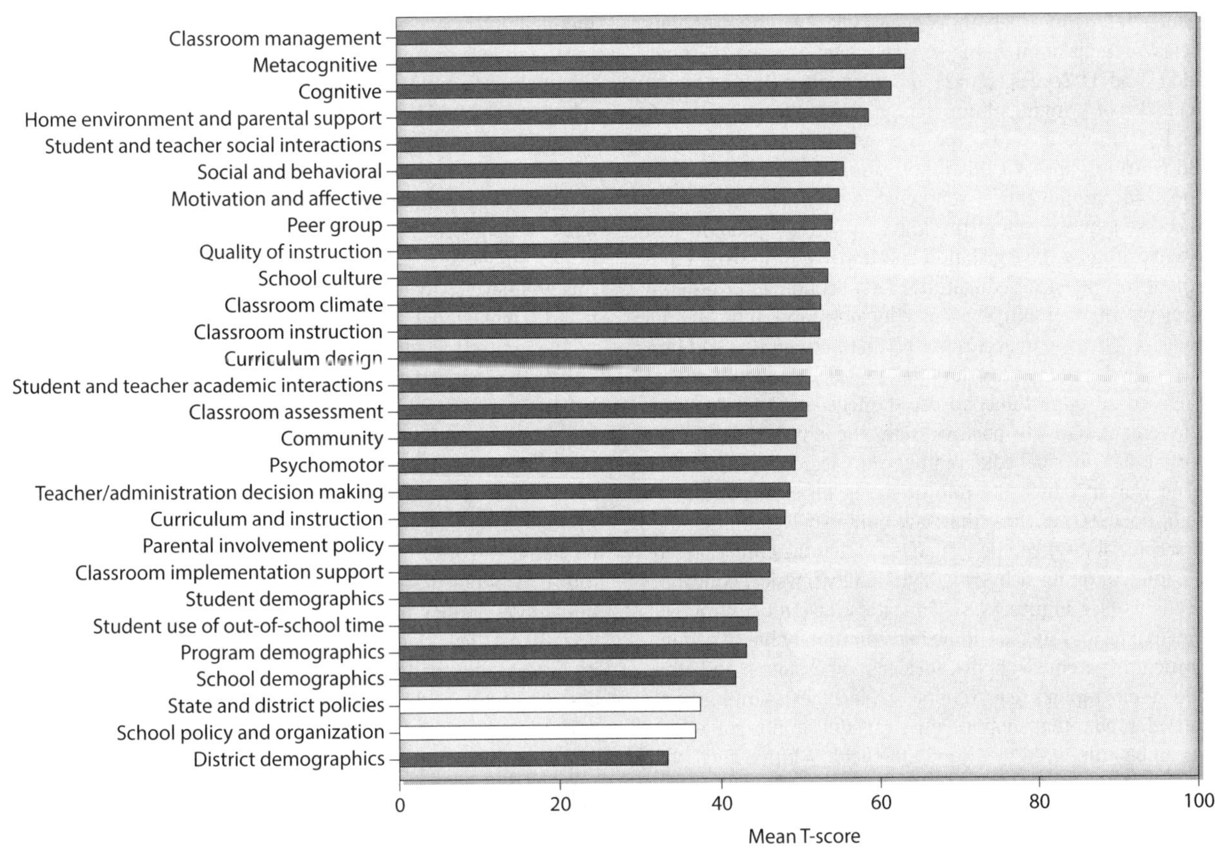

FIGURE 19.7 Educational variables' relative contribution to student learning.
Data from Wang, M. C., Haertel, G. D., & Walberg, H. J. (1993). Toward a knowledge base for school learning. *Review of Educational Research, 63*, 249–294.

consequence of having such policies in place: Time in physical education was inversely related with time allocated to recess and vice versa. It appears that schools may be substituting one form of physical activity for another, as opposed to scheduling the required/recommended amount of time for physical education *and* recess. This finding is important in that it reflects the ease with which "physical education" and "physical activity" often are used interchangeably. There is a fundamental difference between trying to implement policies that support the delivery of physical education and those that seek to increase opportunities for physical activity.

Bringing about policy changes is a long-term process that might take several years of ongoing efforts to inform, educate, and persuade policy makers to support and fund new policies and/or legislation. It also requires key stakeholders (e.g., parents, other related professional organizations, businesses, health organizations) to actively demonstrate support for such efforts. Just because physical education–friendly legislation is enacted does not mean that it results in immediately visible changes in practice. The strength of the policy/legislation is critical in terms of its capacity to bring about changes in behavior (i.e., does it include oversight, funding, and accountability?).

Learning Experience 19.6

Your school manager requests that you join her at a meeting with parents. She asks you to prepare a short 3-minute presentation in which you can provide a clear distinction between physical education and physical activity. Describe how would you do that, and prepare a short one-page supporting document that you can leave with the audience after your presentation. Also, provide a list of four or five questions that you might anticipate from your audience and how you would respond to these questions.

Moreover, school personnel may lack awareness of new policies or legislation being enacted. For example, Graber, Woods, and O'Conner (2012) provided an example of the complexity of bringing about changes as a result of national-level legislation. In 2004, the U.S. government passed the Child Nutrition and WIC Reauthorization Act, which requires schools to implement a school-wide wellness plan. The authors sought to explore the impact of this legislation and gauge if and how the legislation had impacted the work environment of physical educators. They conducted in-depth interviews of over 50 physical educators and their school managers. The researchers reported that both groups had limited knowledge of the plan, and that physical education teachers missed an opportunity to use the legislation for program improvement. On the positive side, the physical educators reported that physical education became less marginalized.

One way in which the role of strong physical education–specific policies (i.e., those that have built-in oversight, funding, and accountability) can be visualized is that they are a prerequisite foundation for delivering high-quality physical education to students (see **Figure 19.8**). Educators have no control over contextual factors such as home and community life (e.g., family structure, parental support, socioeconomic status) and other school demographics (e.g., school size, facilities); however, policy development that supports physical education is something that can be influenced by those in the field. Without such policies, the quality of the physical education experiences would be based on the level of professionalism individual teachers demonstrate on a day-to-day basis, and programs are more vulnerable to reductions or, worse, elimination.

Advocating for Your Program and Profession: Whose Responsibility?

Those in physical education may assume that school managers and other policy makers do not care about physical education programs; however, school managers have enormous pressure on them precisely because of other policies imposed on schools regarding improving academic performance. In addition, they likely (1) lack a clear understanding of what quality physical education looks like and (2) have little awareness of recent developments in physical education curriculum development, the research evidence that supports the need for quality school physical education, or the importance of physical activity from a health perspective. Finally, they were once in physical education as students, and that may be their only frame of reference; this will have shaped their views, biases, and ideologies about it. Who will change their perspectives and opinions?

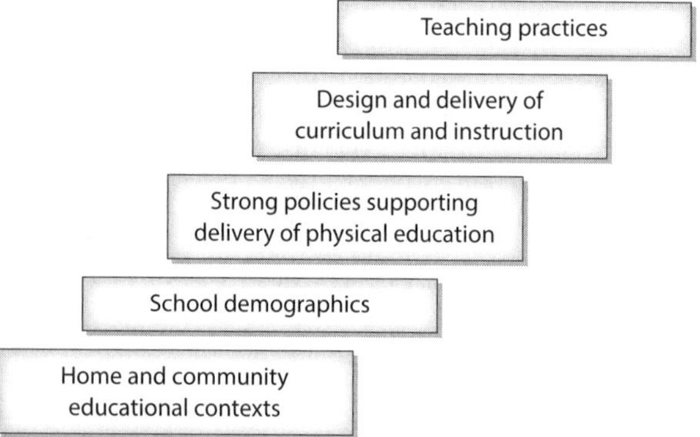

FIGURE 19.8 Contribution of physical education–specific policies to the quantity and quality of school physical education.

It is up to the field of physical education (including teachers) to present policy makers with the evidence that physical education should indeed be a "core" school subject, and how it can contribute to educating the whole child. Just like promoting the program, advocating for policy development is a critical noninstructional function for physical educators in today's education environment. Advocacy occurs both formally and informally. As we argued earlier, formal and informal opportunities play a big role in increasing awareness among policy makers and other groups.

In most developed countries, school physical education programs continue to be seen as an extra, an add-on but nonessential school subject. Subjects like art, music, and physical education are often labeled as "marginalized" school subjects (e.g., Hardman, 2004; Hardman & Marshall, 2009). The context of education today poses a significant conundrum. In many countries, education has witnessed an ongoing stream of reform efforts to improve students' academic performance, resulting in significant shifts in human, time, and monetary resources away from school physical education (e.g., Centers on Education Policy, 2008). At the same time, (1) there is unequivocal evidence of physical activity's benefits, (2) sport is arguably one of the most important and valued cultural phenomena (Siedentop & van der Mars, 2012), and (3) the levels of overweight and obesity have increased substantially in those same developed countries (e.g., World Health Organization, 2010). This has been attributed to such factors as changes in the types and amounts of food that people consume, the manner in which food is processed and consumed, and dramatic environmental changes that have effectively squeezed much of people's physical activity out of daily life. A burgeoning area of research has shown that:

> *. . . increased physical activity is an excellent public health intervention in that a physically active lifestyle has a positive impact in the prevention and treatment of a wide variety of chronic diseases, has unique and independent positive effects on physical and mental functioning and quality of life, acts synergistically with other behaviors to improve health, and contributes to the health and well-being of children and adults of all cultures and ethnicities throughout their lifespan. (Haskell, Blair, & Bouchard, 2012, p. 411)*

Importantly, school physical education programs are one of only a few approaches with sufficient evidence showing they can effectively increase the physical activity levels of children and youth (e.g., Centers for Disease Control and Prevention, 2001; Pate et al., 2006; Woods, Tannehill, & Walsh, 2011). This places school physical education programs squarely in the middle of all the other efforts throughout society aimed at helping all citizens come to value and lead physically active lives. Suffice it to say that school physical education is in a position where it must do all it can to demonstrate how it truly is a core subject within the broader mission of schools. The various program promotion strategies noted earlier are a key part of any advocacy efforts. In addition, physical educators can employ several additional strategies to support program advocacy efforts. They include (1) becoming a member of professional organizations, (2) attending professional conferences and workshops, (3) working together with professional colleagues in the area, (4) making connections with others who have similar goals and interests, (5) developing an advocacy action plan, and (6) actively participating in voicing support or opposition to policy proposals.

Become a Member of Your Professional Association

Becoming a member of one's professional organization and contributing to its advocacy efforts is another strategy that teachers can employ. National organizations such as the American Alliance for Health, Physical Education, Recreation, and Dance (see www.aahperd.org), the Association for Physical Education (see www.afpe.org.uk) in the United Kingdom, Physical and Health Education Canada (see www.phecanada.ca), the Physical Education Association of Ireland (see www.peai.org), and the Australian Council for Health, Physical Education and Recreation (see www.achper.org.au) are important players in advocacy efforts at the national level. In certain countries there may also be regional and state/provincial organizations that engage in advocacy. Professional organizations typically provide (1) information and workshops on current advocacy initiatives, (2) updates on the status of actual legislative proposals, (3) advocacy toolkits, and (4) guidelines, tips, and other resources aimed at helping individuals with advocacy efforts at the local level. In addition, professional organizations will develop and post official position statements on key issues aimed at defining proper professional practices in physical education and sport. Examples might include statements on professional conduct by physical educators, use of physical activity as punishment, recess for primary school–age children, and use of performance-enhancing drugs in sport.

If and when policy makers are considering a legislative policy or mandate, they need to hear from those in the profession on whether the proposed policy or mandate should be supported. National associations of physical education can help lobby for passage of legislation that supports school physical education and physical activity for all school-age youth.

Learning Experience 19.7

Find the website of a national-level professional organization in physical education. Determine the extent and type of advocacy-specific resources and information that the organization provides to professionals in the field, and then do the following:

1. Determine what, if any, current legislative/policy efforts are being supported by the organization.
2. Select two or three appropriate resources that you can use to let your voice be heard specific to that effort.
3. Develop a letter, email, or other means of voicing your support for the proposed legislation or policy.

Attend Professional Conferences and Workshops

Along with becoming a member of one's professional organization(s), attending the organization's conferences and workshops offers physical educators opportunities to stay abreast of developments in the physical education and physical activity policy arena. Teachers will have greater access to the various advocacy resources that they can employ, especially at the local level. It also allows teachers to network and assist each other by sharing advocacy-related information and strategies.

Learning Experience 19.8

Develop a list of five regional, national, and/or international organizations and agencies (along with their contact information) and retrieve the formal policy statement and/or formal recommendations for your state/province and/or country.

Read them with care and prepare a 4-minute coherent presentation for local constituents (e.g., parent organization, school administrators) highlighting the document content and why school physical education should play a central role. Also, develop a one-page summary of the document that provides your audience with the key messages.

Work with Professional Colleagues: You Are Not Alone

Continuing professional development (CPD) is a central component in improving teaching and practices in schools. Effective professional development practices are characterized by opportunities for development; teacher learning being continuous, active, and allowing for reflection; teachers taking ownership of the process; teachers learning collaboratively; and support from school management (e.g., Armour & Yelling, 2007). Increasingly, schools are allocating more time for teachers' professional development. Consequently, many of the professional development activities may lack meaning for physical educators and do not meet their needs (Armour & Yelling, 2007).

Unfortunately, in many cases there is not a person or office that coordinates professional development efforts specific to physical education. Moreover, today's schools are increasingly focused on helping students improve academically, and professional development efforts are pointed in the same direction. Thus, program promotion and advocacy aimed at making physical education more visible and credible on school campuses represents a clear need and would make a powerful CPD target. We know of several cases across various countries where professional physical educators have taken the initiative and developed their own professional learning communities (PLCs). They commit to meeting on a regular basis on days where they are expected to engage in professional development. Only then is there a chance that teachers (and the field as a whole) can form a united front to address the various policy-related issues that confront them. A united front becomes the foundation for bringing about policy development and change.

The success of the periodic meetings hinges on teachers stepping up and being willing to share and learn. As a group, teachers could work together and develop a strategic advocacy plan (see "Develop an Advocacy Action Plan" later in this chapter) that would include specific goals and map out a calendar of activities that would help meet the goals. For example, school managers and other policy makers are likely poorly informed about such topics as current evidence of quality physical education, the benefits of physical activity, the contribution schools can make to the health of children and youth, the importance of recess, and the association between physical activity (and physical education) and students' academic achievement. Thus, educating and informing key constituents (i.e., parents, other teachers, school managers, policy makers) could be made the focus of professional development.

Seek Connections with Those Outside the Field with Similar Goals and Interests

Advocacy is not just the responsibility of individual teachers. Those involved in preparing physical educators, as well as the field's professional organizations, are also key players in this effort. In fact, as can be seen in **Box 19.4**, globally there is broad support from local, regional, and national organizations and government agencies (e.g., Daugbjerg et al., 2009). Many countries now have policy statements, position statements, and/or national recommendations that directly target promotion of physical activity, and many include support for increasing the quantity and quality of school physical education.

Regional and local health organizations are also important potential advocacy partners, especially given the current emphasis on promoting physical activity from a public health perspective. For example, local physicians and surgeons are potentially powerful allies in efforts to ensure the health of children and youth.

National foundations (e.g., Robert Wood Johnson Foundation) have provided significant funding support to programs such as Active Living Research (ALR; see www.activelivingresearch.org/toolsandresources/all) that support the promotion of physical activity. ALR frequently publishes policy or research briefs and other reports that summarize key research evidence around topics; these can be used in support of program promotion and advocacy efforts.

Develop an Advocacy Action Plan

There is substantial variance in the presence, type, and number of physical education–related policies across states in the United States (National Association for Sport and Physical Education and American Heart Association, 2012) and in other countries. Policies or mandates specific to physical education programs and physical activity that schools would/might need to adhere to may include requirements such as the following:

- Physical education as a required subject in the school curriculum
- The amount of physical education in minutes per week
- Curriculum (i.e., is a specific model required?)
- Certification requirements of those delivering the program
- Substitutions/exemptions for physical education (i.e., can other subjects or activities such as band or interscholastic sport be used as substitutes for meeting physical education requirements?)
- Content standards (are there sanctioned standards?)
- Class size limits (is there a maximum number of students allowed in a class?)
- Report cards (is physical education required to be listed among all other subjects?)
- Assessment of student learning for all students in a state, province, or country
- Fitness testing for all students
- Number of minutes of recess per day/week
- Number of minutes of physical activity per day while at school

Any advocacy effort should take into consideration its financial impact. For example, seeking to get a law passed requiring 150 minutes of formal physical education per week

BOX 19.4 Sample Organizations and Agencies Supporting Promotion of Physical Education and Physical Activity in Children and Youth

Australia	
Australian government	www.health.gov.au/internet/main/publishing.nsf/Content/health-pubhlth-strateg-active-index.htm
England	
PE and Sport Strategy for Young People	www.ssp-websolutions.co.uk/PESSYP_small.pdf
Association for Physical Education	www.afpe.org.uk
U.K. Physical Activity Guidelines	www.gov.uk/government/publications/uk-physical-activity-guidelines
Ireland	
Active School Flag	www.activeschoolflag.ie
Irish Sports Council	www.irishsportscouncil.ie/Participation/Local_Sports_Partnerships
Coaching Ireland	www.coachingireland.com
Get Ireland Active	www.getirelandactive.ie/get-info/links
Physical Education, Physical Activity and Youth Sport Research Centre	www.ul.ie/pepays
Physical Education Association of Ireland	www.peai.org
Scotland	
Physical Activity and Health Alliance	www.paha.org.uk
Let's Make Scotland More Active	www.scotland.gov.uk/Publications/2003/02/16324/17895
United States	
Action for Healthy Kids	www.actionforhealthykids.org
Active Living Research	www.activelivingresearch.org
Alliance for a Healthier Generation	www.healthiergeneration.org
Obesity Society	www.obesity.org
American Academy of Pediatrics	www.aap.org
Institute of Medicine	www.iom.edu
Centers for Disease Control and Prevention, Division of Nutrition, Physical Activity, and Obesity	www.cdc.gov/nccdphp/dnpao
National Coalition for Promoting Physical Activity	www.ncppa.org
President's Council on Fitness, Sports and Nutrition	www.fitness.gov
Global	
World Health Organization	www.who.int/dietphysicalactivity/en

and having the program delivered by teachers actually certified in the subject has an enormous financial impact. Especially in times of economic downturn, such legislation has little chance of passing. However, requiring schools to provide a certain number of minutes of active recess is much less costly, and thus might be more palatable to policy makers.

Learning Experience 19.9

Using the previous list, determine whether your school district, state, province, or country has any formal policies or laws in place regarding any of the listed topics. List the actual policies in place. For the policies that are in place, determine whether they are being adhered to. What are the implications of those missing (i.e., not in place)? Finally, what would be the likely financial impact of getting more physical education–friendly policies/laws passed?

For example, if one wanted to propose legislation that requires primary students to receive 150 minutes of physical education per week that is taught by a certified physical educator, what would be the economic consequences for an urban school system with 25 primary schools?

It should be clear that program advocacy is an ongoing process, with a strong proactive approach. Organizing one or two special events or presentations to policy makers per year will likely not carry sufficient impact. Developing a sustained yearly plan of action will help your program stay more visible to the public. Moreover, teachers can be more effective in such efforts if they work together and plan for a deliberate and ongoing advocacy campaign targeting the key constituents. By collaborating with other organizations that also focus on the health and well-being of children and youth, physical education can form a more united front to bring about new (or change existing) policies that support physical education. School managers, who never hear from physical educators about the importance of their subject until proposals are considered for reductions in staff and/or time for physical education, will see right through this and view any last-minute effort to "save" the physical education program as simply a way to save their teaching jobs.

Box 19.5 displays an advocacy assignment that prospective preservice teachers (PSTs) undertake during their final teaching placement as a means to give back to the school in an area they have viewed as critical for physical education. Developing and implementing such a plan can be a focus for professional development meetings where teachers in the region join together. By working as a group, teachers can ensure that the messages, presentations, and other materials used in advocacy are consistent.

BOX 19.5 Advocacy Plan Assignment

Based on your school ethnography and experience in your teaching practice school, develop an exciting physical education advocacy plan to impact an area you view as critical for physical education to move forward. Identify the purpose of the plan and the audience you intend to reach through your advocacy. Articulate clearly how you intend to carry out this advocacy plan, sharing what you expect will be the timeline you will follow. Provide materials that you will use in this effort.

Whenever possible, physical educators should also consider inviting faculty of a physical education teacher education program in the region. They typically also have responsibilities to advocate for school physical education to policy makers. They should also be aware of where the gaps are in the local, regional, and national policy profile for physical education. Thus, they are important allies in any advocacy efforts.

Actively Participate in Voicing Support for or Opposition to Policy Proposals

Whenever there is a legislative or policy proposal being considered by elected local, state, or national policy makers, it is important that their constituents voice their support or opposition to such proposals. Communication with policy makers on such matters can occur through (1) letter writing or email campaigns, (2) scheduling face-to-face meetings with individual policy makers, and (3) testifying before committees or boards that ultimately will vote on the proposal. Most professional organizations now have web links (e.g., "Legislative Affairs") where members can gain access to templates of letters (or emails) that can be filled in by concerned professionals. In the case of regional, state, or national legislators, their contact information can be easily obtained from the Internet (e.g., see www.aahperd.org/naspe/advocacy/governmentRelations/govt101.cfm).

When you meet face-to-face with policy makers (e.g., school boards and legislators), they will expect that you have a "want." Face-to-face meetings with individual policy makers will typically not last for more than 8–10 minutes. **Box 19.6** offers some basic guidelines for such meetings. It is imperative that you prepare for your meeting and that you can answer possible questions that the policy maker may ask. Moreover, be sure to provide the policy maker a summary of pertinent information that supports your case (e.g., fact sheets, research briefs).

If and when the opportunity arises to speak before a legislative committee or a school board, preparation for this

> **BOX 19.6 Do's and Don'ts for Face-to-Face Meetings with Elected Policy Makers**
>
> *Be sure to:*
>
> - Know your issue inside and out.
> - Study, study, study! Know the history and background of the policy maker.
> - Plan, plan, plan! Know what your talking points will be, and be sure you stay on point (i.e., avoid straying to other issues).
> - Clearly identify yourself as a constituent.
> - State your credentials as an expert in your field.
> - Be specific in what legislative action or support you seek.
> - Provide accurate summaries and reliable data using one- to two-page fact sheets.
> - Be positive and friendly, regardless of whether the policy maker appears unsupportive.
> - Be sensitive about time. Do not expect to have much more than about 8–10 minutes. Meetings with constituents frequently get cut short for other pressing matters. Remain courteous!
> - Treat staff with the same level of respect as you do the official.
> - Compliment the policy maker or staff on positive actions.
> - Admit if you don't know an answer, but promise to follow up.
> - Leave your name and contact information.
> - Send a handwritten thank-you note.
> - Follow up with any additional information needed.
>
> *Be sure to avoid:*
>
> - Arriving without an appointment (although dropping in unannounced may be acceptable if you simply seek to drop off your information with staff)
> - Being late (*call* the office if you are running late—*do not text!*)
> - Missing a valuable opportunity to meet with staff members if your legislator is unable to keep your appointment or cuts your time short
> - Being confrontational or overly partisan
> - Trying to discuss more than one issue
> - Getting too comfortable or casual
> - Forgetting to use proper forms of address
>
> Modified with permission from "Do's and Don'ts for Face-to-Face Meetings with Elected Policy Makers." © 2013 American Alliance for Health, Physical Education, Recreation and Dance. www.aahperd.org/naspe/advocacy/governmentRelations/upload/Tips-on-Meeting-with-your-Elected-Officials-9-11-09.pdf

should be equally thorough. Whenever policy or legislative proposals are being considered by such bodies, public meetings are scheduled during which any individual or organization representative can testify and speak for or against the proposal. It is important that any person looking to speak at such occasions is aware of and follows the protocols in place for such meetings. For example, these types of testimonies usually are limited to no more than about 4 minutes. Thus, having a clear message that can be communicated succinctly is a must. Practicing such formal presentations ahead of time to a friendly audience and having someone critique the draft statement are good strategies to ensure that your message comes across as intended.

CHAPTER SUMMARY

Decisions made by school managers/school system managers/legislators directly influence the quantity and quality of physical education provided in schools. Educating and persuading policy makers is arguably the most important type of advocacy in which the field as a whole and teachers can and should engage. Historically, however, physical educators have not viewed this as a professional responsibility. Yet, if they plan effectively and proactively, physical educators can be powerful advocates by educating/informing parents, classroom colleagues, school administrators, students, and policy makers on (1) the latest evidence about the critical role and function of physical education, (2) the many health benefits of physical activity, (3) the economic benefits of physical activity, (4) the importance of providing maximum opportunities for physical activity throughout the school and beyond regular physical education lessons, and (5) the relationship between physical education/physical activity and academic achievement.

We cannot and should not assume that these policy makers have a clear understanding of what quality physical education looks like, the recent changes in curriculum development, and the research evidence that supports the need for quality school physical education. Remember, too, that they themselves were once in physical education as students. For most, that is their only frame of reference, which has shaped their views and biases about physical education. It is up to all involved in the field of school physical education (teachers, professors, and professional organizations alike) to present policy makers with evidence that shows why physical education should indeed be a "core" school subject and how it can contribute to educating the whole child. Increasingly, academics and professional associations have become active in advocacy. To date, however, such efforts have not yet been powerful enough to persuade policy makers to support policies and legislation that makes a difference in the provision of school physical education. The hope is that as a result of global concerns regarding the overweight and obesity levels of children, youth, and adults, and the related consequences, decision makers may be more open to supporting school physical education programs with strong policies and laws.

1. Physical education has been a part of schools in most countries for over a century.
2. Time allocated for physical education has been squeezed because of ongoing educational reform efforts and economic factors.
3. Physical education does not occur in school alone; the 20th century saw the emergence of sport and later the fitness movement, each providing the public with a wide variety of choices for physical activity that can contribute to one's health.
4. Beyond the field itself, school physical education is enjoying widespread support from various government agencies and related professional societies.
5. Program promotion and advocacy play a critical role in the job of physical educators.
6. The public, including school managers, school board members, district superintendents, and government education officials, are unfamiliar with trends and the current knowledge base surrounding physical education and physical activity.
7. Program promotion has three fundamental purposes: (1) increase the program's visibility on and beyond campus; (2) inform parents, school managers, and the public at large about the good things that happen in the program; and (3) improve/maintain the program's credibility.
8. For promotion efforts to be successful, programs must be able to demonstrate what they accomplish, and teachers must maintain currency with trends and developments in the field.
9. Promotion of student and program accomplishments can be communicated to the public and stakeholders using the following strategies: (1) formal presentations, (2) informal information sharing, (3) newsletters and website announcements, (4) inviting key people to visit the program, (5) using local print and television media, (6) connecting with community organizations, (7) fundraising, and (8) special demonstration events.
10. The ultimate goal of advocacy in physical education is to develop new or change existing policies that support its delivery.
11. A policy/law aims to direct people to act in accordance with a set of rules specific to the setting (i.e., rules of conduct).
12. Policies/laws can be set at different governance levels (i.e., school, school district, state/province, national). Policies/laws at one level are superseded by related policies or laws at the next higher level.
13. Teachers in the physical education program can set their own program-level policies; however, they must be within the bounds of policies at the next higher level (i.e., school level).
14. Although well-designed and implemented policies/laws that support physical education do not by themselves guarantee quality experiences for students, they do constitute a foundation for them.
15. There is a growing body of evidence showing that policies and/or laws specific to physical education programs and physical activity levels can make a direct impact.
16. Policy development/change is a long-term process aimed at building support for physical education– and physical activity–friendly policies/laws.
17. Program advocacy is a responsibility of not just physical educators but also PETE faculty and professional organizations within the field.
18. Advocacy strategies that all physical education professionals can employ include: (1) becoming a member of professional organizations, (2) attending professional conferences and workshops, (3) working together with professional colleagues in the area, (4) seeking connections with others outside the field who have similar goals and interests, (5) developing an advocacy action plan, and (6) actively participating in voicing support or opposition to policy proposals.

REFERENCES

Armour, K. M., & Yelling, M. (2007). Effective professional development for physical education teachers: The role of informal, collaborative learning. *Journal of Teaching in Physical Education, 26*, 177–200.

Barroso, C. S., Kelder, S. H., Springer, A. E., Smith, C. S., Nalini Ranjit, B. S., Ledingham, C., et al. (2009). Senate bill 42: Implementation and impact on physical activity in middle schools. *Journal of Adolescent Health, 45*(Suppl.), S82–S90.

Cawley, J., Meyerhoefer, C., & Newhouse, D. (2007). The impact of state physical education requirements on youth physical activity and overweight. *Health Economics, 16*, 1287–1301.

Center on Education Policy. (2007). *Choices, changes, and challenges: Curriculum and instruction in the NCLB era.* Washington, DC: Author.

Center on Education Policy. (2008). *Instructional time in elementary schools: A closer look at changes for specific subjects.* Washington, DC: Author.

Centers for Disease Control and Prevention. (2001). Increasing physical activity: A report on recommendations of the Task Force on Community Preventive Services. *Morbidity and Mortality Weekly Report, 50*(RR-18), 1–14.

Daugbjerg, S. B., Kahlmeier, S., Racioppi, F., Martin-Diener, E., Martin, B., Oja, P., et al. (2009). Promotion of physical activity in the European region: Content analysis of 27 national policy documents. *Journal of Physical Activity and Health, 6*, 805–817.

Evenson, K. R., Ballard, K., Lee, G., & Ammerman, A. (2009). Implementation of a school-based state policy to increase physical activity. *Journal of School Health, 79*, 231–238.

Giovino, G. A. (2012). Patterns of tobacco use in the United States. Surveillance and Evaluation Net Conference Series, CDC Office on Smoking and Health. Available from www.ttac.org/resources/pdfs/062712_Patterns_Tobacco_Use-handout.pdf

Graber, K. C., Woods, A. M, & O'Conner, J. A. (2012). Impact of wellness legislation on comprehensive school health programs. *Journal of Teaching in Physical Education, 31*, 163–181.

Hardman, K. (2004). An up-date on the status of physical education in schools worldwide: Technical report for the World Health Organization. Available from www.icsspe.org/sites/default/files/Kenneth%20Hardman%20update%20on%20physical%20education%20in%20schools%20worldwide.pdf

Hardman, K., & Marshall, J. (2009). Physical education in schools: A global perspective. *Kinesiology, 40*(1), 5–28.

Haskell, W. L., Blair, S. N., & Bouchard, C. (2012). An integrated view of physical activity, fitness, and health. In C. Bouchard, S. N. Blair, & W. L. Haskell (Eds.), *Physical activity and health* (2nd ed., pp. 409–425). Champaign, IL: Human Kinetics.

Johnston, L., O'Malley, P., Bachman, J., & Schulenberg, J. (2010). *Youth, education, and society—Results on school policies and programs: Overview of key findings, 2009*. Ann Arbor, MI: Survey Research Center, Institute for Social Research. Available from www.yesresearch.org/publications/reports/schoolreport2009.pdf

Lauer, H. (2006). *The new Americans: Defining ourselves through sports and fitness participation*. Fort Mill, SC: American Sports Data.

Le Masurier, G. C., & Corbin, C. B. (2006). Top 10 reasons for quality physical education. *Journal of Physical Education, Recreation and Dance, 77*(6), 44–53.

Lounsbery, M. A. F., McKenzie, T. L., Trost, S., & Smith, N. J. (2011). Facilitators and barriers to adopting evidence-based physical education in elementary schools. *Journal of Physical Activity and Health, 8*(Suppl. 1), S17–S25.

McCullick, B., Belcher, D., Hardin, B., & Hardin, M. (2003). Butches, bullies and buffoons: Images of physical education teachers in the movies. *Sport, Education and Society, 8*, 3–16.

McKenzie, T. L. (2012). Personal communication.

McKenzie, T. L., & Lounsbery, M. (2009). School physical education: The pill not taken. *American Journal of Lifestyle Medicine, 3*, 219–225.

Mendes, E. (2011). *One in four Britons smoke, are obese*. Available from www.gallup.com/poll/147023/One-Four-Britons-Smoke-Obese.aspx

National Association for Sport and Physical Education (NASPE). (2008). *Comprehensive school physical activity programs* [position statement]. Reston, VA: Author.

National Association for Sport and Physical Education. (2009). Tips on meeting with your elected officials. Available from www.aahperd.org/naspe/advocacy/governmentRelations/upload/Tips-on-Meeting-with-your-Elected-Officials-9-11-09.pdf

National Association for Sport and Physical Education & American Heart Association. (2012). *2012 shape of the nation report: Status of physical education in the USA*. Reston, VA: American Alliance for Health, Physical Education, Recreation, and Dance.

Ogden, C. L., Carroll, M. D., Kit, B. K., & Flegal, K. M. (2012). Prevalence of obesity and trends in body mass index among US children and adolescents, 1999–2010. *Journal of the American Medical Association, 307*, 483–490. DOI:10.1001/jama.2012.40

Organisation for Economic Co-operation and Development. (2010). Health at a glance: Europe 2010. Available from www.oecd-ilibrary.org/social-issues-migration-health/health-at-a-glance-europe-2010_health_glance-2010-en

Pate, R. R., Davis, M. G., Robinson, T. N., Stone, E. J., McKenzie, T. L., & Young, J. C. (2006). Promoting physical activity in children and youth: A leadership role for schools. A scientific statement from the American Heart Association Council on Nutrition, Physical Activity, and Metabolism (Physical Activity Committee) in collaboration with the Councils on Cardiovascular Disease in the Young and Cardiovascular Nursing. *Circulation, 114*, 1214–1224.

Pentz, M. A., Brannon, B. R., Charlin, V. L., Barrett, E. J., MacKinnon, D. P., & Flay, B. R. (1989). The power of policy: The relationship of smoking policy to adolescent smoking. *American Journal of Public Health, 79*, 857–862. DOI: 10.2105/AJPH.79.7.857

Sallis, J. F. (2010). We do not have to sacrifice children's health to achieve academic goals. *Journal of Pediatrics, 156*, 696–697.

Sallis, J. F., & McKenzie, T. L. (1991). Physical education's role in public health. *Research Quarterly for Exercise and Sport, 62*, 124–137.

Schmidt-Millard, T. (2003). Perspectives of modern sports pedagogy. *European Journal of Sport Science, 3*(3), 1–7.

Siedentop, D., & van der Mars, H. (2012). *Introduction to physical education, fitness, and sport* (8th ed.). St. Louis, MO: McGraw-Hill.

Slater, S. J., Nicholson, L., Chriqui, J., Turner, L., & Chaloupka, F. (2011). The impact of state laws and district policies on physical education and recess practices in a nationally representative sample of US public elementary schools. *Archives of Pediatrics and Adolescent Medicine, 166*(4), 311–316. DOI:10.1001/archpediatrics.2011.1133

Thomas, K. (2004). Riding to the rescue while holding on by a thread: Physical activity in the schools. *Quest, 56*, 150–170.

Trust for America's Health. (2012). Issue report: F as in fat: How obesity threatens America's future. Available from http:/healthyamericans.org/report/100

Wang, M. C., Haertel, G. D., & Walberg, H. J. (1993). Toward a knowledge base for school learning. *Review of Educational Research, 63*, 249–294. DOI: 10.3102/00346543063003249

Woods, C. B., Tannehill, D., & Walsh, J. (2012). An examination of the relationship between enjoyment, physical education, physical activity and health in Irish adolescents. *Irish Educational Studies, 31*, 263–280.

World Health Organization (WHO). (2010). *Global recommendations on physical activity and health*. Geneva, Switzerland: Author. Available from http://whqlibdoc.who.int/publications/2010/9789241599979_eng.pdf

Glossary

academic achievement Performance on a formal test covering academic content (e.g., math, physical education, science, social studies).

accountability The practices teachers use to establish and maintain student responsibility for appropriate conduct, task involvement, and outcomes. This comes in different forms, including written or performance tests that students complete for grades, teacher feedback, praise and reprimands, their active supervision, challenges and competitions, public recognition of performance, and keeping records of performance.

active supervision An umbrella set of strategies that a teacher uses at various times within the lesson, during teacher presentation of tasks, demonstration of skills, student group work, whole class instruction, independent practice, or individual performances. Includes back-to-the-wall, proximity control, with-it-ness, selective ignoring, learning names, overlapping, and pinpointing.

active teacher Believes that he or she can make a difference with students, develops a management system that helps students stay on task, plans and implements an instructional program that is action oriented, motivates students and holds them accountable for performance, and does so within a class climate that is supportive and respectful.

active video games Also referred to as "exergames." An activity combining exercise with electronic game playing. Examples include Dance-Dance-Revolution, Wii, and X-Box Kinect.

activity reinforcers Reinforcers in the form of students' favorite activities or privileges. In primary physical education settings, activities such as jumping rope, shooting baskets, playing soccer, or privileges like getting to be first in line or assisting the teacher with equipment are all potential activity reinforcers. In postprimary, opening or closing the lesson with a related activity of choice may serve as an activity reinforcer.

Adventure Education An experiential learning model that provides learners with the opportunity to challenge themselves physically and mentally, work cooperatively as a group to solve problems and overcome risks, and gain respect for, confidence in, and trust in themselves and their peers. Key concepts of the model include full value contract, challenge with choice, experiential learning cycle, and processing/debrief.

advocacy Any effort aimed at informing, persuading, and/or changing existing beliefs or views with the intent to support new or change existing formal rules/mandates/legislation.

alternative assessment An umbrella term for all forms of assessments requiring students to generate a response. Different from a one-time, formal assessment.

antibias teaching Achieved by the application of effective, caring teaching skills that allow students to understand that they bring differences to the setting. The goal of antibias teaching is to address these disparities in ways that allow for a growing tolerance, respect, and appreciation of diverse perspectives.

apprenticeship of observation A theory developed by Lortie (2002) that posits that among prospective teachers, conceptions of teaching as work begin to emerge during the primary and post-primary years of schooling. These conceptions may well contribute to entrenching traditional teaching practices, while at the same time preventing deliberate and informed changes in practice.

assessment A variety of tasks and settings where students are given opportunities to demonstrate their knowledge, skill, understanding, and application of content in a context that allows continued learning and growth.

assessment "for" learning Occurs at the site of learning, shares learning goals and success criteria, supports learning through feedback, fosters self-assessment and independence, and leads to improved learning.

assessment steps Encourage students to engage with a challenge and determine what they would like to be able to do related to this challenge before considering how they could best pursue these goals on a week-by-week basis.

assessment wheel Encourages the student to record, reflect on, and map their learning related to a unit's big picture goal and to assess their progress towards this goal.

authentic assessment Reflects real life, is performed in a realistic setting, and mirrors what students do outside of school.

authentic outcome An outcome that requires a performance in a context similar to the one in which the knowledge, skills, and strategies will eventually be used.

backward design A method where curriculum design begins with the exit outcomes and proceeds backward to the entry point to ensure that all components are directly related to achieving the outcome.

behavior and management feedback Information provided to the student in response to behavior with the intent of reinforcing, correcting, reducing, or improving a particular behavior that is impacting student learning. It includes prompts, hustles, desists, and praise.

behavior management The formal and planned application of specific, and evidence-based techniques based on the behavioral principles of reinforcement and punishment.

best available knowledge The most current/up-to-date evidence available that can be used in support of stated claims, beliefs, and positions.

boundaries In terms of a policy, this refers to how tightly or loosely the accountability for implementation is applied and how explicit or ambiguous the requirements are for its implementation.

bullying Unwanted, aggressive behavior among school-age children that involves a real or perceived power imbalance. The behavior is repeated, or has the potential to be repeated, over time (www.stopbullying.gov). This can include actions such as threats, physical/verbal attacks, spreading rumors, or public embarrassment.

caring pedagogy Protects children and youth and invests in their ongoing development. Creates the conditions within which children and youth protect the rights and interests of classmates and behave in ways toward their peers that show caring and respect.

change agent An educator who intentionally or indirectly causes or accelerates social, cultural, or behavioral change in an education setting.

check for understanding Questions and/or strategies used to determine if students understood and retained directions and instructions.

checking for student understanding In the management and instructional task system this involves ensuring students understand what they are to do, how they are to behave, and critical elements of a skill or steps in a practice task prior to being disbursed.

checklist A list of statements, dimensions, characteristics, or behaviors that are basically scored as yes or no, based on an observer's judgment of whether the dimension is present or absent.

clarity and ambiguity Related concepts that refer to the degree of explicitness and consistency in how policy/legislation is written. Poorly written policies/legislation are those that include language that provides more latitude in terms of whether to implement them.

classroom activity break Time allocated for physical activity during instruction of academic subjects in classrooms, with the goal of increasing total daily physical activity and/or integrating physical activity into academic content.

classroom ecology The study of the behavior of teachers and students within the various systems in their class environment.

common content knowledge (CCK) Knowledge needed to perform an activity (e.g., soccer, dance). Typically acquired in the process of learning to play and playing a game/performing an activity.

community and club sport Sport or any physical activity within the framework of a sport club or community organization.

community of practice "When you see a group of teachers sharing and critically interrogating their practice in an ongoing, reflective, collaborative, inclusive, learning-oriented, growth-promoting way" (Stoll & Seashore Louis, 2007, p. 2).

competent bystander Students who appear to be actively engaged in the instructional tasks but actually avoid most real involvement.

Comprehensive School Physical Activity Program (CSPAP) A program, overseen and directed by the physical education teacher, aimed at maximizing physical activity opportunities for all students, school staff members, and students' families and members of the surrounding community.

Concepts-Based Fitness and Wellness Focused on the process of physical activity rather than the outcome of students' achieving physical fitness, this model is designed around themes and concepts in three categories (foundational, behavior change, and wellness). These are introduced through a series of classroom-focused concept days that are applied and reinforced through activity days.

consequence An event that follows a particular behavior. Consequences may be positive or negative. In physical education environments, they provide the "reasons" for behaving that students need so they can learn new and appropriate forms of behavior.

constituents People who have a vested interest in and concern about particular issues, programs, and the like.

content standards What students should know and be able to do at a particular developmental/grade level.

contingency Relationship between the situation or context (also referred to as the antecedent), the behavior, and a consequence.

continuing professional development (CPD) Lifelong teacher learning; it includes a range of educational experiences designed to enhance teachers' professional skills, knowledge, understanding, application, and capabilities throughout their careers.

continuum of teacher education The stages through which a teacher passes in their career: initial teacher education, induction into the profession, and early continuing professional development.

cooperative learning (CL) A special variation of small group work that requires the involvement of all members of the group. CL uses questioning to stimulate students to solve problems, think creatively, negotiate, compromise, adapt, and evaluate as they create solutions. CL strategies include (1) pairs–check; (2) jigsaw; (3) think–pair–share; and (4) problem-based learning.

criterion-referenced assessment Relates performance to a given standard, allowing the teacher and student to document how well a student is mastering certain skills.

critical friends Typically two people who trust and value each other's viewpoints and are willing to work together to share, critique, and challenge one another to produce personal and professional growth.

Cultural Studies Developed to meet the needs and interests of students from various backgrounds, cultures, socioeconomic levels, and communities. The intent is to develop young people as questioning, curious, and critical participants in sport and physical activity coming to understand how some young people are marginalized by a lack of activity opportunities available in their school and community.

culturally relevant education Provides students with the opportunity to engage in activities that prepare them to live in a culturally diverse society. Includes a curriculum that cultivates meaningful, affirming, and equitable learning environments, whereby all students are valued members of the educational community.

curriculum All planned learning for which the school is responsible and all the experiences to which learners are exposed under the guidance of the school. Curriculum is also used interchangeably with the terms program and syllabus when a specific school subject, such as physical education, lists selected activities and experiences planned to achieve student-learning outcomes.

curriculum guide A formal district/regional document explaining the objectives to be achieved in a subject and the activities thought to contribute to those objectives. Also often referred to as a curriculum syllabus or a graded course of study.

curriculum model Provide the framework within which instruction takes place. They are focused, themes-based, reflect a specific philosophy, define a clear focus around the content, and aim toward specific, relevant, and challenging outcomes.

curriculum plan An overall view of all a teacher intends students to experience over a number of years (as part of their physical education experience).

cyber-bullying A newer form of bullying using various technologies such as texting, the Internet, and social media.

development–refinement cycle The process by which a curriculum is developed, tested, refined, and further tested in a variety of school settings.

Developmental Physical Education A set of models designed around the individual learner with the intent of meeting each learner's developmental needs and unique growth patterns within a holistic education emphasizing cognitive, affective, and psychomotor outcomes.

device staying power The degree to which use of a technology device or program is sustained over time.

differential reinforcement The teacher ignores the inappropriate behavior while at the same time reinforcing other more desirable behaviors. There are multiple applications of differential reinforcement, including differential reinforcement of incompatible behavior (DRI), differential reinforcement of alternative behavior (DRA), differential reinforcement of low rates of behavior (DRL), and differential reinforcement of other behavior (DRO).

digital natives The generation of youth that has grown up during the emerging era of digital technologies.

direct instruction Provided by the teacher to a whole class or small groups, followed by guided and independent practice in a positive and supportive learning environment set with high, realistic expectations for students for which they are held accountable. Lesson pacing is brisk and teacher controlled, with students getting many learning opportunities and experiencing high success rates. Also referred to as active teaching.

discipline (as a noun) As in "This is a class that is disciplined"; a class with few if any instances of inappropriate behavior and ample examples of pro-social behavior among students.

discipline (as a verb) Application of a consequence deemed a negative consequence; implies and focuses on punishment.

ecology An interrelated set of systems in which changes in one system affect the other systems.

ecology of physical education Ecology is typically made up of a number of systems (managerial, instructional, and social) that interact with each other so that a change in one system influences what happens in the other systems. Just as the natural environment we live in can be understood as an ecological system, so too can teaching/learning in physical education.

educational reform Five characteristics of educational reform have been identified as (1) standardization in education, (2) focus on basic student knowledge with an emphasis on literacy and numeracy, (3) teaching for predetermined results, (4) the involvement of the business world in designing and implementing educational reform efforts, and (5) high-stakes accountability systems that have evolved internationally.

educational technology Use of technology in support of teaching and/or learning.

effective task communication When tasks are communicated in such a way that students will attend to and comprehend the information the teacher presents and that information is sufficient for students to initially do the task as described.

employee fitness/wellness programs Programs developed for improving employees' health and wellness in a school system. Program sessions are typically held during after-school hours. Participation may involve incentive programs that result in a reduction in employees' health insurance premiums.

equipment dispersal Having strategies and class routines to guide distribution of equipment (dispersal and return) and how it is used throughout the lesson.

event task Simulates real life; allows multiple solutions and responses; is important, relevant, and current in an attempt to stimulate student interest; and can be completed in a single time frame.

extending–refining cycle Rink's model for developing progressive instructional tasks; it consists of the informing task (initial task), refining tasks (to improve quality), extending tasks (to make the task more difficult), and applying tasks (to employ skill/strategy in authentic ways).

extracurricular sport Competitive and noncompetitive physical activities (including dance) outside of the formal physical education curriculum but offered within the institutional framework of school.

feedback Information provided to the performer in response to a performance with the intent of reinforcing learning, keeping the student focused on the learning task, informing and motivating the student, facilitating learning, and monitoring the student's responses to a task. Both behavior and content feedback can be auditory, visual, written, an outcome, or feelings.

formal assessment Tend to be standardized and controlled types of assessment.

formative assessment Intended to provide feedback to impact the ongoing instructional process, demonstrating that learning is taking place.

FOS principle "Focus on the student"; a principle established to encourage the teacher to place the student at the center of all decisions.

games teaching Incorporates teaching through questions to encourage students to think critically about tactical problems, appropriate skills, and when to use them.

governing policy A statement/guideline set forth to represent a change in the governance system that directly affects the education (and thus physical education) system.

grades Report a student's performance by attaching a mark to indicate the level of performance. The grade is generally calculated by averaging the results of several different assessment measures that occur throughout a grading period.

group contingency The presentation of a reinforcer (i.e., reward) contingent upon the behavior of an individual in a group, a segment of the group, or the group as a whole. Variations of this technique include dependent-, independent-, and interdependent-group contingencies.

grouping for activity The strategies a teacher uses to group students for activity that consider group size, group structure, and procedures for selecting groups to facilitate student learning.

guided discovery Characterized by convergent thinking where students respond to a series of task questions/challenges that help them progress toward a specific goal with one correct response.

guided practice A period of group practice during which the teacher (1) corrects major errors in performance, (2) reteaches if necessary, and (3) provides sufficient practice so students can move on to participate in independent practice successfully.

Health and Wellness models Focused primarily on giving students the knowledge and skills to make independent decisions on physical activity, and the desire to choose to develop and maintain lifetime physical activity as opposed to a sedentary lifestyle.

Health Optimizing Physical Education (HOPE) Designed for young people to gain skills and knowledge for participation in physical activity in order to gain health benefits across the life span. HOPE includes the five components of a comprehensive school physical activity program (CSPAP): quality physical education, school-based physical activity opportunities, school employee wellness and involvement, physical activity in the classroom, and family and community involvement.

Health-Based Physical Education (HBPE) Focused on young people valuing a physically active lifestyle and choosing to participate in appropriate activities that promote health and well-being. Key to this model is that it represents a pedagogical model intended to provide guidance to schools.

health-optimizing physical activity Any physical activity that requires the energy equivalent to or more than that needed for a brisk walk.

in-service education/training A common form of professional development for teachers to help them improve their knowledge and practice. In-service training usually is one size fits all, offered to teachers of all subject areas in one workshop, designed by outside agencies or to meet an administrative agenda, and mandatory.

inclusion teaching Involves students engaging in learning tasks that have multiple levels of performance and allow students choices in selecting their entry levels.

independent practice Provides the learner the opportunity to integrate new content and skills into what they have previously learned, practicing until they become confident while the teacher actively supervises. For students to integrate new tasks into previously learned material and to practice the tasks so they become automatic.

induction program Designed to support the induction of newly qualified teachers into the teaching profession.

informal accountability Off-the-record practices teachers use to establish and maintain student responsibility for task involvement and outcomes.

informal assessment Tend to be less-structured assessments that are integrated into the learning process.

instant activity A worthwhile and meaningful activity set up for students as they enter the gymnasium.

instructional adaptations These modify a task to make it more or less difficult to accommodate both students who are not challenged enough and students who are struggling with achieving tasks.

instructional alignment When there is a match/consistency among learning outcomes, assessments that determine if students reach those outcomes, and the instructional practices that provide students the opportunity to achieve success.

instructional model Guides the planning, organization and teaching of knowledge and learning experiences. How the teacher organizes and delivers instruction and provides practice to students. Each model has a different role for the teacher and students, and how teachers and students interact with one another.

instructional skills and strategies Aimed at achieving a short-term learning goal; they guide student involvement with content throughout a lesson and are characterized by teacher and student tasks.

instructional task system Composed of all the learning tasks in which teachers ask students to engage, such as taking part in skill practice drills, playing in games, doing structured fitness activities, or team building; these activities are designed for more social or affective outcomes coupled with the associated accountability mechanism(s) employed by the teachers.

journals Allow students to reflect on and share their thoughts, feelings, impressions, perceptions, and attitudes about their performance, an event, an assignment, or other learning experiences.

learning community Exists when students feel valued and supported by their teacher and classmates, are connected to one another, and are committed to each other's learning, growth, and welfare. Students eventually grow to care about each other's successes and failures.

learning experiences The tasks students do to learn and practice content for cognitive development, social development, and physical development.

learning student Is cooperative, eager to learn, enthusiastic about the opportunity to learn more, and responsible for his or her own behavior; enjoys learning and practices purposefully to improve, and is helpful to peers who are similarly engaged in learning.

lesson closure The end-of-class time when teachers bring together the parts of a lesson to make it whole for students, to make sure students understood the important elements learned in the lesson, to re-establish the importance of the lesson elements, and to assess and validate students' feelings relative to the lesson.

lesson plan Related to the unit plan, this determines what will be taught and how a teacher plans to deliver instruction and practice in a lesson.

listserv A program that automatically sends messages to multiple email addresses on a mailing list.

main-theme curriculum model Characterized by a narrow activity focus that serves as the organizing center for the program, allocates time for students to achieve important outcomes, has a clear sense of a more limited good and arranges sequences of activities to achieve that good.

managerial episode Each managerial task constitutes an episode of time and behavior that begins with some event (most frequently a signal or instruction from the teacher), and ends when the next instructional event or activity begins.

managerial skills and strategies Those skills and strategies that help the teacher maintain flow in the lesson, provide organizational structure, and ensure students have the opportunity to participate in learning tasks, interacting with the content to promote their learning.

managerial task system Composed of all the different managerial tasks that frequently occur, such as entering the gym, taking roll, transitioning, organizing for instruction, student (re-)grouping, dispersing equipment, staying on task, following the class rules for behavior, and so on, coupled with the associated accountability mechanism(s) employed by the teachers.

managerial time The cumulative amount of time students spend in managerial tasks, that is, all the organizational, transitional, and non-subject-matter tasks in a lesson.

members in good standing Students who attend class, are on time, wear the appropriate uniform, behave well, and earn a high grade in the class as a consequence.

mentoring Traditionally involves two professionals (usually a mentor and a mentee) working together for the purpose of the mentor providing guidance to the mentee. More recently, mentoring is viewed as a form of professional development shared between two or more colleagues working together for the development of each other.

momentum The smoothness with which the various segments of a lesson flow together. A lesson with momentum has no breaks, no times when activities or transitions slow down the pace.

multimodel curriculum An overarching physical education program developed around selected curriculum models at particular points in time that allow significant outcomes at each level and for every child.

negotiation between task systems Efforts between teachers and students where the demands within one task system are reduced (e.g., the instructional task system) in exchange for student cooperation within another (e.g., student social task system). For example, teachers may allow for certain kinds of student social interaction to gain the necessary cooperation in performing substantive learning tasks.

negotiation within task systems Any attempts by students to change the assigned subject matter learning task, to change the conditions under which tasks are performed, or to seek changes in the performance standards by which task completion is judged by making them easier or more challenging.

non-instructional responsibilities Required tasks and activities, beyond teaching the scheduled classes, that teachers are expected to complete that contribute to the school's mission.

norm-referenced assessment Arises when the teacher and/or student compare performances within a group; common when conducting the more traditional forms of assessment such as skill tests and fitness tests.

objectives Statements of instructional intent that include situation (condition), task (behavior), and criteria that will guide student learning.

observation Likely to be the most frequent assessment measure, in which a teacher provides feedback, manages the classroom, and informs teaching practice. Students can also be encouraged to observe and assess a peer's performance.

ontingency contracts In collaboration with the student, the teacher creates a document in which the contingent relationship is explained between the expected student behavior and the delivery of a specified reward (a reinforcer). Also referred to as a behavior contract.

operating platform Software that directs the operations of a computer, controls and schedules the execution of other software programs, and manages storage, input/output, and communication resources. Examples include Windows for PCs and OS X Mountain Lion for Apple devices.

outcomes What students are expected to do and know as the result of participating in the program.

outcomes-based curriculum A curriculum in which specific outcomes rather than general objectives form the basis of the curriculum.

Outdoor Education Uses the natural environment as the context for experientially enjoying the outdoors and gaining understanding and appreciation for the environment; built on three types of learning: physical skills, environmental awareness, and interpersonal growth.

pace The degree to which the lessons move forward at a steady tempo.

paraprofessional Also referred to as an aide or a para-educator, this is an adult assistant who is not a certified teacher, but who performs many duties in support of a teacher, ranging from helping individual students to assisting with organizational tasks. Commonly assigned to individual students with special needs.

peer assessment Where students observe, make appropriate judgments, and record or provide feedback to their peers.

peer teaching and reciprocal teaching Characterized by students being arranged in pairs or triads, focused on achieving together the goals of guided practice prior to engaging in independent practice.

peer tutoring Used with all young people, and often when teaching students with disabilities. There are two types: (1) when a higher-skilled student tutors a lower-skilled student, and (2) classwide peer tutoring (CWPT) in which all students serve as both tutors and tutees.

performance assessment Requires students to create something using problem solving, critical thinking, application skills, reflection, or other learned skills to demonstrate learning.

performance standards These tell teachers and students how well the student has to perform to meet the standards; that is, how good is "good enough" for that level.

physical activity Any movement activity undertaken in daily life, ranging from normal active living conditions to intentional moderate physical activities, to structured physical fitness and training sessions or dance.

physical education Competitive and noncompetitive physical activities taught as part of a formal school curriculum intended for every student attending school. Physical education applies a holistic approach to the concept of physical activity for young people, recognizing the physical, emotional, cognitive, and social dimensions of human movement.

pinpointing When the teacher stops the class to emphasize or focus on a point by having the class observe one or two students who are working successfully, asking them to demonstrate for the class.

plan-dependent teacher One who invests a significant amount of time in planning effective units and associated lesson plans.

plan-independent teacher One who works from mental recall of previous planning and experience with the activity being taught.

plenty of perfect practice Practice that is pertinent (appropriate for the abilities, interests, and experiences of students), purposeful (lessons are kept on task in a climate that is both safe and challenging), progressive (skills and strategies are organized in ways that lead to sequential, significant learning), paced (activities are sequenced, difficult enough to be challenging yet allow successful practice), and participatory (students are constantly active and learning is equitable for all students).

podcast/vodcast Audio and/or video broadcasts that a user can download from the Internet and play on computers and most other handheld devices.

policy A set of rules aimed at governing the behavior of people within a particular setting (e.g., class, program, school, school system, state, country). "Stronger" policies are those that come with consequences, oversight, and funding. If one or more of these are not present, they are considered "weaker" policies, with the consequence that the policy is less likely to be followed.

policy makers People in positions who review, consider, and vote on proposed new (or changes to existing) formal rules, mandates, and/or legislation. Examples include school managers, school system board members, and local, provincial/state, or national legislators.

portfolio A collection of student work that documents the student's effort, progress, and achievement toward a goal or goals.

positive practice The teacher has students engage in an appropriate behavior a specified number of times as a consequence of misbehaving. Although technically a punishment procedure, it does carry with it an educative dimension in that the appropriate behavior is practiced repeatedly. Also referred to as overcorrection.

premack principles Access to a highly desirable activity is contingent on completing a task that is undesirable and named after David Premack who first coined this contingency. Also referred to as Grandma's rule.

preventive class management The proactive (rather than reactive) strategies teachers use to develop and maintain a positive, predictable, task-oriented class climate in which minimal time is devoted to managerial tasks and optimal time is therefore available for instructional tasks.

primary prevention For physical educators, this means helping children and youth learn how to be responsible for their own behavior and then to act responsibly and helpfully toward their classmates.

pro-social behavior Student behavior that enables achievement of educational and personal growth goals in settings such as physical education lessons.

problem-solving approach Characterized by divergent inquiry that places the learner at the center of the content to be learned, draws out their individual creativity, involves discussion among peers, and stimulates abstract thinking in order to respond.

professional development Formal and informal learning experiences designed to enhance professional career development. Involves gaining the skills, qualifications, and experience that allow teachers to progress across their career.

professional development plan A tool teachers use to reflect on their current practice, set goals for improving that practice, and identify a timeline and the means by which that improvement will take place.

professional physical educator Intends for students to learn, plans for and monitors student enjoyment and progress, manages students to decrease disruptions and increase learning time, organizes learning experiences to match student abilities, and is motivated to be competent and caring.

program promotion Any effort aimed at informing, educating, or building awareness in others about aspects of the physical education program. Analogous to marketing.

progressions Learning tasks that move students from less complex and less sophisticated tasks to more difficult and complicated tasks.

prompt An extra reminder aimed at ensuring that the behavior occurs. Can be verbal, auditory, tactile, and/or visual. Occurs right prior to the occurrence of the behavior. Also called cues.

pseudo-accountability Students who are members in good standing and put forth effort to engage in the assigned instructional tasks. The associated level of accountability is directed at effort or participation. Such students get high marks, regardless of the quality of performance.

punishment Presentation of a consequence, aimed at reducing or eliminating future instances of the same behavior. If the behavior indeed occurs less frequently it can be said that this consequence was punishing in nature. Conversely, if the behavior persists, it would not be a punishment.

questioning techniques Strategies teachers use to clarify student understanding, assess student learning, prompt discussion, seek student insight and perspectives, and encourage students' considering new ideas and content and its application to their lives.

rating scale Indicates the degree or quality of the criterion to be met.

recess/activity break Time during the school day allocated for free play by students. Typically scheduled during mid-morning and mid-afternoon.

reflection For a teacher, this is the process of thinking back on a lesson, the teaching of the lesson, and the students' response to the lesson to allow preservice and practicing teachers to consider their practices and the learning of their pupils in order to make improvements.

reinforcement Application of a positive consequence, aimed at ensuring continued or increased occurrence of that behavior. Applying a negative consequence (also referred to as "punishment") is aimed at reducing or eliminating the inappropriate behavior.

reward costs A punishment technique where students lose previously earned points or privileges as a consequence of misbehavior. Also referred to as response cost.

risk Associated with policy, this refers to the interaction among the ambiguity within the policy, the difficulty of implementing it, and the degree of accountability associated with it.

routines Part of the framework of an effective and positive management system. Routines specify procedures for performing tasks that are repeated frequently throughout the class.

rules Part of the framework of an effective and positive management system. Rules identify appropriate and inappropriate behaviors and the situations within which certain behaviors are acceptable or unacceptable within the class.

school–university partnerships Typically take the form of a formal partnership arrangement between higher education institutions and schools to provide structured support and guidance to student teachers during teaching practice. Recently, school–university partnerships are expanding to include a shared perspective on professional development for professionals in both the school and the university context.

scoring criteria Included in a scoring rubric/guide to judge a performance or product.

scoring rubric Defines the criteria by which performance or product is judged. Sometimes referred to as a scoring guide.

screen time Time spent being sedentary while looking at a computer or television screen.

sedentary behavior Time spent lying down, sitting, or standing still.

self-assessment When students are given the opportunity to assess and modify their own performance, acknowledging that students first need to be taught how to do this.

self-instructional models Allow students to progress through a sequence of learning activities without the physical presence, direction, or supervision of a teacher. Models include (1) individualized instruction, (2) contracting, and (3) personalized systems of instruction (PSI).

service learning (SL) Designed for students to learn about social issues, improve social and interpersonal skills, and develop leadership and positive civic qualities while planning and delivering a service to the community in response to an identified need. Types of SL include (1) direct SL, (2) indirect SL, (3) research-based SL, and (4) advocacy SL.

set induction/ establishing set When the teacher informs the class of what is planned for the day's lesson.

shared-use agreements Formal agreements between a school (or school system) and an outside organization that stipulate the use of a school's physical activity facility during nonschool hours (i.e., evenings and/or weekends).

Skill Theme approach Both a curriculum and instructional model with the content of physical education and the pedagogy. Content is organized by skill themes and movement concepts, with children first becoming familiar with movement concepts such as space awareness, effort, and relationships, followed by fundamental movement themes learned first in isolation and then combined with other skills and movement concepts in more complex and variable settings such as games, dance, and other physical activities.

skills tests When designed in an authentic way, can determine performance level and provide feedback to learners.

small-group teaching A descriptor for a variety of models where the intent is for students to work in small enough groups that will allow all students to work on and achieve a clearly defined task carried out without the direct and immediate supervision of the teacher.

Social Issues models Initially designed to provide alternative activities that meet the needs and interests of young people by involving them in the curriculum process and inviting them to explore social issues that influence physical activity opportunities, political issues impacting sport, or health themes such as nutrition, obesity, or smoking that impact participation in physical activity.

social marketing Use of commercial marketing strategies with the goal to change people's health behavior to improve personal welfare and that of society.

social reinforcers Verbal and nonverbal forms of attention from the teacher (and/or peers) contingent on the occurrence of desirable behavior/performance.

specialized content knowledge (SCK) Knowledge needed to teach an activity (e.g., aerobics, strength conditioning). Typically not acquired through playing/performing.

sport All forms of physical activity (including dance) that, through casual or regular participation, expresses or improves physical fitness and mental well-being and forms social relationships.

Sport Education Intended to provide authentic and rich sport opportunities to all students within the context of physical education, helping them develop as skilled and competent sport participants with the skills and understanding of strategies necessary to participate in sport successfully. Characteristics include seasons, affiliation, formal competition, record keeping, culminating event, and festivity.

station teaching A subcategory of task teaching where students rotate among stations to experience different learning tasks that are not progressive in nature.

student log A record of performance on specific behaviors or criteria over a given period.

Student-Centered Inquiry Designed to change schools and physical education to facilitate the learning of all young people through engaging students, seeking their input, listening to and responding to their ideas, and inviting them to participate in the design of the curriculum as a means of empowering them to take responsibility for their own learning.

student-mediated instruction Includes such models such as (1) peer or reciprocal models, (2) small-group instruction, (3) teams, (4) cooperative learning models, (5) problems-based learning, and (6) service learning.

student-social task system All social interactions that students seek with peers during the lesson coupled with the associated accountability mechanism(s) employed by the teachers (Examples include having fun with a friend during the practice/completion of the learning task, going completely off task with fellow students to engage in some behavior that is social in nature but viewed as disruptive by the teacher.)

summative assessment Provides a final judgment on learning, determining whether learning has or has not happened.

supervision A central teaching function performed by the teacher throughout the class period. It refers to the practices teachers use to establish and maintain student responsibility for appropriate conduct, task involvement, and learning outcomes.

Tactical Approach to Teaching Games A consolidated, applied and teacher-friendly approach to teaching games that progresses students through three phases: game form (representation or exaggeration), tactical awareness (what to do), and skill execution (how to do it). The model emphasizes questioning students to cause them to think critically to solve tactical problems focused on what you want them to achieve (tactical awareness, skill execution, time, space, risk).

tangible reinforcers Reinforcers that come in the form of stickers, pencils and the like. Any tangible item can potentially serve as a reinforcer, if it something that students desire.

task A set of operations/actions used to achieve a specific goal.

task boundaries Refers to how tightly or loosely the teacher applies accountability to task completion and how clear and unambiguous the requirements are for task compliance and completion.

task clarity and ambiguity Two interrelated concepts that refer to the degree of explicitness and consistency in how teachers define tasks and the expected performance A fully explicit task defines (1) the conditions students are to perform under, (2) the performance expected, (3) some standard by which to judge the performance, and (4) the consequences for performance.

task modification Any effort by students to change the assigned managerial or subject matter learning task easier if it is too difficult, or more challenging if it appears too easy.

task presentation Explicit verbal communication and effective use of accurate visual demonstrations and modeling to allow students to gain information on what, why, and how to complete a skill or task and gain content about concepts, principles, skills, and tactics that they do not currently possess.

task risk The interaction among the ambiguity of the task, its difficulty, and the degree of accountability applied to it. Ambiguous tasks produce increased risk for students until they determine that the tasks are either not difficult or carry little, if any, accountability with them. In contrast, a difficult task with strong accountability results in a high degree of risk for the student.

task teaching Organizing the learning environment so that all students can engage in a set of progressive learning tasks simultaneously without changing stations.

teachable moment A moment during teaching when the teacher recognizes that a departure from the lesson focus may have benefits for students.

teacher-mediated instruction Can be delivered (1) directly through group-oriented active teaching models, (2) indirectly through task or station teaching, or (3) indirectly through self-instructional models.

teacher's interactive behavior Key to good management, this is the result of a teacher's clear, proactive behavior that involves instruction and practice.

Teaching Games for Understanding (TGfU) Initially designed as an alternative method for teaching games that emphasized students' finding solutions to problems posed to them in game play situations. Now a six-stage model (game play, game appreciation, tactical awareness, making appropriate decisions, skill practice, game play), TGfU places the student at the center of learning in a problem-based context.

Teaching Personal and Social Responsibility (TPSR) Based on the belief that the most important thing we can teach students is helping them take responsibility for their own development and well-being and supporting that of others through shared power and gradually shifting responsibility for their learning from the teacher to the student. TPSR has eight components: core values, assumptions, levels of responsibility, program leader, daily program format, embedding strategies, problem solving, and assessment.

teaching practice/student teaching An extended period of time in which a student teacher is placed in a host school to practice teaching prior to graduating from teacher education.

teaching strategies General skills and strategies that a teacher uses to facilitate learning within both the managerial and instructional task systems.

teaching through questions Challenges students to engage in cognitive processing, explore alternatives, and formulate a response to a question/problem rather than merely replicate a performance.

team A special type of small group, teams allow students to take responsibility for their own experiences; thus, in some ways it is a form of self-instruction.

time-out A frequently used punishment technique aimed at reducing future occurrences of the problem behavior, by removing the student from the class activity for a short period of time as a consequence of misbehaving or breaking a class rule. Technically, time-out is the removal of the chance to earn positive reinforcement.

traditional assessment Tends to refer to the use of motor skills and fitness as a form of assessment where the main goal is to train students' physical abilities and performance.

transitional task The time when students move from one activity to another (e.g., teams changing courts, moving between stations in a fitness lesson, making substitutions in games, changing the demands of a group task in dance, partner balance task in gymnastics).

transitioning Moving students from one learning task to another through who, what, where, and when statements.

unit (unit of instruction) plan Related to the curriculum plan, this specifies what a teacher plans for a content area to achieve the learning goals, assessments, and instruction in an aligned way over a number of weeks.

verbal desist A verbal reprimand aimed at having the student cease the unacceptable/inappropriate behavior.

video gaming Electronic and interactive games played using computers or computer consoles.

web browser Software program that allows users to explore, retrieve, and present information resources on the World Wide Web. Examples include Apple Safari, Microsoft Internet Explorer, and Mozilla Firefox.

Wi-Fi Short for "wireless fidelity", this refers to wireless networking technology that enables computers, tablets, and the like to communicate using a wireless signal.

wiki A website that allows users to add and update content on the site using their web browser. (The word has its roots in the Hawaiian phrase "wiki wiki," which means superfast.)

Index

Note: Page numbers followed by *b*, *f*, or *t* indicate material in boxes, figures, or tables, respectively.

D

F

G

H

I